Ferret Husbandry, Medicine and Surgery
Second Edition

For Elsevier:

Commissioning Editor: **Joyce Rodenhuis**
Development Editor: **Rita Demetriou-Swanwick**
Project Manager: **Nancy Arnott**
Designer: **Stewart Larking**
Illustrations: **Deborah Marizels**

Ferret Husbandry, Medicine and Surgery

Second Edition

John H. Lewington, B.Vet. Med., MRCVS
Member of the Australian Veterinary Association (AVA);
Member of the American Ferret Association (AFA); World Ferret Union (WFU); South Australian Ferret Association (SAFA); New South Wales Ferret Welfare Society (NSWFWS); Ferrets Southern District Perth (FSDP)

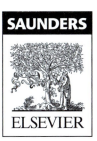

Edinburgh London New York Oxford Philadelphia St Louis Sydney Toronto 2007

SAUNDERS

An imprint of Elsevier Limited
© Elsevier Limited 2007. All rights reserved.

No part of this publication may be reproduced, stored in a retrieval system, or transmitted in any form or by any means, electronic, mechanical, photocopying, recording or otherwise, without the prior permission of the Publishers. Permissions may be sought directly from Elsevier's Health Sciences Rights Department, 1600 John F. Kennedy Boulevard, Suite 1800, Philadelphia, PA 19103-2899, USA: phone: (+1) 215 239 3804; fax: (+1) 215 239 3805; or, e-mail: *healthpermissions@elsevier.com*. You may also complete your request on-line via the Elsevier homepage (http://www.elsevier.com), by selecting 'Support and contact' and then 'Copyright and Permission'.

First published 2000
Reprinted 2002
Second edition 2007
Reprinted 2008

ISBN-13: 9780702028274

British Library Cataloguing in Publication Data
A catalogue record for this book is available from the British Library

Library of Congress Cataloging in Publication Data
A catalog record for this book is available from the Library of Congress

Notice
Knowledge and best practice in this field are constantly changing. As new research and experience broaden our knowledge, changes in practice, treatment and drug therapy may become necessary or appropriate. Readers are advised to check the most current information provided (i) on procedures featured or (ii) by the manufacturer of each product to be administered, to verify the recommended dose or formula, the method and duration of administration, and contraindications. It is the responsibility of the practitioner, relying on their own experience and knowledge of the patient, to make diagnoses, to determine dosages and the best treatment for each individual patient, and to take all appropriate safety precautions. To the fullest extent of the law, neither the Publisher nor the Authors assume any liability for any injury and/or damage to persons or property arising out of or related to any use of the material contained in this book.

The Publisher

ELSEVIER your source for books, journals and multimedia in the health sciences
www.elsevierhealth.com

Working together to grow libraries in developing countries
www.elsevier.com | www.bookaid.org | www.sabre.org
ELSEVIER BOOK AID International Sabre Foundation

The Publisher's policy is to use paper manufactured from sustainable forests

Printed in China

Contents

Acknowledgements vi
Contributors vii
Preface to second edition viii
Preface to first edition ix

Part 1 Husbandry 1

Chapter 1 Classification, history and current status of ferrets 3
Chapter 2 External features and anatomy profile 15
Chapter 3 Accommodation 34
Chapter 4 Nutrition 57
Chapter 5 Reproduction and genetics 86
Chapter 6 Ferret-polecat domestication: genetic, taxonomic and phylogenetic relationships by Bob Church 122
Chapter 7 Ferret handling, hospitalization and diagnostic techniques 151

Part 2 Medicine 167

Chapter 8 Viral, bacterial and mycotic diseases 169
Chapter 9 Ferret gastrointestinal and hepatic diseases by Mark E. Burgess . 203
Chapter 10 Parasitic diseases of ferrets. 224
Chapter 11 Diseases of special concern 258
Chapter 12 Diseases of the ferret ear, eye and nose 289
Chapter 13 General neoplasia. 318
Chapter 14 Endocrine diseases 346
Chapter 15 Managing ferret toxicoses by Jill Richardson 380

Part 3 Surgery 391

Chapter 16 Anaesthesia and radiology 393
Chapter 17 Ultrasonography in ferret practice by Cathy A. Johnson-Delaney . 417
Chapter 18 General surgery by R. Avery Bennett and Geoffrey W. Pye 430
Chapter 19 Ferret vasectomy, orthopaedics and cryosurgery 440
Chapter 20 Ferret emergency techniques by Anthony Lucas 458

Part 4 Special Anatomy 465

Chapter 21 Ferret dentition and pathology by Bob Church 467

Appendix 487
Index 503

Acknowledgements

'Since I was a small boy I have never been without ferrets. They are extremely useful for anyone keeping other animals which might attract the odd rat; and they also make good pets.'

Phil Drabble, The Book of Pets, 1975

I owe a great debt to those veterinarians, past and present, here and overseas, who contributed data, observations on ferret cases, copyright permissions on useful tables, diagrams, etc. There are many non-veterinarians who have done the same for both editions.

Stalwarts of the first edition, Susan Brown, Judith Bell, James Fox, Howard Evans, along with Avery Bennett, Geoffrey Pye and Anthony Lucas, all of the USA, were essential contributors.

New chapter contributors of great merit and expertise include veterinarians of the USA, Cathy Johnson-Delaney, Mark Burgess and Jill Richardson. Mike Murray, Dan Johnson and Max Conn, respectively, allowed me to use their data on laparoscopy, cryosurgery and eye lacrimal duct flushing techniques.

Non-vet anthropologist, Bob Church, has submitted two detailed chapters (Chs 6 and 21): 'Ferret-polecat domestication: genetic, taxonomic and phylogenetic relationships' and 'Ferret dentition and pathology'.

Further genetic information relating to breeding ferrets has been supplied by:

Fara Shimbo, horse breeder and former ferret breeder, Colorado USA; Brett Middleton, geneticist, Assistant Research Scientist, Animal & Dairy Science, University of Georgia; Sukie Crandall BA, ferret owner and co-moderator at Ferret Health List USA, Adviser, International Ferret Congress; Christina Bernard, ferret owner and author, Tasmania, Australia. Not forgetting my wife, Margaret Lewington, BSc, for her assistance in organizing the genetics section.

Tom Willard, nutritionist of Performance Foods, has given expert advice on USA ferret nutrition.

The artistry of Sabine van Voorne, Michael Simmons and Debby Squance is still apparent.

I am grateful for the ready supply of ferret images from veterinarians Greg Rich, Mark Finkler, Tom Kawasaki, Deborah Kemmerer-Cottrell, Dean Manning, Michael Davidson, John Gordon and Amy Kapatkin. *Disclaimer*: Every effort has been made to acknowledge copyright holders for some of the other images in this book, however some are very old images for which the source is now lost.

Other new overseas veterinarians sending ferret cases and images were Yasutsugu Miwa, Chris Lamb, John Chitty, Chris Hanley, Reni Gandolfi, Alessandro Melillo, Hanneke Moorman and Joerg Mayer.

New non-veterinary input came from Dmitry Kalinin (Russia) and Sally Heber (USA).

Special thanks go to Dr Jennifer Richardson of Murdoch University Veterinary School for help with computer images; thanks also to the Murdoch University library staff and the assistance of Professor Graham Wilcox, Professor of Virology and Russell Hobbs, parasitologist, Murdoch University School of Veterinary and Biomedical Sciences, in updating the taxonomy of viruses and parasites, is gratefully acknowledged.

I thank Joyce Rodenhuis, Commissioning Editor of Veterinary Medicine, Rita Demetriou-Swanwick, the Development Editor, Veterinary Medicine Books and Lyn Taylor, Copy Editor, at Elsevier for both their help and encouragement.

Last but not least, thanks and love to my wife Margaret for constant support and stern editing, notwithstanding the vague remark as the book went to press, 'Dogs have masters, cats have servants, but ferrets have slaves'. I am still not sure what she was getting at…

Contributors

Major contributors: Veterinarians:

Chapter 17
Cathy Johnson-Delaney, DVM, DABVP-Avian
Eastside Avian and Exotic Animal Medical Center
Kirkland
Washington
USA

Chapter 9
Mark Burgess, DVM
Southwest Animal Hospital
Beaverton
Oregon
USA

Chapter 15
Jill Richardson, DVM
Director of Consumer Relations
The Hartz Mountain Corporation
Secaucus
New Jersey
USA

Chapter 18
Avery Bennett, DVM, MS, Diplomate ACVS
Phoenix
Arizona
USA
with
Geoffrey Pye, BVSc, MSc, Diplomate ACZM
Senior Veterinarian
San Diego Zoo
California
USA

Chapter 20
Anthony Lucas, BSc, BVMS (Hons), MACVS, MVS, PhD
Carthage
Indiana
USA

Non-veterinarian contributors:

Chapters 6 and 21
Bob Church, BA (Arch), BA (Zoo)
2008 Evans Rd.
Columbia
Missouri 65203
USA

Various contributions by

Fara Shimbo
Hygiene
Colorado
USA

Preface to second edition

When preparing the 2007 edition of *Ferret Husbandry, Medicine and Surgery*, I wanted to keep the 'chatty' nature of the initial material of a book wholly devoted to the Mustelidae represented by the domesticated polecat, the ferret. New subject material has been generously supplied by like-minded people interested in the welfare of the little 'critters'.

The first edition grew out of my association with my first ferret, Fred. I set out to introduce veterinarians who were not yet involved with *Mustela furo* outside the USA, as the pet was becoming popular worldwide.

I put a practitioner's view, as I do now, to someone newly presented with a ferret to examine and to bridge the gap between ferret owner, with working or pet ferret and the veterinarian. The basic concept is the place I consider the domesticated ferret holds as one of the three carnivores sharing the home of man. Figure P.1 sums it up.

The Western world has exploited the ferret, as in its use in medical research, but has also taken the animal to its heart as a pet. However, pet ferrets have succumbed to a variety of maladies, specifically ferret adrenal disease complex (FADC), insulinoma, neoplasia, cardiomyopathy and gastroenteritis problems. These may be attributed to a husbandry, nutrition and even genetic background as shown in this text. Ferret genetics is just being unraveled and requires funds to move forward.

The pet ferret deserves a better healthier life in the future with reduced incidence of maladies, otherwise it may move into an endangered species chapter of a biology textbook.

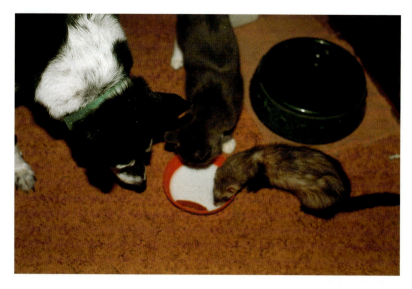

Figure P.1 Cheetah, the dog. Mishka the cat and Sophie the ferret, around a bowl of milk.

Preface to first edition

In 1973 I was a recent migrant to Australia and had never seen a ferret in the UK. Ironically I had been a medical laboratory technician before becoming a veterinarian and dealt with many animals in TB work but never ferrets. Ferrets, as we now know, are good 'models' in biomedical research today in the USA. A Dutch kennel man at the practice in Perth knew I admired otters and was bemoaning the fact that there were none in Australia, except in the zoo. One day he came in and presented me with an 8-week-old piece of furry, nippy quicksilver of a beastie, which I passed from hand to hand like electrified jelly! A male ferret! From working ferret stock! 'Make a pet of that', he said and left.

So I did. Some years later I am still associated with the relatives of Fred, our first pet ferret.

This book sets out to inform the veterinary practitioner on the broad spectrum of conditions relating to Fred's kind, the domestic ferret (*Mustela putorius furo*) regarding basic husbandry, medicine and surgery. It is in essence a personalized account of keeping ferrets and strives to give the ups and downs, the pitfalls and emotions attached to dealing with these fascinating animals by someone who worked up from a scratch knowledge of the subject.

Dedication

This book is dedicated to Fred, Pip, Teddy, Robbie and friends.

Part One

Husbandry

CHAPTERS

1 Classification, history and current status of ferrets 3
2 External features and anatomy profile 15
3 Accomodation 34
4 Nutrition 57
5 Reproduction and genetics 86
6 Ferret-polecat domestication: genetic, taxonomic 122
  and phylogenetic relationships by Bob Church
7 Ferret handling, hospitalization and diagnostic techniques . . . 151

Classification, history and current status of ferrets

CHAPTER 1

'They have become so utterly dependent on man that if they are lost they soon die, because they do not know how to care for themselves.'

Harper Cory. Ferret. Mammals of the British Isles, 1941

The ferret (*Mustela putorius furo*) was named by Linnaeus in 1758 and is a domesticated polecat. The European polecat (*M. putorius putorius*) is the likely ancestor but there is some argument about whether the domesticated ferret is derived from the European, Asiatic, Siberian or Ethiopian polecat. The first is considered most likely, with polecats native to the UK and Europe. *Mustela putorius* (Fig. 1.1) has been deftly described by Miller in 1912.[1] He divided the subgenus *putorius* into three species in the Old World and one in America. The two Old World species occur in Europe. It has been stated that the best way to avoid confusion in the nomenclature of ferret and polecats and arguments about heredity, is to continue to use the traditional names which are in common use, i.e. ferret being *M. furo* and polecat *M. putorius* (C. King, Waikato University, NZ, pers. comm. 2005). The genetics of ferret domestication have been studied (Ch. 6).

The family Mustelidae includes some of the most interesting small- to medium-sized carnivores of the animal kingdom and they are most efficient hunters. The domestic ferret's keen hunting ability comes from this lineage.

The ferret has evolved as a separate subspecies from the polecat, *M. putorius*, through the domestication of its kittens (Table 1.1). Man has partly domesticated some other mustelids, such as badgers, skunks and otters, at some time. An interest in ferrets can lead to an interest in their relatives. Books like *Badgers at my Window* by Phil Drabble, *An Otter in the House* by Dorothy Wisbeski, or *Tupa Tupa Tupa* translated by Peter Knott, on a wolverine in Finland, are a delight to read. Fara Shimbo of Colorado once boarded Nataska (*Mustela eversmanni*) from Russia, which was destined to be used as a surrogate mother for the American black-footed ferret recovery (Fig. 1.2). She said Nataska's fur was so soft that it made her own ferrets' fur feel like steel wool. Figure 1.3 is an image of a Kolinsky or Siberian weasel (from Dmitry Kalinin of the Russian Ferret Society). He is wild but a few centuries of domestication could make him an ideal pet!

Domestication of the mustelids is a fascinating idea as the family contains some of the most efficient killers in the animal kingdom (Ch. 6). It is considered in the UK that the smaller members: weasels, stoats and mink are untameable but this is not always the case: Phil Drabble in 1975 spoke of taming both stoats and weasels when they are 8 weeks of age.[2] Steve Scot, of Leeds, UK, rescued a 2-week-old weasel from a cat in 1981, and hand-reared and tamed it.

The early description of ferrets compared them in size with weasels. In 1774, Oliver Goldsmith described them as 1 foot (30 cm) long; 4 inches (10 cm) longer than *M. nivalis*. He described their colour as commonly cream but added that they were also found in all colours of weasels; white, blackish, brown and part colours.[3] 'The white kind has reddish eyes and the ferret has a longer tail than the weasel'. Goldsmith added that as a native of Africa, the ferret disliked the rigour of the English climate and needed to be kept with care and shelter (Ch. 3). Thomas Bewick in 1790 described the ferret as having 'eyes red and fiery and whole body colour is a very pale yellow'.[4] Its nose is sharper than

CHAPTER ONE

Classification, history and current status of ferrets

Table 1.1 The ferret family tree
The ferret family
CLASS: Mammalia, ORDER: Carnivora 'Fissipeds', FAMILY: Mustelidae, SUB FAMILY

Mustelinae	*Mephitinae*	*Lutrinae*	*Melinae and Mellivorinae*
Weasels, stoats polecats	Skunks	Otters	Badgers
Mink	Honey badgers		
Martens			
Grisons			
Wolverines			

THE MUSTELINE SPECIES			
European common weasel		*Mustela nivalis*	
Least weasel		*M. nivalis rixona*	
Stoat, or short tailed weasel		*M. erminea*	
Long tailed weasel		*M. frenata*	
Tropical weasel		*M. africana*	
Colombian weasel		*M. felipei*	
European polecat		*M. putorius putorius*	
Ferret		*M. putorius furo*	
Steppe polecat		*M. eversmanni*	
Black footed ferret		*M. nigripes*	
Mountain weasel		*M. altaica*	
Kolinsky, or Siberian weasel		*M. sibirica*	
Yellow-bellied weasel		*M. kathiah*	
Back-striped weasel		*M. strigidorsa*	
Barefoot weasel		*M. nudipes*	
Indonesian mountain weasel		*M. lutreolina*	
American mink		*M. vison*	
European mink		*M. lutreola*	
Marbled polecat		*Vormela peregusna*	
Zorella, or African polecat		*Ictonyx striatus*	
North African banded weasel		*Poecilictis libyca*	
African striped weasel		*Poecilogale albinucha*	
Grison, or huron		*Galictis vittata*	
Little grison		*G. cuja*	
Patagonian weasel		*Lyncodon patagonicus*	
Pine marten		*Martes martes*	
American marten		*M. americana*	
Japanese marten		*M. melampus*	
Fisher, peckan or Virginian polecat		*M. pennanti*	
Sable		*M. zibellina*	
Stone, beech or house marten		*M. foina*	
Yellow-throated marten		*M. flavigula*	
Nilgiri		*M. gwatkinsi*	
European wolverine		*Gulo gulo gulo*	
North American wolverine		*Gulo gulo luscus*	

Table adapted from: The ferret family. In: Val Porter and Nicholas Brown's *The Complete Book of Ferrets*. Bedford: D&M Publications; 1997, with permission.

that of the weasel and the foulmart (*Mustela putorius*). The ferret's length was put at 14 inches with a tail of 5 inches. Harper Cory in 1941 called the ferret, 'an albino derived from some wild species of polecat'.[5]

As indicated earlier, the genetic history of the present day ferret has been a subject of conjecture. The dark form of ferret resembles the polecat but is sometimes called a fitch-ferret or polecat-ferret to

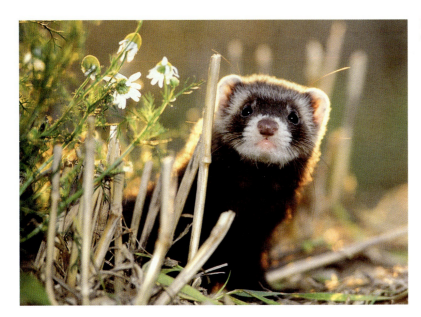

Figure 1.1 European polecat (*M. putorius*). (Photo by Rollin.)

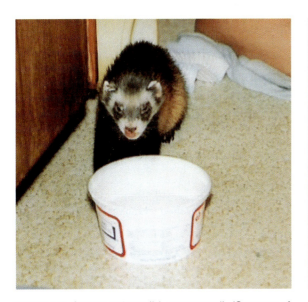

Figure 1.2 Steppe polecat (*M. eversmanni*). (Courtesy of Fara Shimbo.)

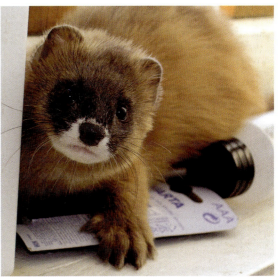

Figure 1.3 Siberian weasel (*M. sibirica*). (Courtesy of Dmitry Kalinin.)

distinguish it from the pink-eyed white ferret. There was some thought that the dark ferret derived from a cross between a wild polecat and an albino ferret but this has not been proven. Domestication takes time, so if we consider that dogs have been domesticated for around 10 000 years, cats about 5000 years and ferrets around 2000 years, man has done very well in his association with *M. furo*.

General ferret history

In ancient times, ferrets were mentioned by Aristophanes (c.450 BC) and Aristotle (350 BC). It is considered that the first accurate account of ferrets used for controlling a plague of rabbits in the Balearic Islands was by Strabo (c.AD 200). Ferrets were initially domesticated around the Mediterranean. The rabbit originally occupied northwest Africa and Iberia and it is reasonable to assume that the ferret was domesticated in the same area to obtain rabbits as a human food source.[6] There were early records of the Romans having ferrets in their villas to deter rats and mice but it was later thought that the Egyptian mongoose had filled that role. The mongoose was better at ratting, while the ferret seemed to have resulted from domesticating polecats for the purpose of hunting rabbits.

The fate of the ferret and rabbit have been intertwined in history. As man took the rabbit as a domesticated food source northwards through Europe, the ferret went too. The rabbits were kept on islands, in warrens or enclosures and Pliny (AD 23–79) mentions both the rabbit and the ferret. In Spain, Isidore of Seville mentions ferrets in 600 AD. The German Emperor, Fredrick II, is supposed to have used ferrets in 1245. In Asia, around the same time, 1221, Genghis Khan used ferrets for hunting. There was a manuscript of a *Livre de Chasse* of Gaston Phebus, Comte de Foix, who ruled in southern France and northern Spain around 1387, which showed ferreting with muzzled ferrets and the use of purse nets. From then on, working ferrets have not looked back and thankfully, the use of muzzles has long since been abandoned.

In the Middle Ages, ferreting was combined with falconry, whereby the ferret would be sent into a burrow to chase out prey, which would then be swooped upon by the falcon.[7] They were, in the Middle Ages, also used to keep vermin away from dining halls; a lady might have kept a small ferret in the sleeve of her gown to release on sight of a rat. The ferrets were smaller than they are today; their size has improved due to better nutrition (Ch. 4).

It is interesting to note that the first appearance of an albino ferret in Britain is not recorded but around AD 1551, a pink-eyed white ferret was described quaintly as being 'the colour of wool stained with urine'. Albino ferrets are frequently not white but yellow-tinged, while black-eyed white ferrets may have dark hairs in the coat in varying patterns (Ch. 5). In the Renaissance period, women were labelled as witches if they practised herbalism and talked to their black cat or pale ferret. Ferrets also featured in folklore, e.g. the Irish believed milk was blessed if it was lapped by a ferret. In the French Courts of Louis XIV and XV, a card game and a courtly dance were invented around *le furet*.

In Victorian times, the cat came into its own as a domesticated pet and the ferret was not far behind. Though not welcomed into the family home as such, there are tales of the docility and tameness of the species, with farm suppliers and carpenters outdoing each other in making the most lavish and sumptuous ferret hutches, which were sold at exorbitant costs (see Fig. 3.1).[7]

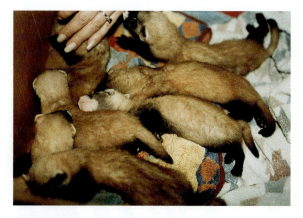

Figure 1.4 Black-footed ferrets (*M. nigripes*). (Courtesy of Mary van Dahm.)

Until recent advances in molecular biology, it has been quite difficult to say with certainty that the ferret actually came from the European polecat (see Ch. 6).[8] There are several contenders, such as the steppe polecat (*Mustela eversmanni*) from Asia and possibly a hybrid of this, the European polecat in Eastern Europe. The exact relationship of all these, including the American black-footed ferret (*Mustela nigripes*) still remains uncertain, since it has been recently shown that they may, under laboratory conditions, produce fertile offspring from a hybrid mating (Fig. 1.4).

Many will know that the American black-footed ferret nearly became extinct because of the decline of their natural food, the prairie dog, due to farming. A captive breeding programme for the remaining few, who are still at risk, is a warning for other mustelids if mankind continues to alter the balance of nature.[9] At the present time, many US zoos are involved with black-footed ferrets.

Examples of world ferrets

United Kingdom

Ferrets were introduced into the UK possibly by the Romans, who used them for ferreting, and also at the time of the Norman Conquest. There are several famous paintings and tapestries, which show ferrets in use with royalty or the landed gentry. The rural working classes started using ferrets probably around the year 1300. In the British Library, there is a picture showing two women putting a ferret to a netted rabbit warren or 'bury'. In 1384, King Richard II issued a decree permitting one of his clerks to hunt rabbits with ferrets, and in 1390 issued another statute prohibiting ferreting on Sundays. Ferret interest was maintained in the UK and Europe through the centuries and there is speculation that the 'ermine' in the portrait of Queen Elizabeth I, by Nicholas Hilliard, could have been a pet ferret rather than a stoat (Ch. 5).

Ferreting for rabbits remains popular in the UK, continental Europe, Australia and New Zealand. Much poaching mythology remains associated with ferreting. A century ago, poaching rabbits using ferrets was still regarded as a serious offence. Garments were home-made by rural working classes to enable ferrets to be carried surreptitiously and probably led to the ghastly idea of 'keeping ferrets down one's trouser legs'! Freshly-killed rabbits could be secreted under the folds of the garments to avoid detection by bailiffs and gamekeepers. Punishment of transportation to Australia was the sentence for lesser charges than ferreting. Ferreting in poachers' subculture has been called 'the business' for centuries. According to Hodgkin, in the 1486 classic *The Boke of St Albans*, the collective names for 'the compaynys of beestys and fowlys' include 'a flflight [sic] of doves', 'a bery of conyis' and 'a besynes of ferrets'. The 'bury' is still used to describe rabbit (coney) burrows and the term 'business' is still used in parts of rural England in describing ferreting for rabbits.[8] The UK ferret population is stable and ferrets are now serious companion pets alongside dogs and cats in the UK. They are included in the Pet Travel Scheme (PETS) regarding export/import requirements (Dr J. Chitty, pers. comm. 2005).

At the present time, the 'Vincent Wildlife Trust' UK, is carrying out a survey on the distribution of polecats and the presence of feral ferrets. As at June 2005, they had verifiable evidence of 389 possible polecats with external features suggesting 328 were pure and 61 with some evidence of ferret in their coat colour. (A wild male polecat was photographed after breaking into the ferret enclosure of the Hampshire New Forest Otter, Owl and Wildlife Park (*VWT Newsletter*, July, 2005).)

There has been an increase in pet ferrets in the UK since the beginning of the twenty-first century. This has been put down to people not finding it easy to keep cats or dogs, e.g. single working people in apartments. Pet ferret numbers could now run to millions (Dr J. McNicholas, pers. comm. 2005).

Europe

France

The French pet ferrets are well served by *Le Club Francais des Amateurs du Furet* as can be seen by the symposium held in Malakoff, Paris in April, 2005. A hall with purpose built open pens was used for a gathering of 60 ferrets and owners. Already micro-chipped, the ferrets were checked thoroughly by a veterinarian before being photographed, displayed, walked, talked to and played with, amid their enthusiastic owners and overseas guests (S. Bridges, NFWS, pers. comm.).

Netherlands

The presence of several ferret organizations shows how popular ferrets are in the Netherlands.

The most important ferret organization in the country has about 600 members with 2–4 ferrets each. Pet ferrets became popular 15 years ago; before that they were used primarily for hunting. Ten years ago fur ferrets were introduced into the country, bred for size and fur. People used these gene lines but the need for various coloured ferrets led to imports from America. It has become apparent that an increase of adrenal gland disease and insulinoma has arisen in ferrets under 6 or 7 years old over the last 10 years. Bringing ferrets in from New Zealand breeding companies, Norway and America, for the breeding of angoras, dark-eyed whites, blazes and other unnatural colours, appears to have made the health of the Dutch ferrets deteriorate to the point where some ferret owners are wondering about the future health of the species (Stephenie Bass, '*Stichting de Fret*', Netherlands, pers. comm. 2005).

Belgium

In Belgium, ferrets were used as working animals and are now mostly kept as pets. Over the last 10 years there has been an improvement in housing, quality of veterinary care and of food. Belgium has fewer pet ferrets than the Netherlands; there are many large pet shops selling ferrets from New Zealand (Wendy Van den Steen, pers. comm. 2005).

Switzerland

Ferrets and polecats are both found in Switzerland. The ferret has been a working animal for farmers and game-keepers for decades (Fig. 1.5). Although popular, pet ferrets are uncommon. The control of ferrets is under the Swiss Federation Act for the Protection of Animals and is quite advanced and very strict (Urs Murbach, Swiss Ferret Fancy Society, pers. comm. 1998). The act applies to wild animals and little difference is made between polecats and ferrets. A permit from the Federal Veterinary Office is required to import, export or to keep ferrets in captivity (there is no mention of domestication). The statutory

CHAPTER ONE
Classification, history and current status of ferrets

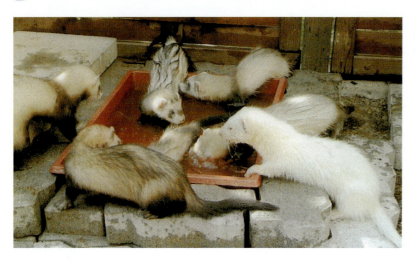

Figure 1.5 Swiss ferrets enjoy splashing around in water bowl on a hot day. (Courtesy of Murbach.)

requirements include a minimum cage size of 2 square metres for two animals; nutrition requirements and the keeping of livestock statistics. If ferrets are kept outside, where free run and playtime with the owner is less likely, a minimum of 4 square metres is needed. The numbers of animals on the premises, the causes of deaths and the names and addresses of the buyer and seller have to be recorded. The owner is not allowed to sell ferrets without permission. The district veterinarian inspects the ferrets and their housing on a regular basis and permission to keep ferrets depends on his reports and they must be renewed every second year. Urs comments that the above only encourages the most serious ferret owners. In some respects, this is a way to produce a responsible pet or working ferret owner and it does give an immediate veterinary input to the animals' welfare. Urs however, considers that Swiss ferrets are generally healthy specimens, live to about 8 years and seldom suffer from the cancers that are seen in other countries.

Spain

The ferret is considered a native Spanish animal used for centuries for hunting wild rabbits, as in the UK. There are also wild polecats in Spain and elsewhere in Europe. The ferrets are divided into three groups of population (Andres Montesinos, pers. comm. 2005). The first is the classic 'captive' ferret population, which are housed in cages and apparently fed with meat only once a week plus eggs and milk at other times. (This apparently keeps them hungry to be hunters, but it is known by UK ferreting groups that ferrets do not need to be hungry to chase rabbits!) Consequently, the working ferrets in Spain are in a bad state of nutrition and suffer worms, distemper and wounds.

The second population group comprises those from working stock, kept in proper domestic conditions and neutered older than 6 months of age. The third population group includes imported stock with early neutering.

Italy

During the last 2–3 years, ferrets have become popular pets in Italy. Pet ferrets are bought from pet shops, private breeders and professional breeders, though the latter are rare. Most ferrets imported by pet shops are from Sweden, Marshall Farms (New York), Canada or New Zealand (Southland Ferrets and Mystic Ferrets). *Note* that all these ferrets are neutered early (6 weeks of age) and descented. Private breeders, with some jills (females) and one or two hobs (males), are becoming more important, breeding every year and selling direct to owners, as in Australia and other countries. These ferrets are better socialized, do not undergo early neutering, and seem to have less chance of getting the problems seen in professionally-bred ferrets from overseas (Alessandro Melillo, pers. comm. 2005). *Note* ferreting is allowed only in Sicily, not on the mainland.

Germany

Pet ferrets in Germany seem mostly to be around Berlin and are mostly indoors. I have a German contact who has a native polecat which comes into the garden, and even has slipped into the house, to see her ferrets or look for food. German pet ferrets seem to suffer from adrenal gland disease, lymphoma and insulinoma (Gisela Hanneke, Berlin, pers. comm. 2005).

Czech Republic

Ferret owners in the Czech Republic may have one or more ferrets free-living in their homes using cat litter trays, with very few living outside and there are no working ferrets. Some ferrets are kept as laboratory animals. They are fed on commercial foods made for cats and ferrets. Adrenal gland disease, insulinoma and other neoplasia exist as major issues (Vladimir Jekl, Brno, pers. comm. 2005).

Hungary

In Hungary, most of the pet ferret population are kept in flats; breeding colonies are kept outside. There are few working ferrets. Pet ferrets are fed on cat food and some on homemade food. Actual ferret food from abroad is brought in but is not often used. The ferret colours described are: wild – dark brown with light brown or white face mask, beige – whole body light brown without face mask and albino, but no black-eyed white. Interestingly, the common diseases are linked with reproduction, e.g. prolonged oestrus (POA). Hungary has two species of wild polecats (*Mustela putorius*, *M. eversmanni*) as members of the indigenous fauna (Professor Gyula Huszenicaza, Budapest, pers. comm. 2005).

Russia

It is recorded that people in the vast eastern Russian regions kept polecats in villages to control rodent numbers. The first ferrets, *Mustela furo* were purchased from the Prague Zoo in 1971 by the USSR. The ferrets adapted to the Russian cold and a breeding colony was established. The new branch of fur farming – polecat farming, started. Using *furo* types to interbreed with farm polecats, a hybrid was developed with improved fur quality and higher reproductive features for the industry. Such hybrids had occurred in Poland some years earlier and were called *thorefretka*, which was in essence a synonym of ferret.

It was not until the end of Perestroika that ferrets were considered as possible pet animals. Pet ferrets are presently mainly purchased from fur farms. The first ferrets were picked out on fur characteristics, i.e. fur quality, size, etc. Friendly temperament was not a first consideration so the animals tended to be on the wild side, but this improved with time. In some cases at first, pet ferrets were not well looked after; they were kept in small cages, fed human food or low quality dog meals and never vaccinated. The situation changed in 2001 when pet ferrets became popular in Moscow, where 68% of pet ferrets live and St Petersburg,

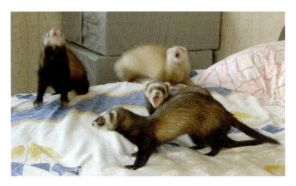

Figure 1.6 Russian pet ferrets bedding down. (Courtesy of Dmitry Kalinin.)

which has 27%. On average, 77% of ferret owners have one pet, 16% have two, while 7% have three or more. One problem has been a lack of veterinary knowledge of ferret needs, but apparently Russian ferrets are healthy (Dr D. Kalinin, pers. comm. 2005) (Fig. 1.6).

Japan

Pet ferrets in Japan are very popular and have been brought in from America (Marshall Farms and Path Valley ferrets) and New Zealand, also some from Canada and Denmark. There is now ferret breeding in the islands. Originally, people wanted a small pet which would not take up space in their small apartment dwelling in the cities. The American ferrets were called 'super ferrets' and commanded prices of US$600 to over US$700 to ferret lovers in Tokyo. Ferrets from Europe were 'non-super ferrets' for not being neutered, etc. but still commanded prices of US$150–400 (Keika Koima, Tokyo, pers. comm. 1999). Since the late 1990s, Japanese veterinarians have become aware of 'American diseases' in the ferrets, including adrenal gland disease, lymphoma and insulinoma (Dr Yasutsugu Miwa, Tokyo, pers. comm. 2005). Interestingly, ferrets are not listed for quarantine in Japan, as the country has been rabies-free for 30 years. Unfortunately, Aleutian disease is now in their stock (Ch. 8).

Australia

Early UK settlers brought game animals with them to Australia as to other colonies. The first rabbits were tame and did not survive but wild rabbits were then imported from Britain. Releasing rabbits into the bush heralded a national environmental disaster, which led to the introduction of working ferrets as biological control agents late in the nineteenth century. Stray or released

CHAPTER ONE
Classification, history and current status of ferrets

Table 1.2 Part of a survey on mammals introduced to southern Australia by the early twentieth century

Common name	Scientific name	Origin	Reason for/route of introduction	Result
Eastern grey squirrel	*Sciurus carolinensis*	North America	Aesthetic	Died out
Three-striped palm squirrel	*Funambulus pennanti*	India	Zoo release	Localized in Sydney, NSW, Perth, WA
Black rat	*Rattus rattus*	SE Asia	Commensal	Widespread
Brown rat	*Rattus norvegicus*	Asian Steppes	Commensal	Widespread
House mouse	*Mus domesticus*	Central Asia	Commensal	Widespread
Ferret	*Mustela putorius furo*	Mediterranean	Hunt rabbits	Did not establish
Gold-spotted mongoose	*Herpestes javanicus auropunctatus*	India, Java, Sumatra	Control of rabbits and rats	Died out
Feral dog	*Canis familiaris*		Commensal	Widespread
Red fox	*Vulpes vulpes*	Europe	Hunting	Widespread
Domestic cat	*Felis catus*	Europe	Commensal	Widespread
European rabbit	*Oryctolagus cuniculus*	Western Mediterranean	Hunting	Widespread
European hare	*Lepus capensis*	Europe	Hunting	Widespread

Adapted from Groves RH, Di Castri F. *Biogeography of Mediterranean Invasions*. Cambridge: Cambridge University Press; 1991, with permission.

ferrets did not colonize the Australian bush as they were a domesticated animal and died out, succumbing to the harsh climate. In Australia, ferrets can be killed by foxes, dingoes, feral cats and hawks. Table 1.2 illustrates these points.

Ferrets were only used against rabbits by ferreting techniques as used in the UK with caged ferrets. Had they imported wild polecats and released them, the situation would almost certainly have been different. The controversy surrounding ferret origins, which raged 60–100 years ago probably helped to avoid a further disaster.[8] In southwest Western Australia (WA), farmers have an ongoing problem with feral foxes, cats, dogs and rabbits, but no feral ferrets. Types and colours of Australian and other ferrets are shown in Chapter 2.

New Zealand

In NZ, in the nineteenth century, ferrets or polecat-ferret hybrids were released into the wild to combat the wild rabbit. The climate was less harsh than Australia's and there were no native predatory mammals, so the animals established with success. Actual working of ferrets (ferreting) was not carried out in early times.

As of 2005, pet ferrets are banned. In 1998, a young ferret happened to stray into another house by a cat door. It unfortunately got into a child's bed and when rolled on, scratched and nipped the child. The press built up the incident to create a 'murderous ferret' drama. Unfortunately, that ferret was put down immediately, although there was no rabies problem; but it stirred things up for the banning of pet ferrets. Many ferret owners protested and even moved abroad to protect their pets but the ban was enforced despite rigorous rallying against it. At the time, feral ferrets (or hybrid polecat-ferrets) were being killed off because of a threat to ground-dwelling native birds and as suspect TB carriers. The NZ pet ferret-loving community is dismayed; house and garden pet ferrets had not previously caused trouble. Could things have been handled differently?

Interestingly, in 1949 a Dr R.W. Balham took five live adult polecats from the bush to the Dominion Museum. Charles McCann wrote about them and the general Mustelidae introduction into the country.[10] The four males and one female were kept in captivity for some time and surprisingly the males were docile and amenable from the start. The jill was nippy but she settled down in time. They were fed on fresh raw meat and it appeared they refused dead bird carcasses, preferring the meat which they had in plentiful supply. Going forward to the 1980s, Bob Jeffares, ferreter and naturalist of Tu Kuiti, was adamant that there were no polecats on either island but only feral ferrets. He considered that with the modern introduction of the rabbit calicivirus, the ferrets, stoats and weasels of NZ were getting more adverse publicity. There was a fear that without easily available prey (rabbits), the mustelids would turn to ground-dwelling birds for food. Perhaps they did in some instances. He disagreed with the overall concept, citing that previous research had shown that if there was an abundance of easy prey, i.e. large rabbit numbers, ferrets would breed most prolifically. Take away the abundance and the population would drop due to a corresponding decrease in breeding; there was a direct relationship between the population of predators and their prey. (Could the feral ferrets have been trapped and domesticated? Even exported for their bloodlines to other pet ferret countries?)

McCann in 1949 was struck by the easy domestication of the polecats he studied and was of the opinion they were from domestic ferret stock gone feral. The names polecat, ferret and polecat-ferret came from various stock introductions and were considered interchangeable. However, he considered it unlikely that the part-coloured polecats in his charge came entirely from escaped domestic animals. In other words, pure polecats had been introduced into the islands and perhaps mated with released domestic ferrets to give various types of coat colour.

Some dates of the introduction of mustelids into New Zealand:

- 1867 – Introduction of 'five ferrets'; another one arrived a year later
- 1882–1883 – Some 35 shipments of 'ferrets' of 1217 animals; only 678 landed. Subsequently, 198 came from Melbourne, Australia
- 1884 – Nearly 4000 'ferrets' were let loose in NZ. Some 3000 in Marlbourgh district alone and about 400 in Otago. The records give no indication of where the 'ferrets' came from or what they actually were
- 1885/1886 – Author, Carolyn King, quotes numbers of 592 weasels and 224 stoats introduced.[11]

It is now considered that collectors went further than London to collect 'ferrets'.[10] Also large numbers of domesticated ferrets were probably not available for export. If they were, it was questionable whether they could survive in the wild state. Polecats are and were rare in the UK so these would possibly have been taken from European stock, crossed the English Channel to London and shipped on to New Zealand. One story is that ferrets *en route* from the UK to New Zealand in early times were allowed to mate with European polecats so that when the ship arrived in NZ, crossbred ferrets were let loose. The ferrets/polecats were thus able to survive in the wild and were referred to as ferrets. George Symons, a ferreter in Otago, NZ, agreed with Bob Jeffares on the point that feral ferrets, when trapped, are easily domesticated and can be used for ferreting. They tame very easily and quickly. Numbers of feral 'ferrets' are now put at around 1 million in New Zealand. The feral ferrets are easily distinguished from stoats and weasels by their larger size and some comparable features are given in Table 1.3.

Pet ferrets became very popular in the years before the pet ferret ban. Colours were sables, pandas, albinos, chocolates and cinnamons but no black-eyed whites or silver mitts. Owners were concerned about anti-ferret feeling due to the feral ferrets; they looked after their pets. It evolved that pet ferrets were banned in the late 1990s due to destruction of native bird life, presumably by ferrets or polecat hybrids on both islands (Fig. 1.7). A prominent NZ pet ferret owner gave reasons why the claims against pet ferrets were misguided (J. Chessum, PAWS, NZ, pers. comm. 1999). He maintained that,

Table 1.3 The ferret compared with the stoat and weasel in New Zealand

	Ferret (*M. furo*)	Stoat (*M. erminea*)	Weasel (*M. nivalis*)
Facial features	'Panda'-like mask with dark/white hair	Brown face, no mask	Brown face, no mask
Body markings and colour	Dark coat with cream-white underfur. Tail large and with black hair. Leg hair dark.	Coat brown in summer with white belly. May be all white in winter. Tail thin and brown with black tip kept in winter. Legs have brown hair in summer.	Coat is brown and does not change like the stoat in winter. Tail thin like stoat and brown, no change in winter and no black tip. Legs also brown.
Body weight (mean g) Hobs Jills	1200 600	324 207	126 57
Body length, tip of nose to end of tail (mm) Hobs Jills	582 480	390 347	270 224

Chapter One
Classification, history and current status of ferrets

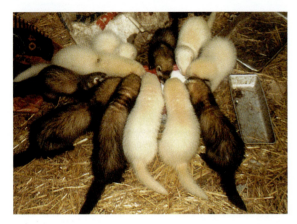

Figure 1.7 Working ferrets in New Zealand pre-1999. *Note* that gathered around the milk bowl are an albino jill with five white kittens, a spayed sable jill and *four feral ferrets*. (Courtesy of George Symons.)

as pet ferrets were sterilized, straying ferrets were not going to have a long-term effect on the feral ferret numbers. In fact, pet ferrets are known to lack good hunting and survival instincts to support themselves in the bush. Pet ferrets, being domesticated, will try to contact human kind in the first instance. If they are rejected, then they may go wild as a stray dog or cat would. The stray ferret usually does not travel far from home and most are found within 1 week.

Ferrets were bred commercially for fur production in fitch farms in NZ from around 1983 but declined in recent years. The original stock were feral ferrets crossed with imported Scottish ferrets; later ferrets were imported from Denmark and Finland to upgrade the pelts (M. Dennis, Southlands Ferrets, NZ, pers. comm. 1998). No further ferrets had been imported up to 1998. It was said that when fitch farms went out of business, the ferrets either escaped or were let loose adding to the feral animal disaster. Two farms went over to breeding ferrets for the pet market overseas; one farm has a 2000 ferret breeding stock (J. Chessum, PAWS, NZ, pers. comm. 1999). The South Island breeding establishment, Southlands Ferrets, Invercargill, produces a number of ferrets sold overseas for laboratory purposes and as pets in the USA and Japan. The North Island Mystic Ferrets Co. in Hamilton advertises pet ferret colours as panda, sable, dark sable, chocolate, cinnamon and albino, available for online sale, not to New Zealand or Australia. It has been suggested by a Netherlands vet that Aleutian disease (AD) may have been introduced into Western Europe from New Zealand. It is somewhat ironic that the NZ Government, paranoid about feral ferrets, would allow at least two ferret breeding establishments to stay in the country but ban serious pet ferret enthusiasts.

America

Ferrets were introduced into North America in colonial times, from those kept for vermin control on board wooden ships and by people who had been using them for ferreting in Europe. Ferrets were also excellent ratters and were better than cats. Some were brought to the Americas from Spain around 1875. The ferret was so successful at hunting rabbits, that some states banned them to protect the rabbit population. Some states like California, Massachusetts and Hawaii banned ferrets completely for fear of losing their native species.

Demand for animal pelts began to include ferrets, along with mink, beaver, etc. and some artists' paint brushes are actually hairs from fitch ferrets.[7] By the year 1915, the town of New London, Ohio, was known as 'Ferretville'; half the ferrets in the USA were bred there. About 2500 breeding females were kept in the area and demand for ferrets numbered close to 200 000 yearly. Ferrets fetched US$2–3 each and perhaps US$5 for a breeding jill. They were sold to hunters, trappers, sportsmen, farmers, elevator and mill men, ranchers and others. A 1943 book by Mr A.R. Harding on *Ferretville* spoke of the 'docility and loyalty of these creatures'. The use of ferrets for hunting rabbits declined over the years unlike in other countries. In recent times, ferrets have been used extensively in the USA and Canada for biomedical research. The pet ferret industry has also boomed. The commercial breeding of ferrets is carried out for laboratory ferrets and for pets and there is some private breeding of pets, of which the estimated population is now over 10 million. Americans love their pet ferrets (Fig. 1.8).

The American way with pet ferrets glamorized them well before ferrets became popular in the UK, Australia and New Zealand, where they are still working animals

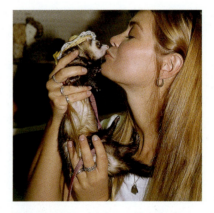

Figure 1.8 American pet ferret with owner. (Courtesy of Greg Rich.)

but now increasingly seen as garden or household pets. Ferrets were banned in a number of American states until the advent of a good rabies vaccine specifically for ferrets and a change of heart that they were not just exotics or wild animals. However, even today, ferrets are banned in California, as they are in Queensland, Australia. There are continuous demands on these states to change the laws against ferrets. With the increased popularity of 'pocket pets', changes should be made.

A lot has been written about American ferrets. Some in-depth study of their behaviour, reproduction, development and inheritance, with her own American pet ferrets, has been given by Fara Shimbo (Ch. 5).[12,13] Their long time vital use in medical experimentation is known. Usually, Marshall Farm's (NY) ferrets are standardized by being sterilized and descented at 6 weeks of age. They have been under some criticism but have been in the ferret market for some time supplying laboratories and in recent years the pet ferret market, and are still a major source of ferrets.[14] The company is conscious of environmental factors affecting ferret health.

Not all medical experimentation in the past led to deaths in ferrets. Dean Manning of Wisconsin, with Judith Bell, did non-lethal experiments with ferrets on blood types and were keen enough on ferrets to take some home as pets after the experiments were concluded. Manning admired the ferret sense of play and can be seen in Figure 1.9 letting the ferrets exercise in the laboratory. The hopeful conclusion is that something else besides animals should be used for experiments in this modern world.

The selling of ferrets de-sexed at an early age is possibly changing for pet ferrets at least in the USA. Early sterilization may well be a ferret health hazard (Ch. 14). The United States Drug Authority (USDA) has been pushed to improve the standards of ferret

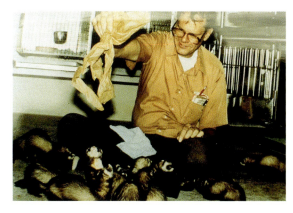

Figure 1.9 Laboratory ferrets at play. (Courtesy of Dean Manning.)

farms, ferret distributors, transportation etc. Basically pet ferrets have been sterilized at 5 weeks of age and then transported to retailers from major breeders. There is a pilot programme now to sell ferrets no younger than 12 weeks of age and delay sterilization (Sukie Crandall, pers. comm. 2005).

South Africa

A South African friend had two pet house-ferrets, which played with the pet mongoose, whose sole purpose was to keep snakes away from the dwelling. Migrants from southern African countries who live in the hills around Perth expressed interest in buying ferrets as pets, because there are a number of poisonous snakes. Unfortunately, the average Australian ferret is not too keen to take on the role of mongoose! Out fer-

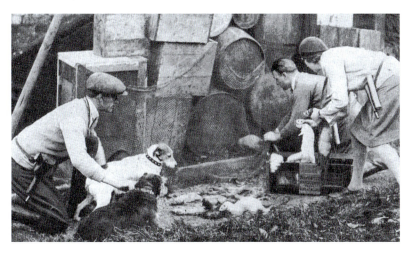

Figure 1.10 Use of ferrets in rat-catching in early 1930s. (*The World of Wonder*, Vol. 4. Edited by Charles Ray.)

reting, if the ferret senses a snake in a hole it will back out in haste with its tail bottle-brushed in alarm! I have only heard of one 'tale of two ferrets' in Spain killing a snake. One ferret teased the snake while the other went for its neck.

As well as protecting humans from venomous snakes and vermin, ferrets have long been used for ratting with the help of Jack Russell terriers, as this 1930s photograph shows (Fig. 1.10). *Note* the rat tally on the ground and both men and women participating in the hunt.

References

1. Miller GS. Mammals of Western Europe (catalogue). London: British Museum; 1912:418–427.
2. Drabble P. Pleasing pets. London: William Luscombe; 1975.
3. Goldsmith O. A history of the earth and animated nature. New York: Arch Cape Press; 1771 (Facsimile 1990).
4. Bewick TA. General history of quadrupeds. Leicester: Windward Press; 1790 (Facsimile 1980).
5. Cory H. Animals of the British Isles. London: Thomas Nelson; 1949. (Previously published as Mammals of the British Isles in 1941).
6. Owen C. Ferret. In: Mason IL, ed. Evolution of domesticated animals. London: Longman; 1984.
7. Shimbo F. The ferret book. Boulder: FURO; 1984.
8. Smith G. The Besynes of Ferettyng. Austral Shooters J Dig 1995:31–135.
9. Carpenter JV, Hillman CN. Husbandry, reproduction and veterinary care of captive ferrets. Annual Proceedings, American Association of Zoo Veterinarians. 1978:36–46.
10. McCann C. Observations on the polecat (*Putorius* Linn.) in New Zealand. Records of the Dominion Museum, NZ; 1995:2, 151–164.
11. King C. The handbook of New Zealand mammals. Oxford: OUP; 1990.
12. Shimbo F. A Tao full of detours: the behaviour of the domestic ferret. Boulder: FURO; 1992.
13. Shimbo F, Maday M. Reproduction, development and inheritance in the ferret. Boulder: FURO; 1994.
14. Brenda (webmaster) (2004) Perspective on Marshall Farms, Ferret Universe. Online. Available: www.ferret-universe.com/marshalls/index.asp

CHAPTER 2

External features and anatomy profile

'I once kept a pet ferret named Stanley. Yet when I would mention my pet ferret to anyone who had not met Stanley, the reaction was almost universally skeptical, "Isn't that some kind of weasel?"'

E.P. Dolensek, DVM. The Penguin Book of Pets, 1978

External features of ferrets

Stray ferrets have been variously described, by unknowing people, as large rats, possums or even some sort of mongoose, despite ferrets now having a high profile in books, on television and in film. When it was released, the film 'Kindergarten Cop' for example, made ferrets more popular in the USA, according to the American Ferret Association.

The dark-eyed and dark-coated ferret resembles the European polecat and has been described as a 'fitch-ferret' or 'polecat-ferret', in contrast to the pink-eyed white (albino) ferret, which is the other traditional colour. It has not been proved that the dark (sable) ferret is a product of a European polecat and white ferret mating.[1] Frances Pitt provided comparative descriptions of the polecat (*Mustela putorius*) and the ferret (*M. furo*) in 1921.[2] The base of the ferret head is narrower than that of the polecat; when viewed from above it resembles an isosceles triangle, whereas the face of the polecat makes an equilateral triangle. The sable ferret's face is interesting for its 'panda' mask look (Fig. 2.1). It is similar to the European polecat, having dark eyes ringed with brown hair and with cream-coloured hair between the eyes and ears, and between the eyes and nose. The eyes are characteristically less prominent than in the native polecat. The nose is white, mottled brown and the ears are small and set close to the head.

When hunting, polecats rely extensively on their sense of smell, even though they have efficient eyes and ears. This is also a feature of ferrets. Like the polecat they have typical cat-like tactile whiskers. Pitt sums up the similarity of the ferret and polecat thus: 'the fitch ferret bears in outward appearance the same relation to the polecat that a half-printed photograph bears to a fully printed one from the same negative'.[2]

Ferrets could be said to have an otter- or weasel-like form. The hobs (males) are more otter-like in shape and size while the smaller jills (females) are more weasel-like. The ferret has short legs with an elongated body. It stands with an arched back and is agile in movement, further arching its back when running. The polecat hob is longer than the adult hob ferret, exceeding 40 cm in body length (head to tail tip), while the hob ferret is smaller at an average of 38 cm. The polecat jill and the ferret jill are typically shorter than the corresponding hobs at around 35 cm (sexual dimorphism). Ferret hobs weigh 1000–2000 g and ferret jills 600–900 g. The birth weight of ferret young (kittens) is usually 10 g (8–12 g range).

The thick blackish-brown outer coat colouring of the 'fitch' or sable ferret is not as dark as the polecat but ferrets living outside tend to be darker. The undercoat is white to yellow against the outer black/brown guard hairs. The colour deepens into black on the legs and tail. Albino ferrets (with unpigmented eyes) and those called black-eyed whites (BEW) are two basic colours (Figs 2.2, 2.3). The genetics of breeding and variations in coat colours are discussed in Chapter 5 along with

CHAPTER TWO
External features and anatomy profile

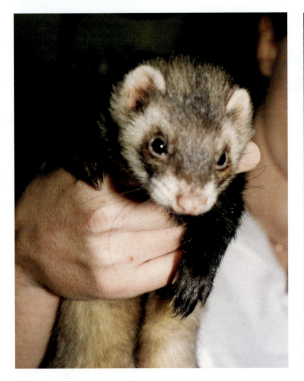

Figure 2.1 Australian sable.

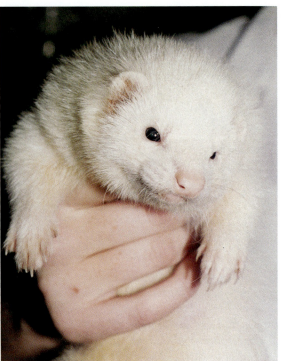

Figure 2.3 Australian black-eyed white.

simple cross-mating possibilities (from Fara Shimbo), in the form of the Punnett Square genotypes. Ferret-polecat domestication is described by Bob Church in Chapter 6.

The mitt ferret (Fig. 2.4) is a grey-coloured ferret with white paws. Mitt, sable, black-eyed white and albino are the basic ferret colours found in Australia.

The pet ferret range of coat colours in the USA

There is a range of 30 coat colour variations recognized at ferret shows by the American Ferret Association and various ferret societies. The Official 2005 AFA Ferret Code of external features describes coat colour and pattern. Eleven basic types can be listed:

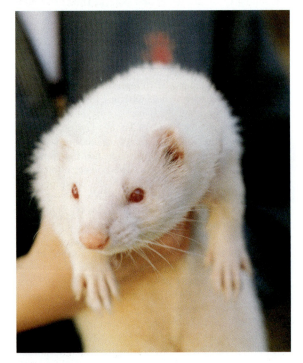

Figure 2.2 Australian albino.

1. Albino
2. Black mitt
3. Black roan mitt
4. Black sable solid
5. Champagne point
6. Chocolate standard
7. Dark-eyed white

External features of ferrets

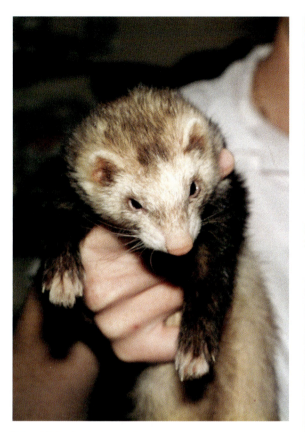

Figure 2.4 Australian mitt.

8. Sable blaze
9. Sable panda
10. Sable point
11. Sable standard.

Except for albino and dark-eyed white (DEW) (our BEW), any ferret can be described using two tables, one of colour and one of pattern as shown in appendix Tables A.14 and A.15. Something of the genetics of coat colour is described in Chapter 5.

Note with the summer moult, sables lighten somewhat. They then darken with the autumn (fall) moult and thicken in coat. This is especially prevalent in ferrets living outdoors, as is usual in Australia, New Zealand before 2000 and the UK, compared with indoor-kept American ferrets.

Colour classification in Russian ferrets is an interesting mix between Russian fitch farms and AFA classifications. The basic genetic colours on a percentage basis are: 81% sable, 15% pastel and 4% albino, with the sable group being variable according to Kalinin.[3] Within sable is the standard sable 46%, dark sable, 4%, pearl, 23%

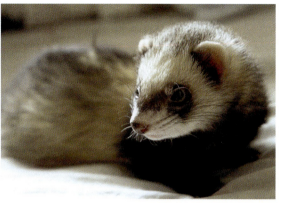

Figure 2.5 Russian sable. (Courtesy of D. Kalinin, Russia 2005.)

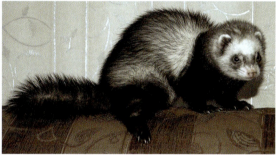

Figure 2.6 Russian pearl. (Courtesy of D. Kalinin.)

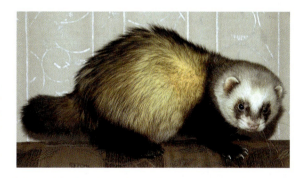

Figure 2.7 Russian goldish. (Courtesy of D. Kalinin.)

and goldish 8%. Their sable and dark sable are coloured from light to dark cream with guard hairs black to warm deep brown (Fig. 2.5); dark sables have a generally darker colour. The undercoats are light to cream but not orange in colour. The mask is V-shaped, not a full or T-bar mask. The Russian pearl (Fig. 2.6) is dark grey; the guard hairs are black with a cold light gray undercoat. Again, the

17

CHAPTER TWO

External features and anatomy profile

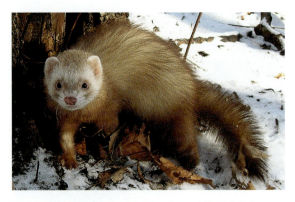

Figure 2.8 Russian pastel. (Courtesy of D. Kalinin.)

mask is a V not a full T-bar mask. The goldish (Fig. 2.7) varies from yellowish to full orange/white with black guard hairs; the undercoat varies from yellowish to full orange. Again the mask is a V, not a full or T-bar. Finally, the pastel (Fig. 2.8) has a colour from light to dark cream with guard hairs light brown and sometimes with an ash-bluish hue. The undercoat is light cream or grey with a V-mask or no mask.[3]

In Italy, most of the pet ferrets are sable or albino but siamese are becoming more common and also silver mitt, black-eyed white and cinnamon. Contacts in Italy have got black sables from Germany. It is possible they might have mink blood introduced to give the self-pattern (A. Melillo, pers. comm. 2005). In Belgium, ferret colours range from fitch (wild colour) to sandy and albino. *Note* some people do not like albinos because

of the red glow of their eyes. The special colours are panda (marked), DEW (our BEW), blaze, polka and angora. These latter ferrets are not considered a good development as they can have deafness and other problems (Wendy Van den Steen, pers. comm. 2005 and see Ch. 5). In Germany, ferret colours range from *'iltis'* (natural or wild) *'harlekin'* (with white feet) 'Siam' or 'I' (yellow) and albino. The *'zimt-harlekin'* is white or yellow with white feet and with black eyes. There is also the panda (white with black hair) or the black self (whole black), which has mink genes but is not common (Fig. 2.9; G. Hanneke, Berlin, pers. comm. 2005). The black self's behaviour is absolutely the same as other ferrets, despite the mink genes, and they will play together and sleep together (Torsten Schulz, Berlin, pers. comm. 2005).

In Japan, there is a full range of ferret colour types from overseas (Yasutsugu Miwa, pers. comm. 2005).

Ferret anatomical features as they relate to general surgery

There are some standard operations which are performed on ferrets (see Chs 18, 19). A general review of some aspects of ferret anatomy will be provided here with reference to ferret conditions and operations where applicable. These include:

1. Sterilization of hob and jill
2. Dental procedures
3. Vasectomy
4. Intestinal FB surgery
5. Adrenal gland neoplasia
6. Insulinoma
7. Removal of scent (musk) glands. (*NOTE*: This operation is *not* absolutely necessary in ferrets to reduce odour and is considered by some to be a mutilation.) Ferrets that stray need to use their scent glands as an 'escape method' when in danger from a dog or cat. In some countries, the practice is actually banned, e.g. Belgium and the Netherlands (Wendy Van den Steen, pers. comm. 2005). In Japan, people were not sure about ferrets which had been bred privately and not sterilized until 6 months of age, as they had been used to Marshall Farm ferrets, which were sterilized and underwent musk gland removal at 6 weeks of age.)

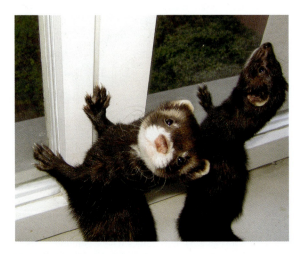

Figure 2.9 Black self female Jadzia Dax has extreme play instinct and looks to go into the garden. Dark 'polecat' male Worf queries when! (Courtesy of Torsten Schulz, Germany, 2005.)

The skeleton

H. Evans and N. An have extensively reviewed the complete anatomy of the ferret (Fig. 2.10).[4] The following picks out a few points of interest to practitioners.

Ferret anatomical features as they relate to general surgery

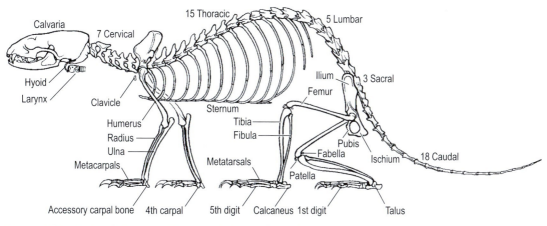

Figure 2.10 The ferret skeleton. (Courtesy of Howard Evans.)

The ferret spine is very flexible, as befits an agile animal whose ancestor, the polecat, ranks among the most efficient of hunters. The ferret carries on the tradition in its ferreting skills. A ferret can turn on itself in a pipe or rabbit warren.

It has been said that the unpaired innominate artery (brachiocephalic) at the base of the neck aids the ferret's agility[5] but there are still two common carotid arteries in the neck and not a single one as implied (H. Evans, pers. comm. 1999).

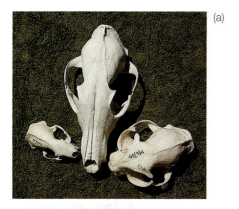

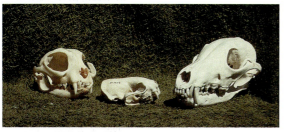

Figure 2.11 (a) Comparative skulls: main pet carnivores, ferret, dog, and cat, dorsal view. (b) Lateral view.

The vertebral formula is: C7, T15, L5 (6), S3, Cd 18.

From Fig. 2.9 it can be seen that the ferret has 15 pairs of ribs with the first 10 pairs attached to the sternum. The first ribs are relatively small, making the thoracic inlet narrow in contrast to other animals for the passage of the trachea, oesophagus and large blood vessels. This can be significant when discussing chest problems. The spinal cord can be subject to damage resulting from fractured vertebrae or disc protrusion. This is a particular risk in breeding jills especially in a heavily pregnant or lactating jill (Ch. 5). Heavily pregnant jills and heavy hobs should be well-supported by a hand under the rump when handling, to guard against excessive strain on the vertebral column. The appendicular skeleton is naturally fine light bone with long bones of matchstick diameter. In accident situations, the long bones may fracture and require pinning with K wire (Ch. 19). It is also possible to use the femur for interosseous blood transfusion (Ch. 20). The ferret resembles the dog in having five toes with non-retractable claws, unlike the cat, and the pet ferret will thus possibly require routine nail clipping.

The skull

The ferret skull shows the characteristics of the carnivore and it can be noted from Figure 2.11 that the ferret and dog have unclosed zygomatic bones to the eye orbit in contrast to the cat.[6] It can be seen from Figure 2.11a that one-third of the ferret skull comprises the short facial region with the brain case relatively large.

Figure 2.12b shows the typical carnivore dentition with large curved canines and strong premolars and molars in the permanent formulae. The dental formulae for the kitten and adult ferret can be given.

CHAPTER TWO
External features and anatomy profile

The kitten's temporary teeth first erupt between the 3rd and 4th week. *Note*: it is possible for a 4-week-old kitten's needle-sharp canines to inflict damage on the jill's mammary glands, leading to mastitis.

Deciduous dentition[7]

Upper
Arcade I $\frac{4|4}{}$ C $\frac{1|1}{}$ P $\frac{3|3}{}$ M $\frac{0|0}{}$
Lower   I 3|3   C 1|1   P 3|3   M 0|0
Total   30 teeth

Permanent dentition[7]

Upper
Arcade I $\frac{3|3}{}$ C $\frac{1|1}{}$ P $\frac{3|3}{}$ M $\frac{1|1}{}$
Lower   I 3|3   C 1|1   P 3|3   M 2|2
Total   34 teeth

The ferret's permanent teeth appear from the 7th week of age, with the upper and lower canines plus the first lower molar appearing first. At about 53 days, the upper molar is seen. This is followed by the second, third and fourth upper premolars, second lower and third lower premolars, which are all present by 67 days after birth. Finally, in the lower jaw the fourth premolar and second molar are present 1 week later.[4] (Further detailed ferret dental anatomy and associated disease are discussed by Bob Church in Chapter 21.)

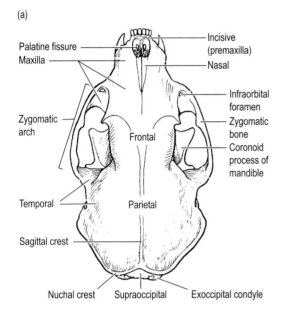

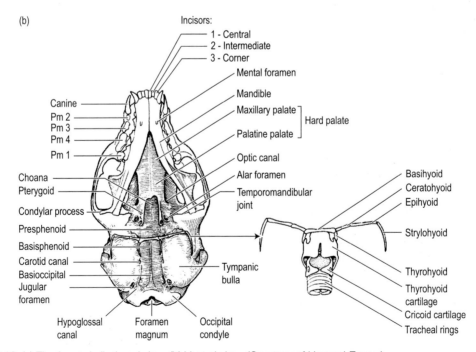

Figure 2.12 (a) The ferret skull, dorsal view. (b) Ventral view. (Courtesy of Howard Evans.)

Ferret anatomical features as they relate to general surgery

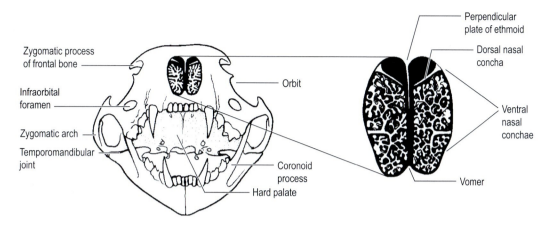

Figure 2.13 Ferret skull, rostral view. (Courtesy of Howard Evans.)

The rostral view of the ferret skull (Fig. 2.13) illustrates the very narrow ventral space in the nasal conchae, through which only a 3.0 French red rubber stomach tube could be passed in an emergency (Ch. 20).

The characteristic carnivore dentition is evident in this view of the skull. The canine teeth shown should remind us that the ferret bite can be very severe and they tend to hang on just as much as a dog! A ferret jaw is powerful enough for them to kill small prey by crushing the skull.

Abnormalities can occur in the dentition. Western Australian ferret kittens have shown supernumerary incisors. In one survey of 350 ferrets from various UK breeders, 26 ferrets had one or two supernumerary incisors.[8] There were three ferrets with broken canines. This was considered at the time an action by ferreters to stop them killing rabbits but is not necessary and today would be regarded as a mutilation. Canine teeth can be fractured in fights or by accidents and modern ferret dentistry can effect a repair.[9] Basic dentistry is now commonly carried out for scaling and extracting teeth under anaesthesia with pet ferrets.

The brain

The neuroanatomy of the ferret brain is discussed in detail by Lawes and Andrews.[10] It is approximately 36 mm long and 24 mm wide and described as a gyrencephalic forebrain when viewed from above; as it overlaps the cerebellum. Studies have been conducted on brain size of ferrets and polecats. In 1982, Smith discovered that Australian ferrets had only about two-thirds of the brain size of their wild polecat cousins, roughly 6 mL compared with polecats at 9 mL.[11]

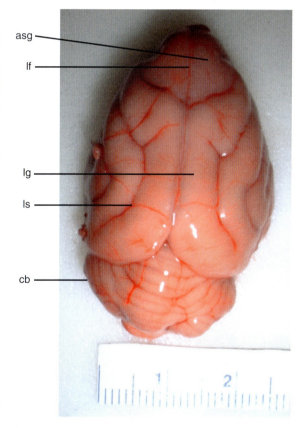

Figure 2.14 Ferret brain, dorsal view: asg, anterior sigmoid gyrus; cb, cerebellum; lf, longitudinal fissure; lg, lateral gyrus; ls, lateral sulcus. (Courtesy of Joerge Mayer.)

CHAPTER TWO
External features and anatomy profile

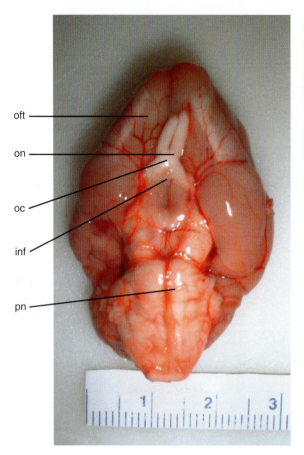

Figure 2.15 Ferret brain, ventral, view: oft, olfactory tubercle; oc, optic chiasma; on, optic nerve; inf, infundibular; pn, pons. (Courtesy of Joerge Mayer.)

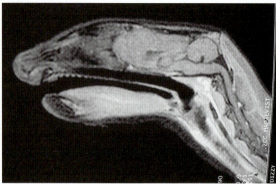

Figure 2.16 Ferret longitudinal section brain and neck (Courtesy of Joerge Mayer.)

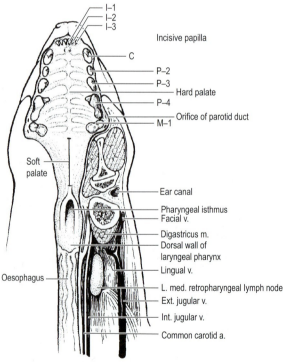

Figure 2.17 Ferret pharynx and structures of interest. (Courtesy of Howard Evans.)

Smith theorizes that his may have a bearing on the ferrets' lack of adaptability to survive in Australian bush conditions.

The average practitioner would perhaps have not seen a ferret brain as shown in Figure 2.14 (dorsal view) and Figure 2.15 (ventral view). Some feature points are indicated. *Note*: the olfactory bulb anterior extension is missing in this specimen.

A ferret brain section including the upper neck as in Figure 2.16 shows some interesting features. The streamlining of the ferret head is obvious as is the large amount of space for the olfactory organ of the nasal sinuses. The relative position of the spinal cord, oesophagus and trachea anatomically can be visualized from this section.

The cribriform plate between the olfactory sinuses and the brain could well be the site of entry to the brain by cryptococcosis yeasts. This disease and others of the special sense organs of the ear, eye and nose are discussed in Chapter 12.

Note in Figure 2.17 the upper dental arcade where the molar appears tucked behind the fourth premolar and is sometimes the site of a root abscess. The jaw musculature is indicated by the cross-section of the digastricus and masseter muscles on the left side. The ferret has a powerful bite, like all mustelids. It has a well-developed masseter muscle originating at the zygomatic arch and inserting on the masseteric fossa, condyloid crest and mandibular angular process. The digastricus muscle originates on the jugular process and tympanic bulla and passes to the ventral border of the caudal portion of the mandible and has the action of opening the jaw (H. Evans, pers. comm. 1998). The major adductor muscle of the lower jaw is the temporalis and is well-developed in the hob. The deep pterygoid muscles, lateral and medial, assist the master and temporalis muscles in the crushing and chewing motion of closing the jaws. The ferret, like the polecat, can clamp its jaws tight on a prey and will not let go. Large strong birds have been known to take weasels, stoats and even polecats aloft when they have been bitten on the foot.

The external jugular vein is one of the main routes for bleeding or giving blood. It lies quite lateral on the neck and is deeper to palpate in a hob with its thickened neck.

The oesophagus can have a dilated transthoracic section defined as a megaoesophagus (this is sometimes also seen in puppies). The musculature of the oesophagus is thin and weak and motility is reduced, leading to typical food bolus collection and regurgitation (K. Rosenthall, pers. comm. 1999). This condition has occurred in ferrets and is now a rarity.[12]

Figure 2.18 indicates that the salivary glands consist of five pairs, the parotid, mandibular, sublingual, molar and zygomatic. These glands can be damaged in fights between hob ferrets; this situation typically occurs in the mating season. The resulting formation of mucoceles will require surgical drainage. Miller and Pickett have described an operation on a zygomatic salivary gland mucocele.[13]

Figure 2.19 provides a ventral view of the ferret head and neck region showing the position of the thyroid and parathyroid glands plus the medial retropharyngeal

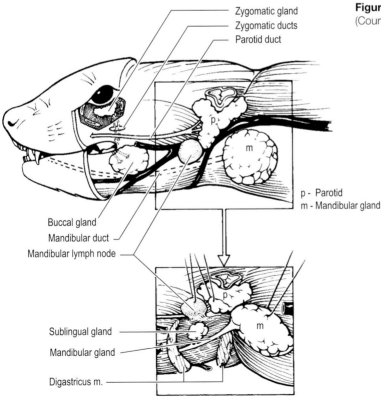

Figure 2.18 Ferret salivary glands. (Courtesy of Howard Evans.)

CHAPTER TWO
External features and anatomy profile

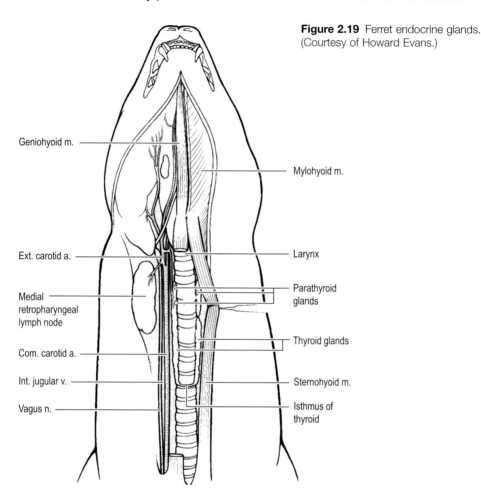

Figure 2.19 Ferret endocrine glands. (Courtesy of Howard Evans.)

lymph node. The latter can be the site of neoplasia as can other external lymph nodes (Ch. 13).

The ferret tongue (Fig. 2.20) is long and freely movable and can be pulled forward to expose the tracheal entrance for endotracheal tubing as in other animals. The lingual frenulum can be the site of grass awn penetrations, especially in working ferrets in summer.

Figure. 2.21a shows the ferret heart and lungs seen *in situ* under ventral view. The heart is found roughly between the 6th rib (indicated) and the 8th rib and for auscultation purposes is more posterior in the chest than first imagined. The heart ligament joining it to the sternum will lose its fatty coat in cases of heart disease and, on radiology, if the heart is actually resting on the sternum, it can be a sign of early cardiac enlargement and disease according to Brown.[14] Figure 2.21b shows internal views of right and left cranial lung lobes, right middle lung lobe, left caudal lobe, right atrium and right ventricle of the heart and lung view of Figure 2.21a.

Note: the ferret lungs have a large volume in relation to body weight, with total lung capacity exceeding a predicted value by 297%. This indicates why the ferret has value as an experimental animal for research into human conditions. A cast of the ferret lung is shown in Figure 2.21c.

The lungs contain excess submucosal glands in the bronchial wall and extra terminal bronchioles, making them anatomically like human lungs.[15] The cellular situation makes ferrets able to be infected by human influenza and canine distemper.

Figure 2.22a,b shows that the ferret left ovary is caudal to the left kidney. *Note* how the uterine horn is related to the ureter. Care must be taken not to damage the ureter or sever it during ovariohysterectomy. The

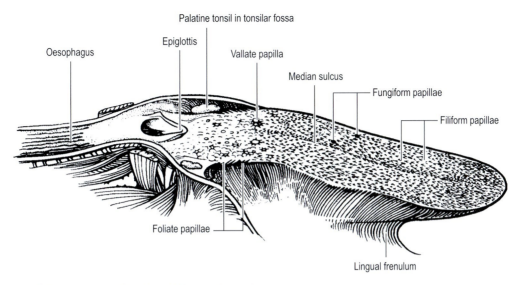

Figure 2.20 Ferret tongue. (Courtesy of Howard Evans.)

heart is seen between the 6th and 8th ribs and is obliquely placed in the thoracic cavity with the apex to the left side.

The thoracic inlet is narrow, as suggested earlier, with the small first ribs.

The thymus gland, which can be associated with juvenile neoplasia (Ch. 13) varies in size depending on the ferret's age. It is situated in the cranial mediastinum just within the thoracic inlet. With the anterior mediastinal lymph node, trachea, oesophagus, major blood vessels, and anterior lung lobe often taking space, any abnormality of even one organ at that point can cause serious interference with chest functions.

Figure 2.23 presents a jill ferret with a normal size vulva that is not swollen in heat. The vulva is hardly visible in the live animal. The left ovary and the quiescent uterine horn can be seen bordered by the descending colon that covers them. This is displaced when trying to find the left ovary during the spaying operation.

The characteristics of the digestive system can be seen where the simple stomach lies on the curve of the liver in the cranial abdomen. It is capable of tremendous swelling and an adult hob ferret has been known to eat 80 g of meat at one time and then slowly digest it overnight. Ferrets are able to vomit and have been used in experiments on the physiology of vomiting relating to humans (A. James, The Chinese University of Hong Kong, China, pers. comm. 1998).

Figure 2.24 shows the small intestine. It is approximately 182.198 cm long and extends from the pylorus of the stomach to the junction with the colon[4] (compare this with the lateral views of Fig. 2.14).

The duodenum, the proximal loop of small intestine, is about 10 cm long. The ileum and jejunum have no apparent demarcation and pass to the large intestine. The large intestine is approximately 10 cm long. There is no ileocolic valve in the ferret and no caecum. Because the caecum is missing, the ileocolic junction is indistinct. However, the junction can be inferred by the pattern of the jejunal artery, which anastomoses with the ileocolic artery. The colon is divided into ascending, transverse and descending portions and ends at the junction with the rectum at the pelvic inlet level. The anus has an internal (smooth muscle) and external (voluntary muscle) sphincter system.[4] It is the external sphincter that encloses the paired musk glands which have openings on either side of the anal canal (like anal glands in dogs and cats) (see later, Figs 2.28, 2.29). The musk glands are approximately 10 mm by 5 mm and their removal (anal sacculectomy) is described (Ch. 18).

Major organs of the ferret abdomen

The liver can be the site of primary neoplasia in the ferret or subject to secondary invasions of malignant cells (see Chs 9, 13).

Figure 2.25a shows the curve of the liver, which fits into the curve of the diaphragm, which is divided into a typical muscular dome with central tendinous area and two crura. The liver is relatively large compared with the average ferret body weight. An 800–1150 g animal could have a liver of 35–59 g; the ratio of liver weight to body weight is 4.3% in ferrets and 3.4% in dogs.[4]

CHAPTER TWO
External features and anatomy profile

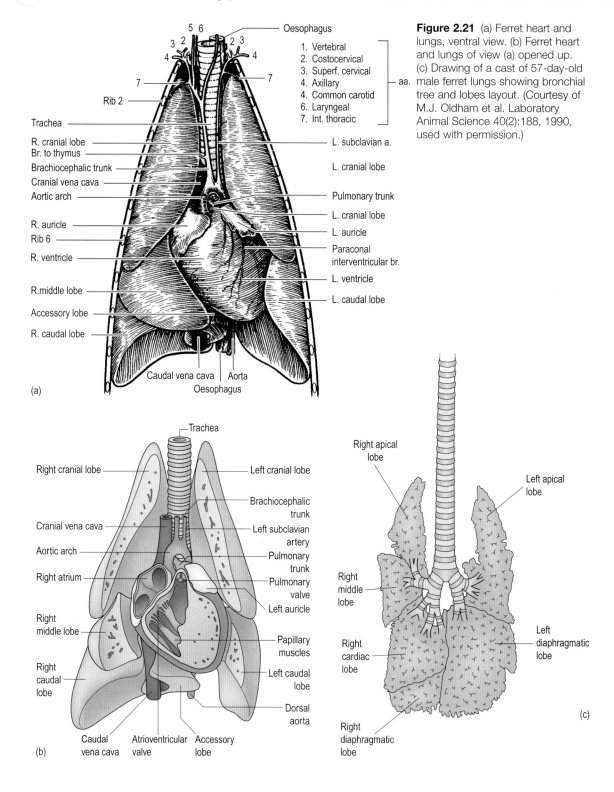

Figure 2.21 (a) Ferret heart and lungs, ventral view. (b) Ferret heart and lungs of view (a) opened up. (c) Drawing of a cast of 57-day-old male ferret lungs showing bronchial tree and lobes layout. (Courtesy of M.J. Oldham et al. Laboratory Animal Science 40(2):188, 1990, used with permission.)

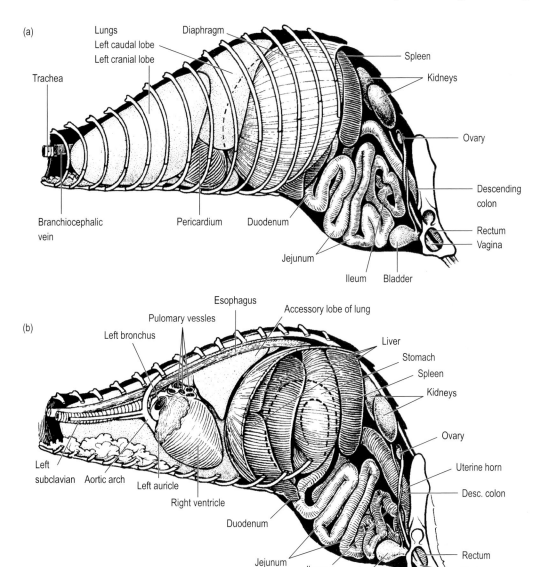

Figure 2.22 (a) The thoracic and abdominal viscera by a superficial left lateral view. Dotted line shows the curve of the diaphragm. (b) The ferret thoracic and abdominal viscera on lateral view showing left lung removed. The dotted lines show the stomach passing to the pylorus dorsally and the duodenum. (Courtesy of Howard Evans.)

The liver has right lateral, right and left medial lobes, a quadrate central lobe hiding the gall bladder and a left lateral lobe.

Figure 2.26 demonstrates the position of the pancreas in the abdomen with the small and large intestine removed. It is an elongate, lobulate, V-shaped organ, usually light pink to bright red in colour. It can be the site of insulinoma cancers in ferrets.

The spleen is a grey-brown organ lying in the left hypogastric area, running parallel to the greater curvature of the stomach. It is crescent-shaped and can become large normally in adults, though also very enlarged as a primary or secondary cancer. The ovaries are seen caudal to their respective kidneys. During spaying of jill ferrets, the ovaries might well be obscured by the presence of fat and thus care must be taken in

CHAPTER TWO
External features and anatomy profile

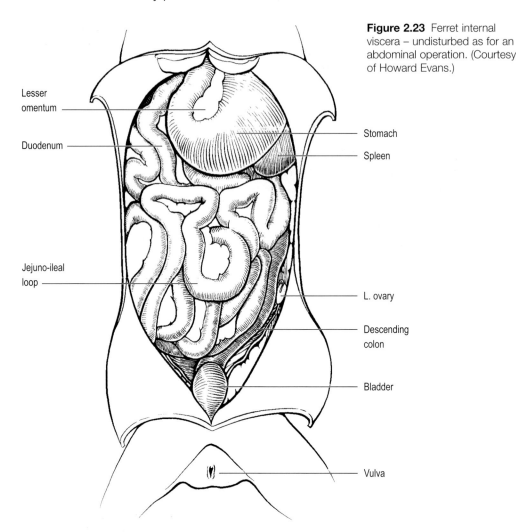

Figure 2.23 Ferret internal viscera – undisturbed as for an abdominal operation. (Courtesy of Howard Evans.)

making sure the full ovary is removed and no remnants are left as these can produce hormonal problems.

The ferret uterus comprises two long tapering uterine horns, which combine immediately in front of the cervix to form a short uterine body as shown. The blood supply to the ovaries, oviducts and uterus is via the ovarian and uterine arteries and attending veins. Both ovarian arteries, as shown, arise directly from the aorta. In addition, Figure 2.26 shows the position of the left adrenal gland, very often associated with adrenal neoplasia, in relation to the left kidney.

Figure 2.27 is an enlarged representation of the positions of the left and right adrenal glands in relation to blood vessels and both kidneys. They are situated adjacent to the upper borders of the left and right kidneys and usually embedded in fat. The exact positions vary with individual animals.[16] The adrenal glands are both subject to hormone-stimulated neoplasia. The left adrenal gland is found close to the left side of the abdominal aorta and caudal to the origin of the superior mesenteric artery. The gland measures 6–8 mm, is oval-shaped and usually has a pinkish colour. It may also have a grooved surface due to the adrenolumbar vein which crosses it to enter the vena cava. The right adrenal gland is more elongated (approximately 8–11 mm long) and is in a more dangerous position in relation to possible surgery. It lies more rostral than the left gland being close to the point of origin of the superior mesenteric artery. It should be noted that the right adrenal gland is always related ventrally to the posterior vena cava, which may overlap the medial half of the gland or overlie it completely making surgery dangerous (Ch. 19). The right adrenal gland may also be grooved by the right adrenolumbar vein.

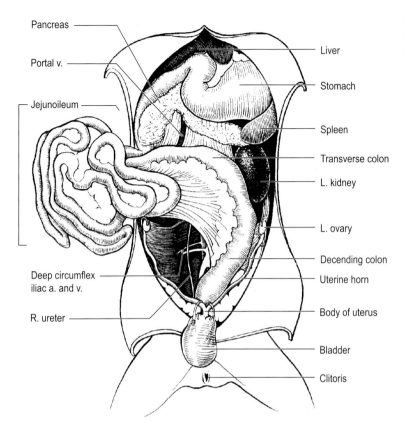

Figure 2.24 Ferret abdominal viscera with intestines displaced. (Courtesy of Howard Evans.)

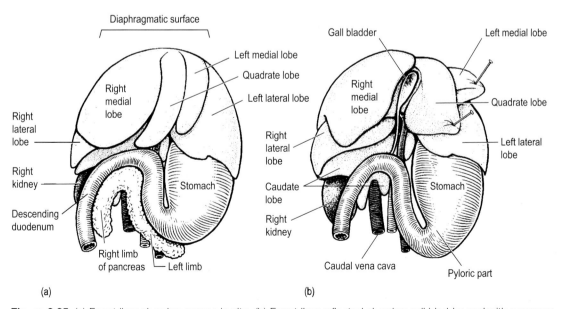

Figure 2.25 (a) Ferret liver showing organs in situ. (b) Ferret liver reflected showing gall bladder and with pancreas removed. (Courtesy of Howard Evans.)

CHAPTER TWO
External features and anatomy profile

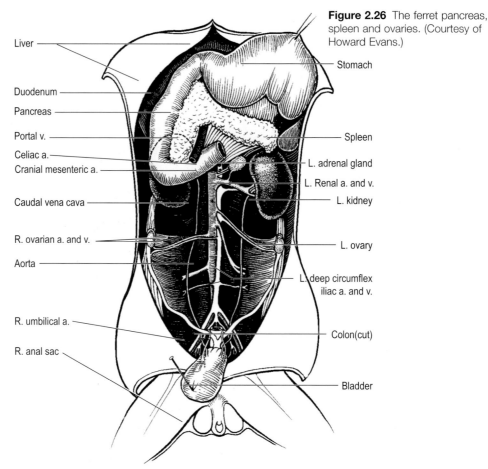

Figure 2.26 The ferret pancreas, spleen and ovaries. (Courtesy of Howard Evans.)

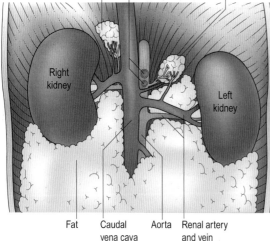

Figure 2.27 Ferret adrenal glands and kidneys. (Courtesy of Lippincott/Wiiliams & Wilkins Co. and Howard Evans.)

The kidneys are both retroperitoneal lying in the sublumbar region on either side of the vertebral column, main aorta and caudal vena cava. They have a classic bean shape (see also Fig. 2.24).

The features of the bladder in relation to the female reproductive system are shown in Figure 2.28 and with the male reproductive system in Figure 2.29.

The bladder naturally varies in size depending on content but when empty, measures roughly 1 cm wide by 2 cm long. The ureters run from the renal pelvis and pass down to the bladder on either side. In this lateral view, *note* the right ureter entering the bladder plus the right uterine horn entering the body of the vagina. *Note* also the position of the musk glands (anal glands). The duct to the rectal sphincter is not indicated but is shown in Figure 2.29.

Figure 2.30 shows a schematic left lateral view of the hob genital and pelvic region blood supply. Castration of hob ferrets is a common operation but a more delicate and equally important operation is that of vasectomy. The treated hob can then be used to take

Ferret anatomical features as they relate to general surgery

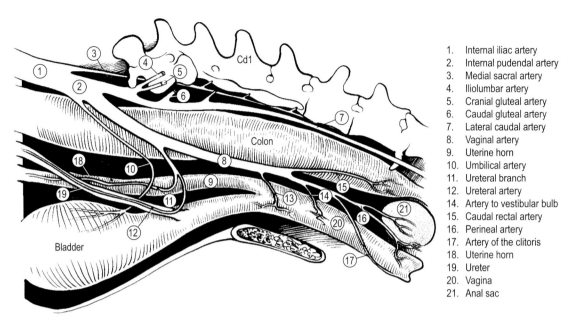

Figure 2.28 The bladder in relation to the jill reproductive system. (Courtesy of Howard Evans.)

1. Internal iliac artery
2. Internal pudendal artery
3. Medial sacral artery
4. Iliolumbar artery
5. Cranial gluteal artery
6. Caudal gluteal artery
7. Lateral caudal artery
8. Vaginal artery
9. Uterine horn
10. Umbilical artery
11. Ureteral branch
12. Ureteral artery
14. Artery to vestibular bulb
15. Caudal rectal artery
16. Perineal artery
17. Artery of the clitoris
18. Uterine horn
19. Ureter
20. Vagina
21. Anal sac

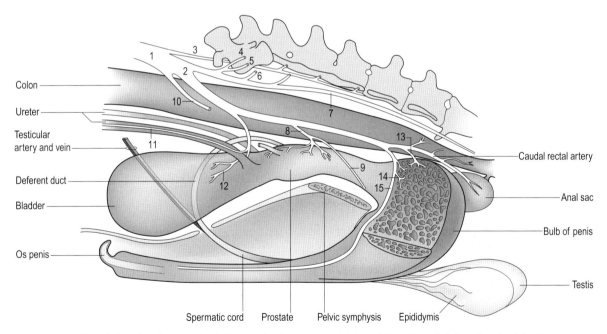

Figure 2.29 The bladder in relation to the hob reproductive system. **1.** Internal iliac artery; **2.** internal pudendal artery; **3.** medial sacral artery; **4.** iliolumbar artery; **5.** cranial gluteal artery; **6.** caudal gluteal artery; **7.** lateral caudal artery; **8.** prostatic artery; **9.** urethral artery; **10.** umbilical artery; **11.** ureteral artery branch; **12.** caudal vesicle artery; **13.** artery of the bulb; **14.** deep artery of penis; **15.** dorsal artery of penis. (Courtesy of Lippincott/Williams & Wilkins Co. and Howard Evans.)

jills off heat, to rest them from breeding without recourse to hormonal injection. The hob genitalia resemble that of the dog in having an os penis or baculum. The baculum of the ferret, and indeed the other mustelids, is a bony strengthening rod as with the dog but has an exterior curled point that makes

CHAPTER TWO

External features and anatomy profile

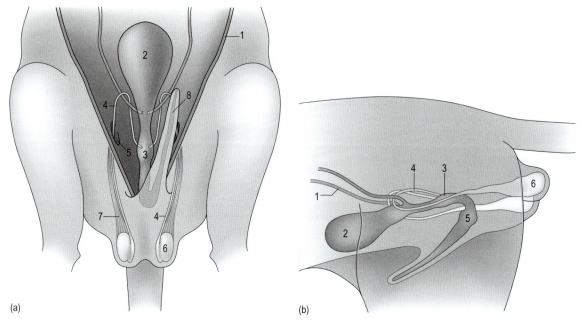

Figure 2.30 (a) Hob genitalia ventral view. (b) Hob genitalia lateral view. **1.** Ureter; **2.** bladder; **3.** prostate; **4.** deferent duct; **5.** inguinal canal; **6.** left testis; **7.** cremaster muscle; **8.** urethra; **9.** bulb of penis. (Courtesy of Lippincott/Williams & Wilkins Co. and Howard Evans.)

urethral catheterization difficult but not impossible (Ch. 20).

Note the position of the prostate gland at the base of the bladder surrounding the urethra. It is not very distinct in the young ferret. At the level of the prostate, the ductus deferens from each side opens into the urethra. Prostatic cysts can develop in association with adrenal gland neoplasia, which can cause urethral obstruction.

Figure 2.30a,b illuminates the layout of the hob genitalia in respect to castration, vasectomy and injuries to the baculum. It is important to visualize the course of the spermatic cord for the vasectomy operation (Ch. 19).

This chapter has attempted to give a general outline of the ferret anatomy relevant to highlighted points of interest and common operations. (For further anatomy details refer to Evans and An[4] in James Fox's book, *Biology and Diseases of the Ferret* (2nd edn.) and for surgery outlines see Chapters 18 and 19 later in this book.)

References

1. Owen C. Ferret. In: Mason IL, ed. Evolution of domesticated animals. London: Longman; 1984:225–228.
2. Pitt F. Notes on the genetic behaviour of certain characters in the polecat, ferret, and in polecat-ferret hybrids. J Genetics 1921; 11:100–115.
3. Kalinin D. Russian domestic ferret: population monitoring. South Australian Ferret Association News 2005; 17(1):11–13.
4. Evans HE, An NQ. Anatomy of the ferret. In: Fox JG, ed. Biology and diseases of the ferret, 2nd edn. Baltimore: Williams & Wilkins; 1998:19–70.
5. Willis LS, Barrow MV. The ferret *(Mustela putorius furo)* as a laboratory animal. Lab Anim Sci 1971; 21:712–716.
6. Wen GY, Sturman JA, Shek JW. A comparative study of the tapetum, retina and skull of the ferret, dog and cat. Lab Anim Sci 1985; 35:200–210.
7. Pass D, Butler R, Lewington JH et al. Veterinary care of birds, rodents, rabbits, ferrets and guinea pigs. Perth, Australia: Murdoch University, Foundation for Continuous Education 1993:65–106.
8. Andrews PLR, Illman O, Mellersh A. Some observations of anatomical abnormalities and disease states in a population of 350 ferrets (*Mustela furo* L.). Z Versuchstierk 1979; 21:346–353.
9. Johnson-Delaney CA, Nelson WB. A rapid procedure for filling fractured canine teeth of ferrets. J Exotic Anim Med 1992; 1:100–101.
10. Lawes INC, Andrews PLR. Neuroanatomy of the ferret brain. In: Fox JG, ed. Biology and diseases of the ferret, 2nd edn. Baltimore: Williams & Wilkins; 1998:71–102.
11. Smith G. Cranial morphology and ontogeny in the ferret. Adelaide: Privately published by G. Smith; 1982.
12. Harms C, Andrews GA. Megaoesophagus in a domestic ferret. Lab Anim Sci 1993; 43:5.

13. Miller PE, Pickett JP. Zygomatic salivary gland mucocoele in a ferret. J Am Vet Med Assoc 1989; 194:1437.
14. Brown S. Basic anatomy, physiology and husbandry. In: Hillyer EV, Quesenberry KE, eds. Ferrets, rabbits and rodents, clinical medicine and surgery. Philadelphia: Saunders; 1997:3–13.
15. Whary MT, Andrews PIR. Physiology of the ferret. In: Fox JG, ed. Biology and diseases of the ferret, 2nd edn. Baltimore: Williams & Wilkins; 1998:103–148.
16. Holmes RL. The adrenal glands of the ferret *Mustela putorius*. J Anat 1991; 95:325–336.

CHAPTER 3

Accommodation

'Many people prefer to let their ferrets run about loose in large huts, houses or in loose-boxes in a stable but this of course is a matter of taste.'

Nicholas Everitt, Ferrets, 1897

Having kept ferrets since the 1970s, I came to consider them equal to dogs and cats as pet or working animals, without knowing about ferrets overseas. When it comes to considering how ferrets are housed, there is a kaleidoscope of ideas in the ferret world, as there is for feeding them. I have endeavoured to give them a habitat encompassing the world of their polecat ancestors and that of the indoor-living dog, cat and indeed the American indoor pet ferret. I am therefore putting forward my ideas on keeping ferrets, with a discussion of the general ways ferrets have been housed in the past and today. I am especially concerned with ferrets in a hot climate.

There was a worry about ferrets 'going bush' in Australia and other countries. In Australia, as explained earlier, they are not adaptable to the climate to establish themselves in the wild, unlike their namesakes in New Zealand. It should be stressed that ferrets do not 'escape' but they 'stray', for they are first and foremost a domesticated animal. Ferrets are however inquisitive and will wander along any interesting scent trail. They should easily find their way back to base, via their own scent trail, but disaster could occur when heavy rain washes away the scent. Storm drains can be a nightmare when it comes to stray ferrets getting down them and going for miles! Ferrets in a 'ferret-proof garden' should be accustomed to part of the entire garden so that it becomes their territory and they are less inclined to wander if given the chance.

People owning single unsterilized pet ferrets will find the ferrets to be more inclined to wander in the mating season and this is the optimum time that ferrets get lost. It is possible to create contentment in ferrets in their enclosed outside environment. In my case, when in practice, I took a number of pet ferrets to work with me each day and, on returning home in the evening, placed them in the back garden. In the interest of ferret bonding with humans, veterinarians should encourage their ferret-owning clients to think likewise. In many cases, the client is well ahead in making the ferret a part of the family, rather than an additional pet.

Basic considerations when discussing ferret husbandry

Ferrets are temperate zone animals but have spread around the world from the UK and continental Europe to the Americas, Australia, New Zealand and South Africa and even recently to Japan, as pet, working or laboratory animals. The *UFAW Handbook* gives the comfort temperature for ferrets as 15–21°C with reference to laboratory animals. Working or pet ferrets are subject around the world therefore to temperature extremes. In Western Australia, possible extreme summer heat is a problem. The temperature can be above 35°C on dry summer days. Dry and hot conditions can be fatal to ferrets as to other animals. Ferrets have no sweat glands and are at risk in temperatures above 30°C. Added to this, there is a range of temperature and humidity over Australia, from tropical to the cool temperate climate in Tasmania.

There are no feral ferrets in Tasmania but they do occur in New Zealand (see Ch. 1). If ferrets are taken to tropical north Australia, they must be kept in air-conditioned premises. Also, if they are kept outside, they would be at risk of heartworm disease (see Ch. 10). If ferrets were feral on mainland Australia, besides the climatic conditions, they would also have predators, e.g. hawks, feral cats, dingoes and foxes. In the UK and continental Europe, ferrets would be more at home with native polecats. In the UK, the incidence of feral ferrets is small compared with the high numbers of feral mink.

In Russia, ferrets have become pets and are kept indoors and outside in sheds. They are larger than American or European ferrets, the body weight of males can be 1.8–3.2 kg and they require space and strong caging. In Japan, ferrets are indoor pets, sometimes kept in small cages, with exercise time out, but some people keep them free in their rooms (Yasutsugu Miwa, pers. comm. 2005). In Italy, the average pet ferret lives 'caged' while the owner is not home and enjoys freedom playing in the house. Many ferret lovers have more than one ferret; the average being 2–3 per household.

Ferret behaviour in groups

A trial was carried out in 2003 on ferret behaviour in pairs with respect to aggression.[1] Personally, over some time breeding ferrets and with ferrets as pets, I have had no real problems of aggressive ferrets. I have had ferrets in a 'colony' situation with one or more hobs with entire jills, neutered males and neutered jills. Within the group, there was an initial squabbling, the older hob pulling the younger around by the scruff, with squealing and perhaps some release of musk glands by the victim, but usually the release of the musk gland is the very last resort. Then the pecking order was arranged between them and the group would then all settle down to drink even from the same bowl. Many times adding a new bought ferret or a taken-in stray to the colony mix caused some chattering and nipping but it soon settled down. Introducing a strange ferret to the group by putting it with them around a bowl of diluted milk helps. I have never kept descented pet ferrets and there has not been a problem with smell. I prefer ferrets to keep their musk glands, as they are an important deterrent if the ferret ever strays and encounters a dog or cat. In the wild, the polecat is a solitary animal and territory would be fought over when hobs met or jills on heat were involved. With pet ferrets, their demeanour is less aggressive than their wild counterparts, as befits the domestication over centuries (Ch. 6).

In some cases the jill, particularly when she is not in heat and is rebuking the advances of a testosterone charged hob, will be aggressive. The hob avoids her attack on him by always turning his back and pushing her away. In a breeding colony naturally the hobs are separated, as breeding stock is valuable. In my garden ferret layout, the numbers of critters have always had space to spread out in what has become their territory.

Ferrets living outdoors

What can you tell your clients about keeping ferrets outside the house? Ferrets have long been considered useful animals in Europe. A remarkable book written in 1897 by Nicholas Everitt, entitled, *Ferrets: their management in health and disease with remarks on their legal status*, puts the keeping of ferrets in perspective. As the UK author wrote at the time: 'Before one can start keeping and breeding ferrets with success it is essential that a fit and proper place be found to keep them in. More often one finds on visiting the lockers of owners of these animals that they are confined anywhere but where they should be. A dark, dismal corner of some draughty outhouse or stable seems a favourite nook for ferret keepers. Any old box, tub, tea-chest or rough bits of board patched together seems to satisfy, and it is wonderful to see how well the animals, in some instances, thrive and multiply in these by no means congenial residences, especially when one considers several manufacturers who will in a few days fix up, at a reasonable cost, any conceivable kind of ferret box, hutch, court or yard that may be desired.' The types of accommodation suggested will be discussed and remarkably, they have not changed much since Nicholas Everett wrote in 1897! This book boasted 42 illustrations, from woodcuts by the author and others. There was one particular illustration of an elaborate combination cote which the author did not actually recommend but gave as one more example of the various hutches, kennels, yards, courts and other ferret homes that could be produced in his time. The fancy combination cote had matchboard sides, backs and divisions, weatherboard roof, painted outside, whitened inside, a wood frame and wire lattice front, wrought-iron bars or netting and the floor wad raised 1 foot (30 cm) above the ground (Fig. 3.1).

Ferrets in the UK, Australia and formerly New Zealand are kept in various kinds of cages, even aviaries, and garden sheds or garages. It has been noted that commercial ferret-breeding establishments and fitch (ferret pelt) farms occur in many countries and add to the ways in which ferrets are housed. The majority of pet ferrets are kept indoors and there are various private breeders for the pet market. One example has quite large cages, some 5 feet by 3 feet (1.5×0.9 m), and stock ferrets at 1–6 per cage. The hobs are kept separated in the mating season. The cages are in an air-conditioned room and the ferrets are allowed to come

CHAPTER THREE
Accommodation

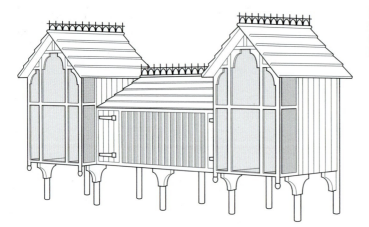

Figure 3.1 1897 Ferret House. Looking at this ferret accommodation could make one think there is nothing more to be said about keeping ferrets!

out and play in rotation (Amy Flemming, pers. comm. 1998).

Any ferrets kept outside must be protected against the extremes of climate. Ferrets in mosquito-prone areas in the USA must be on heartworm prevention and cages must be mosquito-proof. Ferrets are more adaptable to colder climates as are their wild cousins, polecats, weasels and stoats. However, the cold can be intense even for ferrets, and ferret owners in Canada keep their pets in heated basements during the winter (Bell, pers. comm. 1999).

Ferret-proofing the garden

Having ferrets as pets or a breeding colony outdoors demands that if you want them to have maximum controlled freedom, the garden must be secure. There is no doubt ferrets can usually find and squeeze through any defect in a wooden fence or perhaps climb over it. Ferrets in the back garden should have no desire to climb the border fence and should have everything they require in the garden to keep them happy. I have a suburban block with a surround of 'super six fencing' (corrugated fibro-cement sheeting), which is embedded 30–40 cm into the ground, a small length of wooden fencing with a rockery base and a solid wood back gate that is flush with the paving, which makes the back garden secure for keeping ferrets (Fig. 3.2).

My concept of keeping ferrets in the garden running free is that of a 'square within a square'. The first square is what I call a 'ferretarium' (F1) and the second square is the rest of the garden. The ferrets get to know the garden and F1 as their territory and move between the two places where they come to learn there will be shelter and/or food. In addition, there is a smaller ferretarium (F2) which also provides interest for the ferrets. The ferretariums can be closed to secure ferrets in one part of the garden or the gates can be left open so that they can travel from one to the other. The ferrets can develop well-worn paths between their sleeping areas around the garden, like badgers do in their territory. Finally, there is the opportunity to enter the house, which will be discussed later. Thus the ferrets are theoretically drawn away from paying any attention to the outer perimeter fence and the neighbours. The arrangement of the ferretarium setup can be extended to three or four units. Thus ferret cages are not required. I have a small nursery cage for a pregnant jill and an old aviary called 'Fred's aviary' after my first sable ferret Fred. He slept in the aviary before we had a garden fence. Even so, he could be let out in the evening and would come to the family room door to be let in. *Note*: it is good practice when ferrets live outside and come scratching at the door, to pick them up and pet them, even if immediately putting them outside again. This encourages the ferret in the event of really getting lost to go to the nearest house and scratch at the door to be let in instead of wandering off.

I have developed my ferret garden with the addition of fishponds, streams, rockeries, plenty of ground-cover plants and shady trees. This is shown diagrammatically in Figure 3.3, where rockeries and fishponds, two with streams, are in three positions in the garden. The streams run in the evening and there are waterfalls into the ponds. The back garden can be floodlit in the evening. The idea (in theory) is that on a warm evening one sits in the garden, by a pond with cascading waterfalls and tinkling streams and watches the ferrets run around and play.

I use a number of plastic PCV water pipes around the garden for the ferrets to play hide-and-seek in and disappear into if a neighbour's cat gets too curious. The pipes are along the border fence and in the ferretariums and there is a brick ferret maze and a plastic pipe maze. Many of my clients already have been enthusiastic about

Basic considerations when discussing ferret husbandry

①	Main ferretarium - three above-ground sleeping apartments plus summer boltholes
②	Side ferretarium - two above-ground sleeping apartments plus one summer bolthole
B	Summer bolthole position
F	Fred's aviary on south side of house
N	Nursery cage on south side of house
R	Rockery around ponds with all-year plants
P	Fish ponds with koi or goldfish
S	Streams – my ferrets, cat and dog drink from streams
F1	House entry for ferrets via family room sliding door
F2	House entry for ferrets via bedroom back window
⊕	Site of tree
xxx	Plastic ferret pipe runs
∧∧∧	Ferret maze – brick or pipes
▱	Ferret 'dolls' house' for summer accommodation
H	Rabbit hutch convention

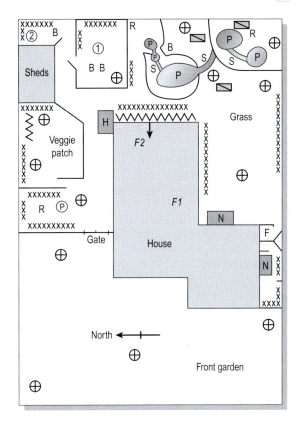

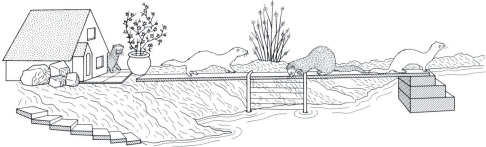

Figure 3.2 Ferret garden ground plan. (Courtesy of Sabine van Voorn.)

such a setup when I have discussed husbandry and shown photos of my garden. It all adds to an interest in ferrets and once started, one can forever improve and change.

With people in other situations, I visualize the possibility of brick-walled gardens or wood-fenced gardens adapted for pet ferrets once the perceived problem of them digging or climbing is overcome. The soil texture must also be considered; having ferrets in loose sand should be avoided. Sinking bricks or chicken wire at a small depth can stop too much digging in the wrong direction, i.e. at the border fence. Ferrets can climb but cannot climb up super six fencing. Of course no wooden planks, etc. should be left leaning at an angle against any fence as the ferret could climb up that and drop into the next garden. With brick walls or wood-fenced gardens, which might give some foothold for an adventurous ferret to climb, putting an overhanging lip facing inwards of brick or wood will deter the ferrets.

In Australia's hot climate, the ferrets tend to sleep during the day and are active in the evening and night. In the winter months, our ferrets are more active but still mostly nocturnal in nature, which pleases the average ferret pet owner who has to work during the day.

CHAPTER THREE
Accommodation

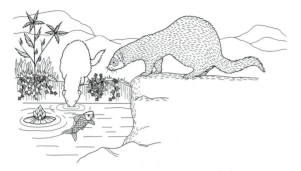

Figure 3.3 Main pond, rockery and ferrets. (Courtesy of Sabine van Voorn.)

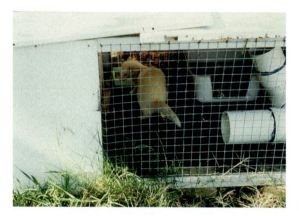

Figure 3.4 Converted rabbit hutch adapted for ferrets.

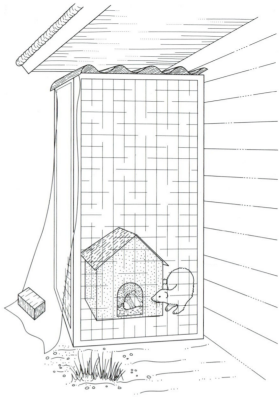

Figure 3.5 Converted aviary. *Note*: the brick to left is holding down shade cloth. Cage includes scats tray and water bowl and door is usually left open. (Courtesy of Sabine van Voorn.)

Ferrets in my garden can live in various types of weatherproof dwelling during the winter months, from a converted rabbit hutch to a converted aviary (Fig. 3.4). It is advisable to have perhaps a converted aviary as an isolation cage for ferrets newly acquired to a colony (Fig. 3.5).

In the summer months, the ferrets are provided with boltholes where they can go underground to stay during the heat of the day. In my ferret garden, one bolthole is situated by a large rockery and the entrance to the bolthole is via two clay pipes going under the waterfall between the cascade ponds and the main koi fishpond (Fig. 3.6). In F1 there are twin boltholes and a single one in F2. It is most important to realize that in our climate the boltholes are essential for summer living outside. They work with the ferrets left sleeping undisturbed in them from early morning to the cool of the evening.

Ferrets can live in the bolthole during the spring, autumn and even winter, when it rains, but it is not considered completely waterproof. The bolthole actually consists of a simple brick-lined hole some 2 feet (60 cm) deep with a paving stone base. The ferrets sleep in the bolthole curled up in old towels and blanket bits

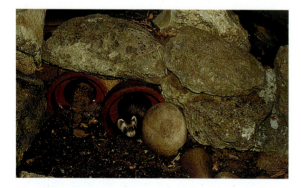

Figure 3.6 Ferret 'Brownie' coming out of bolthole by rockery in the garden.

but in the summer heat they just lie on the cool paving stone floor. Just being 2 feet underground makes all the difference. The ferrets usually stay in 'hibernation' on a hot day and take no water. Small water bowls are knocked over in the bolthole. Large 'cat litter' trays of water are available outside the entry pipes and the area is shaded. They toilet on newspaper in one corner of the boltholes infrequently. I would like to have made the boltholes bigger but the size depended on that of the covering white metal sheet.

Black corrugated plastic pipe has replaced clay pipe in F2 as I found that over the years, the floor of the clay pipe became smooth and with the pipe at an angle, it was difficult for the ferrets to get purchase. A rubber lining path can be slipped down the pipe. The boltholes in F1 can contain a number of sleeping ferrets for the day as seen in Figure 3.7. Once the ferrets were awake

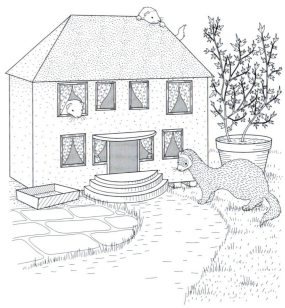

Figure 3.9 Ferret dolls' house in garden. (Courtesy of Sabine van Voorn.)

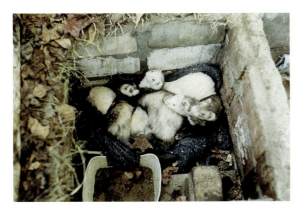

Figure 3.7 Five ferrets sleeping in ferretarium 1 (F1) bolthole (lid removed). *Note*: ferrets only using one of two boltholes; small scats tray.

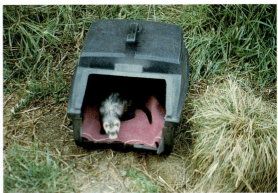

Figure 3.10 Lawn mower grass-catcher as sleeping box for ferrets in garden. Having a handle they can be put anywhere in the garden or ferretarium.

in the evening they played in the garden and bounced around (Fig. 3.8).

I have collected some old dolls' houses to convert to ferret houses and these are put around the garden during the summer months, so that the ferrets can sleep in them during the night (Fig. 3.9). In fact, what you have for the ferret garden to amuse the ferrets is limited only by your own imagination! The cost to set up a ferret garden can be low, as most requirements can be

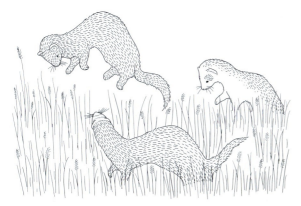

Figure 3.8 Ferrets bouncing around the garden! (Courtesy of Sabine van Voorn.)

obtained from recycled materials. I find that even discarded lawn mower grass-catchers can be converted to summer sleeping quarters, with the addition of an old rug (Fig. 3.10), or lined with newspaper to become a scats (toilet) tray.

Ferretarium 1 (F1)

Referring to the garden plan (see Fig. 3.2) on the east side of the garden by the rockery, housing the summer bolthole, is the main ferretarium (F1) (Fig. 3.11a). In my garden, the ferrets, having free range, can get into F1 by going to the rear of the main rockery and jumping in.

(a)

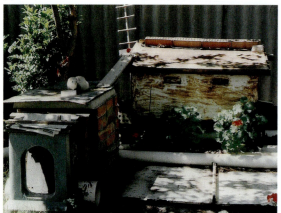

(b)

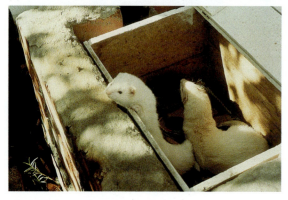

Figure 3.11 (a) Ferretarium (F1) showing large above-ground sleeping compartment at rear. The squares in the foreground in front of pipe are the covers of the two boltholes. *Note* the bricked structure to left, which holds a wood sleeping box. *Note* the converted plastic detergent container in far right corner as a scats tray for the ferrets, usually covered against bird droppings. (b) Two ferrets, Patch and Lucy, in wood sleeping box in brick surround. *Note* the half-curve entrance towards top of photograph.

If the ferretarium gate is kept closed the ferrets can get into it, but once in, cannot get out. I can leave ferrets in the garden last thing at night and know that they will either settle in various sleeping quarters or probably jump into F1 after a time. Once in, they will be secure there all night. Initially, I can have the ferrets sleeping in F1 and feeding there. Once given free range of the garden, they gravitate towards F1 when the gate is left open and the whole area becomes part of their territory. Food can be left in the ferretarium overnight but should be put in a pipe or in the boltholes to protect it from possible night-time cat prowlers! Ferretarium 1 is just low super six fencing with a wooden gate, the fencing being 2 feet in the ground and at least 3 feet standing above. Ferrets cannot jump out of the ferretarium but will come to the side to be picked up. Ferreters like this idea as it makes the ferret aware of a hand coming down to pick it up, as it would when picking up a ferret from a rabbit warren. I have three above-ground sleeping compartments for winter dwelling and two boltholes for summer (Fig. 3.11b and Table 3.1). The two boltholes have white metal covers, which reflect the heat. There is a large old metal dog kennel converted with blankets for sleeping in by the outer fence. To the left is a brick and wood sleeping compartment with a metal cover for protection against wet weather. Having metal structures as sleeping compartments does not matter in the summer because the ferrets will go underground and the above-ground sleeping compartments can be closed up for the season. The above-ground sleeping compartments must be warm in the winter with plenty of old blankets for the ferrets to burrow into and protection from the prevailing wind. Again there is no limit to the ideas for ferretarium accommodation, as long as they keep the ferrets cool in summer and warm in winter. In some countries, either too intense cold or clammy humidity might be more of a problem. The ferretarium, like the whole garden, has generous tree shade against the summer heat.

It is possible to install water sprinkler systems for the summer if there are no water restrictions in place. Shade cloth is useful but does not protect from high shade temperatures in mid-summer. An alternative is to have the ferrets inside during hot days but some people do not want ferrets indoors while others would not have them outdoors. Having trees around the ferret garden serves another purpose than shade: ferrets have an in-built ancestral fear of being exposed out in open space like weasels, stoats and polecats at risk of being taken by a hawk.

Once ferrets are in the summer boltholes, either in the garden or ferretariums, they must not be disturbed in the heat of the day. They tend to 'hibernate' so to speak, with their metabolism slowing and they will stir again in the cool of the evening. When picking up a

Basic considerations when discussing ferret husbandry

Table 3.1 Details of boltholes for ferrets

Boltholes	Top cover: white side of fridge (cm)	Bolthole; internal measurements (cm)	Type of entrance to Bolthole
Twin boltholes (B) in Ferretarium (F1)	66 × 88	50 × 50 × 33	Plastic pipe entrances 120 cm long. Int. diameter 10 cm
Bolthole (B) in Ferretarium (F2)	66 × 88	63 × 45 × 54	Black corrugated plastic pipe in half curved connection 120 cm. Int. diameter 8 cm
Bolthole (B) in garden by fishpond	66 × 88	60 × 40 × 40	Clay pipes in half-curve connection 140 cm. Int. diameter 10 cm

ferret in this condition during a hot day, it is found completely limp and the heart and respiratory rates are hardly distinguishable and one could think they were dead. Water can be left in the boltholes but mostly the ferrets are inert until the evening on hot days.

An ideal situation for a ferretarium might be to enclose an already established lawn area. Ground cover of some kind in the ferretarium, as in the garden, would help to keep the area cool. However, lawns do take a lot of water and we have gone over to native plant groundcovers in order to save water. A suggested plan is shown in Figure 3.12.

The feeding, water and scats tray areas of F1 now have covers against contamination from bird droppings.

I have been concerned about possible mycotic infections from birds (Ch. 12). The scats tray is a discarded plastic container lined with folded newspaper. I use various kinds of plastic scats trays outside, inside the house and at the hospital to get uniformity in toilet training of the ferrets. They are naturally clean and toilet away from their sleeping areas as would polecats. Having ferrets as pets in and out of the house requires making them 'scats tray-wise'. Food and water bowls can of course be put in small lengths of pipe to protect them against contamination. Plastic cat dirt trays are useful for water bowls (Fig. 3.13). The ferrets cannot easily knock them over and in warm weather will sometimes splash in the water (see Fig. 1.5).

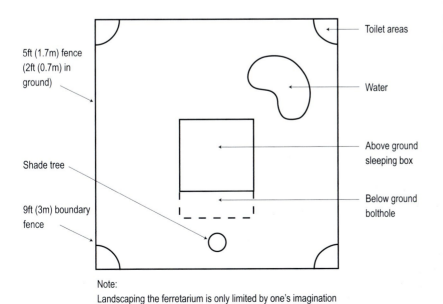

Figure 3.12 A typical ground plan for a ferretarium.

Note:
Landscaping the ferretarium is only limited by one's imagination

CHAPTER THREE
Accommodation

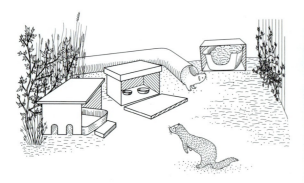

Figure 3.13 The protected feeding, water and scats tray areas in ferretarium 1 (F1). (Courtesy of Sabine van Voorn.)

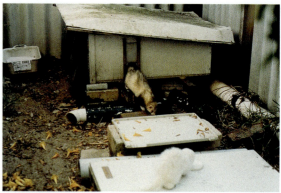

Figure 3.14 Ferretarium 2 (F2). *Note* the ferret leaving above-ground sleeping quarters at rear. *Note* white ferret is on cover of bolthole in foreground. Entrance is to the right by black corrugated pipe. Between sleeping quarters and bolthole is the water supply covered by metal sheet against sun and contaminations. *Note* the scats tray in corner upper left.

Ferretarium 2 (F2)

Ferretarium 2 (F2) (see Fig. 3.2) is set up like F1 but with just one large waterproof above-ground sleeping box with two compartments and a deeper, larger single bolthole for summer living (Fig. 3.14 and Table 3.1). It is protected from the prevailing wind by the garden shed. While I had a number of ferrets, the gate of F1 was kept closed at night, the gate of F2 was left open.

In this way the ferrets had a choice of sleeping in F2 or the garden or moving into F1, so they had a range of movement within the garden. There have never been any signs of the ferrets digging by the border fences to

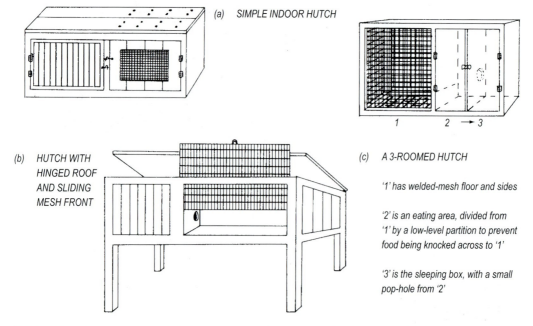

Figure 3.15 (a) Simple indoor hutch for use in ferret shed. (b) Hutch with hinged roof and sliding mesh front on stand. (c) A three-roomed hutch. **1.** Has welded-mesh floor and sides. **2.** Is an eating area, divided from (**1**) by a low-level partition to prevent food being knocked across to (**1**). **3.** Is a sleeping box, with a small pop-hole from (**2**). (From Val Porter and Nicholas Brown's *The Complete Book of Ferrets*. Bedford: D&M Publications; 1997, with permission.)

get out of the garden. At the time of writing, my sterilized hob, Pip uses F2. Ferretarium 1 has been left 'fallow' until I get more ferrets. Pip sleeps all day in the bolthole and wanders down to the house at dusk.

European polecats make use of old rabbit warrens or disused fox lairs to live in. They usually have one chamber as a nest lined with leaves and one area for a larder. I have attempted to give the ferrets a similar

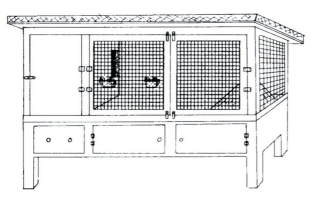

(a) ACCOMMODATION FOR UP TO 4 FERRETS

Dimensions: 6 ft x 2 ft x 2 ft (2 m x 0.7 m x 0.7 m)
Built of tongue-and-groove boarding: bitumen roof with substantial overhang and good slope. Water and food bowls hooked into front mesh. Latrine corner has glass 'splashback' plates.

When the hutch is used for a jill with a litter, glass 6 ins (15 cm) deep is fitted to the mesh at floor level for extra security.

(b) AN INGENIOUS OUTDOOR SYSTEM

The hutch can be used as a linked over-plan arrangement or easily divided into two units.

There is direct access at the rear down into the exercise enclosure at ground level. The enclosure could, of course be extended indefinitely.

Note the sliding tray for easy removal of droppings.

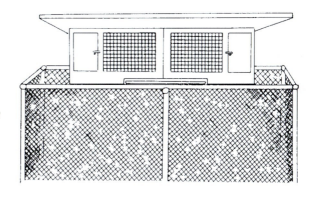

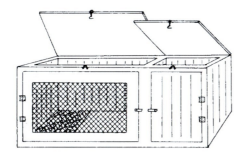

(c) A SPLIT-LID HUTCH

This gives controlled access to either section.

Note the coarse-mesh latrine floor on the left.

Figure 3.16 (a) Accommodation for up to four ferrets. (b) An ingenious outdoor system. (c) A split lid hutch. (From Val Porter and Nicholas Brown's *The Complete Book of Ferrets*. Bedford: D&M Publications; 1997, with permission.)

CHAPTER THREE
Accommodation

dwelling but in the hot climate, they are not encouraged to hoard food for fear of botulism (Ch. 8).

Standard outdoor ferret accommodation

Having described how I like to have ferrets fairly free in my back garden, then the standard general keeping of ferrets can be illustrated. Working and breeding ferrets have been kept in cages and sheds. Pet ferrets have been kept up to now in outside cages of various kinds. North American pet ferrets are mostly indoor ferrets. Private ferret breeders there have various outside ferret accommodation. If ferrets have to be kept in cages, they must be played with adequately to achieve the bonding needed with humans in order to become good workers and domestic pets. The ferret cage traditionally has been based on the rabbit hutch and is still made of wood with wire frontage and hinged doors for access. The ferret hutch could be described as a wooden structure with a wire floor and frontage, while a ferret cage is a wooden sleeping box with a wire ferret run attached.

The wooden sleeping-box part of the ferret cage tends to be warm, but various wire cages are possible with a wooden sleeping box placed separately inside. If

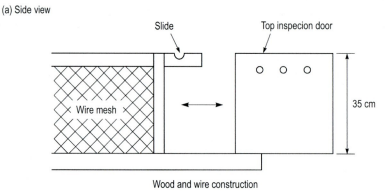

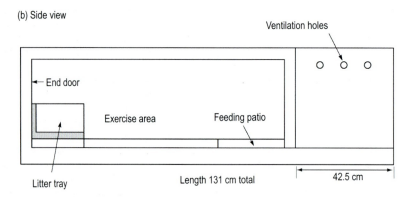

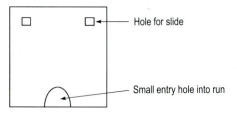

Figure 3.17 Lewington ferret cage (LFC) diagrams. (a,b) Side views. (c) End view sleeping box. The ferret cage has a removable sleeping (whelping) compartment.

possible, young ferrets, especially unweaned kittens, should not have to walk on wire floors, as the wire could harm their feet. Some ferret breeding farms, fitch and mink farms have multiple wire cages with wire floors so that the scats (faeces) will drop through. Ferret hutches in the UK, based on rabbit hutches, usually have complete wire floors or partial wooden floors with a mesh area for a ferret latrine (Figs 3.15, 3.16). For ferrets in cages or living indoors, I prefer a scats tray made from an adapted plastic washing-up bowl with a paper layer. It might be time-consuming to replace soiled newspaper, but it removes the requirement to clean up faeces under the hutch. I found that the wire soon became filthy, was difficult to clean and attracted flies. Ferrets are very clean in not soiling their sleeping compartments. Even 5-week-old kittens will leave the nest to toilet outside (see Fig. 5.12).

The wire for ferret cages should be 2×2 cm heavy gauge non-toxic wire, or 2.5 cm square maximum. If there is a wire floor, it should have even smaller squares and is best covered by a washable board if kittens are caged. There are various UK recommendations for ferret box (hutch) size, e.g. 3 ft (1 m) long by 18 inches (45 cm) deep by 18 inches (45 cm) high, having two compartments, living and exercise, with a roof sloping down to the back. Examples of basic ferret hutches are given in Figures 3.15 and 3.16. These hutch constructions are still used in the original form in many countries.

I see one possible fault in Figure 3.15b, where the entry hole from the sleeping compartment to the exercise area appears to be high up off the floor. This may be alright for agile young ferrets but not for a pregnant or lactating jill. Such an entry hole could cause bruising of the mammary glands and possible mastitis. With the single ferret cage I use for a nursery, the entrance to the sleeping (whelping) compartment is flush with the floor. Another practical point about having pregnant or lactating jills in hutches as in Figure 3.16c is that care must be taken at all times to ensure that the inspection hatch above is secure. A jill agitated for some reason might attempt to force an exit from the hutch, pushing up the inspection hatch and clambering out. With a heavy jill, half in and half out of the hutch, she might well slip a disc or break her back. These things do happen.

Lewington ferret cage (LFC)

My first and only cage suitable for breeding ferrets was adapted from the Brodie Ferret Hutch (Fig. 3.17).[2] An additional idea was to have a sleeping compartment that could be separated from the ferret cage exercise area. The wooden sleeping (whelping) box has a hinged lid, enabling easy inspection and is lockable. The box takes up about 42 cm and the ferret run 130 cm, with a door at the far end, plus a scats tray. It was only designed as an emergency cage and for pregnant jills and those with kittens up to 5 weeks of age. With a jill and kittens in the LFC, the wire floor of the run is covered by recycled ceramic tiles, which are placed with the rough side up. Bedding in the sleeping box is torn-up blankets, towels, sheets, etc.

Note:

1. Sawdust bedding should be avoided as it makes ferrets sneeze.
2. I avoid hay bedding as it may contain harmful grass awns.
3. Straw bedding is possible but I find it messy to clean out and it could contain mites.

The LFC is protected from the weather with respect to heat, rain and wind. It is placed under the house eaves on the southern or eastern side and is out of the sun. It gets the cooling afternoon breeze. In the winter it is protected from inclement weather and further protected with a waterproof sheet if need be, as winter rain can fall in severe downpours.

The LFC must be protected from severe summer heat that can be up to 43°C at times. I have had a pregnant jill or lactating jill with kittens in that situation in the cage. I use the 'Coolgardie meat safe technique' (see below) for keeping them cool in such weather. The system must be set up early in the morning of an expected hot day and must be left all day until the cool of the evening. The rationale is simple but effective. A plastic sheet protects the sleeping compartment from water. Then a large wet blanket is draped over the sleeping compartment and as much of the cage as possible. Next a bucket of water is placed on the sleeping compartment and a wet towel is draped from the bucket to the wet blanket. In this way the cooling by evaporation keeps the sleeping compartment cool throughout the day. The jill and kittens can 'hibernate' in the heat of the day and need not be disturbed. I have not lost any ferrets from heat stress, which is a risk factor for ferrets outside on hot days. Of course having a relatively small cage makes this technique easier to set up. All that is needed is to make sure the ferrets have adequate water and the water bucket is topped up during the day. Increased global warming might be a problem in the future for ferrets living outside.

Ferret owners having outdoor cages use various ideas such as shade cloth and even water sprinklers (Fig. 3.18). Water restrictions can upset the latter technique and it is wasteful in hot weather. Ideas like frozen water-filled bottles have been tried but will require changing and opening the sleeping box to do so defeats the purpose of keeping the ferrets cool. Either use the Coolgardie safe

CHAPTER THREE
Accommodation

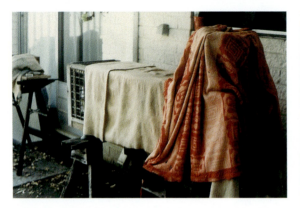

Figure 3.18 A Lewington ferret cage set up against the summer heat. Red blanket covers water bucket and sleeping box. Actual box protected with plastic sheet against water. *Note*: no ferrets around as they are sleeping in cage away from the heat of the day.

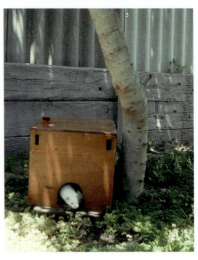

Figure 3.20 LFC sleeping box under tree. Jill and kittens are kept together and can exercise in the evening in garden, ferretarium, or even in house.

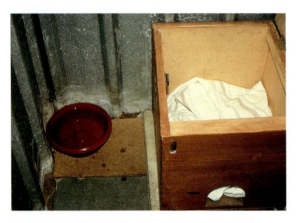

Figure 3.19 LFC sleeping box set up in a ferret's cage.

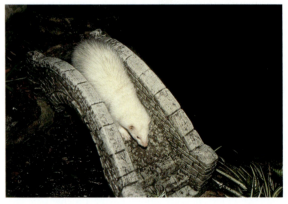

Figure 3.21 Ferret 'Heidi' on a bridge over the stream between ponds at the southern corner of the garden. *Note*: ferns around pond make a good jungle!

technique as described above, keep them indoors or let them go underground. It is tempting to check ferrets throughout the very hot day but better to leave them quiet as long as they are well protected by the technique.

My cage has been used basically for the pregnant jill and when the jill and kittens require more space, the LFC sleeping box can be moved and transferred to a converted aviary (Fig. 3.19).

Thus the jill and kittens stay in the same sleeping box. I think it is important that the kittens still stay with the jill after 6 weeks of age. They remain with the jill until they are sold so they gain maximum attention from her. Using the LFC sleeping box, the jill and kittens can be put in a ferretarium or even just left in the enclosed garden, without upsetting their original 'nest' (Fig. 3.20). A scats tray is placed within easy distance of the box.

The jill will soon take the kittens on 'hunting' trips around the garden. The ferrets can play in the garden and around the fishponds (Fig. 3.21).

Other types of ferret accommodation

There is no doubt that severe cold or wet climates dictate the use of sheds, to keep ferrets in cages or free in the shed. Worker and breeding stock ferrets are kept in cages and sheds in the UK, Europe, New Zealand and some parts of Australia. A New Zealand ferret breeder

Basic considerations when discussing ferret husbandry

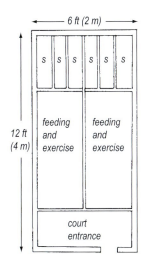

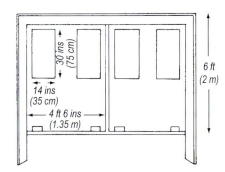

Figure 3.22 (a) Six-berth court. (b) Four-berth court. (From Val Porter and Nicholas Brown's *The Complete Book of Ferrets*. Bedford: D&M Publications; 1997, with permission.)

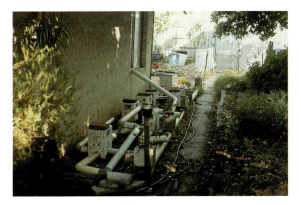

Figure 3.23 Pipe maze with ferrets around and pipe to the window ledge. *Note* the use of Tuckertime boxes as sleeping boxes. These were used overnight in summer.

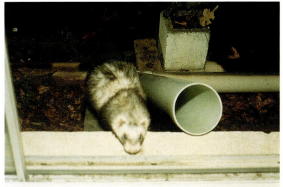

Figure 3.24 Ferret 'Midge' atop a plank by the back bedroom window, which is left slightly open in the evening for the ferrets to come in and out of the house by use of the plank. Ferrets have to slide down the pipe to get out when plank is taken away.

kept his working ferrets on straw in a converted shed with a concrete floor (see Fig. 1.7). He did not experience very hot conditions like Western Australia but had cold winters and snow (George Symons, pers. comm. 1993). A Perth (Western Australis, WA) ferreter keeps his working ferrets in a wooden hutch but with a long pipe deep underground to an exercise yard, which has super six fencing on three sides. The ferrets get away from the heat by sleeping in the pipe (Bert Geddes, pers. comm. 1980). A UK veterinarian who owns ferrets has hers in a sheltered, shaded reinforced mesh-fronted shed and the ferrets can use a walled garden for play. This is a near ideal situation (D. Wells, pers. comm. 1997). In the UK and Europe any ferretarium setup would tend to be muddy in the wet times but the plants would grow! Concreting the ferretarium would defeat the purpose of a natural area for ferrets, but there have been such structures called 'courts' in the UK.

Ferret courts

The courts are made of brick and concrete as a walled ferretarium (Fig. 3.22a,b). They are reminiscent of old single house pig sties. They were designed in the early twentieth century and consist of a number of sleeping compartments and an extensive feeding and exercise area.

James McKay of the National Ferret School, Derbyshire, UK, has courts like aviaries, which measure 3 m × 2.5 m × 2 m high. His hutches (cubs) are wooden and measure 1.5 m × 0.75 m × 0.75 m high. In addition, he has six laboratory-type cages constructed of fibreglass, measuring 1 m × 0.75 m × 0.75 m high. The court system serves a need and keeps ferrets confined. No doubt the courts could have a number of pipes for the ferrets to play in and this could be useful for training working ferrets in being retrieved from rabbit warren entrances.

Plastic pipes are popular for the sport in both Australia and UK of racing ferrets down long tubes. I have indicated the extensive use of pipes in the garden and ferretarium to keep the ferrets occupied and for providing an escape from neighbourhood cats. I had a pipe maze outside the house back bedroom with a 'slide-pipe' going from the maze to the window ledge (Fig. 3.23). The idea was that when I came home from the veterinary hospital with my ferrets, I was able to 'post' them down the slide into the maze and the back garden. I actually got the ferrets to zip down the slide of their own accord!

I also placed a plank from the ground to the windowsill so the ferrets could come in or out of the house (Fig. 3.24). I could open the window, clap my hands and retreat to the living room. After a few minutes there was the patter of little feet down the corridor and ferret faces appeared demanding to be fed. They would do a weasel war dance around the room! I have taken the plank and pipe away now (under orders from my wife, Margaret), but at least it proved a point, the ferrets got wise to the route into the house!

Ferrets living indoors

What can you now tell your clients about keeping ferrets inside the house? 'Our ferret is named Pest and her quarters are built into the cupboard at floor level. Since Pest is housebroken, we no longer latch the door. She is left entirely free, and while she sleeps in her den at night, she often naps in other nooks she has found around the house' (Sara Stein, *Great Pets* 1976). This statement shows how adaptable ferrets are to becoming the companion animal.

American laboratory workers, veterinarians, and technicians attending laboratory ferrets no doubt had the opportunity to take a ferret kitten home. Ferrets have unfortunately been used for experiments for too long a time.[3] Thus a spread of interest occurred in the 'little critters' for their rightful place, after working animals, as household pets. In the USA, the emphasis was mainly on ferrets as household pets, as there were very few who lived outside, but evidently this has changed (Amy Flemming, pers. comm. 1998). The main concern with ferrets outside in the USA/Canada was the fear of them getting rabies from raccoons, etc. and being a human threat.

Besides their popularity in North America, the ferret has become established as a pet in countries around the world. Ferrets will harmonize with dogs and cats, on the whole, as companion and household pets. At one time, I had seven ferrets, one dog and two cats. The ferrets would come into the house and live in the garden and ferretariums. Ferret owners around the world differ in the amount of freedom they can give their ferrets. Ferret owners in America, and even some in Australia now, do sacrifice one room for the enjoyment of their ferrets. Fara Shimbo in Colorado kept ferrets in one room of her house with a pipe maze setup and has written extensively about ferrets and their ways.

Some American enthusiasts, and now even Australian, confess to having between 10 and 20 ferrets in the house. With reference to my ferrets, I used to have one ferret in overnight, two in the garden and four in the ferretarium. In the past, in severe stormy weather, I have had up to 10 ferrets in overnight.

Ferrets are beginning to be kept in apartments in Australian cities where they stay in walled balcony situations, which is ideal as long as the ferret is protected against weather extremes. There must be no way that the ferret can climb the exterior wall to admire the view! 'High-rise syndrome' in the past has occurred in the USA, where ferrets fell from window ledges. Most pet ferret owners in North America do not have ferrets free in the house but in indoor cages. These can vary in complexity with usually a sleeping box, feeding area and scats tray. The cages are of strong wire mesh and can be double-storey with connecting ladders. The original ones were based on laboratory cages. Some ferrets could hurt themselves running up and down wire ladders and I would personally keep ferrets on one level with plenty of pipes to play in, as does Fara Shimbo. She had a moveable ferret cage to put outside the house with a pipe

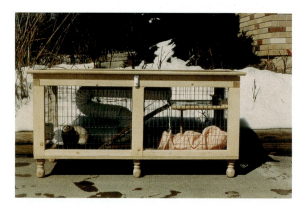

Figure 3.25 Fara Shimbo's ferret cage for indoors and outdoors. *Note* the curved plastic pipe as stairway, better than wire ladder.

ladder to the upper sleeping box (Fig. 3.25). She also had a complete room (as mentioned earlier) given over to ferrets (see Fig. 3.26).

My ferrets have always come into the house. What I have now is a large converted trunk (80 × 40 × 40 cm) as a sleeping box plus a small wire run (80 × 40 × 30 cm) with a scats area (Fig. 3.27). The idea is that the box is big enough to have a rolled blanket for sleeping and enable the ferrets to be in the dark even if the room light is on. One should be aware of ferret adrenal disease complex (FADC) nowadays (Ch. 14) and cut down the long photo-periods for house ferrets. At the moment, my ferret Pip can come into the house in the evening for food and play. However, he can be left in the sleeping box in the dark with a blanket over the run. House lights in the family room are switched off in the evening while we are in the sitting room. He could stay all day in the sleeping box to sleep with the blanket over the exercise run in darkness. He exercises evening and morning or overnight if he is outside in the garden. Ferrets in the house overnight can sleep in the bathroom as shown in Figure 3.28.

Ferrets are easily conditioned to fitting in with the human lifestyle. On the whole ferrets, after playing in the garden and also in the house in the evening, will happily sleep from 10 p.m. to 6 a.m. the next morning, only getting up rarely to use the scats tray and perhaps drink. Once in a routine, they remain comfortable in their sleeping boxes overnight.

The plastic scats trays serve their purpose in the house as they do in the garden and ferretarium. They are placed in corners of the rooms the ferrets are allowed

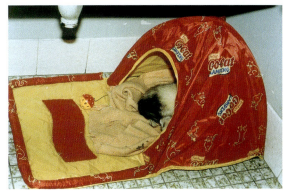

Figure 3.28 Use of cat plastic 'igloo' for sleeping ferret in bathroom under sink.

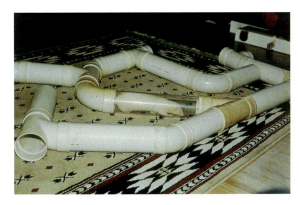

Figure 3.26 Fara Shimbo's indoor ferret pipe layout in one room. *Note* the clear plastic pipe.

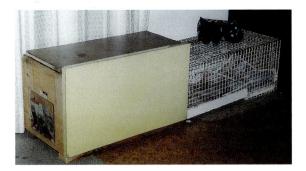

Figure 3.27 Lewington indoor sleeping box and run. Box is long, small end air hole and overall dark to keep ferrets in. A blanket could be used to keep run dark too.

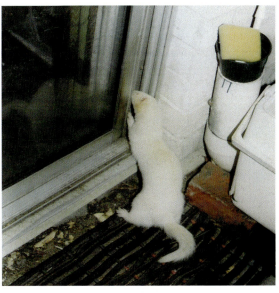

Figure 3.29 Ferret 'Hector' hoping to enter the family room.

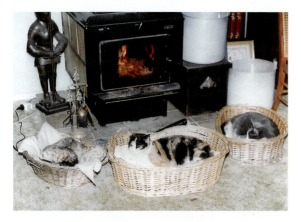

Figure 3.30 Ferret 'Tyke' and cats 'Sophie' and 'Miska' hogging the winter fireplace.

which is in line with ferrets only being able to recognize red (Ch. 6).

At one time when the family room sliding door and the back bedroom window were left slightly open, there would be a constant traffic of ferrets coming and going between the garden and the house. A great deal of ferret behaviour depends on the weather. On warm spring or summer nights they will play in the garden. In the colder times of autumn they will be more active. On a cold wet winter's evening, the ferrets prefer to play indoors. Our cats Sasha and Mishka shared the fireplace with ferret, Tyke (Fig. 3.30). Our dog would curl on a sofa given half a chance and doze with ferret, Snowy (Fig. 3.31).

Ferret rooms and cages

in, and they use them. It is important to keep replacing the newspaper or the ferrets would go elsewhere if the scats tray is dirty. If the ferrets are fed in the house, the ferret owner must be careful they do not stash uneaten food in places like under seats or cupboards.

The ferrets scratch at the family room sliding door to be let in (Fig. 3.29). Once the ferrets are in the house, play can get chaotic. Hide-and-seek with them doing the hiding becomes more of a chore than a game. One useful amusement is the Dizzy Kitty box, which adapts well to ferrets. Young cats are supposed to spend hours trying, with their paws, to get plastic balls out of a cardboard box. The difference with ferrets is that they get completely into the box and bring the balls out in their jaws! They then hide the balls well away from the bemused cat! This is as far as I would go with ferret toys. One has to be aware of ferrets chewing toys and getting foreign body obstructions. I find that Pip is more attuned to play with a red ball than any other colour,

The American way of keeping pet ferrets indoors has now become popular in Australia and elsewhere. Many people now, e.g. Claire, a friend, has given over a whole spare bedroom for her ferrets, Fifi and Fergus (Fig. 3.32). The room is on the cool side of the house, the floor is tiled, the windows have blinds to darken the room during the day and there is a two-tiered ferret cage.

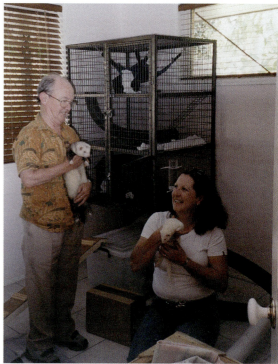

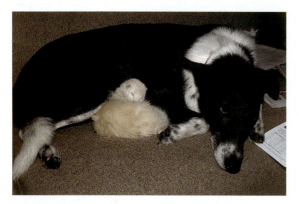

Figure 3.31 Dog 'Cheetah' and ferret 'Snowy' sneaking a nap on the front room sofa until turfed off!

Figure 3.32 A typical Australian ferret room with ferrets 'Fifi' and 'Fergus'.

Basic considerations when discussing ferret husbandry

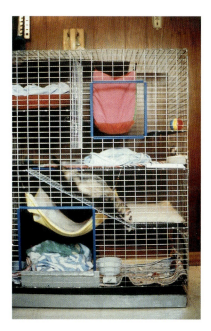

Figure 3.33 Dean Manning's indoor ferret cage. *Note* the hammock and ferret on wire ladder.

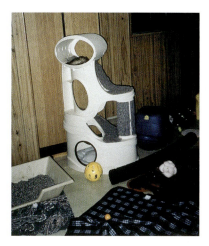

Figure 3.34 Mary van Dahm's basement for keeping ferret indoors. Climbing frame for ferrets and various toys.

Claire is well aware of adrenal problems in ferrets and insulinoma (Ch. 14), so the room is kept dark during the day while she is at work. Lights in the room are not left on unnecessarily. The ferrets are fed a fresh meat diet. She has wire ladders between the two levels of the cage. There is black corrugated tubing for play tunnels in the cage and on the floor. The tubes give a good grip and would not damage ferret feet as wire ladders might. There are hammocks and scats trays in the cage and further scats trays on the floor. The ferrets can be fed in or out of the cage. However, the ferrets get to play in the room and parts of the house in the evening. This is a good example of an indoor setup for pet ferrets; they are safe, secure and protected from the elements. This setup is best for their health and well-being.

One Perth ferret enthusiast has six ferrets indoors in a ferret room but has, for exercise, an outdoor three-tiered cage with hammocks on each level and sensible black-ridged pipes for ferrets to go up and down. The outside cage is not used in high summer. In Wisconsin, Dean Manning, retired researcher, also keeps his pet ferrets indoors using two-tiered cages when they are not out to play (Fig. 3.33). Each cage has one or two scat trays, which the ferrets absolutely use. He keeps several scat trays around the house, which are used 99% of the time. Mary Van Dahm of the Ferret Advice & Information Resource Society, Chicago, has a whole basement set aside for her critters, with cages and play space like a kindergarten (see Fig. 3.34).

In Italy, the most common cages are around $80 \times 40\,cm \times 60\,cm$ high with a shelf, a hammock and a litter box. In multiple ferret houses, they are housed in one big cage (groups of de-sexed or breeders out of season) or in different smaller cages (if in season) or free-range in a ferret-proof room. Some people let their ferrets free-range the house (Alessandro Melillo, pers. comm. 2005). Ferrets are out in exterior cages when the weather is not too hot or too cold as the regional temperatures differ.

Ferrets, laboratories and veterinary hospitals

How would you keep ferrets at your place? 'Ferrets typically have a friendly, inquisitive nature. They tend to urinate and defecate in one habitual area and are easily trained to use a litter box. Being nocturnal creatures ferrets are usually quiet and spend a great deal of time sleeping.' A quote from a modern pet ferret book? No! From *Laboratory Management of the Ferret for Biomedical Research* by Moody et al. in Laboratory Animal Science, June 1985; 35:272!

Much as I hate the idea of ferrets in laboratories, certain normal data is procured from this source (see Appendix Tables). Housing ferrets for research means they are in cages some $60 \times 60 \times 45\,cm$ with grid size of $2.5 \times 1.25\,cm$ mesh with various type floors. They are kept in a temperature range of 4–18°C with kittens kept at above 15°C. In a breeding colony, the kits need to be kept warm once separated from the jills. Researchers are aware that ferrets get heat stress above 30°C. The humidity is usually 40–65%.[4] In a constant indoor environment, the photo-period (hours light:hours dark) is

CHAPTER THREE
Accommodation

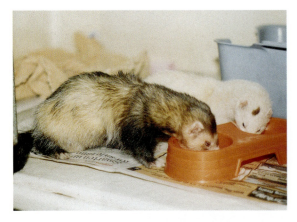

Figure 3.35 Ferrets jill 'Patch' and hob 'Boysie' in hospital cage.

controlled. For breeding colony or lactating ferrets, the ratio is 16:8, the winter cycle is 10:14. Non-breeders have a 12:12 situation. Photo-period length is interesting when considering the adrenal disease problem (Ch. 14).

Unlike most veterinarians, I tended to take ferrets to work with me each morning when I was in practice. One reason was to let clients see ferrets, which many had never seen. In the breeding season, I could sell my ferret kittens from the hospital and at the same time brief buyers about husbandry. The ferrets travelled in the car in 'Pet Voyager 200' plastic cat-carriers, which are the right size to have a scats tray (a small converted plastic lunch box) and bedding for the ferrets. The carriers are stackable. Many ferret owners now use this type of carrying basket for their ferrets. My ferrets were offloaded into the veterinary hospital ferret yard, which was enclosed on one side by a brick wall; the two ends were super six fencing and the only entrance by the laundry door of the building. The yard was mostly grassed, with various sleeping boxes around it. There were no boltholes. Ferrets boarded at the clinic could safely be let out into the yard, which had a mixture of plastic pipes for ferrets to play in. Ferrets at the hospital were of course kept in during the summer heat.

To have my ferrets at the veterinary hospital completed the three ways of keeping ferrets, i.e. in a garden, in a house and in a 'laboratory' situation. The hospital cages were not built with ferrets in mind and had to be adapted. There were cat cages 60 × 60 × 60 cm and dog cages 70 × 80 × 100 cm, all converted to holding ferrets. They were fibreglass, not stainless steel, being some 20 years old, and the original front cage wire was of too large a mesh for ferrets, so 2.5 cm square strong *non-toxic* aviary wire was clipped to the inner side (Fig. 3.35). Galvanized wire can cause zinc poisoning in ferrets (Ch. 15).

The fibreglass cages tend to be cool in summer and warm in the winter; I prefer them to stainless steel cages for any animal. The ferret cage is set up with newspaper on the base, torn up blanket pieces or rolled towelling for bedding with the usual plastic scats tray identical to those I use at home. A plastic water/food bowl is placed to the front of the cage; earthenware bowls can also be used.

Ideally, we should have had a separate ward for ferrets only but we did not get the case numbers to warrant it. Consulting with Susan Brown in the USA, on hospital design for ferrets, she says even as a specialist hospital they have an open plan situation and do not have separate wards for ferrets and rabbits. However, they tend not to put ferrets next to rabbits! They do have an 'isolation' ward for ferrets and a 'hot ward' for ferrets recovering from operations. In winter, we had mobile electric oil-filled column heaters and in summer, mobile evaporative air coolers for the hospital and kennels. *Note*: for ferrets in for observation, a clean plastic scats tray is used for obtaining a urine or scats sample. It is placed in the cage, without paper in it, so that the ferret may oblige with a sample, with no stress to the animal.

There are ferret hospitals in the USA, which use clear Plexiglas-fronted cages. These are usually on the front of stainless steel ferret cages, which contain the usual sleeping area and scats tray for the ferret (S. Brown, pers. comm. 1993). Stainless steel cages tend to be cold and for postoperative ferrets, electric warming pads are installed. I found the use of a small towel in a fibreglass ferret cage is sufficient. Additional equipment for ferret accommodation could be a baby humidicrib converted for sick animals. In the USA, an acrylic intensive care unit for ferrets is used in specialist hospitals (basic hospitalization techniques are covered in Ch. 7; Emergency procedures in Ch. 20).

Mobile racks of cages are now popular for general use in veterinary hospitals and are based on research laboratory cages developed in the 1980s. Specific mobile ferret cages were developed by Wilson and O'Donoghue (1982), in a stack of three rows with cages 49 × 46 × 46 cm high. A double-size cage could be incorporated in a set for a jill and litter. The cages were built of 1.6 mm anodized aluminum sheeting, with the top, front and door of 2.4 mm diameter stainless steel wire mounted on a 6 mm diameter stainless steel wire frame.[5] Removable partitions could be included, made of the same material. The ferrets had sawdust bedding and wood-wool for nesting. A rigid clear plastic screen prevents sawdust being scattered and the cage doors open downwards. The ferrets would naturally pass scats in one corner and cleaning would have to be ongoing. I would think for veterinary hospital purposes, the use of solid metal cages with plastic scats trays would be an easier

Basic considerations when discussing ferret husbandry

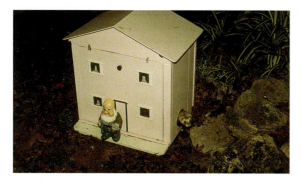

Figure 3.36 A gnome and ferret 'Pandy', at the bottom of our garden!

option, as these can be removed when soiled and replaced immediately by a clean one. If the ferrets try to 'nose' behind the scats tray, the latter could be secured in some form of holder in one corner of the cage. With my fibreglass cages, I used two small bricks to secure the scats trays.

New ferret owners may need guidance as to possible dangers with ferrets being kept outdoors or indoors.

Dangers to ferrets living outdoors

There is no doubt that having pet ferrets living outside can pose problems and it is not due to the gnomes and fairies, sorry, ferrets at the bottom of our garden (Fig. 3.36)! There are also perils for ferrets used for hunting!

Heat stress

This is *the* main concern in Australia, and other hot climate countries, with lethal effects on ferrets. Because

> **Author's practical example**
>
> **Ferret 'Wombat' in 41°C heat in Port Hedland, WA**
>
> An owner's response with no veterinarian around is interesting. Barry said 'I found Wombat completely stiff on his side outside the house, barely breathing. He was picked up and held in a child's paddling pool with his head just out of the cool water for half an hour. Slowly he came to, his body hydrated and his breathing quickened.' *Note*: rehydration salts formula can be used for ferrets. This can be made up or rehydration sachets for infants can be obtained from pharmacies (see Appendices).

Barry Bowden, pers. comm. 1986.

ferrets have no sweat glands they will rapidly dehydrate in temperatures above 30°C especially when stressed by working or being forced to play in the heat. They can be dead within half an hour. Treatment requires rehydration with i.v. or s.c. Hartmann's fluids.

Harmful creatures

Working ferrets may come across poisonous snakes. In open country small ferrets, like stoats and weasels in UK or NZ, could be taken by hawks. Working ferrets can pick up fleas, mites and ticks from the bush and from rabbit warrens and even canine distemper if they come across a sick fox or dingo (in Australia).

Insect bites

The question of insect bites can be puzzling, as the ferret owner rarely actually observes the insect and the bite. In Western Australia, the WA Museum has produced a list of the most dangerous insects which affect people in the State and this can be taken as a guide for ferrets, as indeed also for dogs and cats. No doubt every country has their list of dangerous insects and veterinarians should note them with regard to ferrets.

Western Australian Museum list of dangerous insects:

1. Honeybee: sting can kill in minutes.
2. Red-back spider: bite rarely fatal but causes intense pain and swelling.
3. Trapdoor spider: extremely painful bite (seen in eastern Australia).
4. Marble scorpion: pain from sting can last for hours.
5. White-tailed spider: bite sometimes not felt but can cause symptoms from swelling to ulceration, common in gardens, (personal experience!).
6. Sergeant ant (Bull-ant): powerful painful bite causes swelling, fairly common on dogs' noses in gardens.
7. Sand scorpion: painful bite.
8. Centipede: painful bite, sometimes requiring hospital treatment.
9. Wolf spider: painful bite, more frightening because of its size, as large as an adult hand.
10. Kangaroo tick: bite can be painful, more nuisance than dangerous but might be a vector of arthropod diseases as ticks are in the USA.

Note: 'What might be just painful to humans might well be lethal to ferrets'.

I have not knowingly had ferrets with insect bites in the garden or ferretariums, though we do not use insecticides and the garden boasts numerous spiders, which we hope keep the flies, etc. down. I have done spot checks on the ferret pipes and not found spiders in them. A tennis ball placed in one of the pipes will be found outside it in the morning if the pipe has been used by the ferrets.

Other dangers

A possible case of ferret paralysis due to *Ixodes holocyclus* (paralytic tick) was seen in eastern Australia; this tick is not found in Western Australia.

Mosquitoes can infect dogs, cats and ferrets with *Dirofilaria immitis* and cases have been recorded in Australia (Ch. 10). Having fishponds and mosquitoes, I give my ferrets ivermectin against heartworm.

Fishponds are an essential part of the garden layout but of course ferrets could fall into the water. Ferrets can swim but they are not active swimmers like their UK otter cousins. Care must be taken with aged ferrets and also kittens around fishponds. My ponds are fitted with submersed ferret ladders. Swimming pools can be death traps to ferrets, dogs, cats and children.

Some native plants are considered toxic but ferrets are not fond of chewing plants or berries; fibre is not good for them. On the other hand, Americans are concerned about ferrets living indoors being poisoned by toxic indoor plants. Many countries have National Animal Poison Control Centers to be consulted on pet ferret poisoning cases.[6] Toxicology with regard to ferrets and lists of potentially toxic houseplants and plants in general are covered later (Ch. 15).

What happens to cats might happen to ferrets. In the UK, a cat brushed up against some oriental stargazer lilies.[7] The cat licked the pollen and within hours it went blind, had renal failure and became paralyzed. All lilies are poisonous to cats so watch your ferrets, in case.

Australian native frogs can make ferrets at least foam at the mouth when they attempt to hold one. One of my hob ferrets, Tyke, did just that when he picked up a burrowing frog (*Heleioporus albopunctatus*) and I happened to be around to rescue the frog and wash the ferret's mouth out. Mostly, my ferrets do not get near garden frogs as they jump and leave the ferret standing (Fig. 3.37)!

A ferret death caused by a green tree frog (*Litoria moorei*) has been recorded where a 3-year-old ferret, Ossie, died shortly after biting the frog (G. Ireland, Tamworth, NSW, pers. comm. 1996).

A problem that might increase is that caused by the spread of the introduced poisonous cane toad (*Bufo marinus*) across Australia. One case has been already recorded in Queensland, where a number of dogs are treated annually for cane toad poisoning. A ferret, Bud, was seen attacking a toad and the owner washed the ferret's mouth out. The ferret 'flattened' and there was concern about water in the lungs. There was excessive salivation and upper respiratory wheeze. It was considered that a combination of toad venom and the water treatment caused the listless ferret. The ferret improved during the day, was kept in overnight for observation and found to be alert in the morning. It is difficult to judge the extent of toxicity in this case but the effect did wear off (C. Kidd, Brisbane, pers. comm. 1997). In areas of Australia infested with cane toads, ferret owners should have a well-fenced ferret- and toad-proof garden or keep the ferrets indoors. The cane toad toxin irritates the lips of any animal which bites or ingests it. The victim's nose and ears bleed and there is internal bleeding leading to death. Tadpoles and mature toads are poisonous. At the time of writing, cane toads have advanced into the Kakadu National Park and are suspected of killing even crocodiles.

Ferrets will eat snails, so with garden ferrets there is no need to keep snail bait. I find crushed snail shells in the ferretarium sleeping boxes and boltholes. One danger of snail pellets around is that if ferrets are fed any kind of dry ferret biscuit food they may be inclined to try the bait and could die overnight. Put up with snails and do not put out snail bait is the answer, especially with ferrets living in the garden. Snails, however, are implicated in the life cycle of the cat lungworm, *Aelurostrongylus abstrusus*, not yet seen in ferrets. However, another species of lung worm has been seen in mustelids in the USA.[8]

On rare occasions, the fungus *Cryptococcus neoformans* from bird droppings can affect ferrets in warm climates and is deadly (Ch. 12). Even some species of Mycobacterium have been recognized in ferrets (Ch. 8).

Garden chemicals should be banned if you have garden ferrets, in case of contamination in their food or play areas. Natural garden fertilizers should be used, with compost bins. However, ferrets love to dig into

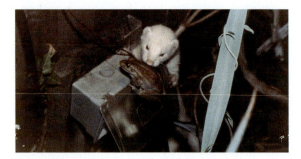

Figure 3.37 Ferret 'Susie', looking at a garden frog. In the next instant, the frog jumped away leaving a perplexed ferret!

compost bins from underneath and will eat worms, etc. if the bin is not sealed off!

The garden shed with paints, oils, etc. should be well sealed so that inquisitive ferrets cannot get in and upset something. My present hob, Pip, is as quick as a flash to explore the smells in the shed so I work in it while he is safe in the ferretarium.

Garden rat bait should never be used. I had a case of ferret poisoning with Talon which required vitamin K dosing and use of apomorphine s.c. and s.c. fluids over a day. The ferret had been on biscuit ferret food and chewed a poison pellet. There is also a risk of ferrets eating mice or rats recently poisoned by bait. One jill ferret when spayed developed a haemorrhage 2 h postoperatively and was treated with i.v. vitamin K. The vet was later told that 2 days previously, the jill had eaten the stomach contents of a dead mouse (R. Sillar, Casino Vet. Clinic, NSW, pers. comm. 1997).

One occasion, after 3 weeks away on holiday, we found extensive rat droppings in the garden shed and a dead rat in an outside water barrel. As our cat, Mishka, and ferrets Pip and Squeak, had been boarded out did the rats feel able to move around freely? We had no recurrence of rat problems until quite recently (2005) when Mishka and Pip killed a rat each. I believe the rabbits and guinea pigs caged outside next door might attract rats to their feed pellets. I never feed our animals outside.

Ferrets can climb but not usually straight up like their agile pine marten cousins or cats. They might get up a tree or wall with a particularly rough surface. One ferret owner had a pencil pine in a courtyard and the pet ferret found a way to climb its tight-knit interior branches, got to the top of the courtyard wall and jumped over. Usually ferrets climb trees that grow at an angle. Being somewhat shortsighted and more used to nocturnal activity using nose and ears, ferrets can be confused at heights and may be injured jumping down. Ferrets can jump from a solid surface, so sleeping boxes in a ferretarium should be well away from the side fences or the side fences should be made higher. There is a possibility of injury if ferrets misjudge distance. I have had ferrets jump from the top of a brick column 40 cm high to a window ledge 40 cm above to get into the house by an open window. With active hobs there should not be broken wire mesh around for them to climb, as it has been known for them to injure the penis and baculum (see Fig. 16.7).

Dangers to ferrets living indoors

In the house, ferrets can get into very small places such as behind wardrobes, refrigerators and washing machines. Getting into the latter unnoticed can lead to a disaster. A ferret of mine, Sophie, got into a top-loading washing machine and into the space between the washbowl and the side of the machine. It was only by putting the machine on its side and leaving the top open that she eventually came out! Front-loading washing machines are worse as they are easier to get into. A ferret has been recorded as surviving by a miracle, a full wash cycle (G. Jenkinson, Mandurah, WA, pers. comm. May 1999); however, others have not been so lucky.

To help avoid these problems, plenty of distractions for the ferrets for play should be provided around the house, as around the garden, A wholly ferret room with pipe mazes as used by Fara Shimbo in the USA could be an attractive idea to suggest to prospective pet ferret owners. Ferrets could chew electric cables but are not chewers like rats and I have never come across it with the numbers of ferrets I have had in the house. Usually ferrets around and in the house deter rats and mice. Wiping electric wiring with a bitter solution is recommended. Ferrets can chew

Author's clinical examples

1. A 3-month-old ferret, Frank, in a northern mining town, Tom Price, WA, could easily die in the summer heat. Kept indoors in air-conditioned comfort he managed to chew a used ear plug, probably attracted by the ear wax smell, and died of an obstruction before he could be taken to a vet 300km away. Rona lost another ferret to possible spider bite in 2004. The ferret caught wolf spiders and was found dead with the only signs being ulceration of the mouth (Rona Rastinger, pers. comm. 1999).

2. A mining town in Canada had a severe problem with pet ferrets eating foam earplugs until they became more careful with their pets (Vannevel, Ontario, pers. comm. 2005).

3. An 8-month-old sterilized hob, Grommet, one of my jill Patch's last litter, ate a small piece of netting, used to protect fruit trees from birds; the material had got burnt and probably looked like a toasted worm. Grommet developed signs of intestinal blockage and required surgery, which was successful (A. Kelly, Cannington Vet. Hospital, WA, pers. comm. May 1999).

4. I had a sick adult sterilized hob pass a 50×140 mm part of a toy rubber elephant's foot, on the consulting room table, which was a relief to him, the owner, and myself!

5. One of my jills, Smudge, in her pseudopregnancy moments, would pinch washing up sponges and hoard them in a garden bolthole. She never chewed them but I presume took them as her sponge babies!

many things that are dangerous: leather, rubber shoes, Styrofoam packaging, sponges, cotton wool, rubber balls, etc. Pet ferrets in the USA seem to be hooked on chewing and get intestinal blockages, which send them back more than once to their veterinarian. Advise against giving ferrets dog, cat or children's toys of any material, let alone ferret toys!

There is much concern nowadays about the effects of the internal house environment on the health of people and their pets.[9] The pet ferret has a nose close to the ground. It is feasible that they can get irritated respiratory pathways just by sniffing in house dust. In a study in Seattle, 25 houses out of 29 checked had high levels of toxins and mutagens in rugs. The common irritant can be formaldehyde from new carpets.

In the indoor cage situation, I feel that urine vapour can be an irritant if the scats tray is not changed frequently. Sneezing and coughing can occur. The scats tray should be as far away from the sleeping quarters as possible, which is not always easy from a space point of view. House ventilation is therefore very important and all household chemicals capable of producing irritant vapours should be stored well way from ferrets.

Keeping ferrets in working sheds or garages or cars should be avoided. Lead, cadmium, mercury and arsenic are considered suspect pollutants in a closed environment.

In humans, indoor air pollution gives chronic headaches, fatigue, itchy or watery eyes, nasal or throat infections. *Note*: the ferret lung at cellular level is very similar to human. The house ferret is primarily susceptible to respiratory trauma so that sneezing and coughing is the first sign of something wrong, which also might be wrong for the human in the same atmosphere!

Ferrets can get under the feet very easily. Ferrets can appear in the house at speed and apparently from nowhere. One tends to walk slowly and not heavily around ferrets. I have seen cases of ferrets injured by being trodden on by bare feet, so shoes could be a disaster. My present hob, Pip got under the heel of my Wellington boot when he was a kitten, which broke his humerus (2003).

In the house rocking chairs should be immobilized with ferrets around and care taken that they do not burrow into the interior of an easy chair. More than one pet ferret has suffocated that way.

Ferrets can learn to open an almost closed sliding door. I had a 6-month-old jill ferret, Jennie, and a Jack Russell male, Patch, of similar age (Fig. 3.38). Together in a passage, with an almost closed sliding door to the family room, Jennie quickly spotted the possible opening. She opened the door by pulling at it with both front paws while lying on her side. This was repeated a number of times and Jennie always outsmarted Patch! Who says ferrets do not bond with other species?

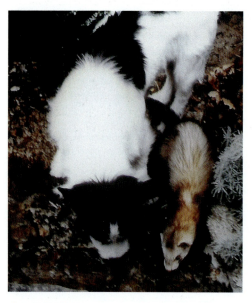

Figure 3.38 Dog 'Patch' with ferret 'Jennie' drinking from the stream.

References

1. Staton V, Cromwell-Davis SL. Factors associated with aggression between pairs of domestic ferrets. J Am Vet Med Assoc 2003; 222:1709–1712.
2. Brodie I. Ferrets and ferreting. London: Blandford Press; 1978.
3. Thornton PC, Wright PA, Sacra PJ, et al. The ferret, *Mustela putorius furo*, as a new species in toxicology. Lab Anim 1978; 13:119–124.
4. Fox JG, ed. Biology and diseases of ferrets. Laboratory animal medicine, 2nd edn. American College of Laboratory Animal Medicine; 2002:483.517.
5. Wilson MS, Donnoghue PND. A mobile rack of cages for ferrets, (*Mustela putorius furo*) Lab Anim 1982; 16(3):278–280.
6. American Ferret Report. The spring gardener: potentially toxic plants. American Ferret Report 1997; Mar/Apr:20.
7. The West Australian. Cat danger. Perth: The West Australian 7 May, 2005:22.
8. Dinnes MR. Medical care of non-domestic carnivores. In: Kirk RW, eds. Current Veterinary Therapy. Philadelphia: Saunders; 1980:710–733.
9. Pitcairn RH, Hubble Pitcairn S, eds. Creating a healthier environment. In: Natural Health for Dogs and Cats. Emmaus: Rodale Press; 1995:104–113.

CHAPTER 4

Nutrition

'Jumbo was called Jumbo because he was so large. In the prime of life he weighed four and a half pounds, which is a great weight for a ferret.'

Frances Pitt, Friends in Fur and Feather, 1946

I am giving in this chapter, my personal experience of feeding ferrets, plus a general review of feeding ferrets in the USA, Australia, New Zealand, the UK, Europe and Russia. Practitioners will be asked not just what to feed ferrets but how much and that can be a controversial subject. It is essential to remember that ferrets are obligate carnivores and require a meat diet with a high percentage of high quality protein, high percentage fat and relatively low percentage carbohydrate and a low fibre content.[1] Ferrets should *not* be fed a vegetarian diet. Figure 4.1 shows why. With high vegetable protein, ferrets are liable to get bladder stones, poor coat and skin features, eosinophilic gastroenteritis (which involves wasting, diarrhoea, ulceration of the skin and ear tips and swollen feet), poor growth of kittens and decreased reproduction.[2]

Feeding ferrets in the USA

Captive black-footed ferrets (*Mustela nigripes*) were fed raw rabbit (ground muscle and bones), dry pelleted mink food, dried beef liver, vitamin E and unlimited water.[3] The nutrition of the American domesticated ferret, whether laboratory-reared or as a house pet has evolved over the years. There is ongoing concern with nutrition in all species – including humans.

The first commercial estimations of ferret feeding requirements were made at Marshall Farms, New York, which led the way, engaging in rearing thousand of ferrets mostly for biomedical research and also later for the pet ferret market which has expanded.

Nutritional requirements of different carnivores have been compared with dietary levels required by ferrets and the composition of commercial diets that appear adequate for ferrets have both been tabled.[4] The dietary requirements of ferrets are met by various commercially prepared foods on the USA market and their composition is based in part on dietary findings from laboratory-fed ferrets, farmed ferrets (fitch farms for pelts) and the basic mink farm diet.

Marshall Farms recognized that natural ingredient diets are more palatable for ferrets than commercial preparations from the work of Dr Stillions, who devised a natural ingredient diet (Agway Marshall Ferret Diet) in the 1980s.[4] The original diet for Marshall Farms included dog food cereal with beef tripe and beef lungs but this did not prove satisfactory in the long term because of inadequacies in the protein sources and it is no longer used. Also, the meat, liver, lung and tripe, was obtained from slaughter houses, etc., so there was a risk of parasites infecting the ferrets which was not a good idea as they were going on to laboratory use (J. Bell, pers. comm. 1999). However, the dietary ingredients are still listed but only for comparison with other ferret foods.[4]

The feeding of large numbers of ferrets needed to be streamlined for cost and ease of feeding, so the trend went to feeding a dry food, based on mink diet. The Marshall Premium Ferret Diet (Kelly Feeds), which is fed to laboratory and breeding colonies and sold commercially in the USA was put together by Hartsough

CHAPTER FOUR

Nutrition

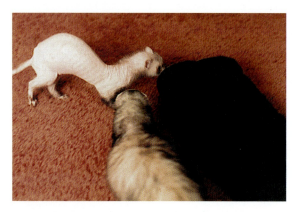

Figure 4.1 Bald sable ferret rescued from owner who fed it vegetarian food. The ferret showed poor growth and baldness. It dramatically improved on a meat diet. (Courtesy of Fara Shimbo.)

Table 4.1 Marshall Premium Ferret Diet: guaranteed analysis

Crude protein	not less than 38.0%
Crude fat	not less than 18.0%
Crude fibre	not less than 3.5%
Moisture	not more than 10.0%
Ash	not more than 6.5%

Source: R. Scipone, Marshall Farms, pers. comm. 1999.

and Bell from a mink diet in 1990 (J. Bell, pers. comm. 1999). The Marshall Premium Ferret Diet is an ad lib dry diet with a guaranteed analysis as shown in Table 4.1. Scipone of Marshall Farms lists the ingredients of this diet as the following: chicken by-products, herring meal, corn, cod fish, animal liver, dried beet pulp, brewers dried yeast, cane molasses, salt, sodium propionate (a preservative), DL-methionine, L-lysine, taurine, vitamin A acetate, vitamin D_3 supplement, niacin, biotin, choline chloride, folic acid, thiamine mononitrate, pyridoxine hydrochloride, BHA (a preservative), vitamin B_{12} supplement, menadione sodium bisulphate complex (a source of vitamin K), D calcium pantothenate, manganese oxide, inositol, ascorbic acid, iron sulphate, copper sulphate, zinc oxide, cobalt carbonate, potassium iodide, sodium selenite. Note that the crude fibre is given at not less than 3.5%, which is not in line with at least one particular American nutritionist who advises fibre content of ferret foods should be 2% or less (T. Willard, pers. comm. 1999). However, Marshall Farms maintain good ferret growth and reproduction with their formulation according to Scipone.

Fox et al. indicated the diet for ferrets, housed for research, in relation to a protein meat source as protein/fat requirement.[5] The diet is 30–40% protein and 18–20% fat for non-breeding adult males and females. There is a minimum of 35% protein with 25% fat for breeding males and females while for jills at peak lactation the minimum is 35% protein and 30% fat for healthy ferrets. Laboratory ferrets are fed ad lib which is not my way (see later).

Note: one USA veterinarian recommends a diet with 42–55% protein, 18–30% fat, 8–15% carbohydrates and fibre low at 1–3%. To avoid insulinoma, snacks and sugary treats must not be given (M. Finkler, pers. comm. 2005).

In Table 4.2, Bell has recorded the actual fibre percentage and not the label guaranteed value. At Marshall Farms, all ferrets are on a diet with ad lib feeding provided by food hoppers attached to the cages.[6] Private breeders in the USA also use the Marshall Farms Premium type of ferret food for convenience with large numbers of ferrets (Flemming Farms, pers. comm. 1998).

Note: the original mink diets used for ferrets contained a high fish content, which is not acceptable to ferrets, unlike some other mustelids, e.g. otters and mink. The modified mink diets were made around 40% protein and 20% fat. According to Bell, when breeding colony kittens were 3 weeks old, the above diet was mixed with water and had extra beef tallow added to raise the fat content to 30%. It was fed in a paté form.

Note: ferret kittens' eyes do not open till they are 4 weeks old but they can smell the wet food and leave the nest to get it from the food dispensers.[6] The jills and kittens were fed the diet ad lib until the kittens were weaned. The diet for mature ferrets should contain at least 30% protein but for young growing ferrets, up to 6 months, plus pregnant and lactating jills, the percentage should be 40%. Abnormalities can occur in weaned kittens receiving less than 30% protein.[7] At Marshall Farms young kittens saved for research or breeding continued to have a wet diet available until they were 12 weeks old and then a different dry diet was fed to weaned ferrets ad lib, which was also based on chicken, with 34% protein and 18% fat.[6] The young ferrets stayed on this diet until they entered the breeding colony at 4.5 months for jills or 9 months for hobs and then they returned to a higher protein diet. The fat requirements for adult ferrets should be 18–30%, while a minimum of 25% is required for lactating jills and kittens up to 6 weeks of age. For non-breeding adult ferrets, the fat level is considered best at 18–20%.[6] For energy consideration, Fox and McLain maintain that ferrets require to consume daily 200–300 kcal/kg body weight and they suggest that a value of near 5000 kcal/kg calorific density would be

Table 4.2 Comparison of constituent nutritional values of some American foods used for ferrets

Major nutrients (%)	Marshall Premium Ferret	Purine High Density Ferret	Iams Kitten Food	Totally Ferret	Science Diet Feline Growth
Crude protein	39.8	39.0	34.9	36.5	34.3
Crude fat	20.2	20.5	23.1	23.3	24.8
Crude fibre	2.2	2.6	1.43	1.4	2.8
Moisture	4.2	10.0	7.28	7.5	7.5
Ash	7.4	6.5	5.53	6.5	5.4
Carbohydrate	26.2	21.4	27.8	24.8	25.2
Amino acid (%)					
Arginine	2.52	2.05	2.44	2.4	2.0
Cystine	0.45	0.59	0.75	0.44	
Glycine		1.73			
Histidine	0.91	0.61	0.81	0.95	
Isoleucine	1.67	1.44	1.49	1.30	1.25
Leucine	3.09	3.2	2.51	2.55	3.29
Lysine	2.74	2.02	1.96	2.40	
Methionine	1.18	0.85	0.74	1.05	0.73
Phenylalanine	1.64	1.48	1.37	1.4	
Tyrosine	1.32	0.76	1.04	1.10	
Threonine	1.9	1.31	1.45	1.50	
Tryptophan	0.33	0.29	0.35	0.38	0.25
Valine	1.99	1.77	1.88	1.72	
Serine		1.26			
Aspartic acid		2.02			
Glutamic acid		4.04			
Alanine		1.61			
Proline		1.94			
Taurine	0.25	0.24	0.23	0.24	0.24
Linoleic acid	3.0	2.76	4.50	4.5	4.09
Minerals percentage unless otherwise stated					
Calcium	1.2	1.4	1.19	1.28	1.2
Phosphorus	1.05	1.25	0.95	0.88	0.89
Ca:P	1.14:1	1.12:1	1.25:1	1.49:1	1.35:1
Potassium	0.75	0.56	0.90	0.68	0.59
Magnesium	0.10	0.12	0.085	0.092	0.10
Sodium	0.55	0.40	0.60	0.42	0.32
Iron (p.p.m., mg/kg)	360	320	284	240	
Copper (mg/kg)	30	24	30.2	24	
Manganese (mg/kg)	70	72	63	80	
Zinc (mg/kg)	145	232	200	240	

CHAPTER FOUR
Nutrition

Table 4.2 Comparison of constituent nutritional values of some American foods used for ferrets – *cont'd*.

Major nutrients (%)	Marshall Premium Ferret	Purine High Density Ferret	Iams Kitten Food	Totally Ferret	Science Diet Feline Growth
Iodine (mg/kg)	2.6	2.0	2.1	2.0	
Selenium	0.3	0.6	0.25	0.35	
Vitamins					
A (IU/kg)	35,100	25,100	16,400	25,000	24,556
D (IU/kg)	2200	3700	1620	1800	1305
E (IU/kg)	155	250	150	300	515
C (IU/kg)	20		19	75	
K (ppm, mg/kg)	1.2	3.2		2.0	
Riboflavin (mg/kg)	25	20	17	55	
Folic acid (mg/kg)	1.5	4.3	3.63	3.0	
Niacin (mg/kg)	95	110	140	120	
Thiamine (mg/kg)	12.8	56	32	45	
Biotin (mg/kg)	0.60	0.48	0.9	10.2	
Pantothenic acid (mg/kg)	25	26.2	53	35	
Pyridoxine (mg/kg)	12.5	17.5	25	35	
Inositol (mg/kg)	95			100	
Energy values					
Metabolizable energy (ME) (kcal/g)	3.89	4.0	4.58	4.35	4.58
% ME from protein	45	43	34	37	33

Table modified after Bell.[1]

required for growth and reproduction.[4] Marshall Farms produce young adults that are on average heavier than the ones I have seen in Australia. A body weight graph is shown in Figure 4.2.

Bell is of the opinion that the criterion of a good ferret diet is that it can maintain a ferret colony and support their reproduction needs and this depends on the quality of the ferret diet, of which there are many commercially available in the USA.[1] She has given examples of some premium dry cat food and pelleted ferret diets that meet the criteria in respect to high protein and fat content and preferably low carbohydrate and fibre content. The main source of calories for ferret energy is fat, which when metabolized in the body releases twice as much energy as either protein or carbohydrates. The major possible ferret foods can be compared with the Marshall Farms basic for breeding, research and pet ferrets as shown in Table 4.2. The major diet components and the amino acid profile of proteins are listed plus essential mineral and vitamin supplementation. The calcium–phosphorus ratio for ferrets should be 1:1 at least and with the diets highlighted in the table, vary from 1.12:1 to 1.45:1.

For Marshall Premium, Purina and Totally Ferret®, analysis was on the average of the actual batch content and not the guaranteed analysis on the label. *Note* the guaranteed ingredients on commercial foods give only the proportions of crude protein, fat, fibre and moisture but no indication of the quality of the ingredients.[1] For Iams and Science Diet, the label guaranteed analysis was used, with minimum crude protein and fat and maximum fibre, moisture and ash.

Note: some other diets do not meet the standard of the five examples given, as the base chicken meal is considered inferior in having too much indigestible protein, e.g. feathers, more bone, less meat,[1] and the diet becomes deficient in essential amino acids. The American diets illustrated are able to produce from 3.9–4.58 kcal of metabolized energy per gram.

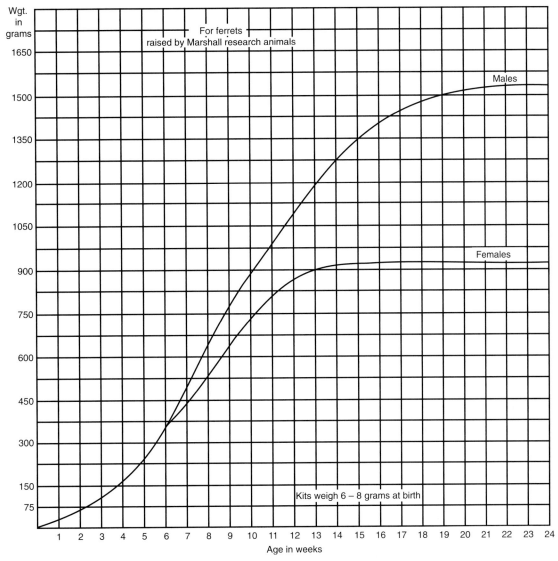

Figure 4.2 Graph of the body weights of ferrets reared at Marshall Farms, New York in 1993. (Courtesy of Dr J. Bell, pers. comm. 1993.)

A point is made that ferrets, like other mustelids, have a relatively short digestive system, with the jejunum division not being distinct and lacking an ileocolic valve.[1] Internally, there is a change from jejunum villous mucosa to ileum smooth mucosa (Ch. 2). It is considered that the food intestinal transit time is short in ferrets because of this anomaly, some 3–4 hours in adults and less in younger animals, being about 1 hour for neonatals. It is considered that ferret food can pass through the gut too quickly for efficient absorption to take place.[1] This apparently justifies the ad lib feeding of ferrets. Bell considers there is an inefficiency factor with the ferrets' short intestine and they need a diet high in protein and fat and low in fibre to compensate. I have never fed solids to my ferrets ad lib and have had no detrimental results. It could be suggested that if food is taken continuously, as in a laboratory situation, the intestinal transit time could be shortened from the natural one occurring in ancestral polecat types, which would only obtain food when they made a kill, probably irregularly.

The intestinal surface enzymes are low in ferrets compared with other animals, so this contributes to poor absorption. For example, a milk drink will produce soft faeces within an hour due to lack of enzyme time action. I have given milk to my ferrets in the morning and they got fatty but firm scats later on but not necessarily within the hour. Another view by an expert on small wild mustelids regarding the gut transit time is that small mustelids have a rapid metabolism, so food passes though quickly and they have few fat reserves. It is not the gut length that makes them constantly hungry and vulnerable to food shortages but their hyped-up metabolism (Carolyn King, Dept. Biological Science, University of Waikato, NZ, pers. comm. 1999). My original ferrets carried some fat and appeared not to be hungry all the time.

Ferrets can evidently only digest simple carbohydrates because the intestinal flora differs from other mammals in having a less concentrated anaerobic flora due to the smaller large intestine. Thus the pancreas can respond life-threateningly to increased sugar intake in the form of excessive sweet treats. Indeed, a rich carbohydrate intake is said to lead to a reduction in essential protein and fat and produce disease problems. It is stated that fat ferrets do not acquire medical problems because of overweight if the diet is well-balanced and no sugar treats are added.[7] Ferrets will evidently eat their caloric requirements but, being on a poor quality diet with high sugar treats, as some USA ferrets have been in the past, they become relatively protein-deficient and have poor coats. Possibly, ferrets in a permanent indoor living situation in the USA would have poor coat health anyway, as they are not getting the environmental stimulation from seasonal weather as ferrets living outside in all weathers do. American pet ferret owners are advised to feed cat supplements such as Nutri-Cal (Evsco) and use liquid Linotone, a small animal coat conditioner comprising linoleic and linolenic acids.

Commercial ferret foods

Commercial diets available in the USA in 1999 and exported worldwide are varied in quality and some have been shown in Table 4.2. The recommended commercial ferret diets available at least in the USA are shown in Table 4.3. Besides these makes, there are numerous pet foods available, e.g. ferret diets, which can be brought online.

Note: Table 4.2 compares diets but there is no mention of protein or nutrient quality. There are multiple specifications on each ingredient that can vary enough to cause specific nutrient deficiencies from batch to batch, e.g. there are at least five different grades of chicken or poultry by-products. These can go from very poor to very high quality as determined by amino acid composition and digestibility. Chicken meat used in the pet food industry actually comes from the remains of human food filleting operations and is thus made up of 40% or more connective tissue such as cartilage. The protein is high in non-essential amino acids such as proline and is poorly or almost not digested at all by pet ferrets or cats.

A query has been made whether pet store chow is adequate for ferret nutrition.[8] It is stated by Bell that cheap pet-shop food or generic cat food is not good for ferrets, as the products contain a ground corn base and ferrets are not good at digesting high fibre diets.[1] Ferrets should also not be fed soy flour and soybean meal. It is known that supermarket cat dry cat foods are palatable because the biscuit is coated with animal fat but they are nutritionally lacking for any age of ferret. If there are a number of cereal-based additions to the diet besides the meat by-product, there may be more plant protein than animal protein present, which is not good for ferrets.[1] Ferret owners should avoid these products, also dog food, home formulations containing too much vegetable matter, vegetarian diets and too many sweets! It has been stated that pet ferrets can be maintained on commercial cat food supplemented with table scraps.[9] Bell is of the opinion that ferrets fed unsupplemented dog food will eventually die, either by malnutrition or by infection of the bowel and possibly the respiratory system brought about by a depressed immune system.[1]

Some interesting comments on feeding American ferrets in relationship to gastrointestinal disease problems are given by Mark Burgess in Chapter 9.

Table 4.3 Ferret diets available in the USA with label fibre (%)

A: Diets for growth, pregnancy & lactation	B: Diets for maintenance
	Any diets of group A or these below
Hill's Feline p/d, Science Diet Feline Growth Fibre 1.1%	Hill's Feline c/d, Science Diet Feline Maintenance Fibre 0.5%
Iams Kitten Food fibre 1.43%	Iams Cat Food fibre 1.63%
Performance Foods Totally Ferret fibre 2.0%	Totally Ferret for Older Ferrets fibre 2.0%
Marshall Farms Premium Ferret Diet fibre 3.5%	Pet store Ferret Chow fibre %?

Table after Finkler.[8] Note: Hill's Feline p/d diet not now in Australia.

One can now compare 1999 guaranteed fibre values for dog and cat foods with 2005 values. My 1999 survey of local supermarket pet food label-guaranteed fibre content, showed tinned dog and cat food ranging from 0.2–3.0% and 0.4–1.0%, respectively and dry dog and cat food ranging from 2.6–5.0% and 3.0–3.50%, respectively. In 2005, the guaranteed fibre for tinned food for dogs and cats was 0.7–5.2% and 0.5–1.0%. With dry food, the readings for dog and cat were 2.7–5.0% and 2.5–5.0%.

Remembering the Scipone crude fibre value of not less than 3.5% and the Bell assertion that actual fibre value, not label value is important, an interesting case can be given of possible nutritional problems in ferrets. Bell maintains that an increased fibre intake increases the volume of the faeces with ferrets, as it would with dogs and cats, but will initiate in the ferret a relative protein calorie deficiency whereby the ferret cannot obtain enough of the low density food to keep up its vital maintenance requirements.[1] This of course is in contrast to Marshall Farms' experience with relatively high-fibre diets. However, one could speculate that the possible effects of fibre on the intestine might not show up in relatively short-lived laboratory ferrets. Those sold for the pet market would have a change of diet anyway.

There is an interesting point made by Bell, quoting unpublished data, that soft foods contribute to early dental disease in ferrets under 3 years of age.[1] Giving dry crunchy foods can prevent it. I have found dental tartar with wet meat foods but I prefer the latter diet for ferrets, with some bone inclusion such as chicken for teeth cleaning. Working ferrets on meat/bone diets are found to have good teeth.

The Performance Food Company (PFC, USA) has developed a possibly ideal balanced ferret food. Tom Willard, President of PATH Nutritional Consultants, has brought out interesting points regarding their product Totally Ferret and ideas on ferret nutrition.[10] PFC is the only serious ferret food manufacturing company doing nutritional trials. The ferret has nutritional requirements similar to other true carnivores but there are some essential differences. The cat for instance, is unable to convert beta-carotene to vitamin A, which is essential for growth, sight, and muscle coordination; ferrets can carry out this conversion and are used as research models in human nutrition investigations for this and other reasons.

He comments that there at least 10 companies besides Totally Ferret (TF) with varying degrees of quality. He suggests that Marshall's diet is closest to TF in nutritional quality with the others of lower quality and most with not even a complete and balanced diet for the maintenance of adult ferrets (T. Willard, pers. comm. 2005).

Feeding a poor diet can predispose an animal to poor health and in extreme cases, cause nutritional disease or imbalances. Urolithiasis in cats is an example of a nutritional disease that can be prevented with proper nutritional balance and formulation. *Note*: ferrets appear to be as sensitive as cats to factors causing urolithiasis. Special diets are advised for ferrets. Urolithiasis is a major problem of sterilized ferrets in the USA associated with poor diet (Ch. 11). In Australia, one case of urolithiasis was recorded with a ferret on dry cat food (McDonald, pers. comm. 1998). Bell gives examples of two diets unsuitable for ferrets being associated with urolithiasis and poor reproduction results in ferret colonies.[1] She maintains that the poultry meal of one diet was of low quality, though this cannot be assessed from the analysis or the ingredients list. The problem is that low quality indigestible protein, even feathers and hooves, with too much bone but little muscle meat is added. The outcome is a dangerous deficiency in the total amino acid makeup of the food.

A well-balanced quality diet will build and maintain an effective immune system, a strong muscular and skeletal framework and support the proper functioning of all the internal organs, which will sustain ferrets lifelong.

Carnivores require some 60 nutrients, which are subdivided into seven major categories: proteins, fats, simple carbohydrates, complex carbohydrates, vitamins, minerals and water.

Proteins

Proteins are complex biological compounds made up of individual building blocks called amino acids, 20 organic compounds made of carbon, hydrogen, nitrogen, oxygen

Author's clinical example

A teenage client in 1998 owned three adult ferrets, two jills and a hob, and insisted on feeding them tinned dog food (nameless). It was cheap. I managed to convince him, over the phone, not having seen the ferrets, to at least feed the supplement Animalac (Troy) in addition. All went well until he left home and his parents fed the ferrets. They used dog food but he had neglected to tell them about the Animalac addition. A short time afterwards, I was presented with a hob ferret, which had lost weight, was curled up and moaning in acute abdominal discomfort, also two not-so-sick jills. I kept the ferrets, Boysie, Patch and Lucky, as the teenager did not want them. I immediately put them on to a fresh mince diet and gave Animalac ad lib, with hand feeding to the hob. They recovered and I could only presume at the time that the combination of high fibre and relatively low protein in the dog food was the original cause. It could be surmised that the milk supplement 'coated' the bowel against the 'irritation' of a heavy fibre content. The trio of ferrets passed away in 2003–4.

and two containing sulphur. The protein strands are hundreds of thousands of amino acids long, coiled and packed together into every cell of the body. It is the number and sequence of amino acids that give each protein its unique function and properties.

The ferret requires at least 10 of these essential amino acids to be provided in the food as they cannot be made in the body. These essential amino acids are found most abundantly, and in the correct proportions to the carnivore's own body requirements, in foods made from other animal proteins, e.g. chicken, chicken by-products, meat, meat by-products and animal source proteins, like eggs, fishmeal or casein.

Experimentally, an arginine-free diet resulted in hyperammonaemia and encephalopathy in young ferrets in just 2–3 hours after feeding.[4] It is considered that ferrets, like other animals, eat to meet the requirements of the limiting amino acids and thus could eat more food than would be required to satisfy the needs of other amino acids.[1] The excess food is metabolized and used for energy. The nitrogen waste is excreted by the kidneys and shows up as high blood urea nitrogen (BUN) indicator in healthy ferrets, showing they have an excess of protein. However, the physical condition of the ferret will suffer in situations where the protein is below 30%. If it were possible to make sure the limiting amino acids are given adequately in a lower protein diet, it would be feasible to keep ferrets on as good a plane of nutrition as if their diet contained a standard minimum 35% crude protein.[1]

One of the lesser known amino acids, taurine, which has been found to be essential for other carnivores, is now suggested to be a requirement in ferret diets. It is essential for effective function of platelets, lymphocytes, retinal rods and cones, brain cells, and heart muscle.[11] Taurine is synthesized in the liver from dietary sulphur-containing amino acids (SAA) found in animal proteins, i.e. meat, liver, poultry, animal byproducts and fish meal. Ferrets are not usually fish eaters but some add fish to their diet (J. Usher, pers. comm. 2005).

Fat

Fat is required by carnivores daily as a primary source of energy. It supports their active lifestyle, breeding, showing or simply playing. Animal fats are more digestible than vegetable oils in most carnivores. Like proteins, fats are made up of individual units. These units are called fatty acids linked together in strands. There are over 70 known fatty acids that are found in all the body fat, oils and lipids. Some are unique to plants while others can only be found in animal fats. They contain over 2.25 times more energy per gram than either proteins or carbohydrates.

Carbohydrates

Simple carbohydrates are not required to meet specific dietary requirements for ferrets but will provide metabolic energy, which can spare or substitute for some energy from fats and protein. There are over 70 different saccharides in thousands of carbohydrate types.[12] One simple carbohydrate, starch, is necessary in preparing ferret foods to properly manufacture and give pellets shape and texture. In the case of Premium Foods, the constituents are all fully cooked in an extrusion process where the starches are hydrated and heated to over 200°F whereby they are completely cooked. The ferrets apparently prefer the crunchy texture and shape (like bones?) of the starch in the finished product. *Note*: the foods cooked at a lower temperature, which does not completely cook the starches, are called pelleted foods and are long and slender pellets looking like rabbit food. They are poorly digested, not very tasty or palatable to ferrets and also give loose stools (scats).

One American authority worried about the possible effects of fibre in the dry diet on ferrets. She also felt that dry food was not all that beneficial for ferrets' teeth (S. Brown, pers. comm. 1999). The fibrous portion of any prepared foods from complex carbohydrates, should be low or non-existent, as ferrets, without a caecum (as indicated earlier) cannot digest fibre well. High fibre of 3% or more in the diet causes digestive upsets and stool (scats) problems. It is possible that fibre irritation of the ferret bowel may stimulate ulceration and possibly bowel neoplasia in time. Fibre content should never be above 2% in ferret foods.[13] (Notice again this idea contrasts with the findings at Marshall Farms, NY. Remember that vitamins and minerals should be contained in premium ferret foods to meet dietary demands. These are also illustrated in the analysis table by Bell (Table 4.2).)

Vitamins

Vitamins are metabolic regulators and are required in very small daily quantities relative to proteins, fats and carbohydrates. There are 15 known and required vitamins which are involved in all of the thousands of metabolic pathways that convert food nutrients into body nutrients.

Vitamins are of two kinds and listed by Willard[12]:

1. *Fat-soluble*: Vitamins A, D_3, E and K. (*Note*: fat soluble vitamins can be stored in the body fat, but excessive levels can cause toxicity effects.)
2. *Water-soluble*: The B vitamin group including thiamine (B_1), riboflavin (B_2), pyridoxine (B_6) plus cyanocobalamin, (B_{12}). Also water soluble are niacin, pantothenic acid, folic acid, biotin, ascorbic

acid (C), choline and inositol. (*Note:* choline is a nitrogenous alcohol and an important methyl donor while inositol is a sugar alcohol. Neither are true vitamins but have vitamin-like properties and are used in premium and super premium dry and semi-moist diets.)

Minerals

Minerals, like vitamins are involved in most of the body's metabolic processes and mineral levels and balance is extremely critical in all carnivore diets. Imbalances between the 16 or so known essential minerals can cause major problems and initiate many diseases and debilitation abnormalities in the pet. Osteochondrosis in dogs is an example of a calcium imbalance disease.

Minerals are also of two kinds[12]:

1. *Macro-minerals*: required in greater proportions in the diet; calcium, phosphorus, sodium chloride and magnesium plus sulphur which is combined with other nutrients. These are often called 'structural minerals' as they are concentrated in bone and muscle.
2. *Micro-minerals*: called trace elements and required in minute but important levels: zinc, iron, copper, iodine and selenium plus cobalt, chromium and molybdenum which are usually combined with other nutrients and never added to the diet in the pure form. Additionally, fluoride, nickel, vanadium, silicon and tin are necessary but in minute and organic form in the diet.

WATER: Must always be in plentiful supply with all nutritional ferret diets and protected from contamination.

In studies with ferrets and cats, Willard has shown that diets high in animal protein such as chicken, poultry or other meat proteins will produce acidic urine – below 6.4. For the well-being of the cat or ferret, utilization of a high quality animal protein in the diet appears to be the best way to lower urine pH, thus reducing the risk of lower urinary tract diseases.

The work of the Performance Food Company is encouraging for ferret nutritional needs. Veterinarians advising on ferret diet should consider the points of a diet tested on ferrets with a guaranteed analysis and specific ingredients. Ferret foods like Totally Ferret should show full ingredients and availability of the diet for ferret growth, gestation, lactation and maintenance. *Note* that pelleted ferret foods are usually modified mink foods and fed to fitch ferrets in pelt farming organizations. They smell of fish, which most ferrets are not particularly keen about and are certainly not

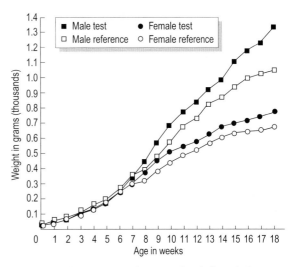

Figure 4.3 Average growth curve of male/female ferrets on Totally Ferret®.

suitable for pet ferrets. Good quality chicken, poultry, pork or beef fat are generally the best way to improve palatability at the lowest cost. Willard states that with a guaranteed percentage analysis, a good ferret food should have at least 36% protein, 22% fat with 2% or less fibre. It should be suitable for ferret growth, pregnancy and maintenance as with foods specific to dogs and cats.[13] *Note* an average growth curve for male and female ferrets on Totally Ferret is shown by the graph in Figure 4.3.

It is considered that older or aged ferrets will do well on the above diet but can gain weight as their activity greatly decreases. Bell puts a ferret maintenance diet at 30–35% crude protein and 15–18% fat. I find that older pet ferrets on virtually ad lib feeding with dry ferret food can put on weight regardless. For older ferrets, it is suggested that a lower protein range of 31–33% and 16–18% fat might be better suited but evidently this has not been proven in current feeding studies. The active ferret needs to be kept active as it grows older, otherwise it can tend to obesity, especially if the owner finds it difficult to cut down on the ferret's food. I think ferrets living at least some time outdoors, or working ferrets, have an advantage over indoor ferrets, especially where the latter are mostly kept in cages. Activity of the ferrets will depend on climate. In Western Australia, the hot summers dictate only evening or night activity for ferrets, otherwise there is a high risk of heat stress. Added to this, the ferret is naturally nocturnal. This can be changed by having ferrets in a mild climate or in a house situation where they are played with during the day and sleep more at night. To obtain a weight reduction in heavy ferrets, there cannot be an increase in fibre content of the diet, as with dogs and cats, due to the stated detrimental effect of fibre on ferrets. It is suggested that lowering the protein levels in the diet is the only way to go. However, for ferrets recovering from sickness a good quality protein food is essential.

The ingredient list of quality ferret food should be checked to see that it contains the best sources of protein, fat vitamins and minerals. Sources of good protein for ferrets should be listed as chicken and poultry by-products meal, meat meal, whole eggs, liver, herring meal and animal by-products.[13] It is considered that a high quality simple carbohydrate like rice flour or brewers yeast should be in the food to add texture, being easily digestible. The fat source should be from chicken, other poultry and animal fats, with other fat sources being vegetable oils, lecithin, corn oil or fish oil. The presence of individual amino acids such as lysin, methionine and taurine should be seen to be listed on the packet of ferret food along with the other ingredients.

It is essential according to Totally Ferret® that the product be packaged well to keep it fresh. Of the dry ferret foods, the Performance Foods range seems to be a safe choice if ferret owners cannot revert to fresh meat diets. The American Ferret Association recommends it.

Feeding Australian ferrets

When I started with ferrets in 1971, I came into feeding from a different angle to the ideas expressed by American sources, purely because I was unaware of the American way with ferrets! I started with a general knowledge of feeding dogs and cats. When I got my first ferret, Fred, I turned to a human medical book (1965 vintage edition) and found a bold statement of feeding laboratory ferrets: 'Each ferret requires 4 oz of raw meat (horse flesh, lights, etc. are satisfactory) and 4 oz of fresh milk daily' (4 oz ≅ 110 g).[14]

At the time, having no American text on ferret diet, and knowing them to be carnivores, I followed on from that statement. I see no reason to change. I modified the basic feeding routine for adult ferrets and pregnant and lactating jills with kittens.[15] Details of the nutritional requirements in a breeding colony are given in Chapter 5. I fed my ferrets once or twice daily, with the main concern that food was not left out in the day to spoil in the Western Australian heat (Fig. 4.4). I then learnt, as indicated in the previous section, that ferrets have a short digestive system and presumably need ad lib feeding. I found that did not necessarily apply to how I fed my ferrets. In support, other ferret owner clients feed their pets quite happily twice daily without adverse effects.

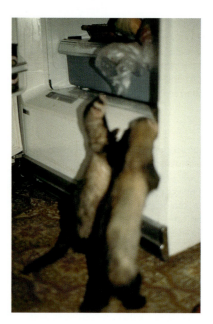

Figure 4.4 Jason and Brownie inspecting the fridge.

Personal ferret feeding procedures

I feed my ferrets at about 7.30 p.m. and again at 7.00 a.m. I used to take them to work to check. They will still pass scats (stools) in the afternoon, over 6 hours since being fed. I can only presume that the digestive system has adapted to the amount of food entering the system at specific feeding times. I was at first giving adult ferrets a basic 'handful' of mince, which worked out about 90–120 g, each night. I gave no solids in the morning but a milk drink, again not measured. The overnight meal had to be eaten or any remains were removed. The milk associated with the meat provided minerals and vitamins plus extra protein and fat; it is known that meat is low in calcium so a diet with meat alone will cause skeletal problems. The milk was changed to a commercial milk supplement when I went into breeding ferrets. With adults, diluted milk or milk supplements can be fed but are not needed constantly as with young ferrets. I estimated a rough weight of food for a 9-week-old ferret at 25 g daily (wet weight) plus a daily vitamin/mineral supplement drink. At the present time, I give my jills 40–60 g and the hobs 60–80 g meat daily; this can vary with the season. It is now fed half at night and half in the morning. Many times the ferrets do not eat all that is offered and they are fed individually so I can keep track.

Having my ferrets outdoors and now also indoors, I am admittedly a bit paranoid about ferrets stashing uneaten food in odd places and it becoming spoilt in our climate! Thus, I tend to keep the feeding down to an approximate set weight. Using dry food would be tempting to overcome this concern. However, dry food stashed away can still go mouldy. In addition, the ferrets do not appear to suffer from an extended time without food. Water is available all the time whether they are outside or inside. I can feed the ferrets half their ration in the morning and not return till late, about 11 p.m. and find the ferrets sleeping unperturbed. They do not then ravenously attack the food given to them; they wake and are active, which is natural for nocturnal animals. In addition, sometimes food offered at 7.30 p.m. is not eaten till much later in the evening; the main thing is that it is eaten. The portion not eaten straight away is eaten the next morning and there is no waste. Thus, ferrets can sleep mostly, but not completely, through the day and then are active in the evening and at night living in the garden. This is best, as I do not want them active in the daytime in hot weather. This idea would, naturally, differ in other climates. Other ferret owners say the same, as when they are working, the ferrets have to be left alone during the day. Leaving the ferrets titbits like a bowl of dry biscuit foods to nibble on between times is not required. Also having dry nibble foods tends to require an animal to drink more water.

Ferret foods

I used to have rabbit for the ferrets when ferreting, but now only rarely. I feed a combination of fatty or steak butchers' mince plus varieties like lamb hearts, lamb or mutton pieces, chicken wings (uncooked or cooked) plus whole eggs at weekends. Sometimes my ferrets get lactose-free milk in the mornings in winter, but mostly they are left water. It is probably better to feed milk diluted on its own or give just a small amount of food with the morning milk. For adults, the milk is more of a treat and not necessary as it is possible with BEW strains to have a metabolic deficiency, which could lead to cataract in later life (Ch. 12). The feeding of pregnant and lactating jills is another matter and considered in Chapter 5.

A friend maintained his breeding and working ferrets on a meat diet consisting of 35% protein, 30% fat and 5% ash and only gave milk to his breeding jills and kittens (Tom Garrick, Sydney, NSW, pers. comm. 1998).

Table 4.4 shows another ferret owner's recipe for ferret meat (Dave Such, Sydney, NSW Ferret Society President, pers. comm. 1998) which was interesting but he still insisted on leaving ferret biscuit available 24 hours a day and it also includes frozen vegetables.

In my opinion, dry food left out for outside-living ferrets in a hot climate would only require the ferret to

Table 4.4 Ferret diet for breeding colony

700 g cheap mince, must be fatty
70 g mixed frozen vegetables (avoid corn)
2 rice biscuits
2 teaspoons of bone meal
1 teaspoonful of calcium powder (breeding season only)
Contents are mixed together and put through a mincer.

Note: ferret biscuits are available 24 hours a day.

drink more water and could be counterproductive to the ferret's health. If biscuits are considered an aid to keeping ferret teeth clean, this has not been shown by some of the ferrets I have seen on that diet. In addition, my sterilized hobs over the years have never shown any cystitis or urolithiasis with blockage, as seen in some American pet ferrets on dry foods.

What is fed to ferrets of course regulates what comes out as scats (faeces). This is probably of no concern with outdoor ferrets but for pet ferrets coming indoors frequently or totally indoor pets the smell and consistency of their scats is important. Mince/lamb combinations usually give low-smelling oblong scats, which are easily cleaned up. Ferrets fed wholly kangaroo meat produce runny scats with a strong odour. Too much fat supplement produces yellowish scats with an offensive odour. Milk can give yellow fatty runny scats unless diluted with water. Lactose-free milk is suitable for ferrets. Liver added to the diet causes slimy scats and should anyway be fed only infrequently. The vegetable matter in the diet (Table 4.4) is of no use to ferrets and it is suspected that plant fibre can be harmful over time, as they have no way of digesting it. As it was put by an American pet ferret owner to veterinarian Judith Bell: 'You put veggies in and you get veggies out'.[1] Vitamin/mineral supplements can be sprinkled over the meat, e.g. Animalac (Troy) or Biolac. I do not use Di-Vetelact supplement now, as I suspect some ferrets could be in danger of getting galactose-induced cataracts but this has not been proved conclusively (Ch. 12).

A variety of meats have been fed to ferrets in Perth, WA. A 1992 survey of 36 ferret owners in the WA Ferret Society found some 66% of ferrets were fed mince, 52% kangaroo meat, 44% rabbit and 16% chicken. These figures include the fact that some owners were feeding a mixture of meats, as I do.[16] Considering other meats, there was a smattering of diced steak, sheep, goat, lamb, fish (surprisingly) as well as heart and liver being fed to ferrets. Some owners were feeding tinned cat food and dog food sometimes and also dog chow or dry cat food. The replies came from both ferreters and city ferret pet owners. Some ferret owners admitted to still feeding the old bread and milk diet and someone fed pig pellets!

If asked for a diet for young kittens and adult ferrets, I would say bring them up on a variety of fresh meats with bone, chicken for fat, chicken necks and wings and even kangaroo pieces or lamb hearts. To encourage adult ferrets to accept a fresh meat meal, one might need to virtually starve the ferret as change may be difficult after a lifetime on commercial foods. It is suggested putting a fatty acid supplement on the meat as a temporary measure to get them to change.[2]

Feeding routines:

a. Feed whole meal in the evening and milk drink in the morning.
b. Feed half meal in evening and half meal in morning plus milk drink.
c. Feed whole meal in evening plus milk and no milk in the morning.
d. Feed whole meal in evening and only water in the morning.
e. Feed half meal in evening and half in the morning with only water.

Routines (a), (b) and (c) refer to feeding pregnant and lactating jills and kittens (see Ch. 5).

Routines (d) and (e) can refer to adult hob ferrets and jills, not pregnant or lactating. This is because if adult ferrets are getting a good meaty/bone diet, plus eggs occasionally, they do not require a milk supplement.

Feeding starts from 6 weeks of age at 25 g plus daily per ferret with equivalent non-lactose milk or vitamin/mineral supplement till adult at 6 months of age. The body skeleton must be serviced before the rest to give the animal a good body frame by making sure the calcium/phosphorus content is kept up. Feeding rabbit to ferrets is a natural way, but surprisingly, rabbit is now a gourmet dish and expensive unless one is a ferreter and gets the ferrets to chase out their own dinner! From 3 months of age, the 25 g daily is increased in stages until 40–60 g is reached for jills and 60–80 g for hobs at 6 months of age. About an equal amount of milk or milk substitute is given with meat, usually in the morning. Occasionally, liver and eggs can be given. Adjustments in food amount are made in the light of hot or cold seasons of the year or jill pregnancy. I have found no need to go above about 80 g of meat for hobs. In July 1999, my two adult hobs averaged 1600 g and five jills averaged 796 g.

Water availability is a must for ferrets; if water is restricted, or forgotten, the ferrets could maintain body condition in normal weather on a diet of wet meat food. However, I would be worried that there might be a dangerous situation with ferrets on dry food with lack of water in a hot climate. This is especially a concern with older ferrets; there could be possible effects on the renal system.

How ferreters (those who work ferrets) feed their ferrets

Working ferrets have a good carnivore diet. I have seen many at all ages in excellent condition, though sometimes dirty from working, with good teeth on their meat diet. Kangaroo shooters with ferrets feed them on fresh kangaroo meat, which is a high protein meat and/or rabbit meat. With a number of ferrets, the colony gets a whole rabbit carcass, which they will devour, leaving little but some skin and the skull (Bert Geddes, Perth, WA, pers. comm. 1982). Ferrets have also been fed on the odd emu! Ferreters I have known fed their ferrets on meaty bones plus liver and whole eggs once weekly or fortnightly. One ferret owner fed his six adult working ferrets with about 450 g meat (kangaroo or rabbit) in a single bowl and gave 1.25 pints of milk daily. He had the milk supply prepared in a blender with a teaspoonful of honey plus knob of butter and warm water. It was poured over the meat as an evening-only meal. The rest was given as a next morning drink. This ferreter also fasted his ferrets 1 day a week, the same as the family and dogs, with no apparent ill-effects (K. Cooper, Perth, WA, pers. comm. 1982). The food fed by Karim Cooper of 450 g for six ferrets could be averaged at 73 g (wet weight) per ferret. (I advocate 40–80 g per ferret.)

Natural feeding

There is a movement in Australia for feeding dogs a more natural 'raw meaty bone' diet instead of tinned or dry food.[17,18] *Note* ferreters have been doing the equivalent with ferrets for years and would be loathe to change! Working ferrets are usually lithe and well muscled without any excess fat, though body fat is put on in the winter by all ferrets living outside. The food intake can be up to 30% more in winter; this would depend on climatic conditions with the ferrets losing weight in the spring. The teeth are usually excellent.

The feeding of dogs and cats on a more natural diet has been promoted in an excellent Australian book by Dr Tom Lonsdale in 2001.[18] He points out that wild dogs and cats can eat raw rabbits and he is concerned with the cooking of any meat or viscera, which decreases the nutritional status of proteins, fats, carbohydrates, vitamins, minerals and micronutrients. He points out the destruction of biologically active cellular enzymes in cooked 'prey'. With the animal (e.g.

dog, cat or ferret) eating cooked material there is no source of cellular enzymes from the meal to assist the digestion alongside the enzymes produced by the pancreas. The pancreas thus has to work on its own and has a bigger task in the digestion process. Could this in the long term become a 'strain' on the domestic animal's pancreas?

It is considered by Lonsdale that the way to get a complete good mix of protein, fat, carbohydrate, fibre, vitamins and minerals without loss of nutritional value is to feed dogs and cats fresh meat and bones. I would suggest this for ferrets also.

It has been advocated, by Dr S. Brown in the USA, that pet ferrets could be fed 'prey animals' such as live mice, rats or chicks to make sure they had a 'natural' meat diet. These 'prey animals' could be delivered to the door by producers. She has pointed out that owners of exotic snakes will feed them mice but balk at giving live prey to ferrets. Of course, the aesthetic reason will stop most ferret owners following through with this suggestion.[2] The idea is pushing ferret nutrition back to the feeding ideas for working ferrets. Frozen rats are another option for in-house ferret meals. It has been pointed out that a large supply of mice or juvenile rats would be needed to keep the average pet ferret happy. The average mouse contains 30 kcal energy source while the average adult ferret requires 200–300 kcal/kg per day. Thus a 1 kg ferret would need 7–10 mice per day (M. Finkler, pers. comm. 2005).

In America, there is the Archetype Diet by Wyson. It is cold processed, containing beef, lamb and chicken meat products in small chunks for ferrets. *Note*: Brown advises that the diets are made from meat suitable for human consumption, which is what I have always done for my ferrets. The food should contain organ meat, muscle, fat and bone. The fat level should be high with no grain or grain products, sweeteners or chemical preservatives.[2] Brown is also against the processed diets that are ferret treat food. She has found they contain no meat products at all but are entirely composed of sweeteners and grains plus some fruits and vegetables. She considers this unacceptable, unhealthy and possibly dangerous to ferrets. She makes the point that owners find it emotionally good to feed treats to pets, be they dogs, cats or ferrets. Ferrets may be said to have a sweet tooth but it is detrimental to the animal if it brings on insulinoma attacks (Ch. 14). Overuse of fatty acid supplementation can cause obesity, which I have found in the past. Brown suggests turning to giving more natural treats to pet ferrets such as raw liver or heart bits, raw egg or even a mouse! (My ferrets may have found their own mice in the back garden.) She refutes the idea that fresh meat makes ferrets more aggressive and I agree with that statement. Ferrets eating natural prey would possibly get some bacterial input but it should boost their natural immunity to disease.

The possibility of additives in meats from the human meat market is addressed by our WA Agriculture Department's Standards for Meat.[19] Minced meat for instance has to have no additives and lean mince is having fat at not more than 100 g/kg. Fatty hamburger mince can be used with combinations of other meats including chicken and rabbit. The chances of food additives of any sort in meat causing ferrets some toxicity is not recorded. The possibility of dangerous food additives in pet food is taken up later in this chapter.

Commercial ferret foods

Some American dry foods, cat, dog and ferret, are available in Australia but we also have an Australian-made biscuit and meal food called Ferret's Choice.

Ferret's Choice

This is supplied as Premium Ferret Biscuits and Premium Ferret Food and the composition of the foods will be of interest generally to veterinarians advising ferret owners on nutrition.

Premium Ferret Biscuit

This has 39% protein, 23% fat base with 3.5% fibre plus moisture 6% and a Ca:P ratio of 3:2.50. The fibre content is thus higher than recommended by Willard and noticeably the same as the American Marshall Premium Ferret Diet. The food is produced from poultry meal, wheat, fish meal, lupin meal, omega 3- and 6-fatty acids, tallow, premium vitamins and minerals, lysine, DL-methionine, taurine and citric acid. Premium Ferret Biscuit is considered an ad lib food and there is a feeding guide. *Note*: it is suggested that the food be mixed with meat or other food.

Premium Ferret Food

This has 36.5% protein, 23.5% fat base with a lower 1.5% fibre plus moisture 9.0% and a Ca:P ratio 1:0.08. This food is produced from fish meal, wheat flakes, vegetable oils, fish oils, skim milk, yeast powder, meat meal, egg powder and oats plus premium vitamins and minerals, lysine, DL-methionine and taurine.

The latter food has a strong fishy smell and seems to me to equate to mink diets used initially for ferrets in fitch farms and breeding colonies in the USA, in which ferrets need to be brought up from kittens to accept fish foods. It is interesting to compare this new ferret food with other foods regarding grams of food to body weight (Table 4.5).

CHAPTER FOUR
Nutrition

Table 4.5 Feeding guide for Premium Ferret Food

Ferret body weight (kg)	Amount fed per day (g)
<0.5	20–30
0.5–1	30–40
1–2	40–50
2–3	50–60

Personally, I would still go for natural meat diets for ferrets. It is considered that too much processed material goes into dry ferret diets and that they are not really that good for teeth care. Evidently, this is the same for dogs and cats on dry diets in the USA (S. Brown, pers. comm. 1998).

Feeding New Zealand ferrets

New Zealand had pet and working ferrets but now only feral ferrets. Ferrets are still bred at Southlands Ferrets and Mystic Ferrets for the laboratory and pet market overseas. Although an unpalatable idea, there was an established fitch farm industry like the mink farming industry. Their ideas for feeding ferrets can be a baseline for discussion on modern pet ferret keeping.

New Zealand fitch farms nutrition

The dietary requirements of past fitch-farmed ferrets are interesting to compare with the American standards of feeding ferrets today. A past review on nutrition states that the fitch (ferret) requires a very high quality diet and it is made up of 50–60% lean meat, 10–20% fat, 5–10% liver and 5–10% bone. *Note*: this mixture was given uncooked and fresh.[20] The meal was adequate for energy, protein, essential fats, mineral and vitamins for ferret optimal growth and production.

Fitch farms obtained their feed from various sources and they were not particularly choosy, e.g.

- Poultry carcasses (eggs removed), poultry offal (liver, gizzard, lung and heart), poultry necks, heads and feet, day-old chicks
- Sink (stillborn) lambs and calves (whole) and cull ewe carcasses (except stomachs and intestines)
- Mutton and beef livers, hearts, kidneys, and lungs
- Horse carcasses (except fat, stomach and intestines)
- Fish whole, fish scrap (heads and racks) and fishmeal
- Cereals (cooked), wholemeal flour, bran
- Commercial vitamin-mineral premixes
- Milk powder, bone flour, eggs (cooked), butcher's crackling.

(*Source*: MAF Wellington, NZ.)

Table 4.6 indicates the ways the basic diets for fitch were set out.

Note: all offal contains high quality protein but there are disadvantages in dealing with it. Intestines contain a large bacterial flora and could spoil food giving acute enteritis to ferrets, e.g. *Salmonella* or *E. coli*.

Ruminant stomach parts used for ferret food must be washed clean of their plant fibre stomach contents as we know the latter are indigestible to ferrets. Mutton from culled ewes and rams is excellent for providing protein, calcium and phosphorus in the ferret but the sheep must be skinned as ingested wool may result in fur balls in ferrets and bowel

Table 4.6 Examples of basic diet of fitch

Ingredient	Level of ingredients (%) weight, as fed					
	Mutton ration		Poultry ration		Fish ration	
	A	B	A	B	A	B
Mutton (skinned carcass, except stomach and intestines)	95	80		20		50
Poultry (entire carcass, eggs removed)			100	40		
Poultry offal (liver, gizzard, necks, heads, feet)		10		40	40	
Fish (entire)				60		
Fish scrape (heads, necks)				10		50
Mutton (or beef) liver	5					
Total	100	100	100	100	100	100

Note: Ration A predominates in one type of ingredient; ration B is a mixture. Addition of cereal, salt and vitamin mineral mixtures is optional. (Courtesy of MAF information.[20])

obstruction. Finally, any horse products used in ferret diets must have any excess of fat trimmed as horse fat tends to become rancid and toxic to ferrets.

Note: When the fitch farms were very productive in New Zealand, the feeding of the ferrets was *once* daily as this produced less wastage. A guide to the daily food requirements for a growing fitch in the old establishments is useful to compare with my feeding ideas and other feeding routines for young and adult working/pet ferrets and is shown in Table 4.7.

Note that there is a drop-off of food intake around 16 weeks of age, but a weight increase is seen in these ferrets. The feed is assumed to be a properly balanced typical meat ration continuing 15% protein (wet matter basic (WMB) and 60% moisture. With the jills, the daily food intake hits 110 g, which was the recommended feeding of laboratory ferrets by Cruickshank[14] and is taken to 130 g in the hobs before being reduced.

Fitch ferrets were assumed to have similar protein requirements to mink. Figure 4.5 shows the growth curve in a NZ fitch farm in 1983 with animals on mutton and beef. The data is given as an example of the growth weights at the time.

Note in Figure 4.5, the separation of jills' and hobs' weight curves appear around the 200 g body weight, compared with the separation on the Marshall Farms graph at around 340 g. The former is at 5 weeks of age and the latter at 6 weeks of age. Both organizations were looking at jills flattening out at a weight of 900 g and hobs at 1500 g.

The introduction of Scottish Highland ferrets to fitch farms showed a higher growth rate of these new bloodlines in Figure 4.6. Considering daily food requirements, it can be seen that at the age 5-week mark the new ferrets were getting 13 g daily, which is less than those ferrets fed as in Table 4.7. Table 4.8 shows this. The growth separation curve between hobs and jills is earlier,

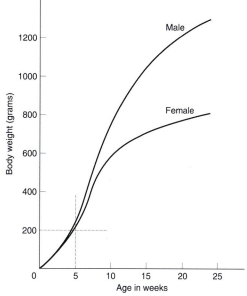

Figure 4.5 Fitch farms in New Zealand: body weights of ferrets. (From AgResearch Ltd., with permission.)

as can be seen in Figure 4.6, however the growth weights peak at a higher level.

The New Zealand review of the suitability of food sources for ferrets highlights some general nutritional problems that might occur in feeding working ferrets or breeders in particular. Notice in Table 4.8, the daily food intake is level for males/females up to 5 weeks after which the males eat more and gain more weight than females. The food intake for males/females levels off from 16–22 weeks of age. This can be an aspect of pet nutrition also.

Table 4.7 Feeding ferret hobs and jills

Age (weeks)	5	7	9	11	13	16	22	26	30
Hobs									
Body weight (g)	240	460	680	840	970	1100	1270	1350	1400
Daily food (g)	20	40	70	90	110	130	120	100	90
Jills									
Body weight (g)	230	400	540	620	680	740	800	840	860
Daily food (g)	20	40	70	90	110	110	90	90	80

From: Fur Farming Fitch (Nutrition and Feeding), with permission.[20]

CHAPTER FOUR

Nutrition

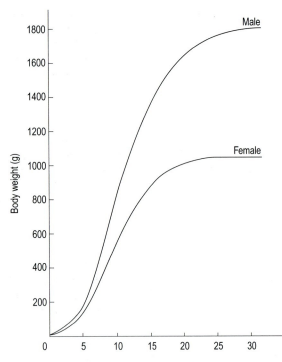

Figure 4.6 Growth curve of standard Scottish Highland fitch, fed mutton ration. (From AgResearch Ltd., with permission.)

Adverse nutritional conditions in ferrets

Veterinarians might take note of the conditions below when giving advice to clients:

Biotin deficiency

The use of cull layers was considered risky, as they might contain raw eggs. Avidin, a factor present in raw egg whites, inactivates biotin. Ferrets could develop a biotin deficiency if the raw egg content was over 20% of the diet.

Clinical signs: Alopecia down the back and general body, which would have to be differentiated from other alopecia conditions. Additionally, there might be hyperkeratosis, conjunctivitis and possibly fatty liver.

Treatment: Removing eggs from the carcasses as routine or adding 55% of yeast or vitamin/mineral supplement to feed. Avidin is destroyed by cooking eggs at 91°C for 5 min and I know of one NZ ferreter who fed cooked eggs to ferrets with no adverse effects (Bob Jeffares, pers. comm. 1997). Biotin is included in dry ferret diets (Table 4.2).

Thiamine deficiency

The intestines of some fish, e.g. Pacific mackerel, could contain thiamase, an enzyme which destroys thiamine (vitamin B_1).

Clinical signs: In mink on raw fish diets the disease was originally described as Chastek paralysis, that is paralysis with symptoms of anorexia, gradual loss of flesh, paralysis and death.[21] It was a disease of fitch farming in NZ. The disease in ferrets shows lethargy and anorexia, which can move to dyspnoea, prostration and convulsions. Treatment must be quick.

Treatment: By i.p. injections of 5–10 mg of vitamin B_1 for 3 days.

Note: In 2005 it was recognized that the use of sulphur preservatives causes thiamine deficiency in cats and dogs.[22,23]

Table 4.8 A guide for daily requirements for growing fitch

Age (weeks)	3	5	7	9	11	13	16	22	26	30
For one male										
Body weight (g)	80	150	400	700	950	1200	1400	1700	1800	1800
Daily protein (g)	1	2	7	12	16	20	24	22	20	16
Daily food (g)	7	13	50	80	110	130	160	150	130	105
For one female										
Body weight (g)	60	120	300	450	650	750	900	1050	1050	1050
Daily protein (g)	1	2	5	9	13	17	20	19	17	15
Daily food (g)	7	13	30	60	90	110	130	130	110	100

Wet matter basis (g). Feed is assumed to be properly balanced typical New Zealand meat-type ration containing 36% protein, 31% fat, 21% carbohydrate and 12% ash (DMB). Fitch are assumed to have similar protein requirements to mink. (Adapted from NRC Nutrient Requirement of Mink; 1968:23; Courtesy of MAF Information.)[20]

Hypervitaminosis

The recommended offal for ferrets (fitch) included liver, lungs, heart, spleen, kidneys, tripe and udder. Remember ruminant liver is very rich in vitamins A, D, E, K and all B vitamins; care must be taken to avoid hypervitaminosis effects due to too much liver over a long period. Adult ferrets can accept a 90% liver diet for short period.

Clinical signs: If liver is given too often, the excess of vitamin A causes exostosis and hip problems in rapidly-growing animals. With young ferrets if just self-feeding exclusively on liver, they can develop paralysis, which leaves them either without the use of their back legs or with curvature of the spine.

Treatment: Use of anabolic steroids in affected cases would tend to speed up growth and use up excessive vitamins in the system. With the young ferrets affected, liver is removed from the diet and they are given injections of 5 mg anabolic steroids plus 30 mg chloramphenicol i.m. that is repeated 3 days later. However, recovery would take over 2 weeks and the kittens might well be permanently deformed.

Yellow fat disease

Entire fish can be used but oil-rich fish, e.g. mullet or tuna, should be supplemented with vitamin E or an antioxidant to prevent yellow fat disease (vitamin E deficiency, nutritional steatitis). This is again a disease of fitch or mink on fish diets and can affect young animals. Most working or pet ferrets do not take to fish foods.

Clinical signs: Sudden, with kittens going off their food and found dead overnight. Ferrets might show a peculiar unsteady gait followed by paralysis and death. The problem can be fish scraps stored away, whereby their high concentration of unsaturated fatty aids becomes rancid as a result of low or deficient quantities of antioxidants.

Diagnosis: Ferret being on a high polyunsaturated fat diet but usually only diagnosed on post mortem with the skin of the abdominal and inguinal regions appearing thickened and pitting to pressure. Watery fluid escapes from a cut surface and the subcutaneous and visceral fat is brownish-yellow.

Prevention: By avoiding fish in the diet or supplementing with an adequate vitamin/mineral product.

Nutritional hyperparathyroidism

Without adequate vitamin/mineral addition to the ferret diet, which is unlikely nowadays, the condition of osteodystrophia fibrosa (nutritional hyperparathyroidism) can occur due to lack of calcium. It was recorded in NZ fitch farms in the 1980s.

Clinical signs: Mostly occurs in rapidly-growing kittens with weight loss, though appetite is good, reluctance to move and inability to support body weight. The ferret assumes a posture resembling a breaststroke swimmer; called 'swimmers' (Ch. 5). The bones are soft and easily broken. Thus it is important that ferret breeders are concerned about bone build-up before body mass, i.e. the frame must support the filling!

Nutritional rickets

In rapidly growing ferrets, as in mink, if the food is deficient in vitamin D, calcium or phosphorus, the condition of rickets can occur. The condition is now rare. Most diagnoses of rickets may be referred to nutritional hyperparathyroidism.

Ferret commercial breeding

New Zealand has two commercial ferret-breeding organizations, which feed their colony ferrets on diets of poultry-based food and fish-based diets with vitamin/mineral supplementation.[24] These diets are comparable with those of Marshall Farms.

Ferreters feeding working ferrets up to 2000

In New Zealand, ferrets were taken out hunting for rabbits and breeding ferrets were fed on a variety of foods. George Symons of Otago kept his ferrets in a barn with straw on the floor and his feeding routine included using Feedmilk, basically a milk replacer for lambs (see Fig. 1.7).

Formulation: Feedmilk powder is made up at the rate of 200 g powder to 1 L warm water. He made up a mixture of 3 L milk powder plus 1 egg plus 2 tablespoons of cod liver oil. George stated that five grown bucks (hobs) will drink 1 L of milk in 24 hours. George reckoned that the milk mixture alone would be sufficient to keep and rear ferrets. Feedmilk has a minimum crude protein of 25%, milk fat 25%, crude fibre nil, but lactose 29%. It contains also vitamins A, D_3, E, K, B_1, B_2, niacin, pantothenic acid, choline, chloride ferrous sulphate, zinc sulphate, cobalt sulphate, silicon dioxide and zinc bacterin (growth promoter). He also fed as an evening meal to each ferret a thumb-size piece of a Dog roll prepared by the local butcher and containing sheep liver, meat, spice, flour and crackling.

Bob Jeffares of Otorohanga had a basic diet for his ferrets of beef from local farmers' crippled cows.[25] His choice of feeding depended on what was seasonally available so that when rabbits were abundant, the ferrets got fed whole rabbit carcasses, that is a complete dead rabbit, unskinned, ungutted. Bob believed in getting all the natural nourishment and vitamins out of the rabbit for his ferret colony. With possums being trapped for fur, he feeds possum carcasses, skinned of course, but still not gutted. He only fed his ferrets shot or trapped possum carcasses rather than poisoned ones but suggested that it should be safe to feed poisoned possums if the head and feet are cut off so that no residual poison remains. Bob suggested rats and mice as ferret food, which is the natural diet of feral ferrets, stoats and weasels. Ferrets can of course earn their keep by eating vermin rats and mice. (Incidentally, mice are considered the best bait for trapping stray or feral ferrets.)

Bob also fed birds to his ferrets. They were best given whole when freshly killed and he also used bird offal including the head and feet. In the duck-shooting season, they provided food for the ferrets and he also culled geese and puketos for local farmers. Eggs are fed to ferrets without problems and he noticed that they usually eat the yolk and leave the white (which contains the biotin inhibitor) anyway. However, whole eggs raw, beaten up with milk and cereal added, cooked and allowed to cool are fed to ferrets, which love the concoction. Bob used goose or turkey eggs, when abundant, as medicines for sick or undernourished ferrets, which is an interesting point. Ferrets are not however fed fish except perhaps eel, which they seemed to enjoy, as otters do. Bob hunted feral goat and this was food for his dogs and ferrets on occasions, but he only fed the heart, liver and kidney offal to the ferrets. He sometimes fed horsemeat, after clearing the fat content, and the horsemeat was fed as part of a balanced diet. He commented that if he was forced to leave his ferrets with friends while he was away, he resorted to leaving tinned pet food for the ferret meals but they tended to avoid it if fresh meat was available! Milk is a stable part of his ferret diet as seen previously with George Symons. He usually fed bottled milk or powdered milk in preference to milk straight from the cow to avoid bacterial infections. Tuberculosis could be present in bovine milk and ferrets could thus become carriers of the disease. Feral ferrets are hunted because of the TB infection possibility but possums are the more likely carriers (Bob Jeffares, Kuiti, pers. comm. 1998).

Feral New Zealand ferrets

A survey of the food habits of feral ferrets has been recorded.[26] It has been found that they take a wide variety of prey and are also carrion-eaters and, through examination of ferret scats, that they eat mice, rats, rabbits, hares, opossums, hedgehogs, frogs, eels and possibly eggs and birds. There is some evidence of eating plants and insects but as ferrets are true carnivores this is probably part of the prey's digestive system. The type of prey eaten had a seasonal variation. The thought of ferrets being carrion-eaters would be a worry to me with pet or working animals where they might pick up infections. However, it might be that the ferret stores food away as a reflection of its ancestors being carrion-eaters in times of lack of food.

Pet ferrets in NZ had been fed high-grade Iams kitten food but then Totally Ferret® (T. Willard, USA) became a big part of the ferret nutrition market. With the reduction of pet ferrets due to the NZ ferret ban that market was lost (John Chessum, President Ferret PAWS, NZ, pers. comm. 1999).

Feeding British ferrets

Ferreters feeding working ferrets

In the UK, the feeding of working ferrets follows the ways of those in Australia and New Zealand, with the emphasis on fresh meat. It is suggested by one author that whole-carcass feeding of ferret colonies should be once or twice a week, with some other food for the rest of the week. Some sort of fresh meat should be fed every day and a balanced diet is of course essential.[27] Basic feeding of ferrets follows the native polecat ideal of an active carnivore diet. (A survey of what wild polecats consume showed that the stomach contents had 35–71% mammals, 6–14% birds, 9–14% amphibian and reptile, 0–14% fish and 0–24% invertebrate tissues present.)

The amount of food fed to individual ferrets or a ferret colony requires thought. Personally, as indicated previously, I feed my ferrets once or twice daily. One author agrees with that but then suggests little and often is better.[27] This idea may however add to the risk of ferrets storing food away like squirrels with possible contamination.

Feeding ferrets in a colony situation

The UK working ferret situation regarding stored excess food will depend no doubt on the amount fed and if the ferrets are fed individually or as a group. One author suggests a wide range of foods as described previously and adds that wild animals may contain intestinal worms, which is a good point.[27] It is noted that dead rats or mice may contain poison, which is a problem to working and pet ferrets that catch vermin. It is up to ferret owners and landowners where ferrets are used to avoid poisons and concentrate on the use of cats, Jack Russell terriers and ferrets to catch their vermin. It is suggested that laboratory animal culls be used as food but there are better sources of food for ferrets. As ferrets respond to small amounts of any chemical toxins, the risk should not be taken. Working ferrets are in the position to be offered many food types but ferreters should check any cattle or sheep livers, which have been condemned for human consumption as they may have liver fluke infection. No ferrets have been recorded as contracting liver flukes to date but there is always a future possibility with anything in the parasite world. Ferreters are advised to use a reliable licensed slaughter man when obtaining foods such as livers, brains, heart, kidneys and spleen. *Note* that contamination of slaughterhouse meat can occur in rare cases. Diseases such as the transmissible spongiform encephalopathies (TSEs), which have been seen in farmed mink, are still possible future dangers to ferrets.

Ferreters consider meat mince as a standby food. They consider however that vitamin and mineral supplementation milk, and commercial vitamin/mineral supplements, are good sources of nutrition and can be given to all ages of ferrets on a meat only diet without 'natural' food such as game. One suggestion is the Welpi milk supplement, which has 27% protein, 18% fat and a good range of vitamins and minerals (Stephanie Cole, pers. comm. 1999). Being easily able to get 'natural' food makes the difference to city-dwelling people who rely on the local butcher and supermarket.

The influence of mink nutrition on ideas about feeding ferrets

Dry foods are available for ferrets in the UK and again they were developed from mink diets in the early 1960s by the British mink industry. The diets had to be modified for ferret tastes. Research continues into mink and ferret food in America and Europe. There are still some 15 mink farms active in the UK but well below the 300 establishments at the height of mink production in the 1950s. Possible interest in the mink trade in the future has not been ruled out but is objected to in many quarters, with agitators releasing caged mink in 1998. The mink became feral and now compete for natural foods against native polecats, stoats, weasels and otters and could be a menace to working ferrets in some situations. The diet for mink has long been another base line for comparison with the feeding of ferrets. Fitch farms were set up using the feeding techniques of mink farms. The use of pelleted feed was basically one of ease of feeding numbers of animals efficiently.[28]

The basic diet for mink, for comparison with ferrets, is now composed of 80–90% fresh ingredients. Farmed mink in the UK and USA have similar diet ingredients, which would include horsemeat, beef liver, whole fish plus the usual foods procured by ferreters everywhere for their ferrets. This might include culled poultry, poultry by-products, fish scraps, cottage cheese and cooked eggs.[28] The fresh ingredients are mixed in a balanced form with a dry meal mix. The dry components include finely ground cereal grain, supplemented with liver or meat or fishmeal. The cereal ingredients are heated in some way because mink, like ferrets, cannot digest carbohydrates well. Being an animal reared for quick growth and fur production, unlike the average pet ferret, mink protein requirements are high compared with other mustelids. Table 4.9 indicates the nutrition and energy requirements for mink, in growth, maintenance, gestation and lactation phases. This can be compared with the nutritional requirements of ferret breeding, fitch farms or working/pet ferrets.

Regarding proteins in the diet, the important sulpha-amino acids, cysteine and methionine, are essential for fur-production animals like mink, just as a complete essential amino acid composition is important for other mustelids including ferrets. For mink, a common food energy guide is that the protein level be 10% above the fat level; thus a minimum of 35% crude protein to 25% fat on a dry matter basis. An after-weaning protein intake of 25% is recommended by the USA National Research Council. However, most diets contain 35–40% protein with 20–25% fat and 25–35% carbohydrate. The carbohydrate is thus very high for rapid animal growth compared with ferret diets.

The various phases of mink development require special nutritional features as for ferrets:

1. Breeding and reproduction requires a lean high-protein diet with cooked eggs, liver and muscle meats.
2. Lactation and early growth sees higher levels of protein added to the high caloric density diet.
3. Late growth period needs diet with 20% fortified cereal addition plus 25% fat and 35–37% protein (on dry matter basis).
4. In the fur production stage, fat content is reduced to 20–22% while lean meats are increased.

The calcium/phosphorus requirements are met by using 35–40% bone-containing products and this is important in ferret rearing in the kitten stage. *Note*: mink farmers give extra salt (0.5% NaCl) for nursing jills to help prevent nursing anaemia due possibly to dehydration factors.

It is considered that vitamin improvement of the mink diet is not required if the ingredients are of high quality and if fresh liver is added. The actual amount of food fed to mink is ad lib but restriction on quantity occurs during the mating season to keep adults trim and fit. *Note*: mink have one mating season like polecats, while ferrets have two seasons or perhaps three in

CHAPTER FOUR
Nutrition

Table 4.9 Nutrition and energy requirements for mink, (%) or amount per kg dry matter

Constituent	Growth Weaning to 13 weeks	Growth 13 weeks to maturity	Maintenance (mature)	Gestation	Lactation
Energy					
Males (kcal ME)[a]	4080	4080	3600		
Females (kcal ME)	3930	3930	3600	3930	4500
Crude protein (%)	38[b]	32.6–38.0	21.8–26.0	38	45.7
Fat-soluble vitamins					
Vitamin A (IU)	5930	c	c	c	c
Vitamin E (mg)	27	c	c	c	c
Water-soluble vitamins					
Thiamine (mg)	1.3	c	c	c	c
Riboflavin (mg)	1.6	c	c	c	c
Pantothenic acid (mg)	8.0	c	c	c	c
Vitamin B_6 (mg)	1.6	c	c	c	c
Niacin (mg)	20.0	c	c	c	c
Folic acid (mg)	0.5[d]	c	c	c	c
Biotin (mg)	0.12	c	c	c	c
Vitamin B_{12} (µg)	32.6	c	c	c	c
Minerals					
Calcium (%)	0.4	0.4	0.3	0.4	0.6
Phosphorus (%)	0.4	0.4	0.3	0.4	0.6
Ca:P ratio	1:1–2:1	1:1–2:1	1:1–2:1	1:1–2:1	1:1–2:1
Salt (%)	0.5	0.5	0.5	0.5	0.5

[a]E, gross energy; ME, metabolizable energy.
Nutrient requirements are based on an energy level of 5300 kcal E or 4080 kcal ME.
Nutrient requirements increase with higher ME levels and decrease with lower ME levels.
[b]Based on average quality protein with calculated digestibility of 83%.
Higher quality protein and higher digestibility decrease the requirement; lower quality protein and lower digestibility increase the requirement.
[c]Quantitative requirements of minerals and vitamins not determined but dietary need demonstrated.
[d]May not be minimum but known to be adequate.
(Table from *The Merck Veterinary Manual*, 8th edn. Copyright 1998, by MERCK & Co. Inc., Whitehouse Station, NJ, USA. All rights reserved. Used with permission.)

commercial breeding farms where the photo-periods can be manipulated. Care must be taken that for the hob mink, the diet is not too restrictive because of their relatively large size and the need to be sexually active. This could equally apply to hob breeding ferrets. Mink farmers consider the jill's lactation period and early growth of the kittens to be nutritionally critical as it would be for ferrets. It is stated that a poor diet at this time would affect the females' health and the kittens' survival and growth.

With jill ferrets, a good quality meat/vitamin/mineral diet is required, like mink. Mink farmers will feed twice or even three times daily during the critical pregnancy and kitten growth period. I tend to feed lactating jill ferrets once or twice daily but allow access to plenty of supplement drink in between with no adverse effects. Thus, helpful advice can be picked up from information on feeding mink for comparison to ferret feeding, bearing in mind that in pregnancy ferrets are confined just as much as mink.

Commercial ferret dry foods in the UK

The UK also has its own brand of dry ferret food, Ferret Complete; produced by James Wellbeloved Company of Yeovil, Somerset in 1994. It is a balanced ferret food with ingredients similar to the Australian Ferret's Choice.

Ferret Complete

The food includes poultry meat meal, ground whole wheat, soya oil, blood meal, chicken digest, herring meal, poultry fat, sugar beet pulp, ground whole linseed, natural potato protein, vitamins and minerals, extract of yucca, preserved with antioxidants natural vitamin E and vitamin C. The dry food has a typical analysis of: protein 36%, oil 19%, fibre 2%, ash 8.8%, vitamins (IU/kg) vitamin A 20 000, vitamin D_3 1500, vitamin E (α-tocopherol acetate) 200, copper (cupric sulphate) 15 mg/kg. *Note*: fibre 2% as Willard recommends.

Feeding guidelines

Ferret kittens from 3 weeks of age

Small amounts of food are soaked till soft in warm water or broth, then gradually decreasing liquid content. Uneaten damp food is replaced by fresh after a few hours. From 4 weeks of age, it is suggested offering only dry food. I would rear 4-week-old kittens with mincemeat soaked with a lactose-free milk as a way of ensuring they get enough calcium.

Ferrets up to 16 weeks of age

I suggest free-feed and allowing ferrets to clean out the bowls every 2 or 3 days to maintain food freshness. At this age, the daily food consumption of the ferrets should be ~7% of body weight (e.g. ~35 g of food for a 500 g ferret).

Adult ferrets

Free ad lib feeding is suggested but to restrict the diet to ~5% of body weight if the ferrets get too heavy (~75 g of food for a 1500 g ferret). For the final 2 weeks of gestation and lactation, free-feeding is suggested without restriction.

Ferret Complete feeding trial

A survey was carried out by James McKay, Director of the UK National Ferret School, using a long-term trial (J. McKay, pers. comm. 1998). The trial was between feeding groups of ferrets: Ferret Complete only; fresh meat only; and a combination of the two. The result was positive for Ferret Complete, linked to the growth of healthy kittens growing into healthy adults.

In an update, James McKay still feeds Ferret Complete to his 103 ferrets and finds litters are good but there is a build up of dental detritus, which he considers no problem with his ferrets, unlike show ferrets where they would be marked down for 'dirty' teeth (J. McKay, pers. comm. 2005). Considering other commercial 'complete diets' for ferrets, he considers they are less than 'complete' and not really 'balanced'. Interestingly, he notes that some ferret owners/breeders are feeding complete foods during the summer but reverting to feeding carcasses during the rabbiting season of autumn and winter. Apparently, some ferret owners consider 'ferret' food as cat food which has been labelled differently! Food for thought!

In addition, some owners of working ferrets consider 'city' pet ferrets no longer 'real' ferrets. Shades of genetics? City pet ferret owners think working ferrets get poor attention and feed their ferrets dry food more

UK clinical example

An interesting case of aberrant behaviour by a sterilized albino hob, Ryan, from a rescue home, occurred in the UK. The ferret was at first very playful and loveable in a new home. Then the son, who owned him, took Ryan away from home when he went to college. After several months away, Ryan became nippy and unsociable and actually began biting people. He was returned to the ferret shelter, where it was obvious Ryan's demeanour had changed and he was very tense, agitated and refused to play or eat ferret food. He would pace his cage and became unmanageable.

A psychologist, interested in ferrets, was asked to assess Ryan's behaviour as a last resort, before he was taken to be euthanized. Observing Ryan, it became apparent that he was interested in eating anything but normal ferret food! He went crazy over trying to get at some chocolate in a bag and was hissing, squealing and trying to bite when someone tried to take it from him. Then it became clear that while Ryan was away with the college boy, he had eaten, and drunk, practically what a student would: burgers, take-away, sweets, soft drinks, etc. Someone said the ferret reminded them of a dog they knew with hyperactivity, dislike of normal food, anxious and desperate behaviour to get into food cupboards for sweet biscuits, sweets, etc.

The psychologist then realized similarities with children with hyperactivity problems associated with eating patterns. Ryan was a ferret junk food addict! It was laughable but he had to go through a de-tox period to get him back onto normal ferret food, which he did, and became again a loving playful pet ferret.[29]

regularly than worker ferrets. Who is winning in the best nutrition stakes?

Other complete ferret dry foods in the UK include Frankie Ferret (Supreme Foods) and Vitalin (Vitalin Pet Foods). The first indicates it contains high poultry meat levels, essential protein 36%, vitamins, minerals plus taurine, while the second has over 40% meat, fresh chicken and chicken meat meal, high levels of omega-3 fatty acids and prebiotic FOS (fructooligosaccharides) plus whole cooked rice considered a good source of natural carbohydrate. Ferrets should get their energy levels from the fat in food. Carbohydrate in the form of cooked rice might be acceptable if fat level is low, as long as pet ferrets do not get 'sweet extras'. Beware insulinoma!

Feeding laboratory ferrets in the UK

The feeding of laboratory ferrets has been changed over the years from fresh meat diets to pelleted foods similar to Marshall Farms and other breeding establishment feeding programmers. In 1965, ferrets were fed 4 oz raw meat (horse flesh, lights, etc.) with 4 oz fresh milk daily.[14] In 1967, the ideal ferret diet was still considered raw horseflesh and milk daily and a meaty rib bone once weekly for 'dental and gingival friction for the prevention of tartar formation in the carnassial region'.[30] The daily meat and milk was given at 4 oz (113 g) and 3 oz (85 g), respectively, with the meat allowance being reduced to 2 oz (56 g) in the non-mating period. No supplements were given of any kind for the growth and reproduction periods. The cost of horsemeat became a factor. The use of horse blood and milk combinations was not satisfactory for weaning ferrets. The use of fish and milk obtained a good rate of growth but was not used on a large scale because of the offensive fish smell. Attempts to have ferrets eat rat or mouse laboratory cubes failed except when the food cubes were softened in warm water.

The then Medical Research Council experimented with a 'Diet 41', which was used in combination with various quantities of meat and/or protein substitute. The Diet 41 in powder form was mixed mechanically with water into a porridge and finely minced meat was added. This was given to laboratory ferrets in court dwellings in the morning and milk was given in the afternoon with water always available.[30] Diet 41 is shown in Table 4.10.

It is interesting that the elimination of the meat from the above diet evidently resulted in a considerable reduction in growth rate and was not recommended. The use of day-old chicks as food for six generations of ferrets evidently produced no signs of dietary deficiency, and was put forward as a possible diet for laboratory ferrets. (In Russia, mink farms were run in association with chick hatcheries for use of waste chicks.) The use of Diet 41 can be compared with my feeding of ferrets normally and also when feeding pregnant and lactating jills (see Ch. 5). My basic diet for mature ferrets has been noted at 40–60 g meat for jills and 60–80 g for hobs, with or without daily milk and variable to the season's wants.

Dr John Hammond, Jr. in 1974 suggested that pelleted diets were convenient and hygienic for laboratory animals.[30] He used pig weaning pellets with 23% protein, 7.5% fat and 1.5% fibre for a large ferret colony. (Fibre again is in the safe range advocated by Willard.) He also tried a laboratory diet for rodents containing 21.3% protein, 3.4% fat and 2.2% fibre. Both diets comprised mixed cereals with fishmeal, added fat plus vitamin/mineral supplement. He included powdered milk and antibiotics. He avoided products that contained copper, which is a growth stimulant for pigs and cautioned against the use of fish meal products for ferret feeding if the fish were herring. The latter are preserved in nitrates, which during the pelleting process might give rise to carcinogens and thus possible cancers in ferrets. (*Note*: Ferret Complete does contain herring meal.)

Andrews and IIman[31] state that commercial dried dog and cat foods have been fed to ferrets mixed with minced beef. Those tried included Sunlight Dog Crumbles, Spratts dog diet, Friskies and Miao Meal Cat Chow, Purina. They point out that bones can be added to the diet (to help teeth-cleaning) and especially if the ferrets are wholly fed on dog food, which in the UK appears to be widely used. It is also stated that various minced meat foods are used for laboratory ferrets and one diet includes a mixture of a high percentage of fish, 30%, along with chicken 20%, plus tripe 15%, lung 10% and liver 5%. The amount of food eaten by ferrets using various diets is tabulated by Andrew and Illman so the g/day can be compared with feeding pet and working ferrets as in Table 4.11.

An interesting statement is made by Andrew and Illman, that: 'It should be borne in mind that, in the laboratory, ferrets (males in particular) are particularly prone to obesity and it may therefore be unwise to allow the animals free access to highly calorific foods'.[31] I concur.

Table 4.10 Composition of diet

Component	(oz)	(g)
Diet 41	1½–2	42–56
Horse flesh	½	14
Milk	1	28

Table 4.11 Examples of various diets tried out on laboratory ferrets in the UK

Body weight (g)	Sex	Diet	Food intake (g)	Comments	Source
1507 ± 67	3 M	Tinned dog food	42 ± 15	Milk supplement	Andrews and Illman[31]
713 ± 126	3 F	Tinned dog food	47 ± 5.2	Milk supplement	Andrews and Illman[31]
1060 ± 60	8 M	Dead rat	60.5 ± 6	Milk supplement	Andrews and Illman[31]
590 ± 30	8 F	Dead rat	37.5 ± 5	Milk supplement	Andrews and Illman[31]
975	2 M	Purina cat chow	60–70	Eaten over 7–8 meals	Kaufman 1980[a]
1923 ± 95.2	6 M	Mink cereal with chicken, fish and offal 66.2% H_2O	236.2 ± 10.14	Free access to food	Bleavins and Aulerich 1981[b]
791 ± 35.5	6 F	Mink cereal with chicken, fish and offal 66.2% H_2O	115.4 ± 9.19	Free access to food	Bleavins and Aulerich 1981[b]

Table from Andrews and Illman, with permission.[31] [a]Kaufman LW. Foraging cost and meal patterns in ferrets. Physiology and Behavior 1980; 25:139–141. [b]Bleavins MR, Aulerich RJ. Feed consumption and food passage time in mink (Mustel vison) and European ferrets (*Mustela putorius furo*). Lab Anim Sci 1981; 31:268.

It has been commented in the UK that 'dry pelleted carnivore diet should be fed, soaked in hot water to form a paste, for pet ferrets'.[32] I could not disagree more! Surely healthy ferrets require a more solid diet? Why not put them on baby food? I can see a certain Tom Lonsdale grinding his teeth if this proposal was put for cat and dog feeding.

Feeding ferrets elsewhere

In Hungary, a comparison of three different commercial diets was carried out with cats and ferrets, apparently to see if ferrets could be used for laboratory trials on cat food rather than cats.[33] Diet preferences and digestibility studies were done using 10 cats and 10 ferrets. The results showed that ferrets were not suitable for cat nutrition trials.

In Russia, about 50% of ferret owners feed self-made diets based on natural products such as meat, eggs, by-products, sometimes fish and supplements. A further 25% use Hills kitten food or Iams kitten food. Some people actually use laboratory mice, rats or chickens. Unfortunately, some persist in feeding unsuitable food such as cheap cat food, dog food, sausage, potatoes, etc. The Russian Ferret Society recommends feeding premium kitten food as good commercial ferret food is very rare in Russia (Dmitry Kalinin, pers. comm. 2005).

Italian ferret owners at the moment feed dry cat or ferret food plus some table food treats such as banana, raisins, apple, or bread (Alessandro Melillo, pers. comm. 2005).

In Belgium, most people with ferrets feed kibble, usually low-quality ferret kibble or cat kibbles from the supermarket or even dog kibble. More 'ferret educated' owners feed Willard's Totally Ferret®, USA, Eukanuba kitten and Hills kitten foods. Recently, ferret owners have started to gain an interest in raw meat feeding and prey feeding (mostly mice and day-old chicks). A commercial frozen food, Carnibest, specific for ferrets can be delivered. My contact feeds her ferrets Innova cat kibble ad lib plus chicken gravy and Carnibest.

The feeding of ferrets in the Netherlands tends to be commercial American cat food lines with Totally Ferret®, Eukanuba kitten, Hills kitten food and Carnbest being advertised (Wendy Van den Steen, pers. comm. 2005).

In Germany, pet ferrets are fed the meat of chicken, turkey or cow (Gisela Henke, pers. comm. 2005).

In Japan, ferret owners use imported ferret foods and Japanese original commercial ferret foods and do not seem to feed a raw meat diet as yet (Yasutsugu Miwa, pers. comm. 2005).

There is a need to improve diet knowledge in many countries.

Which pet food is the best?

This is a broad question on diet which intrigues pet ferret owners as does the question of good dog and cat foods. There has been growing concern about the additions to pet food that might, over the long period, constitute a danger to the health of dogs and cats. Many voices have spoken up about animal diets.[2,10,18,34,35]

A Japanese contact informs me of a possible food allergy in a male castrate angora ferret which had clinical signs of cough, vomiting, diarrhoea, mesenteric

CHAPTER FOUR
Nutrition

lymph node swelling and redness, swelling and skin itch over a 2-year period. It was on Marshall ferret food but the clinical signs improved on changing to Totally Ferret® food plus low dose of prednisolone (Yasutsugu Miwa, pers. comm. 2005).

A Canadian contact has been researching the North American pet food industry since 1990 and has been shocked to learn that it is virtually unregulated. Anything is fair game as far as the ingredients used in pet products. The bottom line is that as long as the food contains all the nutrients required for pets, the source does not matter. She considers there has been a much higher death rate in pets since the inception of the industry. She prefers to feed her pets on lightly cooked meats in homemade diets (S. Martin, pers. comm. 2003). I am one of those who support the notion of feeding ferrets uncooked fresh meat. In fact I have always used meat 'for human consumption' for my pet ferrets.

At the time of writing, my ferrets, Pip (male) and Squeak (female) get, respectively 60–80 g and 40–60 g meat/day as a basic. Meat includes fatty lamb and ox hearts, chicken wings, chicken necks and carcass and weekly eggs. Incidentally, ox heart is tough compared with sheep's and good for teeth cleaning. Apart from the egg meal, the ferrets are fed separately. (Feeding for pregnancy is another story and is discussed in Chapter 5.) Their coats are good, they maintain weight, are active in play and foraging around the garden.

The human food and agricultural industries still use the pet food industry to offload offal, grains, etc. considered unusable for human consumption.[34] According to Lonsdale, there are 165 and 147 common ingredients, respectively for dog and cat food that are listed by the US National Research Council.[18] If ferrets are fed cat food, as is often advocated, the digestibility of these ingredients is important. We have seen previously, the Hungarian trials with ferrets and cats on preference of commercial foods. Grain has increased dramatically in pet food, not just as a filler but for replacing a high percentage of meat.[34] The digestibility of grain regulates the amount of nutrients the animal receives from the food. Ferrets cannot digest grain products easily and this grain fibre food is usually useless and may be dangerous. Ferrets are not rabbits.

Knowing ferrets require high protein, high fat, low carbohydrate and low fibre, what use are these foods to them? Even dogs do not have a great need for carbohydrates, nor cats; as we know the latter are obligate carnivores like ferrets. In fact, all three species do not have high enough levels of digestive enzymes to deal with a high starch meal.[18]

It is pointed out that there is little information on the bioavailability of nutrients for pet animals in pet food ingredients.[34] The Association of American Feed Control Officials (AAFCO) maintain the nutritional factors of pet food at a certain level. There is concern that an analysis of the real bioavailability values of the ingredients within the tin or packet may differ – is it what it says?

The pet food value is the biological rating (index) of protein.[35] The food composition of amino acids is important. Examples can be given: egg has the top value, rated 100, then fishmeal 92, beef and milk 78, rice 75, soybean 68, yeast 63, wheat gluten 40 and so on. From this follows digestibility, which is how the intestine can manage the food type.

In pet food, the term 'meal' refers to the fact that the meat and poultry by-products of human food preparation are not fresh and need to be rendered by heating, whereby fat-soluble material is separated from water-soluble material while the bacterial load is destroyed. In the process, natural enzymes and proteins found in raw ingredients are destroyed and need to be replaced. The plant protein of the meal suffers and is further degraded, yet is still put as part of the total percentage protein on the label.[18]

Dry pet food is made where raw materials are blended to nutritional formulae, fed into an 'expander' and, under steam, pressure, and high temperature, a type of 'popcorn' process occurs. Ingredients of the wet, dry or semi-moist food types are similar, however the protein, fat and fibre may be different.[34] An example is shown in Table 4.2. Bacterial contamination, however, can occur during the drying or when the food is fat sprayed for palatability.

Wet pet food is prepared from ingredients and additives and is canned after cooking. The cans are sterilized in special sterilization units. In some cases, the food can be cooked directly in the can. One of the rules of the AAFCO is that the ingredient, or collection of ingredients, animals, poultry or fish, must be 95% meat. All ingredients in the can should have equal notice on the label of the contents. The ingredients then must at least constitute 70% of the product. It asserts that all-meat diets are considered unbalanced nutritionally. The 'flavour' product of the food must be detectable by a test method and again registered on the label to show source.[34] Judith Bell noted earlier what is recorded on the label is sometimes lacking in detail. It was suggested that processing is simply ignored in nutritional terms. That is the heating, cooking, rendering, freezing, dehydrating, canning, extruding, pelleting, baking and so forth. This was suggested by a USA vet with his own pet-food line.[34]

Food manufacturers are prone to add soy meal to make up the deficiency but this substance causes diarrhoea and flatulence. Soy meal also has phytin, which reacts with calcium and takes the latter out of use. This immediately upsets the calcium balance in the body. The animal protein in the 'meal' could include items as shown in the New Zealand fitch farming nutrition. In fact, although many good types of meat would be acceptable for the carnivore diet, pet food manufacturers use, e.g. abattoir blood, livers, udders and cattle lips.[18]

Fat is the energy source in ferrets, but in general pet food fat is subjected to the same sort of abuse as is protein. Lonsdale notes that wild rabbits are never fat animals. Ferrets do lay down fat for the winter like their wild polecat ancestors. Rabbit meat would contain some fat up to 6.6%. Water would be 71.1% and protein 20.8% (fat would be 22.8% dry weight). Comparing samples of dog and cat food types he illustrates that in two of four cat diets and three of four dog diets the fat levels are well below that of rabbit meat. Fat comes as saturated, monounsaturated or polyunsaturated (i.e. relating to hydrogen/carbon chains).

It has been noted that polyunsaturated fats in high doses can cause disease in NZ fitch farm ferrets and problems have been noted in cats on such diets. The unsaturated fats are easier to digest but fat content of general pet food is reduced by many factors including the initial rendering in production, storage and exposure of food to air whereby oxidation and fat degeneration occurs. The odour from an opened bag of pet food could be rendered animal fat, restaurant grease, etc., which being rancid and not suitable for humans, is passed on to pet foods. Apparently, restaurant grease (in the USA) has become a major component of feed-grade animal fat. The discarded fats are mixed together and stabilized with powerful antioxidants to stop further spoilage and are used to spray over dry kibble or extruded pellet animal foods to add a 'come and eat me' flavour to the product.[34]

With regard to additives in pet food, Lonsdale uses the word 'digest', which represents the result of the fermentation of chicken offal, etc. to use as a flavour and stimulant to palatability. Having worked some time in a poultry laboratory, I know coccidiostatic drugs, etc. can be added to chicken feed. They can remain in the gut. Evidently, cat paralysis which occurred in the Netherlands and Switzerland in 1996, traced back to poultry guts in commercial cat food.[18]

The procedure of feeding pet ferrets in the USA and elsewhere by constant hopper feeding, as with indoor reared chickens and pigs, follows the method of feeding USA laboratory ferrets. I have quoted the old UK laboratory basic ferret diet and feeding. It might have been with USA laboratory ferrets that a constant food supply all day was meant to indicate the animals were well treated. Those using laboratory ferrets might say that the weight and health of the ferrets must remain standard at all times.

The presence of high fibre content in the colon sets up a wet nutrient-rich base for bacterial multiplication which goes into overdrive giving rise to possible diarrhoea, constipation, infections, liver damage, cancer and encephalopathy – in humans. Are some of these symptoms seen in ferrets on commercial cat food even now? Food companies attempt to reverse these signs by using factors in the diet which bind with bacterial toxins, such as fructooligosaccharides, derived from onions, garlic, etc.

High fibre diets have affected dogs and cats and no doubt would affect ferrets and should be avoided. However, one author states that a few of his ferret patients with chronic diarrhoea have improved on higher fibre diet formulae like Hill's Prescription Diet w/d. He suggests the results are because the fibre stimulates gut motility, improves stool firmness and also tends to inhibit bacterial overgrowth (Burgess, pers. comm. 2005).

Note that high fibre and phosphorus-based chemicals can affect mineral absorption to the extent that calcium and trace elements are omitted. Adding extra calcium to the pet food results in the calcium in high levels further inhibiting zinc, copper, iron and iodine uptake. Thus, serious metabolic diseases can arise and no doubt could happen one time in pet ferrets.[18]

It is considered by some that slaughterhouse waste fed to pets increases the risk of cancers and other degenerative diseases.[34] Moreover, there is a worry that pet food manufacturers' methods of heat and pressure do not actually destroy the hormones given to livestock to fatten or increase milk production. These substances, along with antibiotics, could pass to pets.

Note: European dogs are fed a more natural diet and are considered to be healthier than American dogs.[35]

The accurate quota and stability of vitamins and minerals in food is important. Pet-food makers tend to ensure sufficiency by oversupply. There is immediate concern for selenium, which can be highly toxic and evidently, the difference between the toxic dose and that recommended can be narrow (Table 4.2). It is considered by Lonsdale that there is a narrow borderland between insufficiencies and excess in the average pet, which is alarming. He notes the situation can be acute in growing, pregnant and lactating animals plus working and racing animals. This could all reflect on ferrets, pet and working. He is of the opinion that artificial feeding of pets can bring on the problems of oversupply of vitamins and minerals. Animals on natural foods would not be at risk.

One mineral of extreme importance in animal health is sodium chloride (salt). It must be in balance within the living body cells. Naturally, salt is obtained from water and prey.[18] Carnivores do not get salt-craving unlike herbivores on poor salt-deficient vegetation. Salt at about 0.4 % (dry matter basis) in fresh herbivore meat is the optimum for all pet carnivores. Salt is added to dry food as another way to make it palatable; high levels of 1% or more have been seen on dry cat/dog food labels, thus the request for standby fresh water on the label! My ferrets on fresh meat rarely drink water in their cages when feeding. They get water from the food and never have dry ferret foods.

High blood pressure is apparently a factor of salt toxicity with humans where the heart, kidneys, brain and eyes are affected. Possibly likewise with animals? Treatment of pets with diarrhoea or kidney disease would be feeding raw meaty bones. It might be important to have a salty water bowl with a fresh water bowl, as the salt requirements of sick animals will vary.

Additives and preservatives

Other considerations of feeding ferrets are possible additives and preservatives in pet food (Table A.14). Could they be damaging to health? In the Pet Food (FAIR) report it is stated that chemicals may be added to improve the taste, stability and characteristic of the particular pet food, tinned or biscuit.[34] These additions have no nutritional use, they are supposed to improve the palatability of the food and make it more attractive to the buyer.

Note that preservatives that liberate sulphur dioxide and sodium sulphite have been incriminated in causing thiamine deficiency in dogs and cats by researchers in 2005.[22,23] The sulphur dioxide rapidly inactivates thiamine present in normal meat and meat byproducts; pet meat/mince has been a risk. Sulphites in particular have been involved with food intolerance in humans with symptoms such as headaches, irritable bowel action, behaviour disturbances, skin rashes and asthma attacks.[36] Could a possible equivalent occur in pet ferrets? Food additives are not a new concept, being started in ancient times with the use of spices, etc. Preservatives may be added by the supplier of the raw materials or by the pet food manufacturer. Synthetic preservatives like butylated hydroxyanisole (BHA) and butylated hydroxytoluene (BHT), propyl gallate, propylene glycol and ethoxyquin have been added to dry food to make it last in prolonged storage and to preserve fat content.[4] Dogs have been made sick by propylene glycol, which also affects red blood cells in kittens (*Note*: propylene glycol has been used as a solvent for Ivermectin in ferret heartworm prevention medicine. Corn oil can be substituted.) Other preservatives in pet food can be potassium sorbate and sodium nitrite, also ammonium glycyrrhizin and sucrose are used as sweeteners.[35] The long time build-up of such compounds as BHA, BHT and ethoxyquin, possible cancer-causing agents, have not been studied in pet foods so that long-term effects may be harmful.

Lonsdale records that in 1986, ethoxyquin, accidentally given to laboratory marmosets at 10 times the usual rate for 5 days, caused deaths almost immediately. The deaths continued for 3 weeks. In 1997, the manufacturer Monsanto was required by the USA FDA to reduce ethoxyquin in its dog food by half (to 75 parts per million), due to concerns that ethoxyquin had caused skin problems and infertility in dogs. *Note* that in cats, ethoxyquin has never been tested for safety. Lonsdale is of the opinion that the substance is unsafe and should not be added to pet foods. Willard Performance Foods, USA, considers it to be the most efficacious and safest antioxidant used in feeds but it now has to be replaced. Some pet food manufacturers have shown concern for the problems and now use 'natural' preservatives, e.g. vitamins C, E, lecithin, citric acid and oils of rosemary, cloves, etc., to preserve fat in the foods.

Chemical preservatives are found in fishmeal and some vitamin mixtures are added to kill or inhibit bacteria. Unfortunately, the same substances in the animal cells can be toxic, mutagenic or carcinogenic to some degree. In 1997, the World Cancer Research Fund was adamant that preservatives were safe in human foods; nothing was said about pet foods.[18] It is considered that additives produce an acidic pet food, which could have an irritating effect on teeth and the gastrointestinal tract – yet another reason for bowel irritation in pet ferrets on dry foods? A pet may be eating food containing several types of preservatives, which are not disclosed on the label. *Note* that natural preservatives do not have the shelf life of chemical preservatives but are less likely to cause harm in pet groups.

Coal tar derivative dyes can be used for food colouring[35] and of six indicated, Red No. 40 is possibly carcinogenic and Blue No. 2 has been shown to increase, in the dog at least, a sensitivity to fatal viruses. Thankfully, in the 1970s, similar dyes were banned from both pet and human food. Red No. 2 for instance increased neoplasia and birth defects, while Violet No. 1 was carcinogenic for the skin. Lonsdale notes that rats fed on a high oral dose of the dye erythrosine, which reddens food, develop thyroid neoplasia. In food, erythrosine binds iodine, which is then not available to the animal for use.

Reputable pet-food makers do have feeding trials to back up their label claims of a 'complete and balanced' food. It is not possible to compare labels from different companies unless tests are done on a 'dry matter basis'.[34] It is thought that the quality of ingredients of pet foods is variable so that manufacturers have to add vitamins and minerals to make the product nutritious.

Note: bacteria can contaminate slaughtered animal meat sources. The animal could have died of disease or injury besides natural causes and they are wide open for infections of *Salmonella* or *E. coli* organisms. This contamination could be in up to 50% of meat meals. Heat processing destroys the bacteria but not the endotoxins released when the organism die. This is not tested for. Does heat affect the nutritive value?

Grains such as wheat and corn plus cottonseed meal, peanut meal and fishmeal can be affected by mycotoxins. It is suggested that poor drying procedures and storage is a factor. In 1995, the dog food Nature's Recipe was withdrawn as numerous dogs had been having vomiting fits and loss of appetite.[34] The problem was a toxic fungus, which had contaminated the wheat. The most dangerous fungi (producing mycotoxins) can cause weight loss, liver damage, lameness and possible deaths and this scenario can easily be missed in the odd sick ferret which dies of unspecified causes, if the food is not suspect. (I have given an example previously of three ferrets becoming sick on dog food.)

The National Research Council (NRC) required feeding trials for claims of 'complete' or 'balanced' foods. The pet industry found the idea expensive and restrictive so they set up expert committees for canine and feline nutrition, not any consideration for ferrets, using chemical analysis instead of any feeding trials in early 1990s. However, chemical analysis does not consider palatability, digestibility or the biological availability of nutrients in the food. The AAFCO added a 'safety factor', whereby they exceeded the minimum amount of the required nutrients. It follows that the food label had no indication of digestibility or availability of nutrients data.

It is considered a myth that there is one pet food, which will provide a companion animal, dog, cat and probably ferret, with everything for its entire life.[34]

Summary of possible food additive reactions

With regard to dogs and cats the cereal grains are increased in foods and they eat a primarily carbohydrate diet, which would be no value to ferrets. Of course, dogs are omnivores and cats are supposed to be obligate carnivores, like ferrets. Problems have occurred in dogs and cats such as chronic vomiting, digestive problems, diarrhoea and inflammatory bowel disease (IBD). IBD appears chronic in ferrets in the USA, possibly due to dry ferret foods? (see Ch. 9).

Dental disease is an important topic regarding dog, cat and ferret eating habits. With regard to the latter species, Bob Church gives an interesting survey of ferret dental conditions and possible ramifications of eating commercial pet foods, in Chapter 21.

There is also the question of allergy or hypersensitivity to dog and cat foods in the form of diarrhoea and vomiting. The suggestion that dry commercial pet food could carry bacteria and yeasts has been stated.

Interestingly, feeding only one dry food meal a day possibly causes oesophagus irritation via stomach acid regurgitation. Thus, two meals are suggested![34] Can this be extrapolated to ferret feeding?

Remember the lack of taurine in the food has led to fatal cardiac disease in cats and some dogs. Lack of taurine can lead to ferret blindness (Ch. 12). These alarms have led to taurine being added to cat foods but not yet dog food. Not a problem with ferrets on a fresh meat diet with fresh hearts, etc.

We are all aware of the problem of rapid growth of large breed puppies from ingesting excessive calories from manufactured puppy foods. The formula was to promote rapid growth but seemed to be at the expense of bone strength. On a small scale, I fell into the trap, in 1977, of overfeeding and had troubles with ferret kitten lack of mobility and skeletal problems with my first attempt of mating my sable jill, Wendy, with albino hob, Peter Pan. It was a double disaster as it was an unwanted mating between littermates! It resulted in overweight kittens, which could not get up. This led to my concepts on feeding ferrets, especially breeding stock, as will be described in Chapter 5.

It is stated that in the 1970s, in cats, hyperthyroidism resulted from commercial canned food diets.[34] The disease is dangerous, treatment is expensive and usually life-threatening. The cause of the disease is not yet known.

Note that rice- and chicken-based foods have high protein levels of 34% but low fat levels at 13%, which is unsuitable for ferrets. Thus, there is still some concern about commercial pet foods.

Special foods for allergy-prone pets

Hill's Pet Nutrition Company has a low allergen food 'Feline z/d' made for cats with food allergies. Many other cat/dog prescription diets are on the market now to combat deficiency and/or allergy problems.[35] Do we need such diets? Willard is adamant that dog and cat foods should not be fed to ferrets and I agree. Could it be said, as Lonsdale has indicated, that we have been directed into a corner with an array of commercial diets, while ignoring natural foods? Will we need future prescription diets for ferrets? I would avoid the situation completely by feeding a fresh meat diet – figuratively from my own plate!

Critical disagreements on diet

The bone and raw meat food diet is not without its critics (D. Kemmer-Contrell, pers. comm. 2005). It has been found by one Canadian study that 30% of the stools of animals eating these diets contain *Salmonella*. Repeating, personally I feed fresh meat for human consumption to my ferrets and avoid such infections. Of course, with dogs and cats that would be a lot of *Salmonella* going into the soil and ground water. With bone and raw meat diets there are concerns of imbalances with several minerals in dogs and cats. Parathyroid disease causes an increase in blood urea nitrogen (BUN), which measures kidney function, and pitted tooth enamel, which may be due to calcium imbalances. Cervical spondylosis, an abnormal development of the cervical spine leading to walking problems, and neurological tremors have been seen on diets which do not contain choline or acetylcholine. There is even a worry about spontaneous abortions on the diet.

As regards the ethoxyquin controversy, it has been found to be a potent antioxidant; it prevents liver cancer in rats at high levels which contradicts Lonsdale's findings of toxicity and supports Willard's ideas.

Conclusions

The veterinarian confronted with requests for advice on the feeding of ferrets in various situations can see from the foregoing that a lot of work has been done on mustelid nutrition regarding ferrets and mink. The balance of opinion will swing between the natural 'prey' meat diet and the prepared dry 'convenience' diets. The high quality dry ferret diets will be advocated for being easy to give and good for teeth. Natural meat diets of good quality protein will maintain ferrets equally for pet, working and breeding colonies. The use of a fresh meaty bone diet for dogs and cats has been advocated for the prevention of periodontal disease and this concept could well be applied to feeding ferrets.[18] However, they need to be started as kittens to a diet and are difficult to change.

The bottom line is that ferrets are carnivores and I would personally advise feeding ferrets on as natural a diet as possible, having used fresh meat diets over the years. Yes, they do require making up and that is why a dry food 'instant' meal might seem more attractive. Yes, they require eating at the time but they can be refrigerated if not eaten and given later.

The early experience of some veterinarians in the USA was that they were seeing problems in the long run on prepared diets (S. Brown, pers. comm. 1995). These were postulated at the time to be from the fibre content of prepared foods, carbohydrate excess and chemical inclusions of some kind plus stress on the renal system over time. Now reports express concern on general pet foods.[18,34,35] It may be thought that mink, fitch ferrets and ferrets in biomedical research are not expected to live a long life, as would be working and pet ferrets, and perhaps long-term effects of nutrition are of no concern. In Australia, it is still encouraged that practitioners return to the feeding days of a meaty bone diet to avoid the problems that have arisen with artificial foods.[17,18]

Time will tell.

References

1. Bell JA. Ferret nutrition. Vet Clin North Am Exotic Anim Pract 1999; 2:169–192.
2. Brown S. Re-thinking the ferret diet. International Ferret Newsletter. The Netherlands: The World Ferret Union; 2003:6–12.
3. Burns R, Williams ES, O'Toole D, Dubey JP. *Toxoplasma gondii* infections in captive black-footed ferrets (*Mustela nigripes*) 1992–1998: clinical signs, serology, pathology and prevention. J Wildlife Dis 2003; 39:787–797.
4. Fox JG, McLain DE. Nutrition. In: Fox JG, ed. Biology and diseases of the ferret, 2nd edn. Baltimore: Williams & Wilkins; 1998:149–172.
5. Fox JG, ed. Biology and diseases of ferrets. Laboratory animal medicine, 2nd edn. American College of Laboratory Animal Medicine. San Diego: Academic Press; 2002:483–517.
6. Bell J. Breeding and nutrition. Information pamphlet. New York: Marshall Farms; 1993:April.
7. Bell J. Ferret nutrition and diseases associated with inadequate nutrition. Proc North Am Vet Assoc Conf, Orlando, Florida; 1993:719– 720.
8. Finkler DVM. Practical ferret medicine and surgery for the private practitioner. Roanoak: Roanoak Animal Hospital; 1999.
9. Ryland LM, Bernard SL, Gorham JR. A clinical guide to the pet ferret. Compend Contin Educ Pract Vet 1983; 5:25–32.
10. Willard T. A review of the nutritional needs of the ferret. International Ferret Newsletter. The Netherlands: The World Ferret Union 1997; 13:8–10.
11. Fettiman MJ. Trace elements and miscellaneous nutrients. In: Adams HR, ed. Veterinary pharmacology and therapeutics, 7th edn. Ames: Iowa State University Press; 1995:731–733.
12. Willard T. A review of the nutritional needs of the ferret. Internation Ferret Newsletter. The Netherlands: The World Ferret Union; 1998:15.
13. Willard T. Carnivore nutrition incorporating biotechnology into modern pet food manufacturing. Personal prepared paper; 2005:1–13.
14. Cruickshank R, ed. Medical microbiology. Edinburgh: Churchill Livingstone; 1965:1018–1019.
15. Lewington JH. Ferrets: A compendium. Vade Mecum Series C. No. 10. University of Sydney: Post Graduate Foundation; 1988.
16. Pass D, Butler R, Lewington JH et al. Veterinary care of birds, rodents, rabbits, ferrets and guinea pigs. Perth, Australia: Murdoch University Foundation; 1993.
17. Billinghurst I. Give your dog a bone. Lithgow, NSW: Dr I Billinghurst; 1993.
18. Lonsdale T. Raw meaty bones. South Windsor, NSW: Rivetco; 2001:Chs 4, 5, 8.
19. Department of Environmental Health. Standard C1 meat, game meat and related products. Western Australia: DoEH; 1996.

20. Ministry of Agriculture and Fisheries. Fur farming fitch: nutrition and feeding. New Zealand: MAF Information Services; 1983/84.
21. Okada HM, Chihaya Y, Matsukawa K. Thiamine deficiency encephalopathy in foxes and mink. Vet Pathol 1987; 24:180–182.
22. Malik R, Sibraa D. Thiamine deficiency due to sulphur dioxide preservative in 'pet meat'– a case of déjà vu. Aust Vet J 2005; 83:408–411.
23. Singh R, Thompson M, Sullivan N, Child G. Thiamine deficiency in dogs due to feeding of sulphite-preserved meat. Aust Vet J 2005; 83:412–417.
24. Dennis M, ed. Information newsletter. Invercargill, NZ: Southland Ferrets; 1998.
25. Jeffares R. The keeping and breeding of hunting ferrets. Hangatiki, NZ: R. Jeffares; 1997.
26. Roser RJ, Lavers RB. Food habits of the ferret (*Mustela putorius furo*) at Pukepuke lagoon, New Zealand. J Zool 1976; 3:269–275.
27. Porter V, Brown N. The complete book of ferrets. Bedford: D&M Publications; 1997.
28. Fraser CM, ed. Nutrition of mink. In: The Merck veterinary manual, 7th edn. Rahway, NJ: Merck; 1991:1240–1243.
29. McNicholas J. On the couch: saving polecat Ryan! Ferret First 2005; 24:8.
30. Rowlands IW. The ferret. In: Cooper J, ed. The UFAW handbook of care and management of laboratory animals. Wheathamstead: Universities Federation for Animal Welfare; 1967:582–593.
31. Andrews PR, Illman O. The ferret. In: Poole T, ed. The UFAW handbook of care and management of laboratory animals. Wheathampstead: Universities Federation for Animal Welfare; 1997:436–455.
32. Lloyd M. Veterinary care of ferrets, clinical examination and routine procedures. In Practice 2002; February:90–95.
33. Fekete SG, Fodor K, Prohaczik A, Andrasofszcky E. Comparison of feed preference and digestion of three different commercial diets for cats and ferrets. J Anim Physiol Anim Nutr (Berl) 2005; 89:199–202.
34. Pet Food Exposed? The F.A.I.R. Report 2001; IX:1–14.
35. Pitcairn RH, Pitcairn SH. Dr Pitcairn's complete guide to natural health for dogs & cats. Emmaus: Rodale Press; 1995:7–21.
36. Malik R. Preservatives in 'pet mince' as a potential trigger for allergic reactions including asthma and inflammatory bowel disease. University of Sydney: Post Graduate Foundation 2005; Control and Therapy Series 240:1619.

CHAPTER 5

Reproduction and genetics

'Each species has its "characters", some of whom will be easier to deal with, while some other litter mates will be much harder.'

Ian Brodie, Ferrets and Ferreting, 1978

The breeding of ferrets

Nicholas Everitt in his book *Ferrets* 1897, made a statement on the 'points' of the dog ferret.

'After having considered its antecedent repute for health and stamina, we should take note of its points and general appearance. Its body should be slim, lengthy, and muscular, its legs and feet sound and strong, its face sharp, fur clean, glossy and thick, and it should be quick in movement. A stumpy, large headed, dull-looking animal should not be used for breeding purposes; nor should any ferret that is not in soundest health and condition. A periodical mixture of blood is not only to be encouraged, but is essential to success'.

So there you have it – a call for genetic 'strength' even in 1897!

The breeding of ferrets differs from that of dogs and cats in that jill ferrets can become sick if not mated and practitioners must be aware of this when discussing breeding with clients. Ferrets are bred worldwide. In Australia, there are small private groups, which produce ferrets for use as hunting animals and pets. This also occurs in the UK, continental Europe and North America. There are also major breeding establishments for the production of large numbers of ferrets, but not in Australia. Marshall Farms, New York, USA, have produced thousands of ferrets since 1939, mostly for use in biomedical research and some for the pet industry. The original breeding stock included ferrets from the UK and also polecat bloodlines to increase the animals' size in the early days, thus producing a broad initial gene pool (J. Bell, pers. comm. 1993).

There are also private breeders in the USA and Canada who buy-in stock from the UK, Germany, Scandinavia, New Zealand and even Australia. At the present time, the latter two countries cannot import new blood lines and pet ferrets are banned in Queensland, Australia and New Zealand. I hope that these restrictions may in time be reversed, with perhaps a licensing system for pet ferret owners. The Australian Quarantine and Inspection Service (AQIS) was investigating the import risk of ferrets, leading to a possibility of relaxing Quarantine Proclamation 76A, prohibiting the importation of fresh ferret stock but at the time of writing this has not happened.

New Zealand has former fitch farms and commercial breeders, Southland Ferrets and Mystic Ferrets, producing ferrets for worldwide pet and laboratory use. However, with Aleutian disease possibly in these ferret stocks, it might be unwise to buy fresh ferrets from those sources (Ch. 8).

The popularity of television 'Animal Hospital'-type shows have increased interest in ferrets as pets and many people want to get into ferret-breeding. In the UK there have been some television programmes vigorously promoting ferrets, which evidently are bought on impulse. This has led to their later abandonment and the setting up of ferret shelters which still occurs in Australia and is a feature of life in the American ferret world. Possibly, the registration of ferret breeders, as occurs in Switzerland, and/or raising the price of ferrets sold would help

Ferret breeding season

to decrease impulse buying. The price of ferret kittens had gone up in Australia to $60 and even more so in Japan. Mystic Ferrets charge $200–300 while Marshall Farm and Angora ferrets cost $300–600. Many Japanese buy their ferrets more cheaply from Path Valley, Canada.

Ferret breeding season

In the southern hemisphere, the breeding season starts in August and continues until January of the next year. It has been observed in New Zealand that in wild ferrets, the hob testicles enlarge in size and weight in August and both hobs and jills are ready to mate in September.[1] This has been my experience with pet ferrets in Western Australia, with mating beginning in late August and early September and the jills returning to heat 2 weeks after the kittens are weaned.

Photo-periodism, i.e. the changing duration of daylight and darkness, controls ferret mating hormonal responses. The hormone melatonin is involved in activating the sexual spring/summer cycle and terminating the autumn/winter cycle in the ferret-breeding season. Its influence depends on day length.

Decreased day length leads to higher melatonin output during the dark hours. Exposing the ferret to more than 12 hours of darkness maintains higher-circulating melatonin from the pineal gland. The result is a suppression of GnRH and inhibition of pituitary LH with the termination of the breeding season, after which the ferrets gain winter coats and put on fat (C. Johnson-Delaney, pers. comm. 2005).

This was manipulated in large commercial mink or fitch farms for early breeding by subjecting jills to a 14:10 light:dark hours routine. Commercial ferret breeding establishments like Marshall Farms, New York, use the 14:10 ratio to produce 2–3 litters per year (J. Bell, pers. comm. 1993). Jills can produce 6–10 kittens per litter.

The hob ferret responds to short day-lengths and the jill to long day-lengths. The hob ferret matures by 6 months of age and in the sexually mature hob, the testicles become more prominent and noticeable in the scrotum from the time of the winter solstice (Fig. 5.1). They regress in size and position in the autumn and winter. The hob remains in breeding condition therefore over 4–5 months, covering the spring and summer. The jill requires at least 14 hours of uninterrupted daylight in any 24-hour period before she can become responsive to breeding.[2] The natural photo-periods in Western Australia give a mating season from August/September–December/January of the next year.

Signs of heat

The jill shows an increasingly large vulva from the beginning of the breeding season to a fully engorged state when she is ready to mate (Fig. 5.2). This contrasts with the hardly noticeable vulva in the quiescent jill.

Ferret jills, like other mustelids, are induced ovulators, i.e. they need specific stimulation to release the ova to ensure that there is a high probability of the sexual act being positive and not wasteful. This contrasts with other animals which have spontaneous ovulation; the

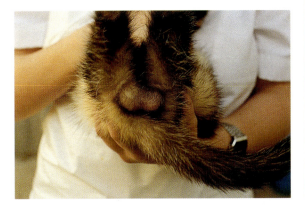

Figure 5.1 Hob showing enlarged testicles in the mating season.

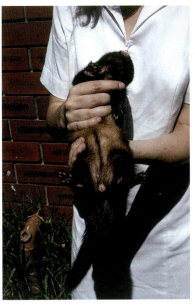

Figure 5.2 Jill showing enlarged vulva indicating she is in season.

CHAPTER FIVE
Reproduction and genetics

females release mature ova without stimulation prior to actual mating.[2] Ferret jills are seasonally polyoestrous and will keep in oestrus, unlike dogs and cats, unless taken out of heat by mating, by use of a vasectomized hob (vassy) or by hormonal injection.

Ferret jill reproductive cycle

The jill comes into oestrus when the vulva is enlarged and mating is best around 7–10 days post-maximum vulva swelling as this is close to the oestrous peak and gives a good chance of pregnancy. Unless the jill is mated she will go into post-oestrous anaemia. The gestation period is usually 42 days. The kittens are born normally fairly quickly. The lactation period is up to 42 days when the kittens are weaned. The jill will come into the second reproductive heat in 14 days. This cycle is shown in Figure 5.3.

The ferret shows similarities and variations in the sexual cycle from other mustelids and it is interesting to compare their sexual season with other mustelids. For instance, the native polecat is sexually active from February to the end of June (northern hemisphere) and has a direct implantation into the uterus like the ferret. It can produce a second litter later in the summer, which is usually caused by the first being lost prematurely. The ferret can have two litters a year whether one litter is lost or not. The weasel, like the ferret and polecat, has direct implantation, differing from the stoat, which has a delayed implantation mechanism whereby the spring ova are kept in suspended animation for 9–10 months. Development only occurs in the following spring when the daylight lengthens. Sexual activity in

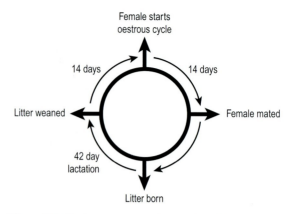

Figure 5.3 Fitch oestrous cycle. (Courtesy MAF Information, NZ, 1984.)

stoats is strictly controlled by changing day length and this control cannot be over-ridden by loss of a litter or an abundance of food. Food is not a problem for domesticated ferrets. On the other hand, least weasels (not common weasels) can have a twice-yearly mating season like ferrets but this is a feature of wild animals only if there is a glut of food available.[3]

Figure 5.4 can be adapted for the southern hemisphere remembering that spring begins in September. The hob and jill should be checked early in the mating season for any signs of illness and possibly vaccinated if it has not already been done. They should both be treated for fleas. I found Frontline Spray useful for numbers of ferrets and it showed no toxicity (Ch. 10). Fleas can be a problem, especially for kittens, if an infestation occurs.

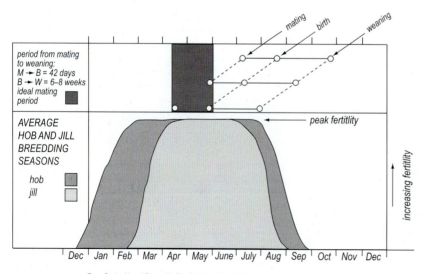

Figure 5.4 Breeding chart for ferrets in the northern hemisphere. (From Val Porter and Nicholas Brown's *The Complete Book of Ferrets*. Bedford: D&M Publications; 1997, with permission.)

88

Hob behaviour in the mating season

The hobs can be kept together in a colony out of the mating season but in season they may well fight and there is usually a dominant male. I found that with father and son, the younger hob would be dominated though he might carry more weight. A new hob will be picked on until the 'pecking order' is re-established. An unsterilized jill will excite the hobs into activity. The hob will sniff around the jill, chattering and following her and sniffing at her scats. The solitary hob runs around with his hindquarters close to the ground and urinates in a trail to show a territory-marking trait. It has now been found that the hobs' and jills' urine contains 30 volatile compounds with 2-methylquinoline unique to the hobs' urine.[4] Quantitative comparison of the 30 compounds shows a significant difference between the hob and jill. It suggests perhaps that ferrets do use urine marking, in deference to anal gland secretion, for sex and individual recognition. *Note*: 10 of 26 compounds in anal secretions from jills and hobs were also found in urine. However, most of the major compounds in anal glands of both sexes were not present in urine. The authors suggest the urine may convey specific signals that differ from those of anal glands. Personally, I was never aware of breeding stock (hobs) expressing their anal glands (except in fear) but they did mark territory like a dog.

Jill behaviour in the mating season

The jill will sniff around the hob's musk glands but until the light stimulation begins to act on her hormones so that she starts producing oestrogens and the vulva becomes very apparent, she will resist the advances of the hob. Oestrogens can be detected in the jill's urine when she is on heat.

It is known for jills and hobs to show affection for each other by licking and grooming. This point was picked up by McCann in observing the sexual behaviour of polecats, the ferret ancestors, in captivity.[5]

Mating behaviour

With the combination of the attention of the hob and light influences, the jill develops a prominent vulval swelling but still does not readily submit to the hob. Mating of ferrets can be rough and noisy. The hob begins to attack the jill by catching her by the scruff of the neck, which causes shrill screams from the jill in what becomes rough foreplay. The jill is dragged around protesting but eventually stays still while copulation occurs

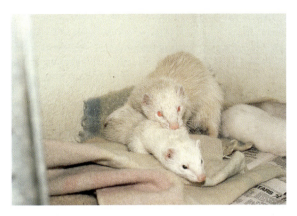

Figure 5.5 Albino hob on top of a black-eyed white jill.

(Fig. 5.5). (*Note*: some jills become tense when being 'scruffed' for examination, possibly due to a memory of mating with a hob.) The best time to breed the jill is about 2 weeks after the first signs of vulval swelling. For the jill ferret's size, the vulva gets tremendously enlarged, moist and there is wetness round her tail and hindquarters from her secretions. The musk glands are not released by either party during copulation. With polecats, this is not always the case.[5]

It is essential for the breeder to handle the jill regularly before and after mating and all through pregnancy, so she will be 'bonded' to allow the breeder to handle her and the kittens from the day of birth. It will be found that the jill becomes very 'loving' to the breeder as she moves into oestrus and this phenomenon also occurs when a jill goes into pseudopregnancy if for some reason she does not conceive.

The jill may shed hair up to the mating time, like she does before parturition, and may moult a bit when she ovulates, which is brought about by the copulation. I leave the hob and jill together for at least 24 hours and like to observe that they have mated at least twice. The mating can be for at least half an hour and the hob and jill can be picked up together when coupled and do not stir.

After mating, the hob is removed and the pair are kept separate during the gestation, parturition and weaning periods. I kept my pregnant jill in a 'nursery cage' and she was handled and petted every day. Some breeders leave the jill or jills in a community situation with other jills until about 2 weeks before parturition. Jills can be kept with sterilized hobs (hobbles) but they should be fed separately. The hob should not be forgotten at this time and should get its share of petting and playing. It is important that when checking a number of hobs in the mating season, to wash your hands between ferrets, as the scent of a competitor may arouse the ferret you are handling. That goes for handling pregnant, or on-heat, jills and active hobs.

CHAPTER FIVE
Reproduction and genetics

Any vasectomized hobs (vassy hobs) should be kept away from pregnant jills or active hobs to prevent trouble. Once the mating season is over the ferrets can be mixed again and usually, after some chattering, scruffing and mild fighting to re-establish the pecking order, they settle down.

The pregnant jill

The jill should be located in a quiet place during pregnancy. I had my nursery cage under the eaves of the house on the east side to protect against weather and heat and for quick observation (see Figs 3.17, 3.18). Noisy dogs can be a problem and cats are curious about ferrets. Some breeders use a shed for the jills and even a room in the house can be sacrificed for the jill. This does give the jill added protection from the weather, noise and even theft of litters! Parturition is usually at 42 days post-mating and the average litter is eight kittens.

Note in Figure 5.6 that the vulval swelling in the pregnant jill has reduced quickly from the prominent swelling of heat. If the mating has not been successful then the vulva reduces more slowly over 5–6 days and the jill may go into pseudopregnancy. The vulva loses its moisture and begins to return to its usual inconspicuous size. The rate of reduction depends on how long she has been on heat and is quicker earlier in the season than later.[2] The jill may well shed some of her coat at this time.

Pregnancy detection

At about 2–3 weeks, the fetuses can be detected by palpation as swellings in the uterus (Fig. 5.7). If only one or two fetuses are present, they may be confused with the jill's kidneys. In general, the kidneys are firmer and less moveable but are however found halfway between the ribs and pelvis in the same area as kitten development. *Note:* jills are difficult to restrain on their backs and are better checked by standing them upright with their feet on the table (Ch. 7). If available, ultra-

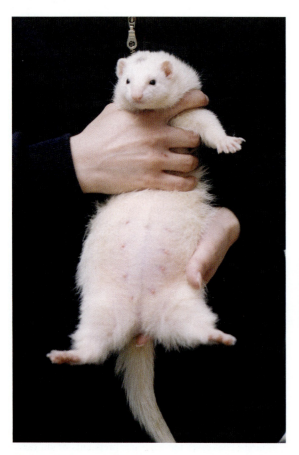

Figure 5.6 Pregnant jill, Patch, notice prominent teats.

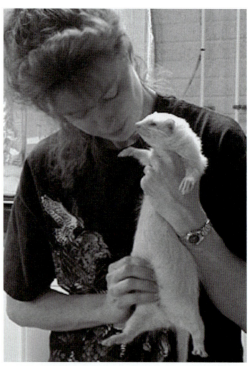

Figure 5.7 Sally Heber of Shady Hollow Ferretry checks mated jill to see if she is falsing or needs medical attention to deliver her kits. (Courtesy of the American Ferret Association.)

The pregnant jill

sound has been found useful for indicating pregnancy even at 10 days post-mating.[6] The development of the mammary glands is not a good indicator of impending parturition. Behaviour of the jill is a better yardstick; she becomes quieter, loses interest in food and will confine herself to the nursery-sleeping box. I had one jill, Patch, who went off her food pre-parturition and took nearly 3 weeks to come back to eating meat. She only accepted milk drinks daily. A jill's nipples appear pink and enlarged with a discharge the day before birth. She will lick the vulva when the kittens are imminent.

The sleeping box should be adequate in size, as in Chapter 3. Marshall Farms have their jills in cages 60 × 90 × 45–60 cm made of 2.5 cm square galvanized wire mesh. They are put in 1 week before the kittens are due and stay there until the kittens reach 6 weeks of age (J. Bell, pers. comm. 1993). It is important that the nursery-sleeping box should have a semicircular entry hole with the base flush to the floor, not a circular entry hole, so that the jill cannot damage its mammary glands going in and out. An inspection lid to the sleeping box must be lockable to stop an agitated jill trying to get out and hurting herself.

Straw is the usual bedding for working ferret jills[2] while commercial ferret breeding farms and research units use wood shavings, a plastic dish pan for a nest box, with a terry towel for the jill. The towel should not be too large as the kittens can get caught in the creases and starve or suffocate. In the fitch (fur) farm situation the whelping box is underneath the ferret cage (Fig. 5.8) and more natural as a whelping area.

In an old laboratory environment, the whelping box (Fig. 5.9) shows the entrance hole is too high which could lead to the jill hurting her mammary glands and getting mastitis; this was corrected. In a good laboratory

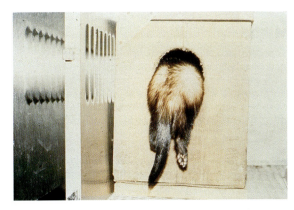

Figure 5.9 Entrance to laboratory nursing box showing poor design for entrance. (Courtesy of Dean Manning.)

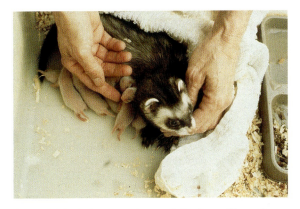

Figure 5.10 Laboratory jill in whelping box with newborn kittens. *Note*: jill allows inspection. (Courtesy of Dean Manning.)

environment, the jill is in a whelping box where she and the kittens can be handled (Fig. 5.10).

I have tended to use small old bits of sheeting, which the jill can curl up in. The sheet is put into the sleeping box as a 'folded handkerchief'. The top 'fold' of the handkerchief is made into a cover, which the jill quickly takes to and curls up. I tried straw but found it too messy for cleaning and there may be a problem of mites in that material.

Ferret parturition

Most pregnant jills I have had seem to carry the full 42 days before going into labour. The jills are handled constantly and allow the handling of kittens from birth. The jills are kept in the nursery cage alone but they can be kept with other jills until about 2 weeks before being due to whelp. Working ferrets have been known to carry on ferreting well into their pregnancy without trouble.

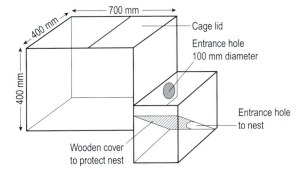

Figure 5.8 Fitch whelping cage. *Note*: nest box was below floor level. (Figure in memory of those ferrets used for fitch farming and research.) (Courtesy of MAF Information, NZ, 1984.)

CHAPTER FIVE
Reproduction and genetics

> **Author's example**
>
> I once gave a ferreter a podgy ferret jill found in the suburbs but not claimed after a couple of weeks of advertising. He wanted another working ferret but I was unimpressed when he said the jill would take to ferreting. He went bush with a friend and they worked the ferrets and evidently the podgy jill took to it like an otter to water! They camped under the stars and in the night heard some squeaks from the carrying box with the stray ferret. They found that she had not only got them some rabbits but produced six kittens as a bonus! We never gave it a thought that she might be pregnant, as she looked a typical roly-poly over-indulged pet ferret!

My ferret whelping box described in Chapter 3 and Figure 5.11 shows ferret jill Jenny's newborn kits.

I left my ferret jills knowing they will probably whelp overnight or early morning. I have had to help one jill who came into whelp prematurely when taken to the hospital.[7] With laboratory breeding ferret colonies, it is suggested that the jill whelping can be a risky business and she should not be left unattended. Many private breeders will leave their jill during parturition in the belief that the jill will attack and kill the kittens if disturbed. The jill usually delivers the kittens over 2–3 hours in laboratory and large ferret breeding establishments. The jill will attend to the placenta of the kittens but only settles down to feed them once all have been delivered.

Manning and Bell consider the whelping should be over in 2 hours but comment that ferrets have a high incidence of congenital abnormalities concerning the head and neck and that dystocia is frequent in laboratory-bred ferrets. A caesarean operation may be needed (D. Manning, pers. comm. 1990). The kittens are born in a sequence of pairs in laboratory ferrets with a few minutes rest between pairs.

My ferrets seemed to have been more leisurely with breaks between single births. One of my early jills, Jenny, had eight kittens between the hours of 12 noon and 7.30 p.m. the same day, without a sound. She certainly did not have them all at one hit. However, if an hour passes without a birth something could be wrong and this may involve abnormalities. It is suggested, if the unborn kitten is close to the cervix then use oxytocin (0.3 mL i.m.) to attempt to move it.

Normally, kittens are born hairless, blind and weigh 8–10 g. The jill will eat the afterbirth, which is beneficial but results in tarry scats for a while. The kittens must suckle shortly after the jill has completed labour to gain the first colostrum. The jill will settle down in a half-curved position on her side and let the kittens suckle on her eight nipples. In situations where there are more than eight kittens I have observed a jill take a satisfied day-old kitten which has fallen off the teat and place the kitten over her back. By the time the kitten has managed to squirm its way back to the mammary glands another kitten has had a chance to feed. The kittens gain a white fuzz of body hair early in the first week, which darkens with time, but a variety of colours from albino to dark sable will develop depending on the parents' genes. Jill 'Sophie' nursed some good litters (Fig. 5.12).

The kittens' eyes open from 4–5 weeks of age while their temporary teeth erupt from 3–4 weeks, with the canines first so that the jill may be subject to trauma to the mammary glands from their needle-like teeth.

The jill will take meat to the kittens from 4–5 weeks of age. Excessive overfeeding of the jill at this time may result in her taking more food to the kittens, possibly resulting in overweight animals. The jill will lose weight feeding the kittens but quickly put it back on after they are weaned. The kittens should become very active from 5 weeks of age and be walking on a flat surface, not wire, to strengthen their legs. I put a board over the wire in the nursery cage to the scats tray, which the

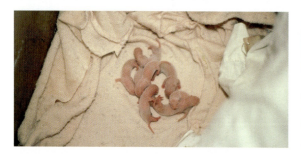

Figure 5.11 Just-born kittens in Lewington nursery whelping box. Jill, Jenny, removed.

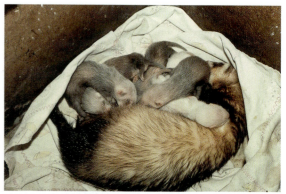

Figure 5.12 Lactating jill, Sophie, with six 3-week-old kittens in Lewington nursery whelping box.

Problems associated with ferret breeding

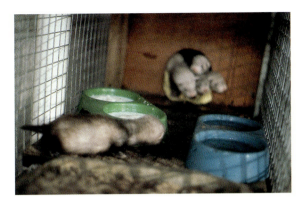

Figure 5.13 Six-week-old kittens leaving Lewington nursery whelping box to toilet on scats tray at end of cage run.

kittens soon learn to use like their mother (Fig. 5.13). Another idea with wire-based cages is to put tiles on the wire but with the rough surface uppermost.

Again, it is important for the breeder to handle the kittens, with the mother, from birth if possible, to give them human contact. The kittens are played with and will 'play-fight' with the breeder, which is a learning experience. If possible, the kittens are given time out in the garden or 'ferretarium' as described in Chapter 3. The kittens can be sold off from the jill from 6 weeks of age but 8 weeks of age is better to allow them to get the most of maternal care. The jill is not separated from the kittens, but the kittens from the jill, as they are sold.

In a ferretarium environment, the jill might well take the kittens underground into the bolthole and will do so if cats come around. Kittens of 7–8 weeks of age would weigh half the weight of the jill but she will still be able to drag them into the bolthole if need be, away from any danger. The kittens will keep close to the mother on any excursions around the ferretarium or garden. The kittens and jill will all be playful and the hob can be brought back in to join the family. The hob will 'play-fight' with the kittens but I have never seen a hob aggressive to the kittens. The jill will come into heat again after weaning the kittens so the hob will probably be more interested in her and they can go on to produce a second litter that season. In Western Australia (WA), the second litter will be produced in the hottest part of the year and once that litter is over, autumn (March) brings a decline in sexual activity of the jill and hob. In the case of laboratory ferrets, artificial photo-periods are induced for 'in-house' breeding as is done in Marshall Farms. The jill may come on heat while nursing a litter and show alopecia but I have never seen it. If it happens in American ferret breeding farms, the jills, if not to be mated, are taken out of heat with hormone injections to prevent possible hyperoestrogenism (J. Bell, pers. comm. 1993).

Problems associated with ferret breeding

Problems with the hob

Hob fertility rises with the increase in testicular size over the breeding season and is shown in the breeding chart, Table 5.1. If the weather becomes excessively hot, as in WA summers, the hob may become sterile. Thus hobs must be:

- kept indoors or in a ventilated shed
- kept in protected cages, as with the 'Coolgardie safe' technique (see Ch. 3)
- allowed to go underground in boltholes during the heat of the day, as seen in a ferretarium.

Table 5.1 A comparative weight chart of the kittens from Jenny (1984), Wendy (1985) and Patch (1998)

Weeks	Jenny	Wendy	Patch	Comment on Patch and kitten
0	8 g (8)	10.4 g (9)	7.2 g (11)	Patch stops eating
1	18 g (6)	23 g (8)	16.4 g (5)	
2	49 g	49.3 g	50 g	Patch eats meat
3	85 g	79.1 g	80 g	
4	121 g	118 g	117 g	Patch with mastitis
5	172 g	170 g	200 g	20 g meat per kit
6	250 g	263 g	270 g	25 g meat per kit
7	324 g (6)	389 g (4)	335 g (2)	
8			425 g (2)	

Numbers in brackets indicate the number of ferret kittens.

Injury to the hob's penis is possible; I had a rampant hob catch its baculum (os penis) in a wire fence while trying to get to a jill with almost disastrous results! Hob and jill should not mate in situations where there are terry towels as bedding. A laboratory hob ferret got its penis tangled in loose threads with constriction of the blood supply and another near disaster! Laboratory hobs have been seen to confuse a roll of toweling in a breeding cage for the jill they are mating with (D. Manning, pers. comm. 1994).

Problems with the jill

Fertility can be a problem with extreme hot weather extremes as seen in WA, so if the jill becomes overheated and her body temperature too high, any fertilized ova will not implant in the uterus.[2] *Note* that if the eggs are already fertilized and implanted, then increased body heat can damage cells of the CNS, resulting in kittens of subnormal weight with cleft palate and hydrocephalus defects. It is stated by one author in the UK that with a daytime temperature of 85°F (29°C) ferrets could mate but the jill will not become pregnant although as long as the nights are cool she will thrive. With a constant day and night temperature of 70°F (22°C) the hob and jill are unlikely to mate.[2] In hot summer climates like WA, the temperature is fortunately usually reduced by a cooling afternoon sea breeze. The night temperatures can fall quickly especially with clear skies. Most ferrets would be nocturnal and mating at night when it is cooler. My ferrets were sometimes kept at the hospital overnight to mate in very hot conditions. Temperature ranges are not a problem in commercial ferret breeding establishments under air-conditioning, unlike ferrets being bred in cages outside.

Pregnancy toxaemia (PT)

Some authors describe pregnancy toxaemia in jills, whereby for some reason they are starved accidentally in the last week of gestation, bringing on toxaemic shock.[8] One reason may be simply a change of diet late in gestation, which puts the jill off its food, even for 1 day. I have not had this condition in my pregnant jills as I have had a set nutrition from mating to parturition.[9] Pregnancy toxaemia occurs in primiparous jills and can sometimes occur with jills with large litters (over 10 kittens). It is thought that with more fetuses, a factor of abdomen size comes in, whereby the uterus takes up the space that would be occupied by an extended stomach.[10] (I had jills with litters of 13 kittens with no toxaemia problems.) With the normal ferret gestation of 42 days the condition can arise in the 10 days leading up to that time.

It is considered that ferret breeders should make palatable food and water available 24 hours a day. I fed jills nightly, or perhaps night and morning, but food is not left out all the time. Milk or milk supplement drink, however, was available plus water. It might be that the milk drink is the reason for my jills' not getting pregnancy toxaemia with large litters. It is known that jills will drink large volumes of water when they are on dry food and will stop eating without adequate water. Dry food, especially in a dry climate, in my opinion, increases the ferrets' need to have water, which they would not need so much when eating fresh moist meat. In the WA climate, the temperature would increase the need for hydration and dry food only adds to the problem. I know that a jill with kittens, when properly protected from the heat (see Ch. 3), will spend the day feeding the kittens and resting up. She will eat and drink in the evening and night while periodically allowing the kittens to feed. My Wendy's 1985 litter of 13 kittens was an example (see Fig. 5.22). Of course, jill ferrets indoors or in commercial breeding establishments would not be subject to the rigours of the climate.

Clinical signs of pregnancy toxaemia occur with the jill becoming lethargic just before the whelping date, being dehydrated and having a 'doughy' feeling to the skin.[10] There might be tarry black scats and the jill may be so dehydrated that the uterus outline, and even the kitten images, can be seen on her abdomen. The jill is in a critical condition and unless immediate treatment by caesarean operation is performed, she can die. The jill will have hair loss, also ketonuria and azotaemia with the blood glucose less than 50 mg/dL and definitely is not a good surgical risk. She may lie on her side, being cold, with glazed eyes.

Laboratory checks on jills with PT are important to establish signs of anaemia, azotemia, hypoglycaemia, bilirubinaemia, high levels of hepatic serum enzymes, hypoproteinaemia and ketonuria. *Note*: the body tries to overcome the hypoglycemia by gluconeogenesis with the jill taking more triglycerides from fat stores, which are hydrolysed to free fatty acids (FFA). The result is that the liver is stressed, as triglycerides are re-synthesized from the FFA, leading to severe hepatic lipidosis. With the increase of FFAs from triglycerides, and a change in the hepatic metabolism from fat synthesis to fat oxidation, ketogenesis occurs. The result is a ketonuria and osmotic diuresis as the ketones move into the extracellular space and elude complete resorption to pass into the urine.[11]

In the USA, ferret breeders are advised to give high-quality nutritional supplements, especially to jills predicted to have large litter sizes. Nutrical (EVSCO Pharmaceutical's Buena, NJ) or Ensure Plus (Abbot Laboratories, Ross Products Division, Columbus, OH) is suggested.[12] In Australia, there is Animalac (Troy),

Problems associated with ferret breeding

Canadian clinical example[11]

A late stage pregnant 1300 g jill from a local ferret rescue shelter, had depression, weakness and anorexia. Her owner had no experience with pregnant jills. The jill was fed on Premium Ferret Food. Presented to the vet it showed a moribund state, recumbency and hypothermy. Its temperature sat at 34.8°C with pulse of 140/min and respiration at 38 breaths/min. It was passing dark brown scats and on palpation of the abdomen, a large number of kits were found. Capillary refill was 3 seconds and blood glucose registered at 3.3 mmol/L (normal range 6.97–10.49 mmol/L). Ketones were found in the urine. With pregnancy toxaemia suspected, fluids were given, a balanced electrolyte i.v. solution, at the rate of 2 mL/L per hour using a 25 gauge needle via the cephalic vein, with additional 10 mL of 5% dextrose. The jill was warmed up and responded after having 150 mg of glucose in 5% dextrose orally. Her condition improved in 1 hour. An emergency caesarean was carried out and 12 live kittens were obtained. The jill then received a full ovariohysterectomy and recovered slowly with intensive care and at 13 days postoperation, she started to eat on her own. In the initial stages, she was force-fed Hill's Science Diet plus water. The kittens were hand fed initially which can be difficult in ferrets. The procedure was to force feed them with a mixture of 3 parts milk replacer and 1 part whipped cream using a syringe and teat cannula. The kittens were fed 4 times daily but were not too responsive. Despite home nursing, all the kittens died by 10 days. Stress could have been a major factor in the pregnancy toxaemia, with the jill being left at the ferret shelter.

Biolac (Smith) and Nutrigel (like Nutrical). The UK has Lactol (Shirley's)[2] and Welpi, and New Zealand breeders use Reliance Feedmilk (see Appendices).

Batchelder et al. have given an excellent account of 10 jills in late gestation and with large litters getting PT.[13] They compare the condition with several animal species including mink. The serious nature of PT is seen by the jill fatalities and the poor prospect of litter survival. Half of the 10 jills were from a research laboratory and half from a commercial breeder. Five jills had litters of over 10 kittens. Two jills were found dead, while two had to be euthanized. Of the six which received supportive treatment, five had hysterectomies but only three survived out of the six. These latter jills were found to have less pronounced azotaemia, hypoproteinaemia, and were not anaemic. Further, they had less liver activity increase. Only a few of the kittens from these survived till weaning. A sad result.

Urolithiasis in the pregnant jill

This is an interesting condition in ferret colonies in America where they have been fed on pelleted dry diet containing plant based protein. Urolithiasis is described as a major urinary disease of ferrets in Chapter 11. No pregnant jills to my knowledge in the UK, Australia or New Zealand have had this condition.

Parturition problems

One UK author[2] states that where the whelping box is too warm at the time of parturition certain problems can occur such as the following:

1. The jill may not chew through the umbilical cords. An odd condition seen in kittens produced in a laboratory or breeding farm, whereby the kittens are born so rapidly that the jill does not get time to chew the umbilical cords and the kittens get bound up in cords and the wood shavings used to line the whelping box.[10] This is another reason for not using such material. I prefer my jills to have a clear whelping box with just light sheeting and a proper scats tray outside in the exercise run (Ch. 3).
2. The jill may fail to produce milk (agalactia) for some reason. The jill, even with a maternal instinct to nurse kittens, may fail to lactate for several days. This can be due to a neighbour's dog constantly barking, which I have experienced with a jill which caused me to stop breeding ferrets for a time. As a result of the milk failure, the newborn kittens appear to suckle vigorously but are not getting any milk. They can be seen to be almost transparent due to lack of milk (Fig. 5.14). It can lead to early deaths of kittens. Having a well-satisfied, contented, even spoilt, jill may eliminate the problem. This is easier to do with one or two pet ferrets than with a large ferret colony or commercial ferret-breeding establishment. There may be stress on a pregnant or lactating jill in a 'crowded' breeding house. The ferret is really a solitary breeder, like its polecat ancestor. The ferret owner, the hob, the jill and kittens should be the only elements of the breeding equation. The hob is left out of the scene until the kittens are weaned.

The keeping of pregnant jills and kittens in hot situations has been discussed in Chapter 3. The nutrition of the jill in the pregnant and lactating stages with a high quality food is essential. It is also paramount that the jill is protected against disease and covered by required vaccinations. The breeding jill should be kept isolated against possible systemic diseases which could affect the reproductive cycle. Bell and Manning have

CHAPTER FIVE

Reproduction and genetics

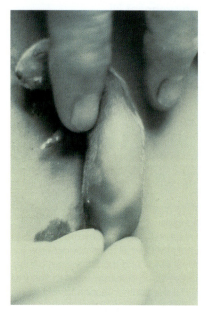

Figure 5.14 Kitten without milk showing an almost transparent abdomen. (Courtesy of Dean Manning.)

recorded reproductive failures in ferrets and mink, after their contamination with the organism *Campylobacter jejuni*[14] (Ch. 9).

Ferret jills are susceptible to human influenza so any affected humans must be kept away from them. If the jill does fall sick in early pregnancy or postpartum, the need for vigorous antibiotic and fluids is essential. With kittens around, they must be separated until the jill is with milk again or the kittens can be weaned off early. Mastitis is one problem which causes agalactia and can be dangerous to the jill's health if not treated promptly.

3. The kittens may die in the womb because the jill fails to give birth (dystocia).

It would appear from talking to veterinarians in the USA, dystocia of some kind is prevalent in some laboratory-kept breeding colony ferrets. Manning and Bell admit that posterior presentation, especially with large kittens, can complicate parturition in their experience with laboratory ferrets. They lost a jill with a vaginal prolapse when it had a large kitten unassisted. It ate the prolapsed tissue with resulting haemorrhage. Their advice is that an hour without delivery of a kitten calls for drastic action. The use of oxytocin i.m. to stimulate labour has been mentioned. If there is a congenital malformation in the neck or spine, then surgery must be done, as the jill will not feed kittens already born until all are expelled. An immediate caesarean is advocated. They also found that cold hungry kittens will not attempt to nurse and will quickly die even if placed with a surrogate mother. Fostering newborn ferret kittens is time-consuming.

For uterine stimulation, another author recommends oxytocin at 0.5–1 mL i.m., which would be a relatively large volume for a small muscle mass in the ferret. Besch-Williford lists possible congenital conditions in ferret kittens as lack of limbs and tail, anencephaly, corneal dermoids, hemivertebrae scoliosis, gastroschisis, cleft lip and palate, open eye and kinked or short tail.[12] When knowing little about ferret parturition, I first used 0.1 mL oxytocin on a ferret jill with dystocia, but on reflection it was too small a dose.[7]

Caesarean section

The jill is anaesthetized with isoflurane or halothane and a midline approach is made as for ovariohysterectomy (Ch. 18). This gives good access to both horns of the uterus and there are no postoperative complications, with the jill able to nurse the kittens. Figures 5.15 and 5.16 show the exteriorization of the uterus and removal of one fetus. The jill in question had no trouble with her first litter. It was given oxytocin for the second litter but failed to respond. The single kitten was 3 days overdue as verified by the fact that when removed from one horn of the uterus it had a hair covering. The jill and kit survived okay. Other jills with one or two kits can be an extra day or two late.

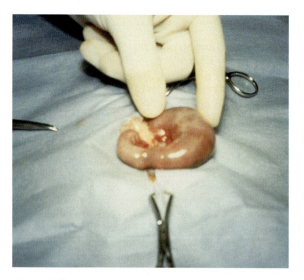

Figure 5.15 Caesarean operation: uterus exposed. (Courtesy of Mark Finkler.)

Problems with older jills at parturition

Author's clinical example

One morning (1989) I had a 1-year-old BEW jill, Susie, which I took to work with me on the 42nd day of gestation, for radiology, as I had never radiographed a jill near term. She was placed with a neutered hob, 'Cub', who knew her and they went to sleep together for the day. I was expecting Susie to give birth in the evening. However, Susie had four kittens without any trouble in the late morning before we got round to radiographing her. Cub slept through the whole thing! She was taken home that evening and reared four kittens perfectly. This shows an uneventful parturition in a jill.

Five years on, a pregnant Susie was taken again to the hospital 3 days before the 42nd day for close observation one hot January day. I was concerned with her age, the heat and the fact that she had developed cataracts (Ch. 12). Up to that time, she had been alone in the nursery cage at home. She was placed that morning with two neutered hobs, Simon and Hoppy, who knew and never hassled her and they promptly went to sleep together. In the early afternoon, Susie suddenly stood up while I was watching her and started moving around the cage making pitiful whimpering sounds while the other two ferrets slept on unperturbed. They were promptly removed! Susie would move around the cage and then, for a while, stop. She was in obvious discomfort and distinct muscular rippling flank movements could be seen. She made no attempt to lie down in the whelping position as jills normally do at parturition. She showed distinct 'flowing' contractions down the flank from diaphragm to pelvis. She then produced one dead kitten by breech birth (Fig. 5.17), with my assistance, plus the afterbirth (Fig. 5.18).

Susie was helped over too long a period of time with oxytocin injections but only 0.1mL s.c. as I was too cautious. I should have gone for a higher dose as previously quoted (D. Manning, pers. comm. 1990). Had I been more experienced I should also have gone for a caesarean operation but I had not experienced dystocia in the ferret before. After the first dead kitten she had two live ones, one 4 minutes after 0.1mL oxytocin s.c. and the other 10 minutes later, unassisted, so I felt more confident. One hour later, after oxytocin, she had another live kitten. One hour later the oxytocin was repeated and she had one more live kitten. So far so good! As Susie usually produced four or five kittens, I took her home that evening. Next morning early, she still had four live kittens but only two apparently feeding. When checked at noon she had had three more kittens but two were dead. She thus had alive three large and two small kittens. The outcome was a total of eight kittens, twice her usual, and she was now 5 years old, with five born alive and three born dead but two of the live kittens died 3 days postpartum. The weights of the three remaining kittens were 13.8g, 14.5g and 11.5g. The weights of the kittens she lost were 9.5g, 9.2g, 9.2g, 4.1g, and 4.1g. The average birth weight of ferret kittens is 6–12g.

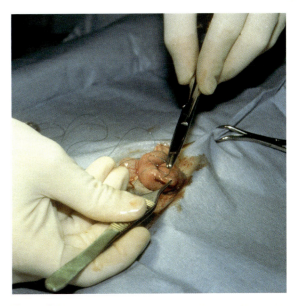

Figure 5.16 Caesarean operation: single fetus delivered with hair on body indicating overdue parturition. (Courtesy of Mark Finkler.)

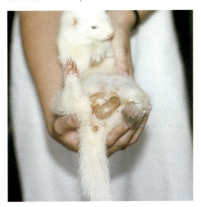

Figure 5.17 Jill, Susie, giving birth to kitten at Craigie Veterinary Hospital (1994.)

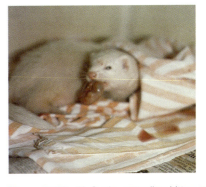

Figure 5.18 Jill, Susie, attending kitten and afterbirth at Craigie Veterinary Hospital (1994.)

There is no doubt that the parturition time was far too long. Some BEW jills can have problems. In addition, Susie had cataracts but this did not seem to affect her licking the kittens and eating the afterbirths. She did attempt to eat the first dead kitten. One USA ferret owner had blind ferret jills that would not deal with the umbilical cord and afterbirth and needed constant attention (A. Marks, Florida, pers. comm. 1990). The initial oxytocin dosage was too low. Susie actually took 20 hours to have eight kittens and was given six doses of oxytocin of 0.1 mL s.c or i.m. over that period. In the bitch, oxytocin causes contractions within 10 minutes and may be repeated at 30–40 minute intervals, but the bitch may become refractory to its effects in time.[11] I do not know this effect in ferrets. This case is given to illustrate the factors of dystocia due to a first large kitten and prolonged use of oxytocin at a low dosage.

In USA breeding establishments, gestation is put at 41–42 days with the primiparous jills being slightly earlier. With litters of one or two kittens they can be overdue which is considered to be due to lack of hormonal stimulation from the fetuses to actually trigger parturition.[10] These kittens usually die around the 43rd day. Dystocia may be caused by the still-growing kittens if labour is precipitated by oxytocin. It is known that in dogs if oxytocin is given before the onset of parturition, it may cause premature placental separation and fetal deaths.[15] If a jill has only one palpable kitten, then at 41 days it is advised that the jill is given 0.5 mg (0.1 mL) prostaglandin F (Upjohn). This is followed in 1–4 hours by 6 USP units of oxytocin i.m. to induce whelping, which usually occurs 2–12 hours after the treatment.[10] If there is no response within 24 hours, the drugs are re-administered or one should go straight to a caesarean operation. The jill is not at risk during the 24 hours but may lose her milk which affects the kittens' survival.

Problems with kittens post-whelping

Some jills get very anxious at parturition and some may experience a prolonged natural delivery, as with Susie. This leads to them not releasing their milk for 12–24 hours, which again happened with my jill. Thus unfed and unattended, kittens will lose weight rapidly and die. They become chilled and hungry with hypoglycaemia and may well be rejected or cannibalized by the jill. It is considered that kittens must be attended to immediately for any chance of survival.

In Susie's case, because of her history of small litters, no immediate hand rearing was attempted. However, orphan ferret kittens are most difficult to rear, except with an immediate change to a willing foster mother which was not available at the time. The technique is that the kittens of both jills are removed for a short time and mixed and then placed with the foster mother who hopefully will accept the additional kittens. She must be observed for any signs of rejection of the new kittens. Hopefully, the underfed orphans will get some good feeds. If the good teat suckers are put with the agalactic jill, the more forceful sucking may stimulate her delayed milk letdown. With no foster mother available, the hand rearing of kittens can take up a lot of time.

Hand-rearing kittens

Mike Jasper, UK, has recorded his experience with working ferrets[2] and Dean Manning, USA, has recorded experiences with laboratory-reared kittens.[16] The attempt in the latter case to hand-rear from birth a total of 36 caesarean-derived or naturally delivered kittens, resulted in only *one* survival past the age of 4 days, although it did survive to be an adult. *Note*: the caesarean operations were done under halothane anaesthesia. It was found that the feeding of orphan kittens less than 10 days of age with exclusively ferret milk is of paramount importance. A way of milking donor ferrets was illustrated.[16] Manning did go on to eventually rear three kittens entirely by hand, out of 50 attempts and put the cost of around the clock attention to the task at well over $30 000! He kept one as a very expensive pet ferret.[17]

Any unattended orphan kittens must first be warmed and treated with i.p. or oral glucose (2.5%) saline, or given i.p. lactated Ringer's solution (D. Manning, pers. comm. 1990). The kittens can be stomach-tubed with fine polished Teflon tubing and given a milk supplement. The jill's natural milk contains a higher proportion of fat than cow, cat or goat (see Appendices). If success in hand-rearing orphan kittens is to be achieved, they need to get the first colostrum milk, then there is a better chance of success with painstaking regular feeding of the suggested supplements. Feeding orphan kittens requires feeding every 2 hours, night and day, initially using eyedroppers. Feeding bottles, used for cat kittens, can be adapted for ferrets. Hygiene must be maintained to prevent disease problems in the susceptible orphan kittens during hand feeding. One can use 30 gauge needles for initial i.p. injections of the newborn kittens using 0.5 mL of an electrolyte (Fig. 5.19).

It is possible that initially after hydration and stomach-tubing for force-feeding, kittens can be returned to the jill but otherwise foster-mothering or hand-rearing are the options. *Note*: the jill will not feed the litter until all are born; consider Susie's case, so any dystocia might not be recognized early. Then the oldest kittens already born may suffer with weakness and chill. It is suggested that such kittens be left under a desk-lamp for warmth or even placed with an non-lactating jill. If more than 6 hours occurs without the kittens feeding, their blood glucose should be raised by force-feeding or fluid injec-

Problems associated with ferret breeding

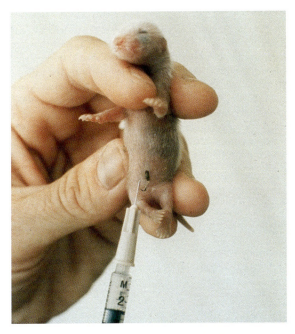

Figure 5.19 Injecting kitten i.p. with fluids. (Courtesy of Dean Manning.)

tion. A vicious circle occurs when the kittens do not feed; the jill lactates less.

When fostered out, the age of the kittens is important because the teats of a jill with very young kittens are very small and teat enlargement occurs as the kittens progress. Therefore very young kittens put with a foster mother with older kittens will find it difficult or even impossible to latch on to the teats. In addition to feeding, it must be remembered that very young kittens are dependent on their mother to stimulate their urination and defecation by licking them around the belly. This can be done for orphan kittens by gently stroking the belly with a finger or cotton bud. If the kittens get constipated, it is suggested that one part in six of heavy whipping cream be added to the milk diet.

Mastitis

This can occur in the acute or chronic form from the 2nd to 5th week of nursing kittens.

Acute mastitis

This occurs where jills with large mammary glands get them bruised in some way. It is important that they do have a large enough breeding box entry, which is flat and flush to the floor, with no ledge on which the jill can hit the glands (see Fig. 5.9). Ferrets in commercial breeding colonies do not have this problem, being in nursery cages. In a ferret compound with jill ferrets squabbling and receiving bites to the mammary glands, mastitis is a possibility. In a jill with kittens, once the kittens' teeth appear from 4 weeks of age, a mammary infection can occur and lead to mastitis.

Symptoms: The mammary glands look inflamed, are swollen and hard. The milk is discoloured or clotted and, in extreme cases, a mammary abscess forms. The infection can spread from gland to gland with the jill becoming more lethargic, dehydrated or even toxic and the acute stage can go quickly to an abscess and then gangrene (Fig. 5.20).

The jill must be separated from the kittens, which are hopefully self-feeding. As stated earlier, the jill starts to bring meat portions into the breeding box for the kittens to suck on and ingest around 4–5 weeks of age. Once the kittens' eyes are open, they can be hand-fed on meat.

Treatment: Immediate use of a broad-spectrum antibiotic is needed before the gland degenerates further into gangrene. It depends on the vigilance of the breeder checking his ferrets regularly to pick up early signs. In New Zealand, occurrence of mastitis (hard udder) in fitch farms had a variable prevalence and was recorded

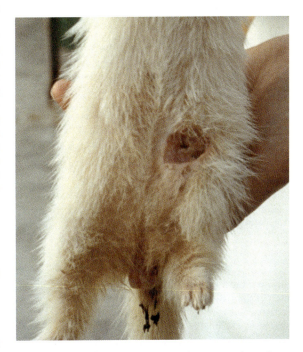

Figure 5.20 BEW jill, Heidi, a stray ferret sent down from Port Hedland for treatment. Mammary gland abscess, from dog bite wound, excised under ketamine/halothane anaesthesia.

CHAPTER FIVE
Reproduction and genetics

Author's clinical example

My BEW jill Patch, (1998) with five kittens, developed acute mastitis when the kittens were just over 4 weeks old and were taking meat with sharp temporary canines. She was found one morning flat on her stomach, listless and not letting the kittens feed. This is the 'flat ferret' syndrome, indicating pain. The posterior two mammary glands were affected, being hot and swollen. Patch was kept away from the kittens, which were put onto a sloppy mince and milk mixture diet. One gland went to an abscess 2 days after I discovered her sick. She had at first an injection of chloramphenicol (0.25 mL i.m.) and was then given clavulanic acid/amoxycillin (Clavulox palatable drops) by mouth (0.3 mL b.i.d.), while a pus culture was taken. This culture showed haemolytic *E. coli*, which proved sensitive to chloramphenicol, so a switch back was made, but giving chloramphenicol injectable by mouth. This involved using sugar water to mix it with because of the bitter taste. A repeat 4 days later found that the *E. coli* was now sensitive to Clavulox, so the combination was continued. The laboratory's explanation of this was the involvement of several colonies of *E. coli* differing in sensitivity, a complicated case. However, after vigorous dual antibiotic cover plus 'milking' the gland daily, flushing the hole in the gland and dressing it with Ungvita (vitamin A ointment, Roche) she recovered in 2 weeks from the time of first noticing the condition. When she was reunited with the kittens, she was wary of them at first, but as they were feeding on their own and not making demands, she accepted them back. It must be emphasized by this example that immediate treatment is required to stop the gland going into the necrosis stage. A veterinarian owned this subject ferret, but how soon would a non-veterinarian ferret breeder recognize the condition and get it treated? Ferret breeders must be advised on the dangerous nature of mastitis in ferrets, or the ferret could be lost for breeding, if not dead. The hygiene and husbandry must be kept up but it is difficult to know how to stop the young kittens nipping the mother's glands. It could occur when the jill is disturbed and gets up quickly possibly scattering the kittens.

on three farms at 3–50%. The treatment in commercial fitch farms, also mink farms, is to foster out or wean kittens, give the appropriate antibiotics and to lance abscesses.[18] On laboratory culture of pus, *E. coli* is common plus pure *Staph. aureus* infections, possibly a skin contaminant.[9] With pet or working ferrets, if the mastitis gets to the gangrene stage it can be removed under general anaesthetic though the glands can be handled without anaesthetic in many cases.

Chronic mastitis

If chronic mastitis occurs when the kittens are say 3 weeks of age, and they have stunted growth from lack of milk, it is considered that they should be removed from the jill for some time to allow the infected milk to pass through the intestine. It is difficult to stop transmission between jill and kittens. The kittens are washed, given oral medication[10] and given supplementary food until they can feed themselves. Chronic mastitis really needs vigorous attention under a general anaesthetic to save the glands and sometimes the jill's life.

Eye infections of newborn kittens

Swollen infected eyelids can occur in kittens with unopened eyes (ophthalmia neonatorum). Some authors consider it due to the jills' dragging the kittens around and causing minute teeth puncture marks in the eyelids.[7] Usually a jill in the nursery box moves the kittens round by 'nosing' them or grasping the scruff of older kittens

Author's clinical example

Lina, a 14-month-old sable jill (1988), had sustained a broken femur a year previously, which was successfully pinned (Ch. 19). She was mated and presented, when her kittens were 5 weeks old, with swollen mammary glands on the right side and the anterior gland prominent. She was typically pyrexic, lethargic and losing condition. She had been on a course of Amoxycillin drops (50 mg/mL) at 0.25 mL b.i.d. but had not responded, with the anterior mammary gland looking very swollen. Lina was given 0.25 mL ketamine i.m. and anaesthetized with halothane by mask. Under anaesthetic the anterior mammary gland was cut open to reveal copious pus. Subsequent culture revealed *Staph. aureus* sensitive to erythromycin, tetracyclines, chloramphenicol and Clavulox. The pus was squeezed out and a 10×10 mm hole left in the mammary gland which was dressed with sulphanilamide. After recovery from the operation, the jill was given 0.25 mL chloramphenicol i.m., which was considered the drug of choice for ferrets, while waiting for the above laboratory results. A daily dressing of the wound, which Lina tolerated, by working pus out and flushing with hydrogen peroxide improved the situation over 10 days in hospital. She was put on twice daily clavulanic acid/ amoxycillin (Clavulox palatable drops, Pfizer) at a higher dosage of the amoxycillin alone at 0.5 mL. p.o. She was then sent home with Clavulox drops and Ungvita (vitamin A ointment, Roche) for the wound, which cleared well. The kittens had been able to feed themselves.

Author's clinical example

Ophthalmia neonatorium

This case involved an 'indoor breeder' having a hob and jill in a large wire American-style cage in the sitting room, with upper and lower sleeping compartment.[19] Against my advice they let the ferrets mate but also left them in the same cage, the hob down and the jill up, though the ladder between the levels had been taken away. The hob still wanted a jill! When the jill had the kittens, she was an agitated first-time mother and the hob of course was interested in what was going on upstairs! Then four, day-old kittens out of eight, were presented, each with one obviously swollen eye which had arisen over 24 hours. They were treated at first by bathing the eye with Optrex (Boots) and then carefully separating the eyelids along the natural suture line using the cutting edge of a 25 gauge hypodermic needle exercising extreme caution against damaging the underlying eye. In fact, the pus holds the eyelids well up from the eye but the needle must not slip down (Fig. 5.21).

The pus was expressed and a cultured swab sample showed haemolytic *E. coli* sensitive to chloramphenicol. The eyes were washed with Optrex and dressed with Chlorsig eye drops (0.5% chloramphenicol, Sigma Co.) and in addition, Optichor eye ointment (chloramphenicol, Ilium Veterinary Products) was smeared around the periphery of the eyelid. *Note*: the kittens were first seen in the morning and returned to clinic in the evening after being returned to the jill for feeding. The hob had been removed to different quarters. The treatment requires to be given twice within 24 hours. If the kittens are left too long without treatment, the swollen eyes cause great discomfort and the kittens could stop sucking, which would be fatal. It has been shown earlier that it is not easy to hand-rear young kittens. The owner was advised on the treatment at home and they were checked 24 hours after the initial examination and had improved but the owner was to treat them for another 2 days. *Note*: the eyelids naturally fuse again until the eyes open from 4 weeks of age.

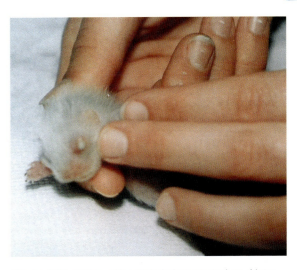

Figure 5.21 Kitten with ophthalmia neonatorium. *Note*: released pus globule.

General ferret feeding has been discussed for adult ferrets in Chapter 4. However, it will be seen right away that there is some difference of opinion on feeding ferrets. This is also the case when considering the pregnant jill, the jill with kittens and the young kittens. In American ferret-breeding colonies, the emphasis is on ad lib feeding of a prepared dry diet. When I started breeding ferrets, I did not have the American information at my fingertips. However, as stated in Chapter 4, I did find an actual daily diet for a laboratory ferret: '4 oz fresh meat daily plus 4 oz milk daily'. The pregnant jill and lactating jill should of course be fed with high quality animal protein and high fat content plus vitamins and minerals. The ideal ferret kitten is one strong-boned initially with a good carriage, which will put on body flesh more during the weaning period and in early adult life.

It is interesting that the 1967 UFAW Handbook (UK) on the care and management of laboratory ferrets states that kittens at 6 weeks of age will consume 2 oz (56 g) of meat and an equal weight of milk per day. A figure for the protein requirement of the young ferret is put at 7% of body weight. For Patch's two kittens at 8 weeks of age and weighing 425 g, that would be 30 g meat daily, which is about right. The feeding of ferrets could be said to have come full circle. My 25 g at 6 weeks of age would increase to 40–60 g daily for a jill and 60–80 g for hobs when mature, plus milk or milk supplement up to that time. In the UK, ferrets are considered ready to be weaned at 6 weeks of age, weighing 300–500 g.[2]

In American commercial ferret breeding, with ferrets on ad lib feeding, the Marshall Farms graph (see Fig. 4.2) shows kittens weighing 6–8 g at birth and 300 g

and dragging them around. However if a jill is alarmed in some way she might well pick the kittens up and move them. Pus causes the swollen eyelids, which must be separated gently to extrude the pus and allow treatment.

Feeding the pregnant and lactating jill plus kittens

Clients will ask 'How much do I feed my pregnant jill and the kittens?'

CHAPTER FIVE
Reproduction and genetics

Author's example
Feeding pregnant jills

After an initial ad lib overfeeding disaster resulting in overweight kittens in an early litter, I had two jills, Jenny and Wendy, who were fed differently. Jenny (2-year-old silver mitt) had a normal 'handful' of meat – around 100 g daily, while Wendy (3-year-old sable) got a measured 110 g (4 oz) daily. Why? I wanted to see how much food it would take to support a pregnant jill and a lactating jill with kittens and the 4 oz (110 g) was a starting point. A 'handful' of meat had been sufficient before with a jill, with a milk drink given daily.

Both ferrets were fed the meat in the evening as usual and consumed it overnight. This was done as a routine against meat spoiling in the hot weather. Unfortunately, the ferret mating season in WA is in the hotter time of the year. The ferrets used the nursery box for their litters in turn and because of the hot climate, meat was not left out during the day. The jills were each given milk early in the morning diluted 50:50 with water (about 220 mL) plus an additional water bowl. The meat as a mixture consisted of fatty mince, some rabbit if available, and an egg weekly: Animalac (Troy) milk supplement was sprinkled as powder over the meat. Thus Jenny was given around 100 g meat daily (wet weight) from mating, while Wendy was given an accurate 110 g and both were fed thus until the kittens got near weaning. Initially not all food was eaten, but progressively more was taken until all was consumed each day.

There was no problem with eclampsia, milk loss or anaemia with these two jills, nor any dystocia. Jenny (mated with BEW Goldie) had a previous litter being fed 'per handful' meat, while Wendy came from the ACT as 'new blood' to be mated with Simon (mitt). A comparative weight chart was kept of the two jills' kittens and weights for the recent jill Patch's kittens have been included also (Table 5.1).

From the Table 5.1 weight chart, a phenomenal weight gain can be seen in the kittens which can double or triple their birth weight in the first week of life. It is essential for the health of the kittens that they get the first colostrum milk like any infants. The ferret weight increase initially should be mostly in the skeleton and it is apparent that the calcium supply for both jills and kittens was adequate with diluted milk plus Animalac and rabbit bones when possible.

With Wendy and her eight kittens, at 6 weeks of age, she returned to being fed 110 g to build her up after the lactation period, while the kittens had 150 g of meat between them, theoretically 18 g for each kitten plus the milk supplement. Wendy's food gradually reduced to around 40–60 g daily. During the 6th week, four of the kittens were sold and in the 7th week postpartum, the remaining four kittens were fed 110 g as a trial together. Thus, around 25 g per kitten with the meat fed only in the evening and the milk supplement drink given 3 times daily could be taken as a base line for feeding weaned kittens. *Note*: in her next litter Wendy had 13 kittens and raised them all (Fig. 5.22)!

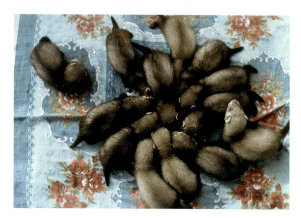

Figure 5.22 Jill, Wendy's second 1985 litter of 13 kittens at 6 weeks of age.

at 6 weeks of age. The graph shows the hobs go on to 1500 g as they mature and level out while the jills go to 900 g before they level out. The growth of Marshall Farms-reared kittens by their usual ad lib method can be compared with my kittens in Table 5.2. Dean Manning and Judith Bell[16] were associated with an attempt at hand-rearing kittens as a method of obtaining gnotobiotic ferrets as shown in Table 5.2. The weight results with their ferret kittens can also be compared with my kittens in Table 5.1.

My small sample of ferret kittens at 6 weeks of age puts them lower than the 'correct' weight at 6 weeks of age, but being lighter can be an advantage for a young animal providing they are getting good quality food. The kittens being fed separately from the jills from around 6 weeks of age were first fed around a communal bowl and then from individual bowls. As shown in Chapter 4, my adults are now fed separately on a wet meat diet.

It is stated by Marshall Farms that their ferrets on the dry diet double their weight from 4–6 weeks and again from 6–8 weeks. This is shown in Figure 4.2 and occurs on my jills' charts from 4–6 weeks of age. It is also stated that if kittens are given less than 30% protein and 20% fat, they grow, but look thin, have poor staring coats and will be susceptible to infection.[8] My young ferrets have shown healthy coats, so presumably were

Problems associated with ferret breeding

Table 5.2 Weight comparisons of gnotobiotic hand-fed kittens compared with conventionally nursed Marshall Farms kittens

Day of life	Body weight of conventionally nursed (g)	Body weight of gnotobiotic hand-fed (g)	Body weight of hand-fed as % of nursed controls
0 (birth)	9.2 (5)	10.9 (13)	118
5	21.6 (5)	11.9 (7)	55
8	35.4 (5)	13.2 (7)	37
11	47.5 (5)	17.1 (7)	36
14	61.2 (5)	23.3 (5)	38
17	84.3 (5)	8.1 (3)	45
20	103.5 (5)	58.9 (2)	57
23	129.1 (5)	77.9 (2)	60
26	155.1 (5)	100.2 (2)	65
29	170.0 (5)	130.5 (2)	77
31	181.6 (5)	147.7 (2)	79

Numbers in brackets indicate the number of ferret kittens.
(This table was originally published within the article entitled Reproductive Failure in Mink and Ferrets after Intravenous or Oral Inoculation of Campylobacter jejuni (Can J Vet Res 1990; 54:432–437). The table is used here with the kind permission of the Canadian Veterinary Medical Association.)

on good protein plus possibly stimulated by the outdoor environment once they were out of the nursery cage and into the garden. The growth curve for New Zealand Fitch ferret kittens (see Fig. 4.3) is much steeper that for Marshall Farms ferrets, indicating a more rapid growth for fur production.

Jill ferrets produce large amounts of 20% fat milk for the kittens between 3–4 weeks of lactation and they can lose condition if fed less than 25.5% fat diet. Again, my jills did lose some weight during lactation but, after the kittens were weaned, soon put it back on again, on a fresh meat diet and mineral/vitamin supplement. Ferreters with nursing jills had an advantage over me by being able to supply rabbit meat plus offal regularly but in recent times rabbit numbers have been depleted by the calicivirus infection. Marshall Farms breeding colonies do well on their diets with 30–40% protein and they know that conception rates and litter sizes will drop if the protein level falls below 30% even for a short time.[8]
My kittens were given meat once daily at night plus milk available either as 50/50 diluted milk or a milk supplement. With commercial ferret breeding at Marshall Farms, the emphasis is on feeding kittens ad lib, which specifies feeding the jill, and kittens of 3–12 weeks of age, a wet diet that is made up by adding water, beef fat and cooked egg to their pelleted food. This makes up the fat content to 30% from 23% plus a protein content of meal at 40%. It is noted that ferret kittens before their eyes open will smell the wet food and climb out of the nursery box to feed from 3 weeks of age (J. Bell, pers. comm. 1993). This differs from my jills taking wet meat into the nursery box when the kittens are 4–5 weeks of age. The wet porridge mixture of the breeding establishment probably does not lend itself to the jill doing that for the kittens.

A Perth ferret breeder fed a selection of ingredients to her kittens, which included boiled chicken, chicken giblets, hamburger mince, fish (sardines) and diced kangaroo. All or some of these ingredients were mixed in a bowl and fed to all kittens 3 times a day but not on a weight basis. Chicken is a good fat source and kangaroo meat a high protein source (Julie Usher, President, Ferrets Southern Districts Club, Perth, pers. comm. 1998). As for vitamin/mineral sources, she used a lactose-free milk or Di-Vetelact, or Calcium Sandoz syrup (latter to be added to milk). I gave up using Di-Vetelact on a long-term basis, as I have had a possible cataract problem in ferrets using it (Ch. 12). She also used Heinz high protein baby cereal and ad lib Supercoat Real Choice dry cat food both of which I would avoid, as the primary food list should adequately cover the kittens' needs.

In my experience with breeding ferrets outside in the WA climate, the routine is to feed the jill and kittens so they eat overnight, *plus* a milk drink in the morning. Fresh water is always available. This system works and is carried out by other ferret breeders.

CHAPTER FIVE
Reproduction and genetics

Author's clinical example

My 1-year-old BEW jill (1998), Patch, was mated with my 1-year-old silver mitt hob, Boysie. She had 11 kittens but lost six in a couple of days; it was her first litter. Patch had been taken in as an unwanted ferret, previously fed on dog food (Ch. 4). She easily became agitated although was not averse to being handled. She had the 11 kittens between 8.30 a.m. and 1.30 p.m., while I was working and not overnight as other jills. She was to be fed 110 g meat plus non-lactose milk during pregnancy, but after parturition she refused all meat for nearly 2 weeks and had only the milk drink. Jills usually go off their food prior to parturition. One UK author advises not to overfeed the nursing jill during the first 2 days after birth of the kittens, as she could develop a mastitis.[2] Patch nursed the five remaining kittens well but to make things more interesting, she developed mastitis when the kittens were 4.5 weeks old and had to be separated from them as described previously in the mastitis section. The five kittens, all hobs, one silver mitt and four black-eyed whites, were reared on mince once daily soaked in the non-lactose milk. (Patch had been seen taking meat into the nursery sleeping box for the kittens the day before she fell sick.) Figure 5.23 shows four of Patch's kittens being fed separately. The kittens first had 50 g meat between five of them plus non-lactose milk, then 20 g each at 4 weeks and 25 g each at 6 weeks.

They were kept at the veterinary hospital during the day and in the home nursery at night. The kittens' eyes opened fully by 6 weeks of age and they became playful and active but still slept a lot. Three kittens were sold at 6 weeks of age and the remaining two at 8 weeks, with three kittens going to be used for ferreting in the country.

The kittens were weighed weekly and Table 5.1 shows the relationship of the five surviving kittens' average weight to those of Jenny and Wendy. The lost kittens had also been weighed. Jills carrying large numbers of fetuses, over eight, would produce litters of smaller weight, under 10 g, and these would be progressively underweight during nursing.[8]

Wendy again mated with Simon, and on a 'per handful' meat diet plus diluted milk had 13 kittens weighing on average 70.75 g at 5 weeks of age, compared to her previous litter weight of around 170 g. At 6 weeks of age, the kittens weighed 110 g against the 263 g for the previous litter, that is 13 kittens against 8 kittens reared. The 'per handful' of meat daily weighed 100 g and this was increased to 175 g daily. The kittens went on to gain weight and were sold at 8 weeks of age, at around 400 g.

Wendy reared her next litter of 12 kittens on a 'per handful' meat diet and milk but ran into trouble with small weight kittens of 109.5 g at 5 weeks of age. Six of the kittens showed a 'spay-legged' condition where their forelegs were not correctly under the chest carriage but splayed out and the kittens had a 'shuffling' movement. These were separated from the rest and given a mineral/vitamin supplement (Di-Vetelact, Sharpe Labs) daily plus calcium powder on their meat nightly. The weak kittens grew stronger by the day and got onto their front legs in the normal way and became active. However, they tended to have a 'swing-out' action of the forelegs, with the legs not completely tucked under the body. At 9 weeks of age, they were able to be sold as active kittens and had no further troubles. This illustrates a complication in kitten development. Besides the diet, the advancing age of the jill might have been a factor causing the condition.

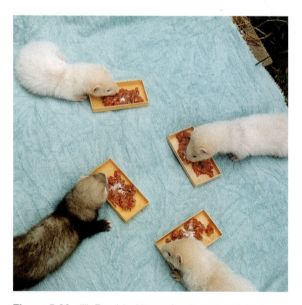

Figure 5.23 Jill, Patch's, kittens feeding on weighed amount of food.

Pseudopregnancy

Lack of conception can lead to pseudopregnancy in jills. The jill's vulva does not immediately decrease in size. With my ferrets, I have rarely experienced pseudopregnancy but many American breeders have. It has been caused by mating with a vasectomized hob. Using human gonadotropin or cystorelin (USA) can give rise to it or by a simple mating with a sterile or weak sperm count hob. *Note*: older males will have greater sperm viability than just-mature males. The pseudopregnancy is not harmful and can be used as a measure to prevent the jill drifting into post-oestrous anaemia (POA).

Jills in false pregnancy behave as if they were pregnant. They put on weight, have mammary gland development and go to a nesting behaviour at the 'whelping' time. They can become very 'loving' to the ferret owner. They store toys, e.g. foam sponges stolen from the kitchen, as 'babies' after 'whelping'.

One of my jills, Susie, in false pregnancy, followed me at heel like a dog. In the ferretarium, she would be taking leaves down the bolthole to make a nursery nest. Once the 'whelping' stage occurs the jill cycles back into normality. If pseudopregnancy has occurred at the end of the mating season, the jill will remain quiescent till the next season. If it is after the first heat, she will come back in heat in 2 weeks for mating.

Breeders can learn the signs indicating pseudopregnancy. The jill grows a beautiful coat at about 1.5 weeks before the 'whelping'. Normal pregnant jills lose their coats about 1.5 weeks before whelping plus developing hairless rings around the teats. The normal pregnant jills grow their coats more slowly than the false pregnant jills.

Pseudopregnancy can be related to implantation failure due to a photo-period effect or to reduced light intensity 1 month before mating. It has been seen in New Zealand fitch farms, being a common occurrence registering 35–70% on some farms.[18] If a recently-mated jill is caged with an unmated jill, the latter gets the hob smell off the mated jill and goes into pseudopregnancy.[2] Commercial ferret/mink farms in New Zealand controlled pseudopregnancy tendencies[18] by:

1. Ensuring maximum light intensity in breeding units in spring and artificially extending light hours in late summer, which are of course practical in housed ferret/mink farms. At Marshall Farms, the breeding rooms have light via translucent panels high on the walls. When the natural light declines during late July until January, the ferrets can be put on a 17-h daylight period using 8-foot fluorescent tubes running the whole length of the building (J. Bell, pers. comm. 1993).
2. The hob ferrets used must be mature before mating and techniques such as testicle size measurement are done. The older hob may become sterile in time.
3. It is possible to sperm-test hobs after each mating.
4. Commercial breeders supplement food with vitamin E to improve fertility (10 g/100 kg of feed).

Important note: Pseudopregnancy may lead to hormonal problems in the jill's future if she is continually missing conception. I have had a sterile jill with an ovarian tumour discovered when she was spayed (Ch. 13). If the jill naturally goes into false pregnancy, perhaps sterilizing the jill or retiring the hob is the practical option for private breeders.

The 'swimmers'

This condition has been seen in Australian ferrets over some time.[20] It is under investigation and there is always the possibility it may be genetic, as the gene pool of ferrets has not been added to since the early 1990s. Normally growing kittens can double or treble their body weight in the first week of life. If for any fault, the skeleton is not up to supporting the burst of growth and consequent increase in body weight as distinct from skeletal weight, the animal is in trouble (Fig. 5.24).

The condition of 'swimmers' or spay-legged kittens has been discussed with regard to my jill Wendy's last litter. In practice, the kittens do not get up. The basis is a lack of strength in all limbs leading to the kitten being unable to bear the weight of the body mass. The general view is that the legs may rotate to a far greater extent than normal and the danger comes from the ribs not being able to support the chest.[20] Breathing is thus impaired by the ribs relatively collapsing and obliterating the chest space. Anoxia occurs and the kittens die within 8 weeks.

The condition could be a type of animal 'rickets' or nutritional hyperparathyroidism with the bones failing to develop strength (Ch. 4). It could also be the jill being overfed with the kittens putting on body weight too soon before the limbs have strengthened up. I had this happen when I was inexperienced with ferrets and our second ferret additions, littermates Peter Pan and Wendy, mated by mistake and produced six kittens. I know now I was overfeeding the jill (and kittens) and she produced kittens too heavy for their limbs. Though

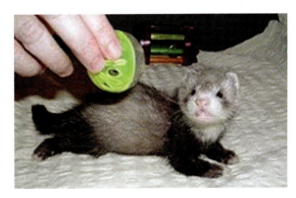

Figure 5.24 'Swimmer' kitten. (Courtesy of Val Hutcheon 2005.)

she was getting plenty of milk and calcium the body protein/fat mass overcame the limb strength. The bones can be soft and easily fractured. Smith has indicated mammals can develop a 'soft bone' syndrome paralleling rickets where their nutrition fails to deliver enough calcium or phosphorus and there might be a genetic fault involved. Osteogenesis imperfecta is the human condition and is apparently genetic. Human breast milk is said to be vitamin D deficient and can leads to rickets in children. Geoff Smith (South Australian Ferret Association) had littermates producing eight swimmer kittens where six died.[20] The surviving two were worked on and survived for 7 years but as cripples. Post mortems on the dead kittens showed the bones had a poor calcium matrix.

Another South Australian ferret breeder recently had a jill, Josie, deliver 11 kittens on 23 December 2005. She was not fully attentive to the kits and four died soon after birth. Six kits appeared normal in size and health but there was one runt jill kit. Over the next 7 weeks, the kits grew normally; the little jill hung on but was two-thirds the size of the others.

On 17 January 2006 she appeared to have seven beautiful sable and sandy coloured kits thriving. Their diet consisted of raw mince, cooked (shredded) chicken, raw chicken wings, a once only helping of 'wet' cat food, diluted milk and diced hearts, all supplemented with calcium. Also some servings of Nutripet vitamin supplement. On 10 February, the breeder noticed a change. Four of the kittens were looking odd and gave the appearance of 'swimmers'. Three were severely affected with spinal curvature and joint abnormality. They gave the appearance of having rickets. Their necks seemed to 'disappear'; their appearance was 'hunched' with limited movement behind. The more severely affected had rapid respirations more than the other kits. They were stressed and weak and though eating, drinking, urinating and defecating, they could not raise their rears to clear the mess. The breeder noted that the 'swimmers' were sables and had what she called 'particularly sweet faces'. She had seen the 'swimmers' condition before and noted the same facial features (Val Hutcheon, pers. comm. 2005).

These kittens differed from my original disaster as they had been moving around to some extent but mine never got up on their four legs. They were put to sleep. I have treated this condition in other kits in the past with some success. I advise a combination of stopping feeding excessive meat to the kittens and giving them just a high vitamin supplement like Animalac as a drink. A small amount of meat can be given with calcium powder mixed in. In addition, the kittens get physiotherapy with a warm water bath swimming and physically moving the limbs under the body as many times a day as possible. The sooner they are seen as 'swimmers', the better. The treatment needs to get results quickly in the growing bones.

I advised the treatment combination and Josie's kittens began to thrive on Animalac (Troy). The kits gradually became stronger over a period of weeks and their respiratory symptoms disappeared. All but one were successful in getting to the scats area and keeping themselves clean.

The kits were started on canned sardines (high calcium) by the breeder and they continued to move about better with the most severely affected one able to move about (with difficulty) but stronger. I would have thought the Animalac alone with calcium powder would have sufficed, but no matter, the kits maintained improvement. However, at 5 months the kits had grown a lot, the spinal curvature was still evident and bow legs and hind leg abnormalities remained but they could all move around quite rapidly albeit unusually.

One can imagine that once the soft body weight was taken off and the stronger bones brought the 'carriage' up from the ground, things were on the mend. Then body weight can be added.

Although hob ferrets are separated from the pregnant jill and lactating jill they can be put with the young kittens later. Thus, Figure 5.25 shows Boysie in his 'castle' with his offspring from a mating with Patch.

There has been some attempt to interbreed pet ferrets with the native wild polecat in the UK (Dr J. McNicholas, pers. comm. 2005). A good idea in theory to perhaps improve the ferret gene pool but it must be remembered that any first crosses are nervous and aggressive, making them useless as pet or working ferrets. Attempts to give pet ferrets a darker colouration,

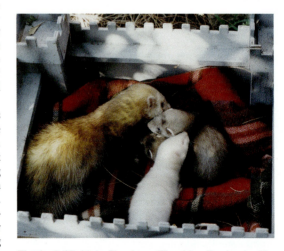

Figure 5.25 Hob, Boysie, sniffing his offspring by jill, Patch, in his 'castle'.

nose pigmentation, etc. are the aims of some breeders. Showing the 'new' ferrets comes generations on! It would need ferret/polecat crosses to be bred for some generations with plenty of handling of kittens to get them up to the present domestication state of pet ferrets. However, Georg Symonds and others, in New Zealand, commented in the past that feral ferrets at least can be quickly re-domesticated.

A profile of ferret genetics on current information

I am not a geneticist, but am attempting to give a general description of ferret genetics from basic breeding ideas. I have bred several litters of ferrets myself in the past. The genetics of skin and coat colour in domesticated animals involving studies with horses, cattle, pigs and cats is well documented by Nes et al.[21] and other researchers, but most genetics research on ferrets is related to their suitability as a model for studying disease in humans, rather than on their coat colour. Knowledge of ferret genetics is improving with the genome (genetic information) of the ferret currently being investigated (C. Johnson-Delaney, pers. comm. 2005). The genomic homology of the domestic ferret with cats and humans has been established.[22] Investigators used a chromosome painting technique to directly confirm chromosomal homology between parts of the karyotype (external appearance of chromosomes) of both the domestic cat and human with that of the domesticated ferret. The data indicated that the ferret had a highly conserved karyotype closer to that of the ancestral carnivore than the cat.

Research work has been carried out on coat colour in commercial mink, *M. vison*, in North America.[23] Mink colour coat varieties are well-established genetically, having been evolved through a selection of variations of colour genes.[21] Thus, the wild genotype for colour, with no mutations, is registered as Standard and colours ranging from dark brown (wild mink found in nature and the colour type 'Wild mink') to the strongly-selected farm mink, Black Standard, which is totally black, due to selection for the dark colour in the past 40 generations. In mink, there are at least three major gene loci for coat and eye colour, mutations which will interact to produce various colour varieties.[24] These major genes are in turn influenced by numerous modifying genes resulting in about 200 possible variants or phases with only a few colours being commercially produced. These are registered as Black Standard, Sapphire, Silverblue, Pearl and Pastel Sapphire. (Incidentally, escaped or released mink, living wild in the UK, are now mostly black with a white spot on the chin. They have bred out most of the other colours that were selectively bred for originally, though there are some pockets of brown mink.)[25]

Unconscious genetic selection occurred from the first instance of man's association with ferrets by using them for hunting. As with any domesticated animal, this was done by taking the young and taming them over time and breeding to keep the line. Interest in early times would have been mainly in the docility of ferrets, their fitness, physique and intelligence (see Bob Church, Ch. 6, for ferret-polecat domestication, with an extensive bibliography).

Study of the genetics of coat colour in ferrets is less advanced than in some other domesticated animal species. It is only recently, due to the popularity of ferrets as pets, especially in America, and the desire for a variety of ferret coat colours for showing, that interest has increased. Private ferret breeders like Fara Shimbo (below), produced practical ideas of coat colouring based on comparative ideas of breeding in other animals.

Basic concepts

The appearance of a ferret is the sum of its observable or detectable characteristics and is called its *phenotype*. It is the expression of its genetic make-up or *genotype*. The genetic information of an individual is carried in the double helical structure of the DNA molecule, which is coiled upon itself many times to form a *chromosome*. Every animal (and plant) has a definite number of chromosomes in each cell. The ferret has 40 chromosomes, of which 20 came in the egg from the jill and 20 in the sperm from the hob, so it has two complete sets of genetic information. (The egg and sperm are known as *gametes*.) This genetic information is organized into *genes*, each of which occupies a particular place or *locus* (plural loci) on a chromosome, so that a particular gene found at a particular locus on maternal chromosome #2 will have a pair at the same locus on paternal chromosome #2. (The two #2 chromosomes are said to be *homologous*, so the ferret has 19 pairs of homologous chromosomes plus the sex chromosomes, XX for a female, XY for a male.)

Each gene codes for a particular protein to be made in a specific way and often at a specific time. The proteins may be involved with the appearance, structure or function of the body and depending on when, how and in what quantity each protein is made, either one or, more usually, several traits may be affected. A particular gene may, through slight molecular changes in the DNA over time (*mutations*), exist in several variants or *alleles*. The genetic information in various alleles may differ, so that different proteins are produced, which may not function in the body in the same way and can have unexpected effects. As each cell has two copies of a gene, the alleles may be the same, in which case it is said to be *homozygous* for that gene, or they may be different, the *heterozygous* condition. Any allele which will make itself evident (i.e. produce its protein) regardless of the other allele of the same gene is said to be *dominant*. An allele, which makes itself known only in the presence of another identical allele, is called *recessive*, because its effects recede behind those of the dominant allele. So dominant alleles will always express themselves in the phenotype and overcome the other recessive alleles. Dominant alleles of genes are represented by italic capital letters and recessive alleles by italic lower case letters.

Sometimes a cross between two different phenotypes produces a third phenotype unlike either parent. Where the parental traits appear to be blended, e.g. black coat crossed with white coat producing grey coat (roan), incomplete or partial dominance is involved. Where both parental traits are seen, but incompletely, e.g. black coat crossed with white coat giving a black-and-white spotted coat, co-dominance is involved.

Coat colour in ferrets arises from a combination of several genes acting together to produce the final colour of the particular animal. *Epistasis* refers to interactions between genes (but not between alleles of a gene). A gene is epistatic when it influences the phenotypic expression of another gene. With many thousands of genes and their possible numbers of alleles, it can be seen that, except in the case of identical twins, each individual carries unique genetic information.

Ferret breeding

As Brett Middleton (Ferret Genetics Forum 2005) suggests, it would have been helpful if ferret breeders in the past had kept accurate records of parentage and important characteristics of the animals such as coat colour, pattern, size, shape, weight, etc. as in other domesticated species. Unless the proper description of pigmentation of both the guard coat and undercoat, as well as skin pigment and markings, is understood, it might never be possible to nail down ferret colours except, maybe, in the broadest of terms (B. Middleton, pers. comm. 2005). He considers that ideas of colour genetics in dogs and horses are not as scientifically established as one might think but are better known than ferret genetics. He points out that horse, cow and dog breeders have the advantage of producing dozens or hundreds of progeny each year for data purposes. Only big ferret breeding establishments such as Marshall Farms or Path Valley have the numbers for extensive trials over many generations.

Another comment on ferret coat colour has been made by Christina Bernard who declares it is not possible to correlate ferret coat colour genes with the colour genes described in other mammals with the possible exception of the albino or C locus. (The basic coat colours have been described in Ch. 2.) For all other colour genes, we can only extrapolate from what is known about colour genes in other species and make intelligent guesses.

Fara Shimbo in Colorado did excellent earlier work on breeding pet ferrets, which is worth looking at.[26,27] Fara had an interest in horse breeding and keen observations from breeding her own colony of pet ferrets. She gives basic ideas about breeding for coat colour. *Note*: ferrets, like cats, have three types of hair covering, smooth guard hairs, awn hairs which are smaller and wavy, and short undercoat hairs. Undercoat colour is inherited independently of the colour of guard hairs, with a few exceptions caused by patterns. Ferrets of any colour (black, sable, chocolate or champagne) may have white, cream, ivory, buff, yellow or maize undercoats. This genetic consideration of ferret coat colour involves the guard and awn hairs only, not the undercoat.

The colour of a mammal's coat and skin is caused by the pigment, melanin, which also occurs in the retina and other layers of the eye, and certain nerve cells as *melanosomes* (pigment granules) in *melanocytes* (pigment cells). In an animal where melanin is completely lacking the coat and skin appear white and the eyes pink as the irises are virtually transparent so the blood vessels in the retina and sclera are visible. Such an animal is an albino; this is a classic variation recognized in Greek and Roman times. Albinos occur in wild animal populations but are seldom seen because they are more conspicuous to predators and have eyesight and hearing problems, so are less likely to survive long enough to breed, but under the protection of domestication they may be preferred as they are easier to distinguish from prey and to retrieve when used for hunting.

C locus – complete expression of colour/albino

This gene exists in all mammals and is responsible for producing the enzyme tyrosinase which controls the synthesis of melanin from the amino acid tyrosine. If a ferret carries two non-functioning alleles (*cc*) on the *C* locus no pigment will be produced (Shimbo). The chain reaction from tyrosine to melanin is not completed and, as the break can be fairly far down the chain, other regions requiring other products are affected, leading to vision and hearing impairment. (In many species, extensive breeding for colour mutation has caused animals who have red eyes and extremely pale colouration, such as the American palosilver mink. The fact that an animal has red eyes alone does not make it an albino – there must be both red eyes and a complete lack of colour to skin and coat.)

If the gene which produces the pigment for colour does not work, i.e. the ferret carries cc, any other genes for colour cannot produce it and the ferret is automatically albino. It would carry a full compliment of pigment cells which contain no pigment because it lacks the enzyme for the conversion of tyrosine to melanin.

The dominant form C is called 'full colour' as discussed by Christina Bernard. In mice, there are at least 103 phenotypic lower series alleles on the C locus, causing other dilution effects to coat colours. Bernard discusses the effects of three of these in changing coat colour.[28]

Chinchilla (c^{ch}): this lightens most coat colours to grey and the eyes are black. Chinchilla is recessive to full colour but dominant to extreme dilution, platinum and albino.

Extreme Dilution Tyr (c^e): here the hair is very light grey and eyes are dark. Extreme dilution is recessive to full colour and chinchilla but dominant to platinum and albino.

Platinum or champagne (c^p): this is seen in ferrets and polecats and is known in the fur trade as 'pastel' or in show ferrets as 'champagne' colour wash.[26] The c^p allele seems to disrupt the chain of pigment formation so that very little pigment is added to the hairs as they grow. (The same effect can occur in other domestic animals by similar versions of the allele, e.g. palomino horses.) The location of the c^p allele on the albino C locus was confirmed in Finland in 1987. The champagne colour c^p is recessive to full colour, chinchilla and extreme dilution but dominant to albino, so that the ferret which carries Cc^p would be coloured normally as is one carrying Cc. A ferret carrying c^pc or c^pc^p would show the champagne colouration.

According to Fara Shimbo, other genes besides the C locus (complete expression of colour) affecting colour in ferrets at various loci include: B locus (brown pigment), D locus (dilution/normal pigmentation of hairs), A locus (agouti/self), I locus (inhibitor/full penetration of colour), S^i locus (Irish spotting/no markings), S^{ab} locus (silver mitt/no silvering), G locus/R locus (grey or 'roan'/ no greying), and M locus (merle/no mottling), all of which Fara Shimbo studied in the early 1990s. Another locus mentioned by Christine Barnard is the extension or E locus.

E locus – extension or MC1R

Melanin occurs in two forms, eumelanin (dark brown and black) and phaeomelanin (red and yellow). This locus controls which of these forms are present – it is the gene for red hair! This gene produces the melanocyte-stimulating receptor (MC1R) which, in the presence of alpha-melanocyte-stimulating hormone (MSH), causes the melanocytes to produce more tyrosinase in order to convert phaeomelanin to eumelanin. If there is no MC1R, the MSH message goes unheeded and the result is gingery-red colouration rather than black or brown. This 'erythristic' variety was documented in wild polecat populations by Frances Pitt in Cardiganshire, Wales, in the early 1900s. The colouration in wild polecats was described as a 'reddish-brown which, when seen in sunlight, shows a kind of faint purple "haze"'. In erythristic ferrets, the exact tint of the fur is best described by the word 'sandy'; the colour tint is confined to the long outer hair, the woolly undercoat being white. She also noted that erythristic ferrets were more difficult to handle than either dark or albino ferrets, and more inclined to 'snap'. She compared this with the hot temperaments of red-haired people and chestnut horses![29]

B locus – brown pigment

This locus codes for the enzyme tyrosine-related protein-1 (TRP-1), which catalyzes the final step in eumelanin production, that of changing brown pigment to black pigment. The gene variant lightens only eumelanin (black)-based colours. The pigment of the hair is brown rather than black with the pigment granules appearing rather smaller and rounder in shape than normal black pigment granules.

Fara Shimbo stated that the dominant allele B produced the full colour, black, in ferrets called sable. The recessive allele b produced the brown pigment, giving the colouration called chocolate in ferrets and cats, mahogany in fur farm ferrets and socklot in mink. It is thought that the chocolate mutation in ferrets came from Scotland via fitch farms (Ch. 4).

D locus – dilution/normal hair pigmentation

This locus codes for the enzyme tyrosine-related protein-2 (TRP-2) where mutations have a dilution effect on genotypes that otherwise provide for an intensely-pigmented coat colour. This effect is not due to a reduction in the amount of hair pigment, in fact mutations at the D locus result in phenotypes that may have more hair pigment than corresponding non-dilute ferrets. The effect is on the distribution of pigment within the hairs. In the dilute phenotype, one- to two-thirds of the pigment is deposited into a few large clumps which have very little effect on light absorption. Diluted black eumelanin appears grey, diluted brown eumelanin appears light brown and diluted red phaeomelanin appears to be cream. It is as if the clumping of the pigment on the hair causes almost microscopic mottling of pigmented areas alternating with areas of no pigment (Fara Shimbo). The hair appears 'blue' if the ferret is black or sable, or 'lilac' if the ferret is chocolate. (*Note*: the *D* locus in mink contains several allelic forms so there is possibly a locus of the same type in ferrets.)

A locus – agouti/self

This determines where and how much dark and light pigment is distributed in the hair. On it depends the banding effect of the guard hair, with dark-coloured tip and base and pale middle. If a ferret carries two non-agouti alleles its hair colour will be solid i.e. without banding. The *A* locus is one of many genes which produce patterns by modifying the way either red or black pigments or both are distributed over the animal as a whole (Fara Shimbo). Seeing the action of the *A* locus in ferrets is typically difficult because of the complicating factor that over most of its body the undercoat of the ferret is visible, making the ferret appear lighter in colour and gradations of topcoat tone more difficult to see.

One pattern marking of the *A* locus is self ferret. Here all the guard hairs on the body, including those of the mask and barrel (body) excepting only the muzzle, ears, and forehead, are the same colour. Black selfs are known from Germany and Spain but a link is suspected to past cross-breeding with mink (see Fig. 2.9). If the undercoat was not visible on self ferrets, they would be solid coloured – solid black, sable, chocolate or champagne. The mask often runs into the throat, and the 'baby bar' remains even in the winter when it would otherwise disappear. The inheritance of self pattern is not clear but appears to be due to a recessive gene '*a*'. Selfs bred to selfs throw about half selfs, and the rest standards and points.

However, it is possible that standards (another allele on this locus) and points seen in such litters are really 'optical illusions' and are all self points. *Note*: in crosses of European polecats, which are black self-coloured, with domesticated ferrets, the result is black or sable self-coloured hybrid kits. True self-coloured ferrets are rare.

The standard pattern allele is completely dominant. It is the most common colouration of ferrets and most common type of pattern in all the other mustelids. It consists of dark areas on the legs, throat and chest and a darker stripe down the back extending to the tail called a 'grotzen'. In standards, the guard hairs of the points, back and neck are black or sable and the hairs of the barrel and belly, and sometimes the mask, are dark umber. Standard ferrets bred to standards throw overwhelmingly standard kits, with some selfs and some points.

The bay point pattern, is the normal colour of the western population of *Mustela eversmanni*, the steppe polecat. The black pigment is restricted to the animal's points and the red pigment of the undercoat shows through wherever it is absent.

Coat colours and shades have been researched for the effects of mutations at *B* and *D* loci using laboratory mice and effects have been seen also in dogs and cats, etc. It is suggested that they affect ferrets too.

I locus – inhibitor/full penetration of colour gene

The function of the gene at the *I* locus is to inhibit or suppress the amount of pigment inserted into each hair, especially in those areas where the hairs are naturally thinner or where, as in the case of the standard pattern, hairs are normally lighter to begin with. Additionally, this is one of the only cases where the undercoat is lighter as well. In self pattern, the entire length of the hair is pigmented down to the root. In the standard pattern, it is pigmented for the upper two-thirds of its length while in the point pattern, produced by the recessive allele i^p, only half the hair is pigmented. Self pattern and point can appear with any colour and are shown below.

S^i locus – Irish spotting/no markings

Shimbo defines common patterns of white markings in definite areas (feet, bib and perhaps some white on the face, head, nape, stomach and tail) as 'Irish spotting' in most domestic animals and 'mitt' in ferrets. Mitt/Irish spotting in horses, dogs and ferrets is recessive, thus crosses of 'four white feet' or 'mitt to mitt' breed true. Mitt can occur in any colour and/or pattern (though will be invisible in an albino). The types are demonstrated in Figures 5.26–5.29 and an Australian mitt is shown in Figure 2.3.

The extent of the mitts, whether they cover just the toes or go up to the wrists, or of the bib, are controlled by multiple modifying factors and thus their inheritance is unclear. There can be head, nape, belly, or tail spots. Almost all mitted ferrets will grey with age, usually between 2 and 4 years. Mitts are inherited independently of colour, patterns and other types of marking according to Shimbo. (Any mitt ferret with a head blaze and mitts which are partial and not evenly margined could be considered as having signs of neural crest variant, see below (S. Crandall, pers. comm. 2005).)

S^{ab} locus – silvermitt/no silvering

Shimbo talked of the silvermitt having only one other analogue in the domesticated animal world, the Sabino

A profile of ferret genetics on current information

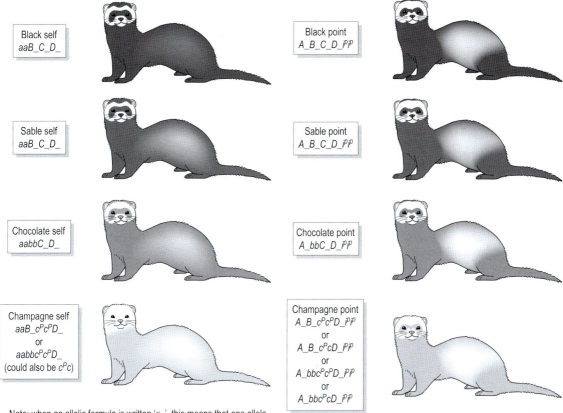

Figure 5.26 The self pattern may appear with any colour as indicated.

Note: when an allelic formula is written '$x\_$', this means that one allele must be x, but it does not matter what the other allele on that locus is.

Figure 5.27 The point pattern.

horse, with the phenomenon being recessive in ferrets. Silvermitt and mitt can occur; both can have white throats. In the mitt the white of the feet stops at the wrist and the edge is clear and distinct, but with silvermitt the white may extend to the elbow. It may run as an irregular line up the inside of the leg.

In the homozygous dominant and heterozygous ferret, no intermingling of white hairs on the body, other than that due to roaning or point pattern, will be seen. In the homozygous recessive ferret, there are four white mitts with indistinct edges, there may be belly spots and tail spots, there will usually be a full bib, and almost always headlight. She talks of silvermitt occurring with any colour or pattern except S^i.

G locus/R locus – grey or 'roan'/no greying

Going white or being nearly white from birth is common among domesticated animals but extremely rare in the wild. *Note*: progressive greying is found in ferrets, dogs and horses but not in cats. In ferrets, progressive greying seems to be a simple recessive, likely *gr*. In most animals, grey/roan is dominant and some alleles on the *R* locus are lethal in the homozygous dominant state.

Note: the Russian ferrets illustrated in Chapter 2 indicate genetic colouring related to the type of melanin present. Putting aside the albino, the pearl (see Fig. 2.6) (silvery) colour is a ferret with little or no phaeomelanin (*C* locus). The goldish ferret (see Fig. 2.7) has little or no eumelanin (*E* locus). The pastel (see Fig. 2.8) can have any colour in dilution (*D* locus) (Christine Bernard, pers. comm. 2005).

Fara Shimbo saw anomalies in the colours of some ferrets: sables with large white markings, apricot-coloured animals with white guard hairs and plum coloured eyes, coffee-coloured ferrets and finally 'red' ferrets who have sable guard hairs but whose underfur is distinctly ruddy. She has noted albinos who remain

CHAPTER FIVE
Reproduction and genetics

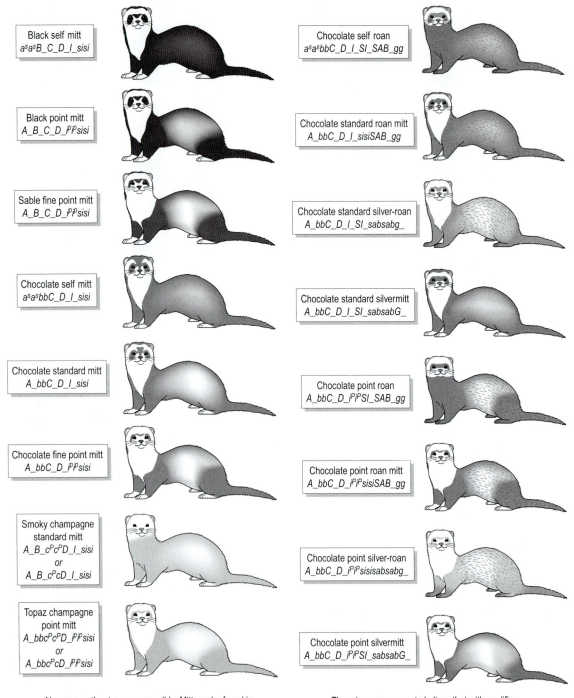

Figure 5.28 Mitt illustrated.

Numerous other types are possible. Mitt can be found in combination with colour and patterns produced at all other loci.

Figure 5.29 Silvermitts, roans, and silver roans add to the types of coat colour.

There is some reason to believe that with modifiers, *sabsabgg* may result in a pigmented-eyed white.

112

white and others who turn to a very deep gold in winter, when every animal gets more colour to their underfur.

Fara Shimbo also noted eye colour features. In the cat, eye colour is inherited independently of coat colour. In the ferret, black/brown/hazel eye colours appear to be influenced by the same genes that control coat colour, i.e. darker ferrets have darker eyes when their eyes are brown. However, presence of any white on the face especially the muzzle, appears to alter eye colour in a regular way. Dark self or standard ferrets often have hazel/green eyes if the white of the muzzle touches the eyelids; chocolate ferrets in like condition may have gray eyes. Interestingly, denim blue or deep blue-green eyes are possible when muzzle white or other head white markings touch the eyelids. It also occurs when the entire head or body is white.

Note that eye colour involves the iris, not the colour of eyeshine. It is best to examine the iris in strong daylight when the pupils will close down and eyeshine is not a confusing factor.

Results of ferret crosses

Fara Shimbo showed the results of some matings involving the C locus and gave examples in the form of the Punnett square. (This was devised by geneticist Professor Reginald Punnett (1875–1967) and is still used by biologists and breeders to predict possible genotypes.)

C locus – complete expression of colour/albino

Albinism in the ferret is caused by the recessive allele c; the completely dominant allele C allows pigment to be produced normally to produce the sable ferret (see Fig. 2.1) where the colours of the ancestor of the domestic ferret, the native polecat, are apparent. The skin, hair and eyes are all pigmented. Ferrets carrying CC (homozygous) are indistinguishable from Cc (heterozygous) ferrets. *Note* that as the recessive c allele is common in ferrets, any ferret has a 2-in-3 chance of carrying it. The only way to be certain that a ferret does not carry albinism is to cross it with an albino. If albino kits are born the ferret is a carrier, if no albino kits occur the coloured parent is probably not a carrier. Albinos mated together always produce only albinos, i.e. they breed true.

The albino cross and other crosses between pigmented and non-pigmented ferrets can be given as basic examples of how this one gene (C locus) can produce different ratios of coloured/albino offspring. If two albinos are bred together, each parent will pass on either of its copies of the allele. In this case, only the recessive c allele is available to be passed on (Table 5.3). If an albino is crossed with a pigmented ferret who is carrying albino (heterozygous), half the litter will be pigmented and the other half albino (Table 5.4). If one parent is homozygous for full pigmentation and the other is albino, all kits will have full pigmentation but will carry albino (Table 5.5). If both parents are heterozygous, half the kits will be heterozygous, one kit in four will be albino and one in four homozygous pigmented (Table 5.6). If one parent is heterozygous and the other homozygous

Table 5.3 Albino x albino (cc x cc)

Parental gametes	c	c
c	cc albino	cc albino
c	cc albino	cc albino

Table 5.4 Albino (cc) x heterozygote (Cc)

Parental gametes	C	c
c	Cc pigmented carrying albino	cc albino
c	Cc pigmented carrying albino	cc albino

Table 5.5 Homozygous pigmented (CC) x albino (cc)

Parental gametes	C	C
c	Cc pigmented carrying albino	Cc pigmented carrying albino
c	Cc pigmented carrying albino	Cc pigmented carrying albino

Table 5.6 Heterozygous (Cc) x heterozygous (Cc)

Parental gametes	C	c
C	CC pigmented	Cc pigmented carrying albino
c	Cc pigmented carrying albino	cc albino

pigmented, half the kits will have each state, but all will look the same (Table 5.7). As with sable and albino ferret crosses, the breeding of champagne pure stock and stock carrying albino or champagne can be visualized. If a homozygous pigmented ferret is crossed with a homozygous champagne, the resulting kits will all be normally coloured but carrying champagne (Table 5.8). If an albino is crossed with a homozygous champagne the kits will be champagne carrying albino (Table 5.9). When two normally pigmented ferrets are bred, one carrying albino and the other champagne, the result is only one champagne kit in four (Table 5.10). When champagne carrying albino $c^p c$ is crossed with albino, half the kits are champagne (but carrying albino) and half albino (Table 5.11).

Table 5.7 Heterozygous (*Cc*) x homozygous pigmented (*CC*)

Parental gametes	*C*	*C*
C	*CC*	*CC*
	pigmented	pigmented
c	*Cc*	*Cc*
	pigmented carrying albino	pigmented carrying albino

Table 5.8 Homozygous pigmented (*CC*) x homozygous champagne ($c^p c^p$)

Parental gametes	*C*	*C*
c^p	Cc^p	Cc^p
	pigmented carrying champagne	pigmented carrying champagne
c^p	Cc^p	Cc^p
	pigmented carrying champagne	pigmented carrying champagne

Table 5.9 Albino (*cc*) x homozygous champagne ($c^p c^p$)

Parental gametes	*c*	*c*
c^p	cc^p	cc^p
	champagne carrying albino	champagne carrying albino
c^p	cc^p	cc^p
	champagne carrying albino	champagne carrying albino

Table 5.10 Heterozygous (*Cc*) x heterozygous (*Cc*^{p})

Parental gametes	*C*	*c*
C	*CC*	*Cc*
	pigmented homozygous	pigmented carrying albino
c^p	Cc^p	$c^p c$
	pigmented carrying champagne	champagne carrying albino

Table 5.11 Champagne carrying albino ($c^p c$) x albino (*cc*)

Parental gametes	c^p	*c*
c	$c^p c$	*cc*
	champagne carrying albino	albino
c	$c^p c$	*cc*
	champagne carrying albino	albino

The importance of the *B* locus (brown pigment)

So far, only the effects of crosses involving one locus have been considered. If both the *C* and *B* loci are considered together, the results can be surprising. It can be noted that the *B* locus affects the production of eumelanin. The dominant form *B* produces the full colour, black or, in ferrets sable; the recessive form *b* produces the brown coloration, called chocolate in ferrets (and cats). Chocolate and champagne are inherited independently. For those trying to achieve champagne colouration in breeding, it is a mistake to think that crossing champagne with chocolate ferrets (hopefully carrying champagne) will result in all champagne kits, in fact the result may be 25% each of champagnes, sables, chocolates and albinos. Suppose we cross a champagne carrying albino (as most champagne do) who is also a sable carrying chocolate (*Bb*, $c^p c$) to a chocolate carrying albino (*bb*, *Cc*). The first parent can contribute the four combination of alleles on the top. The latter parent can contribute only the two combinations below (Table 5.12).

According to Shimbo it is thought that whether a parent ferret is genetically sable or chocolate will determine how the colour pans out when adding the c^p (champagne allele) to the mix. The *B* gene of the sable can modify small pigment precursors so that (*Bb* $c^p c$) produces a taupe or smokey champagne and (*bb* $c^p c$) a 'golden' or topaz champagne. Either or both of these colours can be in a litter born to a chocolate/champagne mating, as shown above.

Table 5.12 Champagne Bb, c^pc x chocolate bb, Cc

Parental gametes	Bc^p	Bc	bc^p	bc
bC	$BbCc^p$ sable carrying champagne	$BbCc$ sable carrying albino	$bbCc^p$ chocolate carrying champagne	$bbCc^p$ chocolate carrying champagne
bc	Bbc^pc Champagne (taupe) carrying albino	$Bbcc$ albino	bbc^pc champagne (golden) carrying albino	$bbcc$ albino

From Fara Shimbo's work above, we can see the range of genetic variation in ferrets, bearing in mind the possible colours and patterns: albino, sable, champagne, chocolate, mitt, silver mitt, etc. where the different alleles produce a 'kaleidoscope' of coat colours.

The names for ferret colours are not always the same in different countries, but here are some results from Italy, where breeder Allessandro Melillo has examples of breeding colour variations with results, including:

1. Silver hob (from silver/siamese) mated with siamese jill resulted in 10 kits: 4 silver males, 2 albino females, 2 light sable males and 2 light sable females.
2. Black self hob (from black self/black sable) mated with black sable (standard sable/black sable) resulted in 6 kits: 2 black sable male and female, 2 very dark black sable male and female plus another black self dead a few hours after delivery and another black sable put to sleep at 5 weeks of age because of megaoesophagus.
3. Black self hob mated with silver panda jill (standard sable/black sable) resulted in 5 kits: 1 black self female (not very dark), 2 sable females, 1 very dark silver female and 1 silver male (darker but with less precise pattern).

Note: the few-day-old kittens from litter (1) in Figure 5.30.

(Christina Bernard has compiled a family tree for her ferret, Teddy, who features in Chapter 8. This can be found in the Appendix as Figure A.1.)

The genetic make-up of the ferret affecting the coat colour, markings, spotting, patterns, eye colouring, hearing, etc. is complex and needs further understanding. As with other animals and humans the field is wide open for more research. Variation in ferret morphology is more conservative than in dogs so that ferrets are probably more akin to cats. Shimbo considered that perhaps research into cat genetics might yield some useful information applicable to the Mustelidae.

The black-eyed white (BEW) or dark-eyed white (DEW) ferret

The colouration known as BEW in Australia is known as dark-eyed white (DEW) elsewhere as their eyes, though always pigmented, are not always black. BEW ferrets have been sought after by those who work ferrets in hunting rabbits, i.e. ferreting. The BEW has the same advantage as the albino of being seen easily in the bush but also is considered to have better vision with pigmented eyes. It is also more attractive than the pink-eyed albino. I have always admired the BEW ferrets and attempted to breed them (see Fig. 2.4). Genetic traits in ferrets have been influenced by environment and selection of specimens over years in the domestication process (Ch. 6). For example, people looked for more docile animals and good breeders. Unfortunately, the BEW appears to carry a lethal gene as the mating of male and female BEW together produces dead kittens.

BEW kittens are possible by mating BEW with sables. I mated a BEW hob, Snowy, with my sable cross,

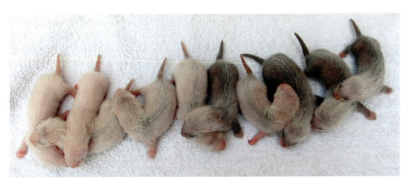

Figure 5.30 Kits from mating of silver hob (from silver/siamese) with siamese jill. (Courtesy of Alessandro Melillo.)

Jenny. *Note*: Jenny had a white face with a pale mask and her eyes had a 'raspberry' tint, certainly a blood glow, when compared with my pure sable ferret, Wendy, with typical black eyes. The result of mating Snowy with Jenny was a litter of eight kittens of which she lost two at birth. The surviving kittens were two sable hobs with white faces, one albino hob, two albino jills and one BEW jill. The BEW jill I called Susie and later mated her with an albino hob, Hoppy. The result was four albino kittens.

BEW, Susie, was later mated with a silver mitt hob, Simon. The results were six kittens, three sable jills, one sable hob and two BEW jills, which had black-flecked tails. One, called Tippy, had a distinctive black tip to the tail while the other was black-flecked all down the tail.

My BEW hob, Snowy, mated to a fitch jill, Queenie, produced ten kittens, eight sable and two BEWs. The BEWs were active and at the time I had no indication they were any more deaf than the sable ferrets, though I did feel that BEW jills were not such good mothers as the sable jills.

These are just examples of how the BEW comes into the breeding patterns of ferrets and are of course circumstantial findings when home breeding. The BEW ferret is somehow derived from the ferret gene pool of coat colour and eye colour genes. The complexity of colour on the genetic level was illustrated by Christina Bernard in considering the albino C locus and the chinchilla colour. She proposes that the dark-eyed white (DEW) might well be a diluted erythristic homozygous chinchilla: d/d, $e/e, c^{ch}/c^{ch}$ or extreme dilution: d/d, e/e, c^e/c^e.[28] The white coat of the albino results from a complete lack of melanin pigment while the DEW lacks melanocytes (pigment cells), but may carry genes for pigment which cannot be expressed, thus any colour or pattern might be hidden under a DEW, e.g. silver mitt or sable. No experimental work has been done on any hereditary pattern in BEWs even though the colour was known before the 1950s. It would be interesting to do some close-up inspections of the irises of BEW versus sable to see if there is any difference; i.e. whether the retinal pigments alone are the reason for the darkness of the eyes or whether the irises are also dark. Fara Shimbo considers dark-eyed white ferrets could actually be blue-eyed.

It has been observed that ferret coat colours can vary during the year – darker in warm seasons and lighter in cold seasons as related to the stoat/ermine condition (Middleton, pers. comm. 2005). In winter, in snowy climates, the stoat, of the same mustelid family, has a white coat due to environmental adaptation to snow cover over centuries. Incidentally, stoats and long-tailed weasels have black tips to their white tails in winter as a defence mechanism against swooping bird predators (King).[3] The complete colour change does not occur in polecats or ferrets, just a lightening of shade, due to a thickening of the lighter-coloured undercoat rather than any change in the guard hairs.

Sensory defects in ferrets

The senses of hearing, vision and smell are essential for hunting animals (Ch. 12). The albino ferret became popular for hunting as ferrets mainly use hearing and smell for scaring rabbits out of warrens. Its eyesight is poor compared with the sable (polecat or fitch) type ferret and BEW ferret as it has the unpigmented tapetum lucidum of the albino gene (however the albino is a robust worker and pet). The extent of visual fields in pigmented and albino ferrets has been compared.[30] Garipis and Hoffmann studied four pigmented and five albino ferrets. It was found by perimetry that for binocular vision, all four pigmented and three of the albino ferrets responded equally well when stimulated along the horizontal perimeter in the central 180° of the visual field. The other two albinos had defective vision in the right hemifield. However, it was apparent when studying them for monocular vision that there was a significant difference between the pigmented and albino ferrets. In pigmented ferrets the visual field of each eye spanned the ipsilateral (temporal) area and most of the contralateral (nasal) hemifield, while the albino ferrets' span of vision was restricted mostly to the ipsilateral hemifield. Thus, there are differences of vision between pigmented and albino ferrets.

Genes and domestication

The classic experiment on animal genetics and domestication was carried out by Dmitry Belyaev and his ongoing team at the Institute of Cytology and Genetics in Novosibirsk, Siberia from 1959 using *Vulpes vulpes*, the silver fox. In general, terms tameness was selected for over many generations of foxes.[31] The team were surprised to find that changes in body size, coat colour and hair length occurred associated with the process of selecting solely for docility – domestication. After 40 years, there are marked differences between the domesticated and wild foxes. The changes were similar to those seen in other domesticated animals. Tameness, yes, but also different coat colours and particularly white patches on the head and feet. Loss of pigment on the head in star-shaped patterns or 'blazes' led to the hypothesis of a 'star gene', tying in the behavioural changes selected for in domestication with piebalding, neoteny, and a host of other changes, many of a visual and auditory nature. In a nutshell, breeding for tameness (reducing the fight/flight distance to zero) produced changes in the timing of brain development that interfered with the migration of pigmented cells during early embryonic development. This resulted in a human-friendly animal but it also resulted in stars, blazes or light-coloured stripes on the head and forehead, white faces, chest blazes, white feet or knees or generalized piebalding. The domesticated foxes tended to have larger litters than the wild ones and there was some tendency to breed more than once a year. Also interesting was the finding that the domesticated fox pups responded to sounds 2 days earlier than wild foxes and their eyes opened 1 day earlier, confirming changes in developmental timing. The 'Star gene' is related to deafness and visual problems and it is noted that Waardenburg's syndrome (see later) is closely associated with piebalding, the outward expression of the 'star gene'.

The changes in any mammal due to domestication, as indicated above, have relevance to what has happened in the ferret. Interest in ferret concerns has been low on the list when considering genetics and effects on animal welfare. Grandin and Deesing have illuminated genetic trends in cattle, pigs and poultry in the farm animal sphere, and in dogs, pigeons, mice, rabbits and mice in the small animal sphere, including laboratory animals but not ferrets.[32] The traits of overall body size, body proportions, coat colour, eye colour, intelligence and behaviour are controlled by many genetic factors put down as 'heritability'; one also has to consider environmental, developmental or nutritional influences. Grandin and Deesing[32] suggest, for instance, there is a definite relationship between depigmentation and changes in behaviour, as studied in foxes. Depigmentation has been associated with deafness in mice; this is also the case in ferrets. Genetically speaking the depigmentation of skin, hair and eyes is a product of the development of the nervous system.

The neural crest

In the very early embryonic life of vertebrates, the neural crest arises from the neural tube. Cells from the neural crest in the fetus make up the body; the whole physical makeup of the animal depends on where the cells go in the genetic plan, what they do and what influences them. The neural crest contains a population of pluripotent cells that originate from almost the entire length of the neural tube and can migrate to various locations in the developing embryo to give rise to several different cell types, e.g. pigment, nerve and cardiac cells. There is now interest in how the movement of cells in the neural crest and their ongoing development may relate to ferret genetics. (The question of sex hormone-producing cells being located in the adrenal glands is also a worry in ferrets, see Ch. 14.)

Melanocytes or pigment cells derive from the neural crest and are responsible for colour distribution on an animal. The cells may not reach the most remote parts of the body so that the lower limbs, chest, belly and under the chin can remain white. This situation is considered common in horses and cattle, dogs and cats, mice and ferrets. Pigment cells and nerve cell primaries for instance can share a common pathway and consequently mutation in genes that affect coat colour can also affect neurological functions (including behaviour), immunological functions, fertility and even appetite according to Christine Bernard.

Cardiac neural crest cells, a subpopulation of the neural crest, are known to play multiple roles during development of the inflow and outflow tracts to the heart and aortic arch. In humans, it is suggested that some neural crest syndromes lead on to cardiomyopathies in the newborn and later. It is thought that cardiomyopathies in the ferret likewise arise from disturbed patterns of heart cell growth. Research on the homeobox gene Lbx1 in regard to normal heart development has been carried out (not on ferrets).[33]

Genes with multiple effects

Several genes are being studied in which mutations cause multiple effects similar to those hypothesized for the 'star gene' and involving the neural crest. Most white markings in domestic animals appear to be related to the KIT gene, an oncogene, which is often referred to as the 'S' (spotting) locus in coat colour genetics (Middleton, pers. comm. 2005).

KIT and KIT ligand

In the field of genetics the c-kit receptor tyrosine kinase gene (KIT) is much discussed.[34] These KIT alleles are important to at least three migratory stem cell paths from the neural crest: pigment cells, haematopoietic stem cells and primordial germ cells. In mice, they cause reduced pigmentation, anaemia and sterility. Yukihiko Kitamura et al.[34] discuss gastrointestinal stromal tumours (GIST) in the cat as a model for molecular-based diagnosis and treatment of solid tumours with the KIT oncogene being expressed by practically all GIST tumours. The KIT oncogene action is further discussed online in such sources as OMIM (Online Mendelian Inheritance in Man), with reference to models in man and animals, basically pigs, bovine and mouse experiments.[35] The relationship of the KIT gene to piebaldism in humans, also mast cell leukaemia, germ cell tumours and GIST is indicated; the genetics work is extensive.

Endothelial receptor type B (Ednrb)

Several different alleles of this gene can cause different levels and distribution of white. A normal-coloured coat is produced by the dominant allele. The 'Irish-spotting' allele can produce white markings on face, neck, chest and lower limbs in dogs. The 'piebald-spotting' allele gives a wider distribution of white. The 'extreme white' allele results in an almost entirely white coat and with it a likelihood of genetic deafness in the animal. The Ednrb gene is responsible for the correct development of the nervous system and mutations of this gene cause a variety of conditions in man and animals, including the Waardenburg–Shan syndrome (WS) of deafness and Hirschsprung's disease of megacolon.

From the above, the white colouration (or almost white phenotype, albino excluded) can be seen as fraught with danger as certain genotypes can produce medical conditions such as deafness, nervous system disorders, infertility, blood disorders intestinal problems and postnatal deaths.

The Waardenburg phenomena according to Fara Shimbo

There are numerous genes involved in the development, structure and functioning of pigment cells. It is possible that any one or more genes could have one or more alleles that result in some degree of depigmentation and thus change ferret coat colour. However, since many or maybe most genes affect more than one trait an allele that causes depigmentation could have another function, harmful or harmless.

The Waardenburg syndrome (WS) was first recognized in humans and deaf blue-eyed white cats. It was also recognized in ferrets with 'badger' or 'Shetland' facial markings and remarked on by Shimbo.[26] In the affected ferret face the eyes are small and widely spaced and often 'pinched' in the inner corner. Mismatched eye colours (odd eyes) occur and a white streak extends back along the head from the white panda face. (Colmara (panda) ferrets showing WS signs have facial markings akin to the deaf Turkish Van cat with the syndrome.) There are often large white spots on the belly and toes. The ferret has severe or total deafness. Mink show a similar condition called a colmira, which is a completely white head also known as panda. Interestingly, colmira mink are called 'deep sleepers' who can be 'even picked up without waking'. According to Fara Shimbo, such ferrets are often deaf and display 'screw neck' whereby some neurological defect causes them to move in an uncoordinated way with a head tilt, which would suggest ear infection at first glance.

Waardenburg's syndrome involves a simple recessive gene at the HuP2 locus in humans and mice. In mink, the gene is called 'V'. *Note*: the gene is said to be of 'incomplete penetrance' as not every homozygous recessive will show all the traits of the condition. However, a mating of an affected hob and jill may show other neurological conditions and developmental defects such as spina bifida and brain defects. Modern genetic investigation reveals that not all white patterns associated with deafness are caused by the same gene associated with WS. In fact, there are five genes implicated in different types of WS; these are listed as PAX3, MITF, EDNRB (see above), EDN3 and SOX10.

Brett Middleton points out the difference between 'depigmentation' and 'white'. If the hair is white but the skin can produce pigment (melanin) then the animal is not depigmented, e.g. samoyed dogs are depigmented, but polar bears are not, as they have black skin. There are a large number of wild species that show areas of depigmentation, e.g. skunks and zebras have stripes, badgers have blazes, some deer have whitetails and giant pandas are black and white; depigmentation in these animals has no associated problems (Middleton, pers. comm. 2005).

The question arises as to why the 'safe' depigmentation genes are not working in domesticated animals? Middleton states that they are not that common in the wild. The question may be answered in the future with a ferret genome survey started in California by Dr Michelle Hawkins. One type of white marking in ferrets which does not appear to involve the neural crest is a complete, clean, bilateral replacement of the standard bib and mitts. That appears to have a different origin and Sukie Crandall states she has not read or heard of any ferrets with this showing medical vulnerabilities in 24 years.

Mutant gene examples

Sukie Crandall, USA ferret breeder, not a vet, has noted one 5-year-old ferret, Scooter, with KIT gene type body-spotting and hypertrophic cardiomyopathy (HCM) which went into wasting until the cardiac disease was found. The KIT oncogene is thus indicated in ferrets and it appears that ferrets associated with this gene have an increased risk of malignances (Wendy Van den Steen, pers. comm. 2005). It is also noted that ferrets with strongly non-bilateral marking, especially around the head, may be candidates for aortic arch malformations as in other mammals.

Depigmentation on the genetic level has given rise to advice to ferret owners not to breed those with head blaze, white heads or extraneous body spotting. This avoids ferrets with polydactyly (presence of supernumerary digits), syndactyly (fusion of claws or digits) or lacking a tail (Sukie Crandall, pers. comm. 2005).

Ferrets with really short limbs and short faces possibly derive from genes for achondroplastic dwarfism, which can be a painful condition although the ferrets usually show good coats. Not to be bred from!

A ferret, Ruffles, with the condition used to have panic attacks and got into self-biting in her first 3 years of life (Sukie Crandall, pers. comm. 2005). The ferret was unable to cope with other ferrets, suffered in the next 3 years from asthma and moved into having insulinoma, cardiomyopathy and also a heart tumour, found on post mortem. *Note*: the ferret, Scooter, with HCM had syndactylism and had multiple operations for GI malformation. He had KIT markings of the body spotting type. Both Ruffles and Scooter were maintained for 6 years of life with tender loving care, but these examples show what conditions can arise from a damaged genetic background.

Two USA ferrets with the KIT markings were found to have developed cystine stones when placed on a high protein diet. One got bladder diverticula and had to have repeated cystotomies, which worked. The ferret remained gaunt for a year, but seemed to recover from the bilateral hydronephrosis and improved in weight and activity level. Evidently, more laboratories are reporting cystine stones in ferrets. With the ancestral stock of pet ferrets in USA fed on a 35% kibble diet, it is considered perhaps a food ingredient problem for ferrets (Ch. 4). It would be interesting to see what these ferrets would be like on a fresh meat diet and feeding once daily. There needs to be more research on the components of the diet in relation to genetics and kidney stone formation, as with other carnivores, both domestic and wild, in which cystine stones have been studied.

Behavioural problems

Depigmentation, including albinism, is also associated with behaviour defects. In other words, not just depigmentation caused by lack of pigment cells, e.g. albino mice are known to be much more 'emotional' or 'reactive' than pigmented mice. Viennese white rabbits are subject to seizures. Pointer dogs suffering from the 'nervous behaviour' defect tend to be highly depigmented. Holstein cows with large amounts of white are more nervous and less productive. White pigs are more likely to suffer from porcine stress syndrome (PSS), which kills them when they are subjected to stress or exertion (Brett Middleton, pers. comm. 2005).

Fara Shimbo remarked on an idiopathic epilepsy in ferrets, which she considered to be caused by a simple recessive gene.[26] She pointed out that an epileptic fit could mimic an insulinoma seizure. The tendency to develop insulinoma is inheritable in some humans and dogs.

A gene with incomplete penetrance causes tail deformities in ferrets and cats (e.g. Manx). The condition is recessive in cats and dominant in mink. Adding aspirin or phenothalein (mutagens) to the pregnant jill's diet exacerbates the condition with kits having short tails or even toes, feet or limbs missing.[26] Other malformations suspected as being genetic are mandibles that cannot fully open and widely-set eyes as seen in WS.

The multiple endocrine neoplasia (MEN) gene in humans has become important with regard to the study of ferrets sterilized at an early age and is discussed in Chapter 14.

The controversial ferret type 'Angora' has been bred in Denmark and exported as pets to the USA, where there is a large group of angora enthusiasts (Wendy Van den Steen, pers. comm. 2005). They are also bred in Holland and sold in Japan and are not neutered. The angora needs to be bred in a straight line or they lose their long hair. Breeding them is difficult (Stephanie Bass, pers. comm. 2005). The angora seems to be genetically damaged, having a high rate of kits with malformations of their skull and nostrils; they have profuse hair growing from their nostrils. Their eyes tend to have a dark background with green flecks (see ferret eye colours). They also tend to have larger litters and are poor mothers lacking in milk.

The unwanted ending ... inbreeding

The modern ferret is becoming increasingly removed from its original genetic pool by breeding, including inbreeding, for certain features. The ferret genetic pool needs refreshment by outbreeding to new ferret lines. The outlook for the Australian scene is that we had a variety of ferret (ferret-polecat?) strains coming in during the nineteenth and early twentieth centuries but no new bloodlines have been introduced for some decades. We have had years of interbreeding with this basic stock, but the danger is genetic weakness and inbreeding effects.

We could consider that there is a population of inbred ferrets in Western Australia (where I live) and another in distant Tasmania where Christina Bernard, with her interest in ferret genetics, lives. We would like to improve Australian ferrets by introduction of new blood lines but quarantine laws do not allow this. The possibility of inadvertent introduction of Aleutian disease, a chronic parvovirus disease, would be devastating (Ch. 8).

Bernard considers that genetic fitness has no correlation with physical fitness and is the overall ability to leave surviving offspring who themselves will be able to reproduce themselves successfully. The signs of inbreeding would show as reduced fertility, increased congenital defects, 'bent-nose' condition, lower birth rate, higher neonatal mortality, smaller adult size and loss of immune system function. Some of these traits had been found in the Russian domestication experiments.

The outcome for individuals with 'weak' genes is a deficient immunological system unable to prevent infection particularly by viruses. Inbred laboratory animals, mice, etc. need to be in a sterile environment. Endangered wild animals, in decreased numbers, are at risk of being wiped out by epidemics due to decreased immunological protection caused by unavoidable inbreeding.[28]

The function of the immune system is to recognize foreign invaders to the body and destroy them by producing antibodies. The ability of the immune system to recognize foreign antigens depends on the genetic diversity of the major histocompatibility complex (MHC) genes. These are positioned close together on one chromosome and are inherited together as a unit called a *haplotype*. The MHC of a ferret is *polygenetic* with many genes and the alleles of each MHC gene are numerous within a population; it is *polymorphic*.

Each ferret has two MHC haplotypes, one from each parent. The alleles of both haplotypes are expressed in a co-dominant manner, so greater diversity between the parents' haplotypes will give the offspring a better functioning immune system. Ferrets in an inbred population, with less diverse haplotypes, are at risk of being unable to recognize and respond to the challenge of infection.

In the wild, the alleles will be numerous and variable adding to the genetic mix of the species concerned. In the event of disease, individuals of the species would survive as they would have the right mix of genes to overcome the infection and would pass that to their offspring, so more and more pathogens would be recognizable. It is considered that over time, the DNA can get stronger by changing or mutation and natural selection working on the changes. In fact, the MHC genes do have a high mutation rate as they are essential for species survival.[28]

Conclusions

From the above information, the state of ferret genetics is an ongoing study. In this resumé, I can hardly give justice to the general work on genetics affecting man and animals. Genetic mutants in embryonic development, as shown above, could lead to cardiovascular disease and other unwanted problems. Brett Middleton has stated, in discussion on the ferret-genetics website, that breeding for certain oncogenes might increase vulnerability to at least some malignancies, especially those most likely to be encountered after the breeding years are past. He points out that unless a species strongly counts on the support of elderly individuals, who are past breeding, for the reproductive success of those who are younger then there is no selective pressure for longevity beyond the breeding years.

Middleton notes that in the USA, and many other places, there is a tradition (going through many, many generations) of domestic ferrets not receiving as much protein in their diet as wild polecats. He states this means that vulnerabilities which would result in early deaths among those who ate a high protein diet, were not selected against, and successful reproduction took place at a far higher rate than would have occurred if the animals had died younger. That alters the proportion of such alleles in the population.

In different orders of mammals, species of similar size do not necessarily have similar life spans. Middleton asserts that members of a species become optimized for the best quality of life related to diet, location, etc. Quality of life and quantity of life may not be the same thing.

He cites a common condition, in some ferrets – insulinoma, where the condition has led to an A/V heart node block. The medications that keep sugar high enough for survival are to some extent actually counter-indicated for the heart condition. He points out that the hypothesis that reducing carbohydrate intake reduces insulinoma is at present hypothetical. This is discussed by Finkler regarding the aetiology of the disease (Ch. 14).

As seen by Crandall's earlier examples, some ferrets are prone to cystine stones on high protein. Middleton points out that a high protein diet would theoretically be good for a ferret regarding the insulinoma but then it might be prone to kidney disease due to the COLA group of amino acids which are high in such a diet. He suggests checking urine pH of ferrets on a high protein diet to make sure it does not go too low (acidic). Cystine precipitates out of urine that is too acidic, unlike the components of struvite stones that form as a result of too much plant material in the ferret's diet and will precipitate out when the urine is too alkaline.

Middleton compares the situation of humans where fat used to be healthy and thin dangerous to health. Now considerations are reversed and this may well be a feature of animals including ferrets. He asserts that there is not enough conclusive information on food and genetics but steps should only be taken to avoid nutritional steatitis (yellow fat disease) or other well-documented problems.

In the dog world, nutrigenomics is a new science exploring the link between food, genetics and disease. Nutrients in the food can assist in prevention of certain genetic diseases of which to date around 450 have been discovered in canines. Studying the canine genome in conjunction with nutrition has brought new breakthroughs with the release of Hill's Prescription Diet® j/d™. This contains eicosapentaenoic acid (EPA), an omega-3 fatty acid (high concentration in fish oil). It can turn off the genes that code for aggrecanase, an enzyme that causes cartilage degeneration (K. Johnson, Hill's Manager, pers. comm. 2005). There is hope to attempt dealing with diabetes and cardiomyopathy. With the ferret genome being investigated in the USA, will similar benefits come to pet ferrets?

I agree with Christina Bernard that pet ferrets have had a rather raw deal, genetically speaking, in becoming so popular. The pet ferret is well off its track as a nocturnal animal. It is placed in a situation where it is in daily play and shown off at pet shows and ferret races. It is fed questionable 'ferret' food; can be in constant longer than necessary light photo-periods, and not allowed to have its usual 20 hours of sleep per day (Ch. 14). Hopefully, while reading this book ferret followers will learn how to change the future and breed healthy ferrets; animals genetically equipped to face whatever life throws at them.

References

1. King C. The handbook of New Zealand mammals. Oxford: Oxford University Press; 1990.
2. Porter V, Brown N. The complete book of ferrets. Bedford: D&M; 1997.
3. King C. The natural history of weasels and stoats. London: Christopher Helm; 1998.
4. Zhang JX, Soini HA, Bruce KE et al. Putative chemosignals of the ferret (*Mustela furo*) associated with individual and gender recognition. Chem Senses 2005; 30:727–737.
5. McCann C. Observations on the polecat (*Putorius putorius* Linn.) in New Zealand. Records of the Dominion Museum 1955; 2:51–165.
6. Peter AT, Bell JA, Manning DD, Bosu WTK. Real-time determination of pregnancy and gestation age in ferrets. Lab Anim Sci 1990; 40:91–92.
7. Lewington JH. Parturition and problems in the aging ferret jill. Control and Therapy Series 147:114–116. University of Sydney: Postgraduate Foundation; 1998.
8. Bell J. Ferret nutrition and diseases associated with inadequate nutrition. Proc North Am Vet Assoc Conf; 1993:719–720.
9. Lewington JH. Ferrets. Vade Mecum Series C10. University of Sydney: Postgraduate Foundation; 1988.
10. Bell J. Preparturient and neonatal diseases. In: Hillyer EV, Quesenberry KE, eds. Ferrets, rabbits, and rodents: clinical medicine and surgery. Philadelphia: WB Saunders; 1997:53–62.
11. Dalrymple EF. Pregnancy toxaemia in a ferret. Can Vet J 2004; 45:150–152.
12. Besch-Williford CL. Biology and medicine of the ferret. Vet Clin North Am Small Anim Pract 1997; 17:1155–1184.
13. Batchelder MA, Bell JA, Erdman SE, Marini RP, Murphy JC, Fox JG. Pregnancy toxaemia in the European ferret (*Mustela putorius furo*). Lab Anim Sci 1999; 49:372–379.
14. Bell J, Manning D. Reproductive failure in mink and ferrets after intravenous or oral inoculation of *Campylobacter jejuni*. Can J Vet Res 1990; 54:432–437.
15. Johnson SD. Canine reproduction. Reproduction: Small Companion Animals Proceedings. University of Sydney: Postgraduate Foundation 1998; 108:69.
16. Manning D, Bell J. Derivation of gnotobiotic ferrets: perinatal diet and hand rearing requirements. Lab Anim Sci 1990; 40:51–55.
17. Manning D. Fostering of newborn ferrets. South Australian Ferret News 5:8–11.
18. Animal Health Division, Ministry of Agriculture and Fisheries, NZ. Diseases of Fitch, Surveillance 1993. NZ: Animal Health Division, Ministry of Agriculture and Fisheries; 1994; 11:2.
19. Lewington JH. Eye infections in ferret infant kittens. Control and Therapy Series. University of Sydney: Postgraduate Foundation 1998; 200:993–994.
20. Smith G. 'Swimmers'. South Australian Ferret News 2005; 17 May:14–15.
21. Nes N, Einarsson EJ, Lohi O. Experience from farm practice. Beautiful fur animals and their colour genetics. Denmark: Scientifur; 1988.
22. Cavagna P, Menotti A, Stanyon R. Genomic homology of the domestic ferret with cats and humans. Mamm Genome 2000; 11:866–870.
23. Rouvinen Watt K. Nova Scotia Fur Institute, 15th Anniversary Book (1984–1999). Canada: Nova Scotia Fur Institute; 2001.
24. US Fur Rancher. Blue book of fur farming. MN: Eden; 1980.
25. McNicholas J. Take a walk on the wild side, meet our ferret's British relatives. Ferrets First 2005 24:10–11.
26. Shimbo F, Maday M. Reproduction, development and inheritance in the ferret. Boulder: FURO; 1994:1–6.
27. Shimbo F. The ferret book, Boulder: FURO; 1993:65–68.
28. Bernard C (as Fret Popper). Various articles. South Australian Ferret Association News 2005; 17: Nos 1–7.
29. Pitt F. Notes on the genetic behaviour of certain characters in the polecat, ferret, and in the polecat-hybrid. J Genet 1921; XI:100–115.
30. Garipis N, Hoffmann KP. Visual field defects in albino ferrets (*Mustela putorius furo*). Vision Research 2003; 43:793–800.
31. Morey D. The farm fox experiment. American Scientist 1994:July/August.
32. Grandin T, Deesing MJ. Genetics and animal welfare. In: Grandin T., ed. Genetics and the behaviour of domestic animals. San Diego: Academic Press; 1999:319–341.
33. Schafer K, Neuhaus P, Kruse J, Braun T. The homeobox gene Lbx1 specifies a subpopulation of cardiac neural crest necessary for normal heart development. Circ Res 2003; 92:73–80.
34. Kitamura Y, Hirota S, Nishida T. Gastrointestinal stromal tumors (GIST): A model for molecular-based diagnosis and treatment of solid tumors. Cancer Sci 2003; 94:315–320.
35. Online Mendelian Inheritance in Man, various authors. V-KIT Hardy-Zuckerman 4 Feline sarcoma oncogenic homolog; KIT. Baltimore: Johns Hopkins University; 2005.

CHAPTER 6

Ferret-polecat domestication: genetic, taxonomic and phylogenetic relationships

Bob Church

'Be a good animal, true to your instincts.'

D.H. Lawrence, The White Peacock, 1911

Ferret domestication

Special problems

The domesticated ferret, *Mustela furo* is an animal with a long history of domestication (roughly 2000–3000 years), yet with little physical evidence to support the process.[1–12] This lack of physical evidence is primarily due to seven disparate factors, all of which must be considered separately when answering questions of ferret domestication. These factors include a lack of skeletal preservation, a lack of data for determining the geographical region of domestication, a lack of ability to archaeologically resolve the skeletal remains of the domesticated ferret from other species in the Mustela genus, a lack of archaeological emphasis on recovery, the close phylogenetic relationships of the polecats, a history of profound introgression between various polecats and the domesticate and the shortcomings of genetic studies. Each factor would make the identification of the domesticated ferret in the archaeological record problematic, but in combination, any determination becomes extremely difficult.

Lack of skeletal preservation

The lack of skeletal preservation haunts the study of domestication for any species, but in the case of the domesticated ferret, it is particularly irksome.[10–13] The problem is not limited to the domesticated ferret, but also to the polecat group in general.[11,14,15] If skeletal elements are to be found, they first must be preserved in a manner that allows recovery.

A major problem in skeletal preservation is that ferret bones are small and are therefore less likely to be preserved in archaeological contexts because they tend to fracture and decompose more rapidly compared with larger ones.[16,17] Even when preservation is good enough for recovery, the bones may be fragmented to such a degree that they are unidentifiable.[16,18] Smaller bones are also more likely to be relocated by moving water, burrowing animals and other biological or geological forces, displacing the elements across a landscape and making the recovery of more than a few parts very difficult.[19,20] Predators or scavengers, including residential domestic canines, can remove, scatter or consume carcasses or bones before they become part of the archaeological record.[21] Humans may have been a major force in the lack of preservation of ferret remains in archaeological sites, perhaps skinning dead ferrets for their pelt, discarding the carcasses in remote locations or feeding the carcasses to other carnivorous pets.

Unknown region of domestication

Not knowing the geographical region of domestication is another problem; if you do not know where an animal was domesticated, how can you recover the remains of early domesticates? This problem almost constitutes a type of 'biogeographical tautology' where you have to know where the remains are located in order to locate the remains.

Suppositions that place the geographical origin of domestication of the ferret in North Africa and Egypt, sometimes suggesting that Egyptians domesticated the ferret prior to the cat, are commonly reported as probable or fact.[22–30] This 'African domestication' hypothesis suggests ferrets originated in North Africa – generally out of Egypt prior to cat domestication – and has remained pervasive even though the idea has been disputed within the ferret community from the beginning.[31–38] Most domestication scientists reject the idea or only mention it in passing.[3–5,10–13,39] One reason for the popularity of the idea that Egyptians domesticated the ferret can be found in A.R. Harding's 1915 book, *Ferret Facts and Fancies*. This book has had a tremendous influence on ferret information in America, where it was the chief reference on ferrets for the better part of the twentieth century. Without citing support, Harding states in the opening paragraph, 'The ferret is a native of Africa. The animal was first domesticated in the northern part of that continent, by the Egyptians, hundreds of years ago'.

The modern version of the 'African domestication' origin hypothesis[24,29,39,40] can be ultimately traced to four basic sources: *British Quadrupeds*,[41] *Systema Naturae*, 10th edn,[42] *Geographica*[43] and *Naturalis Historia*.[44] Most subsequent sources cite one or more of these four. Of these, both Bell and Linneaus cite *Strabo*, so the ultimate cause of the confusion can be traced to a single comment, 'They make a point of breeding Libyan ferrets, which they muzzle and send into the holes'[43] (Vol. II, book 3, Spain, Ch. 2, Section 6. Some translations use the phrase, 'Libyan weasels'). This interpretation of the domesticated ferret's geographical origin has biased centuries of investigations and has caused considerable confusion. In short, part of the difficulty in finding physical evidence of ferret domestication is that early researchers may have been looking in the wrong places.

Where should students of ferret domestication look for remains? The region would have to be a place populated with possible progenitors (*Mustela putorius*, *M. eversmanni*). The remains of steppe and European polecats have never been found in or near Egypt before or during the time of domestication, nor was it likely they ever lived in the region.[9,14,15,45–52] The closest possible populations were reported in northern Morocco[2,53] and in 'the north of Palestine',[54,55] but both references are controversial. Even if true, polecats were certainly in southern Europe, including Italy, Macedonia and Turkey, similar in distance to Egypt as Morocco or northern Palestine. Suppositional arguments of the geographical location of polecats compared with Egypt make little sense in the absence of zoological, archaeological, linguistic and historic evidence. They were similarly close to dozens of period cities, such as Carthage, that could arbitrarily be given credit. Using no other criteria, this would eliminate the possibility of ferrets being domesticated in Egypt simply because polecats were not present during the ferret's window of domestication. The Greeks, Moroccans or Phoenicians could just as easily have domesticated ferrets – if all that is being considered is geographic distance to wild polecats (see [56–67]). While this criterion does not specifically suggest an explicit region where domestication of the ferret took place, it does greatly discount those areas where it could not have occurred.

Inability to resolve skeletal remains from polecats

Even if archaeologists are looking in the correct location for ferrets, there is the problem of identifying them once they are found. Osteological changes caused by domestication are initially quite small or non-existent.[68–73] Additionally, it is difficult to resolve the skeletal remains of the domesticated ferret from other polecats (or between the polecats for that matter), resulting in only tenuous identifications such as *Mustela* sp. or *Mustela* cf *putorius*,[74,75] or identification only to polecat, ignoring possible domesticates.[76,77] This is especially true for the postcranial remains of ferrets and polecats, where only few studies have been published describing their osteology and none on their differentiation.[78–82] While postcranial identification between ferrets and polecats is, at best, problematic, cranial identification can be difficult as well.[83–89] While Lange et al.[90] provide a key to distinguish ferrets from polecats, problems such as the influence of the environment, effects of domestication, diet, sexual dimorphism, cranial variability and the effect of introgression remain to be addressed.[91–96] One exception to the lack of published accounts of identified domesticated ferrets from archaeological sites is the report of remains from the Castle of Laarne in Belgium, dated to the late medieval period.[97]

The problem is that polecats and ferrets are small animals and, during initial domestication, small animals have even smaller changes. If you are studying the domestication of a sheep or dog, early skeletal differences may be measured in a few millimeters, perhaps even in centimeters. Try to investigate the same relative degree of change in a polecat and similar differences may only be a fraction of a millimeter. Factors such as measurement error, sexual dimorphism, neutering, phenotypic plasticity or even nutritional status can result in enough skeletal variation to make such small differences statistically insignificant.

The skulls of polecats and ferrets, which have been studied in great detail for the last century, overlap in size and morphology to such a degree that some individuals cannot be properly identified to species.[57,83,87–92,98–101] If

CHAPTER SIX
Ferret-polecat domestication: genetic, taxonomic and phylogenetic relationships

there are inherent difficulties resolving ferrets from polecats after more than 2000 years of domestication, how much more difficult would it be to resolve early domesticated ferrets? This lack resolution between polecat and ferret osteology – skeletal, cranial and dental – has made the identification of ferrets in archaeological contexts particularly difficult.

Lack of archaeological emphasis on recovery

The search for domesticated ferrets has also been hampered by a historical lack of archaeological emphasis on the recovery, curation and analysis of the remains of small mammals. For a long period of time, archaeology was an investigation of the rich and famous – with more emphasis on gold than goals – and the search for valuable artifacts would trump the investigation of the lives of common people.[17,102,103] As archaeological method and theory advanced, the collection of small bones and teeth became more commonplace, as did the refinement of methods of recovery, identification and analysis.[16,17,102] After zooarchaeology developed as a discipline, the recovery, identification and analysis of animal bones became commonplace, and contemporary archaeologists now attempt to recover the smallest of faunal (and floral) remains for analysis.[16,17,102] Nonetheless, during the early years of archaeology, much evidence was ignored, lost, discarded or left unanalyzed in some museum drawer that might have helped in the understanding of ferret domestication. Some polecat and mustelid bones have been recovered from archaeological and paleontological sites, so the potential for recovery and elucidation exists.[76,77,97,104–110]

Polecat phylogenetics

The close phylogenetic relationship of the polecats has also hampered the investigation of ferret domestication. A great deal of controversy exists regarding the exact relationships between the polecats *Mustela putorius*, *M. eversmanni* and *M. nigripes* and even the European mink, *M. lutreola*.[98,111–120] Part of this problem is due to the need of a comprehensive revision of the genus Mustela using a phylogenetic approach.[111,121–126] Genetic studies are just beginning to illuminate mustelid relationships, although those of the polecats – especially the identity of the progenitor – continue to remain obscure.[6,9,14,46,51,116,118,122–124,127–133] Polecats display a high degree of genetic variability, which may complicate investigations.[134]

Another difficulty is the karyotype of the domesticated ferret and of polecats – and mustelids in general – is highly conserved so that differences within the karyotype that might help resolve relationships are limited.[122,132,135] The polecats are a recent evolutionary lineage, roughly 400 000–600 000 years old.[9,66,118,136] Polecats are thought to have recently evolved from a solitary founding population, radiating from a single Pleistocene refugium.[15,117,128] This would suggest the evolutionary split between the varieties of polecats is relatively recent – one of the reasons why there is a growing trend to view the polecats as a single, rather than disparate, species.[13,116,137–139] It has long been argued that the North American black-footed ferret (*M. nigripes*) is a subspecies of the steppe polecat.[98,114,115,140–142] If so, then these three animals could form a single Holarctic species, following the trend seen in ermine, least weasels, wolves, wolverine, caribou and reindeer, American elk and red deer, moose and European elk and many other species.

One difficulty with subsuming the polecats and ferrets into a single species is the karyotype of the European polecat is $2n = 40$ and that of the steppe polecat and black-footed ferret is $2n = 38$.[6,122,143–145] However, this difference is due to a single Robertsonian rearrangement where there has been a reversal of the ACK 2q+12 fusion that occurred early in the evolutionary history of the clade.[122] While this results in an additional set of chromosomes for the European polecat compared with the steppe polecat, increasing the count from $2n = 38$ to $2n = 40$, the genome itself remains essentially unaltered.[122]

A history of profound introgression

Perhaps the greatest difficulty in the investigation of ferret domestication lies in the history of the domesticated ferret, an animal with a history of profound introgression (hybridization) with polecats. Kurose[9] remarks, 'Remarkably close relationships among the domestic ferret *M. furo*, the European polecat *M. putorius* and the steppe polecat *M. eversmanni* were noticed with 87–94% bootstrap values (named 'the ferret group'), supporting the history that the ferret was domesticated from *M. putorius* and/or *M. eversmanni*'. Similarly, Davison[6] states, 'Ferrets (*Mustela furo*) were domesticated from polecats (*M. putorius*, *M. eversmanni*) over 2000 years ago'. Also, 'The wild source of the ferret remains obscure'. Marmi et al.[116] has a comparable finding, 'Low levels of genetic divergence among European polecat, *Mustela putorius*, steppe polecat, *Mustela eversmanni* and European mink, *Mustela lutreola*, suggest that these species could be considered subspecies within a single species, *Mustela putorius*'.

Part of the difficulty in identifying domesticated ferrets is due to the close relationships between the polecat group, but at least part of the problem is because of a long history of hybridizing ferrets back to polecats.[6,8] Hybridization, however infrequent, mixes the genetic information of the wild types with that of the domesticated forms in ways that are hard to recognize. For example, mitochondrial DNA (mtDNA) is passed through the mother's lineage because she provides the initial cell – with maternal mtDNA – for offspring. A breeder hybridizing a female polecat with a male domesticated ferret could introduce 'wild' information into a domesticated mtDNA lineage, obscuring historic relationships.

Ferrets are commonly hybridized with both species of polecats, *Mustela putorius* and *M. eversmanni*, for a number of reasons, including scientific curiosity or to improve coat colour or hunting characteristics.[6,33,35,37,111,146–156] For whatever reason, this long history of introgression obscures the relationships between the domesticated animal and its possible progenitors to such a degree that the determination of the exact ancestor becomes extremely difficult to accomplish, if such determinations are even possible.

Shortcomings of genetic studies

Historically, if scientists wanted to study the genetics of an animal, their efforts were largely limited to looking at the external shape and numbers of chromosomes – the karyotype. Initial genetic studies suggested the ancestor of the domesticated ferret, *M. furo*, was the European polecat, *M. putorius*.[95,111,141,157] This was because the numbers of chromosomes in the ferret, as well as their relative shapes and sizes, matched those in the karyotype of the European polecat. The two species have a karyotype of $2n = 40$; in contrast, the karyotype of the steppe polecat, *M. eversmanni*, is $2n = 38$. It has been proposed the ancestor of all extant Mustelidae has a karyotype of $2n = 38$,[122] so it would appear the steppe polecat or any other related species, would be disqualified from consideration and the only possible choice would remain the European polecat. This is the basis for the historic argument that the ferret is a domesticated form of the European polecat and why some researchers are so insistent that the ferret's scientific name is *Mustela putorius furo* – in essence, a subspecies of the European polecat.

However, changes in karyotype do not necessarily reflect changes in the genome. The karyotype is the external appearance of the chromosomes in terms of size, number and morphology, while the genome is the information – the genes – carried on those chromosomes. The main difference in karyotypes is that European polecats had a Robertsonian rearrangement that reversed the ACK 2q+12 fusion that occurred early in the evolutionary history of the clade[122] This changed the karyotype, but did little to change the information contained within, which is why ferrets and polecats can hybridize and create reproductively viable offspring.[6,111,146–150,152–156]

Is a different karyotype enough to define a species? It is not unusual for a single species to have geographic variants or subspecies with differing karyotypes. *Akodon cursor*, a neotropical rodent, has 28 different karyotypes.[158] A Turkish mole rat, *Nannospalax ehrenbergi*, has eight different karyotypes.[159] Many other mammalian species have members with different karyotypes, including grey shrews,[160] the house mouse,[161] boars,[162] raccoon dogs[163] and even the weasel.[164] While a majority of species possess karyotypes of a uniform number and morphology, many others do not. It is clear that karyotype number and morphology alone is not remarkable enough to be used to define a species.

Molecular phylogenetic studies have recently supplanted and in many cases seem to have replaced, karyotype studies. These studies generally look at mitochondrial DNA (but are not limited to it) in order to see how many changes exist between two groups of animals such as the polecat and the domesticated ferret. Because changes randomly accumulate over time, it is thought animals with less comparative changes in the genome are more closely related than those having more differences.[165–170] To be able to tell time using these genome differences, the molecular data must be calibrated to an accepted fossil-based time sequence.[118] Thus, any conclusion based on molecular dating is dependent on the accuracy of the fossil dating methods, as well as the proper recovery of the fossils. This is of great concern in a family such as the Mustelidae, where the fossil record is fragmentary or controversial. The accuracy of a molecular clock is only as good as the fossil record on which it is based.

Another problem is sample size; that is, the number of individuals of a single species investigated in a particular phylogenetic study. Some of these studies are based on the analysis of an individual polecat or a relatively few number of individuals.[9,116,118,122,123,133,138] Sample size problems are exacerbated by studies that show polecats demonstrate a high degree of genetic heterozygosity.[134] This forces the dangerous assumption that the sample is representative of the population as a whole.[16,17,165,171] Fagan[172] states (p. 621), 'A sample must be obtained carefully so that it typifies the population without bias, the bane of sampling. Prejudice in the selection process leads to unrepresentative samples and inaccurate population estimates'. There are strong parallels between human and polecat evolution: both having modern forms emerging roughly about the same time, both migrating from a single refugium and both displaying wide genetic diversity. It is therefore likely the sampling problems faced by researchers looking at the genome of polecats would similarly parallel those plaguing anthropologists looking at the human genome (see Powledge and Rose[173] for a review).

CHAPTER SIX
Ferret-polecat domestication: genetic, taxonomic and phylogenetic relationships

The final two problems with molecular phylogenetic studies in ferrets are closely interrelated: the twin problems of domestication and introgression. To date, published studies of the domesticated ferret genome have been in association to its phylogenetic relationship to the polecats and other mustelids, rather than a study of the changes in genome due to human selection.[6,9,117,118,128] This potentially has great bearing on the calibration of the molecular clock used to time the polecat–ferret split; did the process of domestication modify the rate of genomic change? In other words, is the timing of change a reflection of the random accumulation of mutative changes or is it due to inbreeding to preserve human-favoured traits, such as albinism or tameness? Tied to this is the problem of centuries of introgression to both varieties of polecats. Could maternal mtDNA from a recent polecat introgression influence the molecular relationships seen in the phylogenetic studies? Is the timing of change a reflection of an ancient lineage or is it simply because of a history of hybridizing ferrets to polecats to improve hunting characteristics?

This discussion begs the following questions, each with important implications. Could ferrets have been domesticated from steppe polecats, but during domestication had a similar reversal of the ACK 2q+12 fusion experienced by European polecats? Could ferrets have been domesticated from steppe polecats and later introgression with European polecats changed the karyotype? Could ferrets have been domesticated from a European polecat/steppe polecat hybrid? Could ferrets have been domesticated from a western variety of European polecat, transported via trade routes throughout the Mediterranean and hybridized with eastern varieties? Could ferrets have been domesticated from both polecats; the European polecat in the west and the steppe polecat in the east and modern studies have simply been too limited in sampling to detect these differences? Regardless of the questions, answers and implications, it is clear there are shortcomings to the use of the karyotype and mtDNA studies to determine the progenitor of the domesticated ferret and reliance on these types of genetic studies alone cannot provide a satisfactory answer at this time.

Impact of problems on domestication studies

Individually, each of these seven disparate factors would complicate domesticated ferret studies to such a degree that would make any work difficult. Together, they make the study of ferret domestication extremely problematical, which is one reason that the published literature on the subject is so inadequate or non-existent.[1,3,4,5,11,12,36,174–182] A careful review of these sources can be categorized into three basic groups: (1) references that do not mention the ferret, (2) references that superficially mention the ferret and (3) references that attempt to discuss ferret origin, but because of a lack of progress in ferret domestication studies, they essentially cite earlier references. With the exception of genetic studies, very little work has been done to understand how or where polecats became ferrets.

Because of this lack of scholarship, the history of the ferret contains as many myths as truths – myths that are particularly hard to eliminate from the 'common knowledge' of ferrets. Thus, in contemporary literature, a frequently encountered claim is that ferrets have been domesticated longer than cats; a declaration that lacks scientific evidence and contradicts genetic studies, historic documents and zooarchaeological analysis. Likewise, it is frequently suggested that ancient Egyptians domesticated ferrets, that ferrets were domesticated to hunt rabbits and that the introduction of ferrets into Europe was to promote Roman interests. Each of these claims and more, fail to meet the basic requirements of scientific inquiry; that is, the support of evidence. Students of ferret domestication encounter more supposition than evidence and more 'common knowledge' than fact. The legacy of the seven disparate factors complicating the study of ferret domestication is myth and confusion in the public sector and a lack of sustained support in the scientific community.

History of the domesticated ferret

Domestication

Domestication comes from the Latin word 'domus', which means 'of the house and home'. It is generally applied to non-human organisms bred and maintained by humans for food or fiber, companionship, research, hunting, pest control and a host of other uses, including medical and scientific applications. Historically, animal domestication has been a human-mediated symbiotic process whereby natural selective pressures have been replaced by human selection.[4,178,183–187] Domestication is not just the adaptation of an animal (or plant) to better serve human needs, but also the adaptation of human culture towards societal acceptance of the animal.[5,175,186] The domestication process is considered symbiotic in most cases because although the benefits to humans can be considerable, domesticated species benefit as well in terms of protection from predation, medical care, access to nutrients, successful propagation and widespread distribution.[5,186–189] Domestication is considered an important concept in human history – a milestone of civilization.[4,5,70,71,186,190–196] Nonetheless, the concept of domestication remains ill-defined and controversial.[5,70,71,178,185,186,193,194,197]

While there remains considerable debate regarding the co-evolutionary nature of domestication – and to the degree in which animals participate – there are some widely agreed-upon criteria that can be used to define if an animal is domesticated or not. Characteristics of domestication include: (1) human-controlled breeding, (2) providing a useful service or product and (3) some change from the progenitor has been accomplished.[5,39,70,184–186,194,198–200] Tameness is often considered a fourth criterion of domestication in animal species (e.g. Gentry, et al.[184] and references therein). However, feral cats are hardly tame and remain domesticated, while ranch mink are considered domesticated but are rarely tame. Also, it would be difficult to suggest every animal can be tamed – invertebrates or unicellular animals that otherwise meet other criteria for domestication may not be tamable.

Table 6.1 Taxonomy of the ferret

Taxon level	Taxon name	Taxon includes
Kingdom	Animalia	**Animals**
Phylum	Chordata	**Chordates**
Subphylum	Vertebrata	**Vertebrates** Agnatha, Amphibia, Aves, Chondrichthyes, Osteichthyes, Mammalia, Reptilia
Class	Mammalia	**Mammals** Prototheria (egg-laying mammals), Theria (marsupials and placental mammals)
Subclass	Theria	**Marsupials and placental mammals** Eutheria (placental mammals), Metatheria (marsupials)
Infraclass	Eutheria	**Placental mammals** Artiodactyla, Carnivora, Cetacea, Chiroptera, Dermoptera, Hyracoidea, Insectivora, Lagomorpha, Macroscelidea, Perissodactyla, Pholidota, Primates, Proboscidea, Rodentia, Scandentia, Sirenia, Tubulidentata, Xenarthra
Order	Carnivora	**Mammalian carnivores** Caniformia (dog-like carnivores), Feliformia (cat-like carnivores)
Suborder	Caniformia	**Dog-like carnivores** Canidae (dogs), Mustelidae (mustelids), Odobenidae (walruses), Otariidae (sea lions), Phocidae (earless seals), Procyonidae (raccoons), Ursidae (bears)
Superfamily	Arctoidea	**Bear-like carnivores** Mustelidae (mustelids), Otariidae (sea lions), Phocidae (earless seals), Procyonidae (raccoons), Ursidae (Bears)
Family	Mustelidae	**Mustelid carnivores** Lutrinae (otters), Melinae (Eurasian badgers), Mellivorinae (honey badgers), Mephitinae (skunks), Mustelinae (tayras, grisons, wolverines, striped polecats, Patagonian weasels, fishers and martens, ferrets and polecats, mink, weasels and ermines, African striped weasels, marbled polecats), Taxidiinae (American badgers)
Subfamily	Mustelinae	**Weasel-like mustelids** *Eira* (tayras), *Galictis* (grisons), *Gulo* (wolverines), *Ictonyx* (striped polecats), *Lyncodon* (Patagonian weasels), *Martes* (fishers and martens), *Mustela* (ferrets and polecats, mink, weasels and ermines), *Poecilogale* (African striped weasels), *Vormela* (marbled polecats)
Genus	*Mustela*	Ferrets and polecats, mink, weasels and ermines
Subgenus	Putorius	Ferrets and polecats
Species	*Mustela eversmanni* *Mustela furo* *Mustela nigripes* *Mustela putorius*	Steppe polecats Domesticated ferrets Black-footed ferrets European polecats

Ferret–polecat taxonomic relationships.[6,9,14,111,125,126,230]

Of the four criteria of domestication, it seems tameness is the least trustworthy criterion.[5,198]

However, domesticated ferrets meet all four criteria of animal domestication. Ferret breeding has been under human control for centuries – perhaps as long as 2500 years or more.[3,5,6,10–13,118] During that period of time, ferrets have been used for home and agricultural pest control, for food procurement, to string telephone and electrical lines, in medical and scientific research and as companion animals.[3,5,11,12,24,25,26,30–38] Ferrets have undergone a good number of physiological, behavioural and morphological changes, including sustained albinism that shows a change in genetics from their progenitor (see discussion below). As with cats and dogs, ferrets are easily tamed when handled kindly.[25,26,38,201,202] It is clearly evident ferrets are domesticated animals.

Taxonomy

There can be no doubt that the ferret is a domesticated form of the polecat and that it was domesticated in the Old World. Since there are only three extant species of polecats and we can eliminate the black-footed ferret (*Mustela nigripes*) from consideration because it is only found in North America, by default we can infer the European polecat (*M. putorius*) and the steppe polecat (*M. eversmanni*) are the only likely candidates. This is in agreement with current phylogenetic investigations.[6,9,14,46,116,118,122,123,128] Thus, we are able to classify the domesticated ferret to the level of the polecat group, subgenus *Putorius*, without much difficulty (Table 6.1). The determination of the exact polecat progenitor is a bit more complicated.

Historically, zoologists relied on skull comparisons to determine taxonomic relationships and in those studies, since the ferret's skull was most like the steppe polecat, *M. eversmanni*, that species was considered the progenitor.[10,12,13,203] However, as Kharlamova et al.[94] demonstrated, cranial size and shape can be influenced by domestication, calling taxonomic relationships based on skull similarities (or differences) into doubt. Later, after genetics was incorporated into zoology and the karyotype of the ferret was compared with that of the European polecat (*M. putorius*) and found to be similar, that species was proclaimed the progenitor.[95,111,141,157] Modern osteological studies have obscured the issue more than illuminating it; it has been found domestication, diet and caging influences final adult cranial shape in many mammals.[5,68,69,72,94,204–209] Genetic associations are considered to be so indeterminate that a progenitor cannot be reliably ascertained.[6,9,14] It is possible the ferret was domesticated from both polecat varieties or at least has genetic contributions from both species.[9,210] Under these circumstances, many authorities have returned to using the original Linnean binomial, *M. furo*.

One historic test for close species relationships has been the ability of the domesticate to breed and produce viable offspring with the possible progenitor. There is direct and indirect evidence that regardless of karyotype numbers, domesticated ferrets (*M. furo*) can successfully interbreed with both European polecats (*M. putorius*) and steppe polecats (*M. eversmanni*), producing sexually viable hybrid offspring.[6,111,146–150,152–156] By extension, since steppe polecats can interbreed with black-footed ferrets (*M. nigripes*),[211] a good possibility exists that domesticated ferrets and/or European polecats can also interbreed with the endangered species. This means is that relationships between the polecats and ferrets are so close that minor genetic differences, including differences in karyotype, do not prevent successful hybridization.

This finding is consistent with recent genetic work, as already discussed.[6,9,14] This demonstrates the evolutionary differences between these species are minor, suggesting a relatively recent divergence from a common ancestor, again supported by genetic research.[9,15,66,67,117,118,128,136] Indeed, the black-footed ferret, as a separate species, is probably less than 100 000 years old and may be as young as 20 000 years or less.[6,112,118,141,212] Genetic studies have also suggested such a scenario; recent investigation suggests the modern polecat group evolved from a solitary Pleistocene refugium approximately 100 000 years ago.[117,128] Marmi et al.[116] indirectly supports this hypothesis by suggesting a rapid diversification of mustelid lineages. Discussions of polecat remains in the Pleistocene tend to be rather limited, which in part reflects a poor fossil record.[15,75,104,108,212–219] However, it is possible the lack of remains simply reflects that polecats were initially rare – what you would expect if they evolved 100 000 years ago from a single point of origin.

At present, general consensus classifies the polecats as separate species. Nonetheless, there is significant controversy regarding polecat taxonomy. Some suggest the black-footed ferret is a subspecies of the steppe polecat and others suggest all polecats comprise a single Holarctic species and differences are attributable to geomorphic adaptation.[6,13,112,114,116,137–139,141] Marmi et al.[116] states, 'Low levels of genetic divergence among European polecat, *Mustela putorius*, steppe polecat, *Mustela eversmanni* and European mink, *Mustela lutreola*, suggest that these species could be considered subspecies within a single species, *Mustela putorius*'. The natural history of the polecats is strikingly similar. They are all about the same size, share a very similar physiology, produce about the same number of offspring per litter, have similar reproductive strategies, develop similarly, share similar life histories and subsist on prey that typically shelters in burrows or underground (European polecat: amphibians, voles and rabbits; steppe polecat: marmots, gerbils and ground squirrels; and black-footed ferrets: prairie dogs, mice and ground squirrels).[147,220–229] In terms of general differences, the polecats are far more alike than they are dissimilar.

Taxonomists have classified the three polecats – and the domesticated ferret – into the subgenus *Putorius*; in some schemes, the European mink, *M. lutreola*, is also added.[6,112,141,230] Recent work suggests the relationships between the domesticated ferret and the European and steppe polecats are so close that the wild progenitor cannot be determined.[6,9,14,116] Taxonomists are becoming bolder in suggesting the *Putorius* group is a single species.[13,116,137,139] For these reasons, in this work the term 'polecat' should be understood to refer to any or all non-domesticated members of the subgenus *Putorius* (European polecat *M. putorius*, steppe polecat *M. eversmanni*, black-footed ferret *M. nigripes*).

Zooarchaeologists, who investigate the relationships between humans and domesticated animals, are increasingly desirous of a method of nomenclature that would recognize domesticated forms, a practice currently ignored in zoological nomenclature[231] (also see Gentry et al.[184] and references therein). Recently, the International Commission on Zoological Nomenclature has fixed the specific names of 17 wild progenitor species.[184,232] It has been recommended that workers use the scientific names of domesticated forms whenever possible.[184] In the case of the domesticated ferret – because the progenitor cannot be determined – the specific name that should be used is *Mustela furo*; a policy followed here (e.g. Davison et al.,[14] p. 155, Gentry et al.[184], p. 649).

Changes caused by domestication

If all polecats are essentially the same, how then is the domesticated ferret different? Domestication causes documented changes in mammals that tend to be non-species specific. In other words, regardless of the mammal, the changes caused by domestication tend to be somewhat similar.[5,12,174–176,179,180] For example, common behavioural changes include increased acceptance of novelty and a juvenilization of behaviours, physiological changes include an increase in litter size and reproduction and morphological changes include a juvenilization of the skull and altered fur colour and texture. Similar changes occur in most domesticated mammalian species, including carnivores (dogs, cats, ferrets, mink, fox, raccoon dogs, skunks), rodents (rats, mice, cavies, hamsters), lagomorphs (rabbits), artiodactyls (cattle, sheep, goats, pigs, camels, llamas, alpacas) and perissodactyls (horses, donkeys, burros).[5,12,175,176,179,180] How could so many animals, from such disparate locations from around the globe, have such similar changes?

The rule of parsimony or Occam's razor, suggests this is due to similar changes in similar genes rather than a convergence of traits due to different changes in different genes. Because these changes are so similar in taxonomically dissimilar mammals, the simplest explanation is that conserved homogenous genes are being affected. What or where those genes are is still under investigation. For our purposes, we shall consider the genetics of ferret domestication to be a black box. That is, while the exact genetic mechanisms within the box may be unknown, unproved, controversial or in doubt, the results of those genetic interactions can easily be seen and quantified and it is those visible and measurable changes that shall be the focus of our attention.

This discussion will be limited to three basic areas that are impacted by domestication: physiology, morphology and behaviour. It should be recognized that these categories are arbitrary; certainly many (or most) morphological and behavioural changes have their roots in physiology, therefore these categories exist only for the ease of discussion. Physiological differences are those governing body systems and their functions, including raw or 'genetic' intelligence, vision and reproduction. Morphological differences are those displaying measurable variation within the physical attributes of a specific trait, such as fur length and colouration, dentition or body size and proportions. Behavioural differences include learned behaviours, instincts and the interactions between them. Instincts are those stereotypic species-wide behaviours that are not learned but are innately known (although frequently influenced by various environmental factors such as stress, development, maternal care, sibling interaction, etc.) and include predatory, play, curiosity, maternal, sexual, individual distance ('fight or flight') behaviours and more. Again, although I have divided intelligence into emic (internal-genetic-nature) and etic (external-environmental-nurture) categories, this in no way should be understood to infer such a simplistic division accurately reflects how intelligence should be viewed. It is simply an artificial construct meant to show how domestication can affect different aspects of a single characteristic.

Physiological changes

Reproduction

While introgression has probably minimized the differences between the domesticated ferret and the polecats, there are several physiological differences that are readily apparent (Table 6.2).

CHAPTER SIX

Ferret-polecat domestication: genetic, taxonomic and phylogenetic relationships

Table 6.2 Changes in the ferret because of domestication

Category	Generalized change	Specific difference	Ferret	Polecat
Physiological	Reproduction	Increase in size of litter	1–18 (average 8)	2–12 (average 6)
Physiological	Reproduction	Increase in number of litters	2 per season	1 per season
Physiological	Pigments	Depigmentation	Albinism and depigmentation	Generally not present
Physiological	Vision	Colour perception	Reds	Reds and blues
Physiological	Vision	Structural changes	Related to albinism	Generally not present
Physiological	Auditory	Hearing loss	Related to depigmentation	Generally not present
Physiological	Cranial capacity	Decrease in volume	15–20% smaller	Generally not present
Morphological	Cranial shape	Unspecified	Highly variable	Generally consistent
Morphological	Dentition	Crowding	Some minor crowding	Generally not present
Morphological	Body size	Increased size	Increased variability	Generally consistent
Morphological	Sexual dimorphism	Increased percentage	Increased variability	Generally consistent
Morphological	Pelt	Angora	Present	Not present
Morphological	Os penis	Size and morphology	Smaller due to castration	Generally consistent
Behavioural	Social behaviors	Social acceptance	Limited acceptance	Asocial
Behavioural	Personal distance	Fearfulness	Fearless	Fearful
Behavioural	Predatory instincts	Hunting instincts	Generally diminished	Generally consistent

Ferrets have undergone significant physiological, morphological and behavioural differences due to domestication. This list should not be considered all-inclusive. (See text for explanation and references.)

Foremost are the reproductive changes typical of domesticated mammals. This generally means individuals are more promiscuous, there are more offspring per litter and more litters per season. Polecats mate once a year and generally have between 2 and 12 offspring (six on average), while ferrets can mate twice a year or more, producing 1–18 kits (eight on average).[221,233,234] These changes in reproduction may not be as significant as they first appear. Female polecats upon losing a litter will often go into heat and have a second litter that season and female ferrets having a litter removed for commercial reasons may react somewhat similarly.[221,235,236] Also, the female ferret's photo-period cycle is easily disrupted using artificial light, allowing the animal to come into oestrus sooner.[234,237] These two factors alone suggest there is as much – or more – environmental influence as there are changes due to domestication.[155,236–246] Nonetheless, there are enough differences – especially in the increased size of the litter – that suggests changes in the ferret's reproductive physiology have taken place because of domestication.

Albinism and depigmentation

Albinism and depigmentation are profound physiological changes and a good indicator of domestication; albinism is rarely encountered in nature and the maintenance of the condition is historically under human selection. True autosomal recessive albinism is intimately correlated to domestication because human selection maintains the trait.[68,69,72,192] This is especially true in ferrets, where albinism has been a trait favoured by hunters since at least the Middle Ages.[34,40] Albinism is divided into two basic forms, oculocutaneous albinism and ocular albinism, each having multiple types caused by different metabolic or physiological problems.[247–249] While albinism in ferrets is generally of the oculocutaneous type (an autosomal recessive trait due to the disruption of the tyrosine pathway), problems with tyrosine penetrance can lead to depigmentation changes sometimes confused with albinism.[250] In most cases, albinism in ferrets is controlled at a single gene locus; however, sable, chocolate and sandy colourations in ferrets appear to be controlled by at least two loci, probably more.[251–253] The genetics of many ferret colouration schemes are yet to be adequately worked out. In ferrets, albinism is associated with visual and structural changes in the nervous system.[252,254–257]

Vision

Domestication has also resulted in visual system changes, including possible changes in colour vision. The ferret visual system is structurally similar to that of a dog and is considered dichromic[258,259] (also review Yokoyamaa, Radlwimmera[260,261]). Both polecats and ferrets see in shades of gray, but polecats are reported to be able to see into the blues and reds. In comparison, ferrets are apparently more colour-limited than polecats, seeing some reds, but not the other colours.[259,262–264] Visual differences also exist between albino ferrets and their pigmented counterparts in the structure of the brain and the visual pathways.[83,254,263–271]

Hearing

Because albinism causes pigmentation changes in the middle ear and processing auditory information relies on pigmented cells to work properly, it is possible albino ferrets have changes to their auditory system compared with polecats and pigmented ferrets.[266,272–274] Various genes for pigmentation causing albinism, agoutism, brown dilutions, lethal spotting, piebald spotting, pink-eyed dilutions, recessive yellow colourations, steel colouration (dark-eyed whites) and white spotting are known to have complex interactions with genes coding for other traits (e.g. Barsch,[275] Cattanach,[276] Searle[277] and references therein). Certainly, there are established auditory differences in ferrets bred for some depigmented colouration schemes, such as pandas and blazes, who are prone to deafness due to various neural crest disorders or Waardenburg syndrome.[273,278–281] There is very little published on this subject specifically on ferrets, despite abundant anecdotal accounts of hearing loss in ferrets bred for depigmented colouration schemes and further research is warranted.

Cranial capacity

Domesticated ferrets are anecdotally reported to be less intelligent than polecats, both as a result of a decrease in cranial capacity, as well as structural changes within the brain itself – although the idea is controversial.[174,175,198,205,206,208,282–289] This change can be demonstrated by a decrease in the encephalization quotient during domestication (EQ is a rough measure of potential intelligence based on the general assumption that larger brains possessing similar complexity are smarter).[290–292] Cranial capacity is an approximate measurement of the volume of the cranial cavity. If the cranial capacity is measured accurately, the volume can represent brain volume.[293] One problem with EQ is that cranial capacity equals brain volume only in smaller animals, such as the ferret.[209]

The cranial capacity of the ferret is about 15–20% smaller than in polecats, reflecting the typical diminution of brain size during domestication (which lowers EQ).[83,99,205,207,282,294–297] The reduction in size in the ferret's brain can be attributed to a reduction of the telencephalon and isocortex[205,296,298–300] (also see Lockard[301] for comparison). While brain size decreases during domestication, the exact changes are not necessarily the same between species, with differences attributed to the species' evolutionary history.[302] The changes in brain size and structure that occur during domestication do not seem to be reversible, even if the species is allowed to become feral.[302]

Morphological changes

Morphological differences between polecats and ferrets abound and include changes in the skeletal system and dental arcade, body size and shape, fur colouration, length and quality and cranial shape (Table 6.2). These differences are highly variable, ranging from insignificant in one instance, such as post-cranial skeletal changes, to moderately significant, such as body size, to profound in another, such as albinism. Because of the long history of hybridizing ferrets to polecats, many of the changes are relatively minor if compared with changes seen in other species, such as in dogs or cattle.

Cranial morphology

Of the skull morphological differences, the most significant is the width of the postorbital constriction. In ferrets, steppe polecats and black-footed ferrets, the post-orbital constriction is quite narrow, while in European polecats, it is significantly wider.[83,303] Some of this is probably attributable to natural variation[99,204,304] or asymmetry due to environmental impact on muscle function and use.[305] Ferret skulls have significant sexual dimorphism in size, cranial volume and to some degree in external morphometrics.[91,156] Some changes resulting from domestication are masked by various environmental factors, such as diet[93] or hybridization.[101] Breeding ferrets for tameness can likewise have a large impact on skull morphology.[94] Much of the morphological differences are likely attributable to changes in brain size.[205,297]

Dental crowding

Teeth in domesticated mammals are generally more crowded due to facial juvenilization – a shortening of the length of the maxilla and mandible impacting the dental arcade. This is minimal in ferrets, probably due to introgression to polecats.[6,8] Historically the tasks assigned to ferrets have been pest control and hunting, making short-faced ferrets unpopular, so human selection for shorter faces has been minimal. Supernumerary teeth are common.[306–311] Dental pathologies include slight overcrowding, malformed teeth and malocclusion.[221,311–313]

CHAPTER SIX
Ferret-polecat domestication: genetic, taxonomic and phylogenetic relationships

Body size

Initially, domesticated animals have a decrease in body size in relation to their progenitors, presumably due to changes in diet.[5,12] However, reports of ferrets being smaller – or larger – than polecats are mostly uncontrolled, anecdotal and unreliable. The degree of both body size and sexual dimorphism of polecats compared with ferrets appears only slightly less profound (compare Glas[314] with [315-317]). Such changes may be environmental rather than genetic and due to maternal effect, caging, neutering or diet. Because of the long history of hybridization to polecats and the work history of the ferret, it is unlikely selection for body size was desirable or endurable. On the other hand, there are reports that some breeders purposely bred ferrets destined for ratting to be smaller to facilitate entry into small spaces, but such practices were historically discouraged.[35,37,318]

Miscellaneous

Ferrets with a variety of angora fur have been introduced during the last decade and have been reported to show more fearfulness and other behavioural changes compared with typical domesticated ferrets, but the observation has not been qualitatively or quantitatively studied. Some North American ferret associations and ferret farms tend to favour large hobs and are reportedly breeding animals for a larger size. Significant morphological differences exist in the size and shape of the os penis of neutered ferrets that can be attributed to the practice of early neutering, but their contribution to disease has not been researched (Church: unpublished data).

Behavioural changes

Of the three types of changes, the most profound modification in the domesticated ferret is behavioural (see Poole[152] for a review of behavioural differences between ferrets and polecats) (Table 6.2). This makes sense considering ferrets were domesticated to do what polecats already did well – killing small rodents and hunting animals in burrows.[43,319,320] This illustrates a desire to create an animal that was easy to handle, rather than one that would do its job differently. In other words, it is likely that people did not want to change the polecat from what it basically was; they simply wanted a polecat that was predictably safe. Consequently, it is probable polecats were bred for tameness (and possibly for fearlessness and curiosity), rather than colour or body mass. Albinism and depigmentation is a common side effect of breeding for behaviour; see discussion below. In this case, albinism was probably a historic accident rather something being actively sought, but once it occurred, it was selectively preserved.

This is clearly demonstrated by the lack of historic ferret varieties; unlike with dogs, cats, rabbits and a host of other domesticated species, the number of fancy types in ferrets is rather limited. Until this century, ferrets have been generally limited to two basic colour types (albino and sable or polecat-like colouration, with a limited number of colour dilutions) and a shortened continuum of body shapes (ranging from a thin 'whippet' to a stocky 'bulldog'). Ferrets, while clearly exhibiting a range of behaviours that are shared by the polecat group, display some behaviours that are clearly advantageous for working with humans.[152] Some of these are due to learned or environmental factors, not a shift in genetics, making the actual determination of genetic behavioural changes problematic.[321-324]

If the hypothesis that ferrets were domesticated to create a tame polecat is true, presumably for the purposes of pest control or hunting, it could help explain some of the extensive introgression noted between the domesticate and its progenitor(s).[6,9,14,46,117,118] There are two basic types of hybridization events: accidental and purposeful. Accidental introgression occurs when a persistent polecat hob breaks into a hutch containing a ferret jill or when a ferret escapes from captivity. Purposeful introgression requires human facilitation; it is the premeditated breeding of ferrets to polecats for a variety of reasons. In ferrets, historically the paramount reason for the widespread practice of hybridizing ferrets to polecats was to improve their hunting characteristics.[34,35,37,201,202,318,325]

It is possible that because accidental hybridization is generally a random event, the degree of introgression of ferrets into the wild polecat population in a particular geographic area might be helpful to infer the length of time ferrets were held in captivity in that region. For example, assuming random accidental introgression into the wild population, higher percentages of ferret genetic markers might support the hypothesis that ferrets were there for longer periods of time. This may be helpful in determining the geographic centre for ferret domestication, assuming the oldest or most widespread regions of accidental introgression can be shown to correlate to depth of time. At this time, the effectiveness of this approach is somewhat theoretical since wild populations of polecats are becoming increasingly fragmented and entirely extirpated from some regions (for a review of mustelid conservation see Birks and Kitchener,[326] Griffiths[327]).

Gregariousness

Perhaps one of the most commonly cited examples of behavioural changes in ferrets caused by domestication is their oft-reported gregarious nature. Polecats evolved as same-sex exclusionary territorialists where males and females exclude other members of the same sex and where the male territory overlaps the territories of several females (also called a dispersed harem).[151,223,328–330] Many authors of ferret books regard ferrets as gregarious or social animals.[22,26,29] However, because domestication tends to juvenilize existing behaviour rather than creating new ones, it is unlikely domestication has created a new behaviour.[5,12,180,331]

A close examination of ferret behaviour tends to confirm the idea that rather than the creation of a new behaviour, the juvenilization of an existing behaviour (or the retention of a juvenile behaviour) has taken place.[152,329] Many ferret owners and shelter operators that house a large number of ferrets are forced to segregate groups or individual ferrets from each other in order to prevent prolonged fighting. Fighting between these individuals or groups can be protracted, violent and persistent and not at all like the dominance fighting displayed within established groups (review [152,154,329,332,333]). This type of exclusionary fighting is more common in same-sex ferrets, older ferrets, ferrets that have lived alone or those in groups that have been established for some time. In addition, feral ferrets in New Zealand tend to display the same type of exclusionary territorial patterns as polecats, making it unlikely genetic change in this behaviour has occurred.[154,223,334–336]

What has probably happened is that during domestication, the polecat's exclusionary behaviours became juvenilized during breeding for tameness. If so, then other ferrets in established groups are seen as siblings and rather than a gregarious nature being created during domestication, the process resulted in the retention of a juvenile behaviour. This would be more in keeping with the retention of juvenile behaviours seen in other domesticated species.[5,153,174,175,180]

Fear responses

The most dramatic change has been in fear response (the 'individual distance'). Most polecats develop an innate fear of humans, between 1 and 3 months of age, and if obtained before that time and hand-raised, will only display trustworthiness to regular caregivers.[337,338] Yet, domesticated ferrets show little or no fear of humans or novel objects in their environment.[152,339,340]

Behavioural changes are often linked to changes in coat colouration.[252,255,341] Light-coloured heads or white blazes and tail tips, are often associated with gentleness or docility; however, if the non-albinistic depigmentation is extensive, it is likely there will be a negative impact on the nervous system, resulting in visual or auditory impairment, nervousness or excitability, aggression, seizures and other central nervous system problems.[255] Some of these behaviours may be due to factors other than domestication; ferrets may startle easily and display fear responses because of deafness or blindness.

Expression of instinctual behaviours forms a generalized continuum between polecats, polecat-ferret hybrids and ferrets, with ferrets showing the most dilution of expression.[146,150,152,342] Because a correlation exists between the degree of expression of behaviour and brain structure, skull morphology and size can be used to infer non-specific behavioural changes. In other words, while you do not know which behaviour is changed or the degree of change, there is a statistical probability that change has occurred when cranial capacity is reduced.[94] Changes in the expression of curiosity are common (closely related to fear responses), but difficult to differentiate from environmental factors.[339,343,344] Socialization has an important impact on play behaviour, with socially deprived ferrets playing longer and more aggressively than those raised in a social situation.[345]

A portion of a ferret's hunting behaviours remain unaffected by domestication, such as the instinct to bite the most anterior portion of an object and the elicitation of hunting reaction by prey movement; however, much of their hunting techniques require maternal instruction.[346] While visual clues may elicit predatory behaviours, because ferrets primarily rely on olfactory clues, a great deal of hunting success depends on environmental experiences during the 3rd month of a ferret's life.[347] Olfactory deprivation during juvenile development can have a profound effect on adult behaviour.[321]

History of domestication

Early history

The physiological, morphological and behavioural differences found in the domesticated ferret have taken place for roughly 2000–3000 years. Ferret domestication can be traced with certainty to about AD 622 in the writings of the Spaniard Isidore of Seville. There is a high probability the Romans knew of the ferret; Strabo might have mentioned them about AD 17–23 and Pliny the Elder in about AD 77. There is only moderate probability (not certainty) the ancient Greeks mentioned the ferret (or weasel or polecat) several times, first about 750 BC (Homer), then 560 BC (Aesop), 440 BC (Herodotus), 425–392 BC (Aristophanes), 355 BC with Aristotle's works and ending roughly about 320 BC in

CHAPTER SIX

Ferret-polecat domestication: genetic, taxonomic and phylogenetic relationships

the *Characters* of Theophrastus. It is possible the older Greek references are not actually discussing the ferret, but its progenitor or even a generic weasel.[319,348-363]

The Bible

Many histories of the ferret include Biblical references to the ferret as being an unclean animal. A word in *Leviticus* (11:29–30) was translated in the King James version of the Bible (1611) to read: 'These also shall be unclean unto you among the creeping things that creep upon the earth; the weasel and the mouse and the tortoise after his kind [29], and the ferret and the chameleon and the lizard and the snail and the mole [30]'. This passage is the only one in the Bible mentioning the ferret. This reference, combined with the Strabo and Pliny references, was pivotal in creating the supposition that ferrets were domesticated in North Africa. Later, it would be used to support an Egyptian origin older than the domestication of the cat.

Many modern versions of the Bible do not use 'ferret' in this passage, but instead use 'gecko' or 'croaking lizard'; some use 'shrew' or 'hedgehog'. These versions include *American Revised* (1901), *American Standard* (1901), *American Translation* (1935), *Amplified Bible* (1965), *Darby Translation* (1890), *Douay-Rheims* (1609), *English Standard* (2001), *God's Word* (1995), *Hebrew Bible* (1917), *Holman Christian* (2004), *Jewish Bible* (1998), *Lesser Bible* (1900), *The Message* (2002), *Moffatt* (1924), *New American Standard* (1971), *New Century* (1987), *New International Reader's* (1998), *New International* (1965), *New International UK* (1984), *New Life Bible* (1969), *New Living Translation* (1996), *New Revised Standard* (1990), *Revised Standard* (1952) and the *World English Bible* (2004). In the *New King James* version, published in 1982, the word 'ferret' was replaced by 'gecko'.

It is likely the word in question is not a ferret, but a gecko or some other type of lizard. This reference, while having interesting historical value, provides little substance for piecing together the ferret's history of domestication.

Egypt

One of the more frequently encountered hypotheses concerning the origin of the ferret is that they were domesticated in Egypt. This hypothesis is presented in several manifestations – the most common in the ferret community being that the ferret was domesticated sometime prior to the cat. However, the sum of evidence supporting ferret domestication by the Egyptians is underwhelming. There are no zooarchaeological reports, genetics studies, theological support, historical documents, hieroglyphs or biogeographical or ecological evidence that document the presence of either the ferret or polecat in Egypt during the window of domestication. Such ruminations are conjectural suppositions, which, through repetition and decades of reprinting, have taken on a 'truthfulness of familiarity' or 'common knowledge'. Unfortunately, these suppositions are regarded as factual by many in the ferret community despite a singular lack of substantive evidence.

For example, Egyptians generally had a god (or gods) associated with every domesticated animal, yet not a single Egyptian god has ever been found that is linked – in any way – to the domesticated ferret.[47,49,50,364-369] Anubis, the jackal-headed god associated with the underworld, was often associated with domestic dogs; their mummified remains were found in the Anubieion catacombs at Saqqara.[364,367,370,371] Part of the cemetery at Abydos was set aside for dogs and they were buried adjacent to humans (see [366,372] and references therein). Ancient Egyptians commonly mummified domestic cats.[366,373] A review of the literature reveals ancient Egyptians were prone to mummify most creatures. The list of animals mummified by the Egyptians include baboons, jackals, dogs, cats, wild cats, frogs, lions, foxes, rodents, insects, cattle, sheep, weasels, mongooses, gazelles, zorillas, hares, fish, otters, various birds, lizards, snakes, crocodiles, hippopotami and even an egg. There is not contained within this menagerie of beasts a single, verified ferret or polecat mummy.[48,49,50,366,374,375]

As already discussed, there is a lack of theological evidence placing the domesticated ferret in Egypt. The only possible reference in *Leviticus* was probably a mistranslation of an obscure word for a gecko or lizard.[376-380]

Neither are there artistic representations of ferrets on Egyptian hieroglyphs, despite the claim in several popular ferret books; the claim is made, but the hieroglyph itself is never published.[22,23,27-30] A review of the literature shows a singular lack of hieroglyphs that can be positively identified as a ferret, although cats, weasels, zorillas, mongooses, genets and other small carnivores are relatively common. It is possible the confusion stems from the superficial resemblance of the ferret to other Egyptian fauna, such as the mongoose, weasel or zorilla, which are depicted on numerous hieroglyphs.[374,381-389]

There is likewise a singular lack of archaeological evidence. There are no reports of bones or bodies of ferrets or polecats.[390-392] It is true that the lack of evidence might reflect poor preservation or rarity, but such conditions exist for all animals in the same place and time, yet the bones of numerous small and rare species have been recovered, identified and cataloged.[105,106,389,392]

Biogeographical evidence demonstrating that ferrets or polecats were in or near Egypt is lacking. Polecats have reportedly been found in Iberia, Mesopotamia,

Turkey, Lebanon, eastern Palestine and western Morocco, but never in nor close to Egypt.[53,55,393–412] Polecats and ferrets are not included on the published lists of Egyptian mammals.[389,391,403,406,413–422]

There is no place in the world where ferrets or polecats are found in Egypt-like ecological conditions.[179,423,424] The ferret's genetic adaptation to ecological conditions is reflected in its physiology; it is not adapted to an arid ecology because of high water requirements, kidney structure and inability to tolerate extreme heat (e.g. [264,315–317,425] and references therein).

There are only two possibilities; either the ferret was domesticated in Egypt or it was not. If it was domesticated in Egypt, there must have been a reliable source of polecats to serve as the progenitor. If the progenitor – or domesticate – was present, then there should be some sort of evidence from a culture that recorded the details of life on stone and papyrus and yet none exists. It is clear there are serious problems with the 'African domestication' hypothesis.

Mediterranean

The most likely scenario for the domestication of the ferret is that it took place in the southern to southeastern portion of Europe that abuts the Mediterranean, perhaps including portions of extreme northwestern Africa (Morocco). It is probable that domestication was not centred in one area, but was spread out within a region that included major trade routes and agricultural centres so a central point of origin may never be located. This 'circum-Mediterranean origin hypothesis' may partially explain the dearth of archaeological evidence; it is simply too spread out to find easily. There are other reasons that can confuse the issue; consider how many skeletons you find lying around even though there are millions of animals – ferrets were rare during early domestication, so are very rarely found.

Even if ferret domestication was circum-Mediterranean, there are likely to have been some places where the intensity of domestication was greater than in other areas. There are some clues in the historic texts that can help determine who might be more intensely involved in the domestication of the ferret and where and why it occurred. The ancient Greeks were probably involved from a suite of references by Homer, Aesop, Herodotus, Aristophanes, Aristotle and Theophrastus. The references made by Strabo and Pliny to 'Libyan ferrets' might be a reference to Morocco or Carthage or the surrounding environs, suggesting perhaps that the Phoenicians were involved.[426] Those same sources imply that by the time of the Romans era it was already in a domesticated form, so they were not necessarily involved directly. Arguments that the domestication of the ferret could have occurred on the Iberian Peninsula depend on the hypothesis that domestication was for the purpose of rabbit hunting (based on Strabo and Pliny). However, rabbits were not present in ancient Greece or many other areas of Europe at the time of domestication, so it cannot explain references to ferrets in those areas. This suggests the presence of the ferret would have been for other reasons.[11–13]

Domestication is inherently a cultural phenomenon and a look at the interactions of various cultures might lend a clue to the domestication of the ferret. When ferrets were being domesticated, both Greeks and Phoenicians knew of the presence of cats in Egypt and their use in pest control to protect stores of grain. They were also probably aware the Egyptians guarded their cats quite well, prohibiting their exportation, even to the point of returning cats to Egypt if they found them in other countries or putting people to death for the killing of a cat.[5,12,427–430] Egyptian care for the cat might have superficially had religious importance, but there might have been an underlying economic consideration as well. Cats represented mousing technology that increased grain yields, directly influencing the economics of a nation. There is some evidence that a few cats had already entered Greece and other southern European areas as early as 500–300 BC. However, the numbers were small and did not have economic significance.[5,12,427–429,431]

A major requirement for sustained domestication is the economic benefit a culture gains through such efforts.[3,5,12,210,374] For any group to gain economic benefit from the domestication of the ferret, it had to provide either a product or a service of value. In the case of the ferret, possible benefits could have been fur, mousing, ratting, rabbiting and the hunting of other small animals, such as hamsters, susliks or marmots. It is possible the ferret was valuable not just for pest control, but after the death of the animal, the pelt could have been salvaged, doubling the benefits. For the Phoenicians, the benefits of ferrets for pest control aboard trade ships or in shipyard storage facilities, could have been considerable. The Phoenicians had substantial grain production.[426] Ferrets could have been used to protect those stores from the ravages of rodents. The benefits for the Greeks would have been similar. The difference between the two groups is that some historic records exist that support Greek involvement, while in the case of the Phoenicians, there is no supportive evidence yet found.

Greek and Roman references

It is probably not a coincidence the cat was domesticated about 1600 BC, roughly corresponding to the rise of the New Kingdom, precisely to protect Egyptian

CHAPTER SIX
Ferret-polecat domestication: genetic, taxonomic and phylogenetic relationships

grain stores.[5,427–429,431] Admittedly, some controversy exists regarding the earliest remains of the domesticated cat.[5] However, there is a great difference between dating a single cat mandible to 6000 BC and the numerous New Kingdom references to cats about 1600 BC. While is it probable cats were domesticated before that time, proving domestication prior to that date is problematic.[5] Nonetheless, regardless of the exact timing of the domestication of the cat, it is obvious there is a correlation between the protection of grain stores and the acceptance of the cat as an ally in the shielding of those foods.

The Greek involvement in the domestication of ferrets is controversial. It is only supported by the translation of ancient words into modern equivalents and there is no physical evidence that could tie the historic record to the modern animal. Even so, it is probable early Greeks had some involvement in the domestication of the ferret (Table 6.3).

Perhaps the first mention of the ferret's progenitor occurs in the *Battle of the Frogs and Mice*, roughly about 750 BC.[432,433] In this story, a mouse escaped the predation of a polecat or ferret, an obvious reference to a wild mustelid. Contemporary to this reference is the *Iliad*, where the mention of a cap of ferret skin is made – another reference to an animal that is not necessarily domesticated.[434–436] In both of these references, because the context of the story has the animals in a wild situation, it follows the animals are probably not domesticated.

The next mention of an animal that could be the ferret or its progenitor comes from Aesop at roughly 560 BC. There is some controversy about authorship (was Aesop a real person?) and exact date and many versions have been based on translations of translations. If recent translations of the *Fables* are accurate, then Aesop may have mentioned 'house-ferrets' at an early date.[361,362] The house-ferrets in the fables are in a human environment, but are not always depicted as a truly domesticated animal. In the fable, *Of the Ferret and the Man*,[361] the ferret almost seems like an interloper in the man's home. However, in *The House-Ferret and Aphrodite*,[362] the animal is in a clearly domestic situation. It is possible this lack of precision reflects an animal in a transitional state, not wild and yet not quite domesticated.

In the Fourth Book of the Histories, called *Melpomene*, written about 440 BC, Herodotus reports on the wild animals of Libya, 'there are also weasels found in the silphium, very like to the weasels of Tartessos' (Herodotus, Godley,[358] para. 192). The 'weasels of Tartessos' are generally believed to be domesticated ferrets.[359] This is a possible reference to the ferrets mentioned by Strabo and Pliny.[43,44,320,437] This could reflect the possibility that Strabo and/or Pliny used Herodotus as a source of information and their reports are not primary accounts. On the other hand, it could be a confirmation of the other two reports, made more than 400 years before them. If they are ferrets, then it shows a possible domestication hot spot in the western Mediterranean. However, not all are convinced the animal in question is a ferret. Amigues[438] argues the animal is perhaps a genet and that the word for 'weasel' was a generalized term, not necessarily a specific one

Table 6.3 Changes in the perception of the ferret and its progenitor over time

Reference	Author	Date	Term for animal	Connotation
Battle of the Frogs and Mice	Homer	750 BC	Polecat	Wild animal
Iliad	Homer	750 BC	Polecat	Wild animal
Fables	Aesop	560 BC	House-ferret	Habituated to humans
Fourth Book of the Histories	Herodotus	440 BC	Weasels of Tartessos	Tamed or domesticated
The Acharnians	Aristophanes	425 BC	Ferret	Tamed or domesticated
The Wasps	Aristophanes	422 BC	Ferret	Tamed or domesticated
Peace	Aristophanes	421 BC	Ferret	Tamed or domesticated
The Thesmophoriazusae	Aristophanes	410 BC	Ferret	Tamed or domesticated
The Ecclesiazusae	Aristophanes	392 BC	Ferret	Tamed or domesticated
Historia Animalium	Aristotle	355 BC	Ferret	Tamed or wild
Characters	Theophrastus	320 BC	Ferret or polecat	Tamed or wild
Geographica	Strabo	17–23 AD	Ferret	Domesticated
Naturalis Historia	Pliny the Elder	77 AD	Ferret	Domesticated

In a period of approximately 800 years, descriptions of the ferret changed from having a wild connotation to one of domestication. (See text for explanation and references.)

(see discussion below). If this is true, then it questions if the peoples of the western Mediterranean were at a centre of ferret domestication.

Aristophanes was a Greek satirist and playwright who lived from 448 to 380 BC. In *The Acharnians* (425 BC), *The Wasps* (422 BC), *Peace* (421 BC), *The Thesmophoriazusae* (410 BC) and *The Ecclesiazusae* (392 BC), Aristophanes refers at least 10 times to a creature that has been translated as various animals, including a cat, weasel, marten, ferret and polecat. It almost certainly was not a cat, which was not in Greece at the time.[3,5] Most modern authorities reject using marten, preferring instead the terms 'ferret', 'house-weasel' or 'house-ferret'.[348–354] One reason why martens are probably not the animal in question is due to odour. Polecats are called 'foul-martens' and martens 'sweet-martens' due to differences in their body odour; Greek references invariably mention how the animal stinks! Due to the satiric nature of his work, Aristophanes would not have referred to a rare or unknown animal, but one that was common enough for the audience to understand the reference, which was generally one of an animal that steals meat, hunts mice and stinks. These references show an animal that is commonly held in a domestic state, suggesting it was either domesticated or in the process of being domesticated.

Aristotle wrote *Historia Animalium* about 355 BC and mentions an animal that could have been a ferret or polecat.[319,355–357] The importance of the Aristotelian reference is that it implies two versions of polecats can be found: wild and tame.[3,10,12,210] This could indicate an animal in the process of domestication.

In his 320 BC work, *Characters*, Theophrastus discusses various superstitions and mentions those pertaining to weasels.[363] Theophrastus uses the same word as Aristophanes and Aristotle.[319,348–357,363] This can be interpreted as meaning the word was a generic term, such as the current usage of 'mustelid' to describe many different, yet related, animals. It could also mean the animal in question was the same one as mentioned by the other authors, although in this instance, the connotation is probably that of a wild animal.

The next two references of note are from the Roman era, those of Strabo about AD 17–23 and Pliny the Elder about AD 77.[43,44,320,437] As already mentioned, both these references cite the use of what are considered to be ferrets in hunting rabbits. These could be the so-called 'weasels of Tartessos', as described by Herodotus.[359] The main objection to classifying this animal as a ferret is the reference to the creature using its claws to pull the rabbits from burrows, a technique rarely used by the ferret or mongoose, but common to genets.[438] However, in general, these arguments fail to reconcile four basic points: (1) the animals were described as being muzzled, so could not use their teeth for retrieval, but were forced to use other means. (2) Ferrets and polecats, when faced with a prey animal hiding their head by facing away from them and using their body to block the tunnel, will use their claws to scratch at the prey in an attempt to dislodge it from its protective position. (3) Ferrets and polecats, when unable to use their teeth to remove items, will hug or grasp the item with their front paws and scoot backwards, pulling the item with them. It is conceivable this action could be viewed as a use of the claws to pull prey from the burrows. (4) The genet is far more arboreal than the ferret or polecat, is significantly greater in size, has large cat-like ears that would not allow easy access to narrow burrows, cannot turn around within a burrow and so would have to back out and has longer legs that would force the genet to crawl and hinder underground locomotion and prey retrieval. While possible, genets are generally unsuited for hunting subterranean animals such as rabbits. It is more likely that the animal in question was probably species of weasel, such as the polecat or ferret.

The Strabo and Pliny references also state the animal in question was Libyan.[44,45,320,437] At the time of the references, Libya was more-or-less synonymous with north-western Africa and had a great Phoenician influence.[426] This comment, more than any other, has caused those investigating the domestication of the ferret to consider Morocco or North Africa the region of domestication. The problem with accepting this hypothesis is that it presumes the term 'Libyan ferret' actually signifies an animal domesticated in Libya. There is no evidence for this, any more than the term 'Belgian hare' proves hares were domesticated in Belgium (they are rabbits) or the 'English Angora' rabbit comes from England (the angora breed originated in Turkey). Also, Strabo and/or Pliny probably never witnessed the working of these animals, rather reporting information from other sources, possibly even from Herodotus.

There is one piece of evidence that Pliny was probably not discussing weasels. Plautus mentioned a weasel about 200 BC in his comedy, *Stichus or the Parasite Rebuffed*.[439] In that work, which predates Pliny by at least 200 years, the term used by Plautus was 'mustelae'. If Pliny wanted to indicate a weasel, it is likely he would have used mustelae rather than 'viverris'. Viverris is a form of 'viverra', which today identifies another group of animals, but at the time was a Latin designation for a ferret[440] (also see Owen[10] and Zeuner[12]). While there is no clear connection between the animals mentioned by Pliny and Strabo, current consensus suggests it was the domesticated ferret.

What is important about the Strabo and Pliny references is that they accurately describe ferreting, using muzzled animals, to scare rabbits from their burrows. While technology has changed the sport with the addition of nets, shovels, location devices and trained dogs,

CHAPTER SIX

Ferret-polecat domestication: genetic, taxonomic and phylogenetic relationships

the basic method of hunting has remained more-or-less unchanged for more than 2500 years, dating back to Herodotus. The connotation here is the animals used are probably domesticated animals. Strabo specifically mentions they were purposely bred for the task – one of the criteria of domestication.

The Greek and Roman citations are interesting if the pattern of reference – rather than the actual references – is considered. Homer, having the oldest references at about 750 BC, was probably indicating a wild animal. Following the Homeric references were those of Aesop (560 BC) and Herodotus (440 BC), which describe an animal in close association with people, tamed, but not necessarily domesticated. Aristophanes (425–392 BC) makes multiple references to an animal that was clearly living in close association with people, perhaps in the initial stages of domestication, or even domesticated. Aristotle (355 BC) and Theophrastus (320 BC) mention an animal that apparently has a wild and a tame form. Strabo (AD 17–23) and Pliny the Elder (AD 77) talk about an animal bred specifically for hunting subterranean animals – two of the criteria of domestication.

This pattern shows two important events; first, the term for an animal is moving from a generic word to a more specific one; Homer's weasel becomes Pliny's ferret. Second, the association with people and human habitation becomes stronger over time, beginning with Homer's wild polecat pelt to Strabo and Pliny's ferrets bred for the purpose of hunting. Both of these events would be expected if animals were being domesticated within a relatively short period of time; perhaps as short as 500 years.

A greater question is the economics behind the domestication. Does it make sense to domesticate a polecat? What possible benefits exist for taking such an action? One of the more significant events that took place immediately prior to the window of ferret domestication (roughly 500 BC to AD 70) was the incorporation of terrace farming in Greece, resulting in large grain surpluses and an increase in population.[13,172] As in Egypt, these grain surpluses were an attraction to rodents. Unlike Egyptians, the Greeks, as well as the surrounding peoples, lacked domesticated cats or a dependable source of domesticated cats. Greeks almost certainly knew of Egyptian cats and how they were used to protect grain stores. It would not be a great stretch to hypothesize the Greeks utilized a variety of animals in an attempt to protect their grain stores, eventually settling on the ferret.

In Egypt, the domestication of the cat is documented by a tremendous amount of well-preserved archaeological and historic artifacts. Also, the Egyptian culture, preoccupied with eternity, recorded and preserved everything in a manner meant to survive aeons. But, assuming a circum-Mediterranean origin, the climatic and cultural conditions surrounding the domestication of the ferret were different and little survives (or at least has been found) of those initial domestication efforts, save the ferret, itself.

While the ferret's progenitor species is most likely the European polecat, it is probable hybridization with the steppe polecat and/or European-steppe polecat hybrids took place during its long domestication history. This is indirectly supported by the reported use of ferrets by Genghis Khan – about AD 1221 – who came from an area were the predominant polecat was *M. eversmanni*, the steppe polecat.[6,12,441] While little archaeological evidence exists (the oldest confirmed archaeological ferret remains only date to the thirteenth century),[97] there is an increasing amount of genetic, linguistic and historical evidence that is hard to ignore. However, one thing can be regarded as certain; whenever or wherever the ferret was domesticated, it was originally done for a purpose. It was not domesticated to be a pet and probably not for ferreting. For the same reasons the cat was domesticated and probably following a similar Egyptian pattern (excluding the religious aspects), the ferret was probably domesticated to protect stores of grain by killing or driving away mice and other rodents.

Domesticated mammals almost always have progenitors that are social (those that herd or pack together), such as the cow, horse, llama, goat, cavy, rabbit, camels, pigs, sheep, reindeer, dog, etc. It is thought the instinct to socialize is almost a necessary requirement for domestication. Excepting modern domesticated forms like the civet, mink and fox, at least four historic attempts to domesticate nonsocial carnivores were made; the cat, cheetah, ferret and mongoose.[442] Of the four, only the ferret and cat were ultimately domesticated or remained in domestication.[12,13,179] In all four cases, the solitary carnivores were used for hunting; the ferret, cat and possibly the mongoose were used as mousers. Since the ferret was domesticated from a solitary carnivore, the polecat, in much the same way as the cat was domesticated from the wild cat and the ultimate reason was the same (mousing), the original intent was also probably the same. Put simply, if similar types of animals (solitary carnivores) were used for similar types of jobs (mousing), then the intent behind the domestication should also be similar; that is, to protect surplus grain stores.

Domestication – mechanism of change

The mechanism of domestication was, and is, human selection, sometimes called artificial selection. Human selection is a requirement for domestication. In other words, an animal is not domesticated unless humans control their reproduction, even if it is regularly kept for work or as tamed pets, such as Asian elephants. Just like natural selection selects for traits that enable a species to better survive the wild, through controlled breeding, domestication preserves those traits which better serve human needs.[5,183,210,443] As already discussed, changes caused by domestication are remarkably similar across species lines, yet are shared by a large number of taxonomically dissimilar animals separated by millions of years of evolution. For example, horses, dogs, pigs, cattle, cats, ferrets and many other animals all exhibit specific types of depigmented regions on the head, face, tail and feet, commonly called piebalding. They also share similar types of changes in reproduction, facial reduction, coat colours and textures and juvenile behaviours. Most have a stabilized albinistic form and angora variants are common. Yet, they are collectively separated by many millions of years of genetic differences.

Why then all the similarities? What are the chances of different people from different cultures, separated by time and space, to be able to breed so many similar traits in so many different mammals? In domestication, this collection of phenotypic traits are linked to a single, easily recognized and modified behavioural trait.[188,341,443-450] Excluding modern farming practices where non-behavioural traits are of concern (such as fur colour or length or egg-laying ability), domestication tends to select for a specific behavioural trait. That is, tameness or a lack of fear towards humans.

In a single 40-year experiment using the silver variety of red fox (*Vulpes vulpes*), the recognized traits of domestication detailed above were bred into fox by selecting for tameness alone.[443,444,446-450] Belyaev and Trut's work has been mirrored in other species.[296,299,445,449,451-453] The implications are clear; human selection for tameness seems to power the engine of domestication.

There is indirect support of this in older ferret literature. When ferrets were perceived to have lost hunting instincts, they were often hybridized with polecats to strengthen predatory behaviours lost during domestication. This practice was often discouraged because the resulting hybrids were generally unmanageable or untrustworthy.[33-35,325] The behaviours noted in the hybrids showed a loss of the tameness that had been achieved through the process of domestication. Polecats exhibited the most fear towards environmental novelty and humans, ferrets showed the least fear and the hybrids were somewhere in the middle.[152,154,342,345]

It is an easy matter to conclude selection for tameness will influence the expression of behavioural traits, but how does that explain why morphological changes take place, including pie-balding, shortened snouts, differences in body proportions and fur colouration or textural changes? The mechanism is a series of different, but linked genes (polygenes) that are regulated by a single dominantly inherited, maternally affected gene. This gene is called the 'star gene' because it frequently results in a star-shaped white patch of fur on the forehead of many domesticates.[341,443,444,447-449] It is the star gene that is selected for during domestication, which somehow regulates the expression of the other traits.

When selectively breeding animals for docility (tameness), you are, in effect, selecting for the expression of the star gene. What the star gene does is regulate the ontogenesis (or development) of the growing mammal by regulating the functioning of the neural and endocrine systems.[449] Put simply, by selecting for tameness, humans accidentally tapped into the developmental centre of the mammal, altering its neurochemical and neurohormonal development and causing an alteration of developmental timing. This, in turn, had a direct impact on the animal's behavioural, morphological and physiological development. The reason so many of the characteristics of domestication can be expressed in terms of juvenilization is because the expression of the star gene alters normal development, preserving the morphological, physiological and behavioural characteristics of juveniles.[341,443,444,447-449]

The workings of the star gene are not completely understood. Why doesn't it express in wild mammals? Somehow, something occurs while domesticating an animal that activates the gene.[443,444,447-449] It can appear to skip generations or randomly manifest itself without warning. Part of this may be due to maternal effect; mothers with the expressed gene tend to have more offspring that express the phenotype.[443,444,447-449] Confusing the issue, unlike most situations where a double dose of the dominant gene (SS) results in an similar expression as the heterozygous condition (Ss), in the star gene, the homozygous dominant condition can result in a 'double dose' expression (again, for reasons unknown, the double dose expression is not always activated).[444,449]

Mammals, ferrets included, that are homozygous for the star gene can display various developmental neurological problems. These can include auditory problems (including deafness), increased piebalding (depigmentation can be extensive, extending over the chest, belly, hind feet, knees, tail, navel, chin and forehead), hypo- or hyper-excitability and aggression, diminished mental capacity and other problems related to neurological underdevelopment.[443,444,447-449] This can explain many of the anecdotal problems reported when breeding dark-eyed white ferrets, where piebalding is so extensive the ferret appears albino. It may also be a contributing factor for Waardenburg syndrome; even if not directly related, it is likely one influences the other.[454-456]

CHAPTER SIX
Ferret-polecat domestication: genetic, taxonomic and phylogenetic relationships

Since the ferret is a domesticated polecat, bred by humans for mousing (and later, for ferreting), selection was specifically geared to produce an animal that was better suited for human needs. A trait shared by both the ferret and the cat is that they possess an external morphology that has been changed little during domestication. Excluding those modern fancy varieties resulting from a desire to create pet show breeds, both pretty much look like their wild forms in terms of external morphology. Neither have floppy ears, which Darwin saw as one of the hallmarks of domestication.[183] Neither has undergone extensive body size changes. Excluding relatively modern breeding practices designed to create new varieties for the pet market, neither had extensive colouration changes. What was desired was not so much a new animal, engineered to perform a new job, but an animal that would do the same job it was already engineered to do, only somewhat more human friendly. Thus, the predominating selection while domesticating the ferret was for behaviour, not for physical characteristics.

The implications of this are significant. It means the reasons that made the ferret an animal suitable for domestication also result in conditions that make the archaeological identification of them problematic. Because the goal of ferret domestication was probably geared towards creating a tamer animal (a behavioural change), rather than to create an animal to do a different job (a morphological change), physical changes were minor. Centuries of hybridization to polecats have only obscured identification of any possible physical differences between the skeletons of ferrets and polecats. These factors may make the identification of early archaeological remains difficult, if not impossible.

In many ways, the domestication of the ferret paralleled that of the cat (Table 6.4). Ferrets were probably domesticated across a large geographic region, possibly extending from Morocco in the west, to northern Turkey in the east and encompassing most of southern Europe, including parts extending into Asia. It is possible domestication was somewhat intensified in the west towards Morocco. It is probable a more significant degree of intensification occurred in the areas surrounding classical Greece. While ferrets were probably domesticated by a variety of peoples across a wide geographic region, it is likely the Greeks and perhaps to a lesser extent the Phoenicians, were directly involved in the process. It is likely that by the time of Strabo and Pliny, domestication was mostly complete. It is possible early remains of ferrets will never be recovered or properly identified. Nonetheless, a combination of genetic studies, linguistic analysis, careful review of historic documents and future archaeological recovery may ultimately illuminate the origins of the ferret.

Table 6.4 Comparison of initial cat and ferret domestication

Type of Change	Ferret	Cat
Depigmentation	Minor increase	Minor increase
Albinism	Uncommon or unknown	Uncommon or unknown
Litter size	Increased	Increased
Litter numbers/year	Increased	Increased
Body size	Minor increase	Minor increase
Tameness	Increased	Increased
Hunting instincts	Decreased	Maintained
Sociability	Minor increase	Moderate increase
Cranial capacity	15–20% decrease	20–30% decrease
Date of domestication	Approximately 500 BC	Approximately 1600 BC
Distribution	Circum-Mediterranean	Primarily Egypt
Religious significance	Minor or none	Great
Purpose of domestication	Mousing, ratting, rabbiting	Mousing, ratting
Agricultural intensification	Present	Present

Comparison of cats and ferrets, showing the parallels between the domestication of the cat and the ferret. Both are asocial carnivores that were primarily domesticated for purposes of mousing to protect grain stores. (See text for explanation and references.)

References

1. Blandford PRS. Biology of the polecat *Mustela putorius*: a literature review. Mammal Review 1987; 17:155–198.
2. Cabrera A. La patria de *Putorius furo*. Boletín de la Sociedad Española de Historia Natural 1930; 30:477–480.
3. Caras RA A perfect harmony: the intertwining lives of animals and humans throughout history. New York: Simon & Schuster; 1996.
4. Clutton-Brock J. Domesticated animals from early times. Austin: University of Texas Press; 1981:145–149.
5. Clutton-Brock J. A natural history of domesticated mammals. Cambridge: Cambridge University Press; 1999:179–184.
6. Davison A, Birks JDS, Griffiths HI et al. Hybridization and the phylogenetic relationship between polecats and domestic ferrets in Britain. Biological Conservation 1999; 87:155–162.
7. Hyams E. Animals in the service of man. Philadelphia: Lippincott; 1972.
8. Kitchener AC, Birks JDS, Davison A. Interactions between polecats and ferrets in Britain. In: Birks JDS, Davison A, eds. The distribution and status of the polecat *Mustela putorius* in Britain in the 1990s. London: Vincent Wildlife Trust; 1999:84–110.
9. Kurose N, Abramov AV, Masuda R. Intrageneric diversity of the cytochrome b gene and phylogeny of Eurasian species of the genus Mustela (Mustelidae, Carnivora). Zool Sci (Tokyo) 2000; 17:673–679.
10. Owen C. The domestication of the ferret. In: Ucko PJ, Dimbleby GW, eds. The domestication and exploitation of plants and animals. Chicago: Aldine; 1969:489–493.
11. Thomson APD A history of the ferret. J Hist Med All Sci 1951; 6(4):471–480.
12. Zeuner FEA history of domesticated animals. New York: Harper & Row; 1963:401–403.
13. Owen C. Ferret. In: Mason IL, ed. Evolution of domesticated animals. London: Longman; 1984; 225–228.
14. Davison A, Birks JDS, Maran T et al. Conservation implications of hybridization between polecats, ferrets and European mink (Mustela spp.). In: Griffiths HI, ed. Mustelids in a modern world. Management and conservation aspects of small carnivore: human interactions. Leiden: Backhuys; 2000:153–162.
15. Sommer R, Benecke N. Late- and Post-glacial history of the Mustelidae in Europe. Mamm Rev 2004; 34(4):249–284.
16. Lyman RL. Vertebrate taphonomy. Cambridge manuals in archaeology, Cambridge: Cambridge University Press; 1994.
17. Reitz EJ, Wing ES. Zooarchaeology. Cambridge manuals in archaeology, Cambridge: Cambridge University Press; 1999.
18. Davis KL. A taphonomic approach to experimental bone fracturing and applications to several South African Pleistocene sites. Ph.D. dissertation. State University of New York at Binghamton; 1985.
19. Behrensmeyer AK. Time resolution in fluvial vertebrate assemblages. Paleobiology 1982; 8:211–228.
20. Hill A. Disarticulation and scattering of mammal skeletons. Paleobiology 1979; 5:261–274.
21. Behrensmeyer AK Patterns of natural bone distribution on recent land surfaces: implications for archaeological site formation. In: Clutton-Brock J, Grigson C, eds. Animals and archaeology: 1. Hunters and their prey. British Archaeological Reports International Series 1983; 163:93–106.
22. Dustman KD. Ferrets: providing the best home for your ferret. Irvine: Bowtie Press; 2001.
23. Field J, Field M. A step-by-step book about ferrets. Neptune City: TFH; 1987.
24. Harding AR Ferret facts and fancies: a book of practical instructions on breeding, raising, handling and selling; also their uses and fur value. Columbus: AR Harding; 1915.
25. Isaacsen A. All about ferrets and rats. New York: Isaccsen; 1886.
26. Jeans D. A practical guide to ferret care. Miami: Ferrets; 1994.
27. Morton C, Morton EL. Ferrets: everything about purchase, care, nutrition, disease, behaviour and breeding, 1st edn. New York: Barron's Hauppauge; 1985.
28. Morton EL, Morton C. Ferrets: everything about purchase, care, nutrition, disease, behaviour and breeding, 2nd edn. New York: Barron's Hauppauge; 1995.
29. Morton EL, Morton C. Ferrets: everything about purchase, care, nutrition, disease, behaviour and breeding, 3rd edn. New York: Barron's Hauppauge; 2000.
30. Roberts MF. All about ferrets. Neptune City: TFH; 1977.
31. Ash EC. Ferrets and their management. In: Jones CB, ed. Live stock of the farm. Vol. VI: bees, goats, dogs, ferrets, asses and mules. London: Gresham; 1916:157–169.
32. Brodie I. Ferrets and ferreting. Dorset: Blandford; 1978.
33. Carnegie W, Niblett A, Parsey L et al. Ferrets and ferreting. London: Bazaar; 1918.
34. Davies CJ. Ferrets and their management. London: Vinton; 1907.
35. Davies CJ. Ferrets and ferreting: a practical treatise on the training, use and management of ferrets. London: Burlington; 1920.
36. Fox JG. Taxonomy, history and use. In: Fox JG, ed. Biology and diseases of the ferret, 2nd edn. Baltimore: Williams & Wilkins; 1998:3–18.
37. Plummer DB. Ferrets. Woodbridge: Boydell; 1992.
38. Schilling K. Ferrets for dummies. Foster City: IDG Books Worldwide; 2000.
39. Wilkinson PF. Current experimental domestication and its relevance to prehistory. In: Higgs ES, ed. Papers in economic prehistory: studies by members and associates of the British Academy Major Research Project in the early history of agriculture. Cambridge: Cambridge University Press; 1972:107–118.
40. Marchington J. Pugs and drummers: ferrets and rabbits in Britain. London: Faber & Faber; 1978.
41. Bell T. A history of British quadrupeds, including the Cetacea. London: John Van Voorst; 1837.
42. Linné C. Systema Naturæ per Regna Tria Naturæ, Secundum Classes ordines, Genera, Species, cum Charateribus, Differentiis, Synonymis, Locis, 10th edn. Laurentii Salvii: Holmiae Impensis Direct; 1758.
43. Jones HL. The geography of Strabo, Vol. II [translated by Horace Leonard Jones]. Cambridge, MA: Harvard University Press; 1917.
44. Pliny the Elder, Holland P. Naturalis historia: the history of the world, commonly called the natural history of C. Plinius Secundus or Pliny [translated by Philemon Holland, selected and introduced by Paul Turner]. New York: McGraw-Hill; 1964.
45. Cuzin F. Status and present geographical distribution of the wild species of Primates, Carnivora and Artiodactyla in Morocco. Mammalia 1996; 60(1):101–124.
46. Davison A, Griffiths H I, Brookes RC et al. Mitochondrial DNA and palaeontological evidence for the origins of endangered European mink, *Mustela lutreola*. Anim Conserv 2000; 3(4):345–355.
47. El Mahdy C. Mummies, myth and magic in ancient Egypt. London: Thames & Hudson; 1989.

48. Ions V. Egyptian mythology. New York: Peter Bedrick Books; 1982.
49. Janssen R, Janssen J. Egyptian household animals. Bucks: Shire Egyptology; 1989.
50. Phillips DW. Ancient Egyptian animals. New York: Metropolitan Museum of Art; 1948.
51. Sato JJ, Hosoda T, Wolsan M et al. Molecular phylogeny of arctoids (Mammalia: Carnivora) with emphasis on phylogenetic and taxonomic positions of the ferret-badgers and skunks. Zool Sci 2004; 21:111–118.
52. Darlington PJ. Zoogeography: the geographical distribution of animals. New York: Robert E. Krieger; 1957a.
53. Cabrera A. Los mamíferos de Marruecos. Junt para ampliación de estudios e investigaciones científicas. Trabajos del Museo Nacional de Ciencias Naturals, serie Zoológica, No. 57. Madrid: Junta Para Ampliación de Estudios e Investigaciones Científicas; 1932.
54. Tristham HB. Report on the mammals of Palestine. Proceedings of the Zoological Society of London 1866:84–93.
55. Tristham HB. The survey of western Palestine: the fauna and flora of Palestine. London: Palestine Exploration Fund; 1884.
56. Burton M. Guide to the mammals of Britain and Europe. London: Treasure Press; 1976.
57. Heptner WG. Über die morphologischen und geographischen Beziehungen zwischen *Mustela putorius* und *Mustela eversmanni*. Zeitschrift für Säugetierkunde 1964; 29(6):321–330.
58. Long JL Introduced mammals of the world: their history, distribution and influence. New York: CABI Publishing; 2003.
59. MacDonald D. Collins European mammals: evolution and behaviour. London: Harper Collins; 1995.
60. MacDonald D, Barrett P. Collins field guide: mammals of Britain and Europe. London: Harper Collins; 1993.
61. Mitchell-Jones AJ, Amori G, Bogdanowicz W et al. The atlas of European mammals. London: T&AD Poyser; 1999.
62. Novikov GA. Carnivorous mammals of the fauna of the USSR. Israel Program for Scientific Translations, Jerusalem; 1962.
63. Nowak RM. Walker's mammals of the world, 5th edn., Vol. II. Baltimore: Johns Hopkins University Press; 1991.
64. Ognev SI. Mammals of the U.S.S.R. and adjacent countries. Jerusalem: Israel Program for Scientific Translations; 1962.
65. Stroganov SU. Carnivorous mammals of Siberia. Jerusalem: Israel Program for Scientific Translations; 1969.
66. Wolsan M. *Mustela eversmanni* Lesson, 1827 – Steppeniltis. In: Niethammer J, Krapp F, eds. Handbuch der Säugetiere Europas, Band 5: Raubsäuger – Carnivora (Fissipedia), Teil LL: Mustelidae 2, Viverridae, Herpestidae, Felidae (Stubbe M, Krapp F editor of volume). Wiesbaden: AULA-Verlag; 1993:770–816.
67. Wolsan M. *Mustela putorius* Linnaeus, 1758 – Waldiltis, Europäischer Iltis, Iltis. In: Niethammer J, Krapp F, eds. Handbuch der Säugetiere Europas, Band 5: Raubsäuger – Carnivora (Fissipedia), Teil LL: Mustelidae 2, Viverridae, Herpestidae, Felidae (Stubbe M, Krapp F editor of volume). Wiesbaden: AULA-Verlag; 1993:699–769.
68. Davis SJM. The archaeology of animals. New Haven: Yale University Press; 1987.
69. Hesse B, Wapnish P. Animal bone archaeology: from objectives to analysis. Manuals on Archaeology No. 5. Washington: Taraxacum; 1985.
70. Jarman MR, Wilkinson PF. Criteria of animal domestication. In: Higgs ES, ed. Papers in economic prehistory: studies by members and associates of the British Academy Major Research Project in the early history of agriculture. Cambridge: Cambridge University Press; 1972:83–96.
71. Meadow RH Osteological evidence for the process of animal domestication. In: Clutton-Brock J, ed. The walking larder. London: Allen & Unwin; 1989:80–90.
72. O'Connor TP. The archaeology of animal bones. College Station: Texas A&M University Press; 2000.
73. Ginzburg A. The beginnings of domestication: osteological criteria for the identification of domesticated mammals in archeological sites. Israel J Vet Med 1996; 51(2):83–92.
74. Bekken D, Schepartz L A, Miller-Antonio S et al. Taxonomic abundance at Panxian Dadong, a Middle Pleistocene cave in south China. Asian Perspect 2004; 43(2):333–359.
75. Wiszniowska T. Middle Pleistocene Carnivora (Mammalis) from Kozi Grzbiet in the Swietokrzyskie Mts, Poland. Acta Zoologica Cracoviensia 1989; 32(8–15):589–630.
76. Reichstein H. Über Kleinsäuger aus Burg Bodenteich in Bodenteich Kr. Uelzen/Niedersachsen (9.–18. Jahrhundert). Bonner Zoologische Beitraege 1996; 46(1–4):359–366.
77. Riedel A. Animal bones from the Nickelsdorf Roman villa rustica in Burgenland (Austria). Annalen des Naturhistorischen Museums in Wien a Mineralogie Petrologie Geologie Palaeontogie Archaeozoologie Anthropologie Praehistorie 2004; 106A:449–539.
78. Baryshnikov GF, Abramov AV. Structure of baculum (os penis) in Mustelidae (Mammalia, Carnivora). Communication 1. Zoologicheskii Zhurnal 1997, 76(12):1399–1410.
79. Baryshnikov GF, Bininda-Emonds ORP, Abramov AV Morphological variability and evolution of the baculum (os penis) in Mustelidae (Carnivora). J Mammal 2003; 84(2):673–690.
80. Herán I. Contribution towards the morphology of the pelvis in Mustelidae. Zoologické Listy 1962; 11:35–52.
81. Ondrias JC. Comparative osteological investigations on the front limbs of European Mustelidae. Arkiv för Zoologi 1961; 13(15):311–320.
82. Stains HJ. Calcanea of members of the Mustelidae. Part 1, Mustelinae. Bull Southern Calif Acad Sci 1976; 75:237–248.
83. Ashton EH, Thomson APD. Some characters of the skulls and skins of the European polecat, the Asiatic polecat and the domestic ferret. Proc Zool Soc Lon 1955; 125(2):317–333.
84. Buchalczyk T, Ruprecht AL. Skull variability of *Mustela putorius* Linnaeus, 1758. Acta Theriologica 1977; 22(5):87–120.
85. De Marinis AM Craniometric variability of polecat *Mustela putorius* L. 1758 from north-central Italy. Hystrix 1995; 7(1–2):57–68.
86. Herán I. Some notes on the shape and size of the occipital foramen in Mustelidae. Lynx 1972; 13:26–33.
87. Lee S, Mill PJ. Cranial variation in British mustelids. J Morphol 2004; 260(1):57–64.
88. Martinkova A, Janiga M. Quantitative comparisons of cranial shape and size in adults of *Felis silvestris*, *Vulpes vulpes*, *Mustela putorius* and *Mustela nivalis* from the West Carpathians (Slovakia). Oecologia Montana 1999; 8(1–2):32–37.
89. Opatrn? E. Príspevek ke kraniometrii tchoru *Putorius putorius* (Linna) 1758 a *Putorius eversmanni* (Lesson). Acta Universitatis Palackianae Olomucensis Facultas Rerum Naturalium 1827. 1969; 31(11):87–94.
90. Lange R, Van Winden A, Twisk P et al. Zoogdieren van de Benelux. Herkenning en onderzoek. Jeugdbondsuitgeverji, Amsterdam 1986.

91. Glushkova Yu V, Korablyov PN, Kachanovskyi VA. Diagnostic value of the characters for the identification of three mustelid species (*Mustela lutreola, M. vison, M. putorius*). Byulleten Moskovskogo Obshchestva Ispytatelei Prirody Otdel Biologicheskii 1999; 104(1):18–23.
92. He T, Friede H, Kiliaridis S. Macroscopic and roentgenographic anatomy of the skull of the ferret (*Mustela putorius furo*). Lab Anim 2002; 36(1):86–96.
93. He T, Kiiaridis S. Effects of masticatory muscle function on craniofacial morphology in growing ferrets (*Mustela putorius furo*). Eur J Oral Sci 2003; 111(6):510–517.
94. Kharlamova AV, Faleev VI, Trapezov OV. Variation of cranial size and shape in the course of selection of the American mink *Mustela vison* for submissive and aggressive behaviour. Doklady Biol Sci 1999; 367:329–331.
95. Rempe U Morphometrische Untersuchungen an Iltisschädeln zur Klärung der Verwandtschaft von Steppeniltis, Waldiltis und Frettchen. Analyse eines 'Grenzenfalles' zwischen Unterart und Art. Zeitschrift für wissenschaftliche Zoologie 1970; 180(3–4):185–367.
96. Abramov AV, Tumanov IL. Sexual dimorphism in the skull of the European mink *Mustela lutreola* from NW part of Russia. Acta Theriologica 2003; 48(2):239–246.
97. Van Damme D, Ervynck A. Medieval ferrets and rabbits in the Castle of Laarne (East-Flanders, Belgium): a contribution to the history of a predator and its prey. In: Bodson L, Libois R, eds. Contributions à l'histoire de la domestication. Journée d'étude, Université de Liège, 2 mars 1991. Colloques d'histoire des connaissances zoologiques #3. Belgium: Université de Liège; 1992:57–68.
98. Hensel R. Craniologische studien. Nova Acta Leopoldina 1881; 42:167–195.
99. Lawes INC, Andrews PLR. Variation in the ferret skull *Mustela putorius furo*. l. In relation to stereotaxic landmarks. J Anat 1987; 154:157–172.
100. Miller GS. The origin of the ferret. The Scottish Naturalist 1933:153–154.
101. Yamaguchi N, Kitchener AC, Driscoll CA et al. Craniological differentiation amongst wild-living cats in Britain and southern Africa: natural variation or the effects of hybridisation? Anim Conserv 2004; 7(4):339–351.
102. Thomas DH. Archaeology, 2nd edn. Fort Worth: Holt, Rinehart & Winston; 1989.
103. Trigger BG. A history of archaeological thought. Cambridge: Cambridge University Press; 1989.
104. Anderson E. Ferret from the Pleistocene of central Alaska. J Mammal 1973; 54(3):778–779.
105. Aouraghe H. Les carnivores fossiles d'El Harhoura 1, Temara, Maroc. Anthropologie 2000: 104(1):147–171.
106. Bon M, Masseti M. Wild mammal remains from a Roman pit at Oderzo (Treviso, north-central Italy). Boll del Museo Civico di Storia Naturale di Venezia 1993; 44:153–162.
107. Dawkins WB. The British Pleistocene Mammalia. London: The Palaeontographical Society; 1872.
108. La Caverne Marie-Jeanne GA (Hastière-Lavaux, Belique). II-Notes sur les mammifères. Inst R Sci Nat Belg Mem 1980; 177:25–42.
109. Nobis G, Ninov N. Zur Fauna der prähistorischen Siedlung Durankulak, Bez. Tolbuchin (NO-Bulgarien). II Kupferzeit Bonn Zool Monogr 2002; 51:29–59.
110. Prummel W. The faunal remains from the Neolithic site of Hekelingen III. Helinium 1987; 27:191–258.
111. Abramov AV. A taxonomic review of the genus Mustela (Mammalia, Carnivora). Zoosystematica Ross 2000; 892:357–364.
112. Anderson E. The phylogeny of mustelids and the systematics of ferrets. In: Seal US, Thorne ET, Bogan M, Aanderson SA, eds. Conservation biology and the black-footed ferret. New Haven: Yale University Press; 1989:10–20.
113. Dunstone N. The mink. London: Poyser Natural History; 1993.
114. Jones JK, Jr, Armstrong DM, Hoffmann RS et al. Mammals of the Northern Great Plains. Lincoln: University of Nebraska Press; 1983.
115. Kostron K. The polecat of Eversmann, a new mammal from the plains of Czechoslovakia. Acta Acad Sci Nat Moravo Silesiacae 1948; 20:1–96.
116. Marmi J, Lopez-Giraldez JF, Domingo-Roura X. Phylogeny, evolutionary history and taxonomy of the Mustelidae based on sequences of the cytochrome b gene and a complex repetitive flanking region. Zool Scr 2004; 33:481–499.
117. Michaux JR, Libois R, Davison A et al. Is the western population of the European mink (*Mustela lutreola*), a distinct Management Unit for Conservation? Biol Conserv 2004; 115:357–367.
118. Sato JJ, Hosoda T, Wolsan M et al. Phylogenetic relationships and divergence times among mustelids (Mammalia: Carnivora) based on nucleotide sequences of the nuclear interphotoreceptor retinoid binding protein and mitochondrial cytochrome b genes. Zool Sci 2003; 20:243–264.
119. Wozencraft WC. Classification of the recent Carnivora. In: Gittleman JL, ed. Carnivore behaviour, ecology and evolution. New York: Cornell University Press; 1989:569–593.
120. Youngman PM. Distribution and systematics of the European mink *Mustela lutreola* Linnaeus 1761. Acta Zool Fenn 1982; 166:1–48.
121. Dragoo JW, Honeycutt RL. Systematics of mustelid-like carnivores. J Mammal 1997; 78:426–443.
122. Graphodatsky AS, Yang F, Perelman PL et al. Comparative molecular cytogenetic studies in the order Carnivora: mapping chromosomal rearrangements onto the phylogenetic tree. Cytogenet Genome Res 2002; 96:137–145.
123. Hosoda T, Suzuki H, Yamada T et al. Restriction site polymorphism in the ribosomal DNA of eight species of Canidae and Mustelidae. Cytologia [Tokyo] 1993; 58:223–230.
124. Koepfli K-P, Wayne RK. Type I Sts markers are more informative than Cytochrome b in phylogenetic reconstruction of the Mustelidae (Mammalia: Carnivora). Syst Biol 2003; 52:571–593.
125. Wozencraft WC. Order Carnivora. In: Wilson DE, Reeder DM, eds. Mammal species of the world: a taxonomic and geographic reference, 2nd edn. Washington: Smithsonian Institution 1993: 279–348.
126. Zhang Y. Molecular phylogeny of the superfamily Arctoidea. Acta Genet Sin 1997; 24:15–22.
127. Bryant HN, Russell AP, Fitch WD. Phylogenetic relationships within the extant Mustelidae (Carnivora): appraisal of the cladistic status of the Simpsonian subfamilies. Zool J Linn Soc 1993; 198:301–334.
128. Davison A, Birks JDS, Brookes RC et al. Mitochondrial phylogeography and population history of pine martens Martes martes compared with polecats *Mustela putorius*. Mol Ecol 2001; 10:2479–2488.
129. Lushnikova TP. Omelýanchuk LV, Graphodatskii AS et al. Phylogenetic relationships of closely related species Mustelidae interspecific variability of blot-hybridization patterns of Ban-Hi repeats. Genetika 1989; 25:1089–1094.
130. Masuda R, Yoshida MC. A molecular phylogeny of the family Mustelidae (Mammalia, Carnivora), based on comparison of mitochondrial cytochrome B nucleotide sequences. Zool Sci [Tokyo] 1994; 11:605–612.

CHAPTER SIX
Ferret-polecat domestication: genetic, taxonomic and phylogenetic relationships

131. Murakami T. Species identification of mustelids by comparing partial sequences on mitochondrial DNA from fecal samples. J Vet Med Sci 2002; 64:321–323.
132. Nie W, Wang J, O'Brien PCM et al. The genome phylogeny of domestic cat, red panda and five mustelid species revealed by comparative chromosome painting and G-banding. Chromosome Res 2002; 10:209–222.
133. Obara Y. Karyosystematics of the mustelid carnivores of Japan. Honyurui Kagaku 1991; 30:197–220.
134. Lodé T. Genetic heterozygosity in polecat *Mustela putorius* populations from western France. Hereditas 1998; 129:259–261.
135. Cavagna P, Menotti A, Stanyon R. Genomic homology of the domestic ferret with cats and humans. Mamm Genome 2000; 11:866–870.
136. Wolsan M. Evolution des Carnivores quaternaries en Europe centrale dans leur contexte stratigraphique et paléoclimatique. Anthropologie 1993; 97:203–222.
137. Ellerman JR, Morrison-Scott TCS. Checklist of Palaearctic and Indian mammals 1758 to 1946, 2nd edn. London: British Museum (Natural History); 1966.
138. Hosoda T, Suzuki H, Harada M et al. Evolutionary trends of the mitochondrial lineage differentiation in species of genera Martes and Mustela. Genes Genet Syst 2000; 75:259–267.
139. Pocock RI. The polecats of the genera Putorius and Vormela in the British Museum. Proc Zool Soc Lond 1936; 2:691–723.
140. Pleistocene Mustelidae AE. (Mammalia, Carnivora) from Fairbanks, Alaska. Bull Mus Comp Zool 1977; 148:1–21.
141. Anderson E, Forrest SC, Clark TW et al. Paleobiology, biogeography and systematics of the black-footed ferret, *Mustela nigripes* (Audubon and Bachman, 1851). Great Basin Nat Mem 1986; 8:11–63.
142. Kurtén B, Anderson E. Pleistocene mammals of North America. New York: Columbia University Press.
143. Basrur PK. The somatic chromosomes of the ferret. J Hered 1966; 57:110–112.
144. Fredga K. Chromosome studies in six species of Mustelidae and one of Procyonidae. Mamm Chromosomes 1966; 21:145–149.
145. Hsu TC, Benirschke K. An atlas of mammalian chromosomes. In: Hsu TC, Benirschke K, eds. New York: Springer; 1968.
146. Bednarz M. Observations on reproduction in polecat x ferret hybrids. Anim Breed Abstr 1962; 30:239.
147. Denisov EI. Experiment of studying ferret's biology in period of bring up the younglings. Izvestiya Sibirskoe Otdeleniya Akademii Nauk SSSR. Seruiya Biol Nauk SSSR 1985; 2:89–93.
148. Gray AP. Mammalian hybrids: A check-list with bibliography. Technical Communication No. 10 (revised). Edinburgh: Commonwealth Bureau of Animal Breeding and Genetics; 1972:53–55
149. Lynch JM. Conservation implications of hybridisation between mustelids and their domesticated counterparts: The example of polecats and feral ferrets in Britain. Small Carnivore Conserv 1995; 13:17–18.
150. Pitt F. Notes on the genetic behaviour of certain characters in the polecat, ferret and in polecat-ferret hybrids. J Genet 1921; 11:99–115.
151. Poole TB. Polecats. London: Forestry Commission (HMSO); 1970: Record no. 76.
152. Poole TB. Diadic interactions between pairs of male polecats (*Mustela furo* and *Mustela furo* × *M. putorius* hybrids) under standardized environmental conditions during the breeding season. Z Tierpsychol 1972; 30:45–58.
153. Poole TB. Some behavioural differences between the European polecat, *Mustela putorius*, the ferret, *M. furo* and their hybrids. J Zool (London) 1972; 166:25–35.
154. Poole TB. The aggressive behaviour of individual male polecats (*Mustela putorius*, *M. furo* and hybrids) towards familiar and unfamiliar opponents. J Zool (London) 1973; 170:395–414.
155. Ternovsky DV. Biology of Mustelidae. Novosibirsk, Moscow: Nauka Publishers; 1977.
156. Tumanov IL, Abramov AV. A study of the hybrids between the European mink *Mustela lutreola* and the polecat *M. putorius*. Small Carnivore Conserv 2002; 27:29–31.
157. Volobuev VT, Ternovskii DV, Grafodatskii AS. The taxonomic status of the white African polecat or ferret in the light of karyological data. Zool Zh 1974; 53:1738–1740.
158. Fagundes V, Christoff AU, Yonenaga-Yassuda Y. Extraordinary chromosomal polymorphism with 28 different karyotypes in the neotropical species *Akodon cursor* (Muridae, Sigmodontinae), one of the smallest diploid number in rodents ($2n = 16$, 15 and 14). Hereditas 1998; 129:263–274.
159. Coskun YA. new chromosomal form of *Nannospalax ehrenbergi* from Turkey. Folia Zool 2004; 53:351–356.
160. Motokawa M, Harada M, Wu Y et al. Chromosomal polymorphism in the gray shrew *Crocidura attenuata* (Mammalia: Insectivora). Zool Sci 2001; 18:1153–1160.
161. Mitsainas GO, Giagai-Athanasopoulou EB. Studies on the Robertsonian chromosomal variation of *Mus musculus domesticus* (Rodentia, Muridae) in Greece. Biol J Linn Soc 2005; 84:503–513.
162. Rejduch B, Slota E, Rozycki M et al. Chromosome number polymorphism in a litter of European wild boar (*Sus scrofa scrofa* L.). Anim Sci Pap Rep 2003; 21:57–62.
163. Obara Y, Nakano T. Robertsonian fission polymorphism in the northern Honshu Japan population of the Japanese raccoon dog *Nyctereutes procyonoides viverrinus*. J Mammal Soc Jap 1989; 14:19–26.
164. Zima J, Cenevova E. Coat colour and chromosome variation in central European populations of the weasel (*Mustela nivalis*). Folia Zool 2002; 51:265–274.
165. Avise JC. Molecular markers, natural history and evolution, 2nd edition. Sunderland, Massachusetts: Sinauer Associates; 2004.
166. Graur D, Li W-H. Fundamentals of molecular evolution. Sunderland, MA: Sinauer Associates; 2002.
167. Hall BG. Phylogenetic trees made easy: a how-to manual for molecular biologists, 2nd edn. Sunderland, MA: Sinauer Associates; 2004.
168. Hillis DM, Moritz C, Mable BK. Molecular systematics, 2nd edn. Sunderland, MA: Sinauer Associates; 1996.
169. Miyamoto MM, Cracraft J. Phylogenetic analysis of DNA sequences. Oxford: Oxford University Press; 1991.
170. Nie M. Kumar S. Molecular evolution and phylogenetics. Oxford: Oxford University Press; 2000.
171. Grayson DK. The effects of sample size on some derived measures in vertebrate faunal analysis. J Archaeol Sci 1981; 8:77–88.
172. Fagan BM. The Oxford companion to archaeology. In: Fagan BM, ed. Oxford: Oxford University Press; 1996.
173. Powledge TM, Rose M. The great DNA hunt. Archaeology 1996; 49:2.
174. Davis PDC, Dent AA. Animals that changed the world. New York: Crowell-Collier Press; 1968.
175. Grandin T 1998 Genetics and the behaviour of domestic animals. San Diego: Academic Press.
176. Houpt KA. Domestic animal behaviour for veterinarians and animal scientists, 4th edn. Ames, Iowa: Blackwell Science; 2005.

177. Hyams E. Working for man. the domestication of animals. Harmondsworth: Kestrel Books; 1975.
178. Isaac E. Geography of domestication. Englewood Cliffs: Prentice-Hall; 1970.
179. Mason IL. Evolution of domesticated animals. In: Mason IL, ed. New York: Longman; 1984.
180. Price EO. Animal domestication and behaviour. New York: CABI Publishing; 2002.
181. Ucko PJ, Dimbleby GW. The domestication and exploitation of plants and animals. Chicago: Aldine-Atherton; 1969.
182. Zeaman J. From pests to pets. How small mammals became our friends. New York: Franklin Watts; 1998.
183. Darwin C. The variation of animals and plants under domestication. New York: Appleton; 1896.
184. Gentry A, Clutton-Brock J, Groves CP. The naming of wild animal species and their domestic derivatives. J Archaeol Sci 2004; 31:645–651.
185. Herre W. The science and history of domestic animals. In: Brothwell D, Higgs E, eds. Science in archaeology: a comprehensive survey of progress and research. New York: Basic Books; 1963:235–249.
186. Russell N. The wild side of animal domestication. Soc Anim 2002; 10:285–302.
187. Todd NB. An ecological behavioural genetic model for the domestication of the cat. Carnivore 1978; 1:52–60.
188. Budiansky S. The covenant with the wild. Why animals chose domestication. New York: William Morrow; 1992.
189. O'Connor TP. Working at relationships: another look at animal domestication. Antiquity 1997; 71:149–156.
190. Armitage PL. Domestication of animals. In: Cole DJA, Brander GC, eds. Bioindustrial ecosystems. Amsterdam: Elsevier Science; 1986:5–30.
191. Bökönyi S. The development and history of domestic animals in Hungary: the Neolithic through the Middle Ages. Am Anthropol 1971; 73:640–674.
192. Clutton-Brock J. The walking larder: patterns of domestication. In: Clutton-Brock J, ed. Pastoralism and predation. London: Unwin Hyman; 1989.
193. Clutton-Brock J. The process of domestication. Mammal Rev 1992; 22:79–85.
194. Clutton-Brock J. The unnatural world: behavioural aspects of humans and animals in the process of domestication. In: Manning A, Serpell JA, eds. Animals and human society: changing perspectives. London: Routledge; 1994:23–35.
195. Crabtree PJ. Early animal domestication in the Middle East and Europe. In: Schiffer MB, ed. Archaeological method and theory, Vol. 5. Tucson: University of Arizona Press; 1993:201–245.
196. Ducos P. Defining domestication: a clarification. In: Clutton-Brock J, ed. The walking larder: patterns of domestication, pastoralism and predation. London: Unwin Hyman; 1989:28–30.
197. Ratner SC, Boice R. Effects of domestication on behaviour. In: Hafez ESE, ed. The behaviour of domestic animals. London: Baillère Tindall; 1975:3–19.
198. Fox MW. The dog: its domestication and behaviour. New York: Garland STPM Press; 1978.
199. Haber A, Dayan T. Analyzing the process of domestication: Hagoshrim as a case study. J Archaeol Sci 2004; 31:1601.
200. Ingold T. Animal domestication. In: Levinson D, Ember M, eds. Encyclopedia of cultural anthropology, Vol. 1. New York: Henry Holt; 1996:60–64.
201. McKay J. Complete Guide to Ferrets. Shrewsbury: Swan Hill Press; 1995.
202. McKay J. The ferret and ferreting handbook. Ramsbury: Crowood Press; 1989.
203. Miller GS. Catalogue of the mammals of Western Europe. London: British Museum (Natural History); 1912.
204. Lynch JM, Hayden TJ. Genetic influences on cranial form: variation among ranch and feral American mink *Mustela vison* (Mammalia: Mustelidae). Biol J Linn Soc 1995; 55:293–307.
205. Röhrs M. Cephalization, telencephalization and neocorticalization within the Mustelidae. Z Zool Syst Evol 1986; 24:157–166.
206. Röhrs M. Domestikationbedingte Hirnänderungen bei Mustelidaen. Z Zool Syst Evol 1986; 24:231–239.
207. Röhrs M, Ebinger P, Weidemann W. Cephalization in Viverridae, Hyaenidae, Procyonidae and Ursidae. Z Zool Syst Evol 1989; 27:169–180.
208. Röhrs M, Ebinger P. Wild is not really wild: brain weight of wild domestic mammals. Berl Münchener Tierärztliche Wochenschr 1999; 112:234–238.
209. Röhrs M, Ebinger P. How is cranial capacity related to brain volume in mammals? Mamm Biol 2001; 66:102–110.
210. Hemmer H 1990 Domestication: the decline of environmental appreciation. Cambridge: Cambridge University Press.
211. Williams ES, Anderson SL. Vaccination of black-footed ferret (*Mustela nigripes*) × Siberian polecat (*M. eversmanni*) hybrids and domestic ferrets (*M. putorius furo*) against canine distemper. J Wildl Dis 1996; 32:417–423.
212. Youngman PM. Beringian ferrets: mummies, biogeography and systematics. J Mammal 1994; 75:454–461.
213. Kuhn-Schnyder E, Rieber H. Handbook of paleozoology. Baltimore: John Hopkins University Press; 1986.
214. Kurtén B. Pleistocene mammals of Europe. London: Weidenfeld & Nicolson; 1968.
215. Nilsson T. The Pleistocene: geology and life in the Quaternary Ice Age. Stuttgart: Ferdinand Enke Verlag; 1983.
216. Owen PR, Bell CJ, Mead EM. Fossils, diet and conservation of black-footed ferrets (*Mustela nigripes*). J Mammal 2000; 81:422–433.
217. Reynolds SH. A monograph of the British Pleistocene Mammalia, Vol. II: British Pleistocene Hyænidæ, Ursidæ, Canidæ and Mustelidæ: Mustelidæ. London: The Palæontological Society; 1912.
218. Romer AS. Vertebrate paleontology, 3rd edn. Chicago: University of Chicago Press; 1966.
219. Youngman PM. The Pleistocene small carnivores of eastern Beringia. Can Field Nat 1993; 107:139–163.
220. Forrest S. Life history characteristics of the genus Mustela, with special reference to the black-footed ferret, *Mustela nigripes*. Black-footed Ferret Workshop Proceedings 23.1–23.14. Laramie: Wyoming Game and Fish Department; 1985.
221. Hayssen V, Tienhoven A Van, Tienhoven A Van. Asdell's patterns of mammalian reproduction: A compendium of species-specific data. Ithaca: Cornell University Press; 1993.
222. Lodé T. Activity pattern of polecats *Mustela putorius* L. in relation to food habits and prey activity. Ethology 1995; 100:295–308.
223. Lodé T. Conspecific tolerance and sexual segregation in the use of space and habitats in the European polecat. Acta Theriology 1996; 41:171–176.
224. Lodé T 1997 Trophic status and feeding habits of the European polecat *Mustela putorius* L. Mammal Rev 1758:177–184.
225. Miller BJ, Anderson SH. A behavioural comparison between induced estrus and natural estrus domestic ferrets (*Mustela putorius furo*). J Ethology 1990; 7:65–73.
226. Miller BJ, Anderson SH. A comparison of mating behaviour between black-footed ferrets (*Mustela nigripes*), domestic

ferrets (*M. putorius furo*) and Siberian polecats (*M. eversmanni*). Zoo Biol 1990; 9:201–210.
227. Sheets RG, Linder RL, Dahgren RB. Food habits of two litters of black-footed ferrets in South Dakota. Am Midl Nat 1972; 87:249–251.
228. Vargas A, Anderson SH. Growth and development of captive-raised black-footed ferrets (*Mustela nigripes*). Am Midl Nat 1996; 135:43–52.
229. Wildt DE, Howard JG, Morton C, Bush M. Reproductive studies of the domestic ferret as an investigational model for the black-footed ferret. Proceedings of the American Association of Zoo Veterinarians; 1987.
230. Wilson DE, Reeder DM, eds. Mammal species of the world: a taxonomic and geographic reference, 2nd edn. Washington: Smithsonian Institution Press; 1993.
231. Jeffery C. Biological nomenclature. London: Edward Arnold; 1973.
232. International Commission on Zoological Nomenclature 2003 Opinion 2027. (Case 3010). Usage of 17 specific names based on wild species which are pre-dated by or contemporary with those based on domestic animals (Lepidoptera, Osteichthyes, Mammalia): Conserved. Bull Zool Nomencl 60:81–84.
233. Atherton RW, Curry P, Slaughter R et al. Electroejaculation and cryopreservation of domestic ferret sperm. In: Seal US, Thorne ET, Bogan MA, Anderson SA, eds. Conservation biology and the black-footed ferret. New Haven: Yale University Press; 1989:177–189.
234. Fox JG, Bell JA. Growth, reproduction and breeding. In: Fox JG, ed. Biology and diseases of the ferret, 2nd edn. Baltimore: Williams & Wilkins; 1998:211–227.
235. Jezewska G, Maciejowski J, Tarkowski J. Genetic and environmental determination of reproduction results in the polecat. Scientifur 1995; 19:111–113.
236. Ternovsky DV, Ternovskaya YG. Ecology of mustelids. Novosibirsk. Moscow: Scientific Siberian Press; 1994.
237. Amstislavsky SY, Ternovskaya Y. Reproduction in mustelids. Anim Reprod Sci 2000; 60/61:571–581.
238. Bissonnette TH. Modification of mammalian sexual cycles; reactions of ferrets (*Putorius vulgaris*) of both sexes to electric light added after dark in November and December. Proc R Soc Lond 1932; 110:322–336.
239. Forsberg M. Seasonal breeding and the significance of light. In: Tauson A-H, Valtonen M, eds. Reproduction in carnivorous fur bearing animals. Nordiska Jordbruksforskares Förening, Rapport Nr. 75. Copenhagen: Jordbrugsforlaget, Nordisk Kulturfond; 1992: 17–38.
240. Harvey NE, MacFarlane WV. The effects of day length on the coat-shedding cycles, body weight and reproduction of the ferret. Aust J Biol Sci 1958; 11:187–199.
241. Herbert J. Light as a multiple control system on reproduction in mustelids. In: Seal US, Thorne ET, Bogan M, Anderson S, edd. Conservation biology of the black-footed ferret. New Haven: Yale University Press; 1989: 138–159.
242. Lagerqvist G. Reproductive features in the ferret (*Mustela putorius*). In: Tauson A-H, Valtonen M, eds. Reproduction in carnivorous fur bearing animals. Nordiska Jordbruksforskares Förening, Rapport Nr. 75. Copenhagen: Jordbrugsforlaget, Nordisk Kulturfond; 1992: 87–95.
243. Mead RA. Reproduction in mustelids. In: Seal US, Thorne ET, Bogan M anderson S, eds. Conservation biology of the black-footed ferret. New Haven: Yale University Press; 1989: 124–137.
244. Moshonkin NN. Potential polyestricity of the mink (*Lutreola lutreola*). Zool Zh 1981; 9:1731–1734.
245. Murphy BD. Reproductive physiology of female mustelids. In: Seal US, Thorne ET, Bogan M, Anderson S, eds. Conservation biology of the black-footed ferret. New Haven: Yale University Press; 1989: 107–123.
246. Valtonen M. Comparative aspects of reproductive physiology in domestic animals. In: Tauson A-H, Valtonen M, eds. Reproduction in carnivorous fur bearing animals. Nordiska Jordbruksforskares Förening, Rapport Nr. 75. Copenhagen: Jordbrugsforlaget, Nordisk Kulturfond; 1992: 1–15.
247. King RA, Hearing VJ, Creel DJ et al. Albinism. In: Scriver CR, Beaudet AL, Sly WS et al. eds. The metabolic and molecular bases of inherited disease, 7th edn., Vol. III. New York: McGraw-Hill; 1995: 4353–4392.
248. Searle AG. Comparative genetics of albinism. Ophthalmic Paediatr Genet 1990; 11:159–164.
249. Witkop CJ Jr, Quevedo WC Jr, Fitzpatrick TB et al. Albinism. In: Scriver CR, Beaudet AL, Sly WS et al. eds. The metabolic basis of inherited disease, Vol. 2. New York: McGraw-Hill; 1989:2905–2947.
250. Long CA, Hogan A. Two independent loci for albinism in raccoons, Procyon lotor. J Hered 1988; 79:387–389.
251. Graphodatsky AS, Tenovskaya YG, Ternovsky DV et al. Cytogenetics of albinism in ferrets of the genus *Putorius* (Carnivora, Mustelaidae). Genetika 1978; 14:68–71.
252. McLain DE, Harper SM, Roe DA et al. Congenital malformations and variations in reproductive performance in the ferret: effects of maternal age, colour and parity. Lab Anim Sci 1985; 35:251–255.
253. Syed M, Ronningen K, Nes NN. Inheritance of coat colour in ferrets. Acta Agric Scand 1987; 37:85–88.
254. Balkema GW, Drager UC. Impaired visual thresholds in hypopigmented animals. Visual Neurosci 1991; 6:577–585.
255. Grandin T, Deesing MJ. Genetics and animal welfare. In: Grandin T, ed. Genetics and the behaviour of domestic animals. San Diego: Academic Press; 1998: 319–346.
256. Pontenagel T, Schmidt U. Untersuchungen zur Leistungfähigkeit des Gesichtssinnes beim Frettchen, *Mustela putorius* f. furo. L. Z Säugetierkd 1980; 45:376–383.
257. Tjalve H, Frank A. Tapetum lucidum in the pigmented and albino ferret. Exp Eye Res 1984; 38:341–351.
258. Jackson CA, Hickey TL. Use of ferrets in studies of the visual system. Lab Anim Sci 1985; 35:211–215.
259. Wen GY, Sturman JA, Shek JW. A comparative study of the tapetum, retina and skull of the ferret, dog and cat. Lab Anim Sci 1985; 35:200–210.
260. Yokoyamaa S, Radlwimmera FB. The molecular genetics of red and green colour vision in mammals. Genetics 1999; 153:919–932.
261. Yokoyamaa S, Radlwimmera FB. The molecular genetics and evolution of red and green colour vision in vertebrates. Genetics 2001; 158:1697–1710.
262. Gewalt W. Beitrage zur kenntnis des optischen differenzierungsvermogens einiger musteliden mit besonderer berucksigtigung des farbensehens. Zool Beiträge 1959; 5:117–175.
263. Jeffery G, Darling K, Whitmore A. Melanin and the regulation of mammalian photoreceptor topography. Eur J Neurosci 1994; 6:657–667.
264. Whary MT, Andrews PLR. Physiology of the ferret. In: Fox JG, ed. Biology and diseases of the ferret, 2nd edn. Baltimore: Williams & Wilkins; 1998: 103–148.
265. Calderone JB, Jacobs GH. Spectral properties and retinal distribution of ferret cones. Visual Neurosci 2003; 20:11–17.
266. Creel D, Garber SR, King RA et al. Auditory brainstem anomalies in human albinos. Science 1980; 209:1253–1255.

References

267. Creel DJ, Summers CG, King RA. Visual anomalies associated with albinism. Ophthalmic Paediatr Genet 1990; 11:193–120.
268. Garipis N, Hoffmann K-P. Visual field defects in albino ferrets (*Mustela putorious furo*). Vision Res 2003; 43:793–800.
269. Hoffmann K-P, Garipis N, Distler C. Optokinetic defects in albino ferrets (*Mustela putorius furo*): a behavioural and electrophysiological study. J Neurosci 2004; 24:4061–4070.
270. Morgan JE, Henderson Z, Thompson ID. Retinal decussation patterns in pigmented and albino ferrets. Neuroscience 1987; 20:519–535.
271. Quevedo C, Hoffmann K-P, Husemann R et al. Overrepresentation of the central visual field in the superior colliculus of the pigmented and albino ferret. Visual Neurosci 1996; 13:627–638.
272. Gill SS, Salt AN. Quantitative differences in endolymphatic calcium and endocochlear potential between pigmented and albino guinea pigs. Hear Res 1997; 113:191–197.
273. Moore DR, Kowalchuk NE. An anomaly in the auditory brain stem projections of hypopigmented ferrets. Hear Res 1988; 35:275–278.
274. Ueki A. Oculocutaneous albinism with horizontal pendular nystagmus and sensory hearing loss. Jibi Inkoka Tokeibu Geka 1988; 60:75–80.
275. Barsh GS. The genetics of pigmentation: from fancy genes to complex traits. Trends Genet 1996; 12:299–305.
276. Cattanach BM. The Dalmatian dilemma: white coat colour and deafness. J Small Anim Pract 1999; 40:193–200.
277. Searle AG. Comparative genetics of coat colour in mammals. New York: Academic Press; 1968.
278. Keats BJ. B Genes and syndromic hearing loss. J Commun Disord 2002; 35:355–366.
279. Piebaldism OJ-P. Waardenburg's Syndrome and related disorders. Dermatol Clin 1988; 6:205–216.
280. Read AP, Newton VE. Waardenburg syndrome. J Med Genet 1997; 34:656–665.
281. Tomita Y, Suzuki T. Genetics of pigmentary disorders. Am J Med Genet 2004; 131:75–81.
282. Darlington D. The convoluted pattern of the brain and endocranial cast in the ferret (*Mustela furo* L.). J Anat 1957; 91:52–60.
283. Doty BA, Jones CN, Doty LA. Learning-set formation by mink, ferrets, skunks and cats. Science 1967; 155:1579–1580.
284. Hodos W. Comparative neuroanatomy and the evolution of intelligence. In: Jerison HJ, Jerison I, eds. Intelligence and evolutionary biology. New York: Springer; 1988:93–107.
285. Hughes RN. Responses by the ferret to stimulus change. Br J Pyschol 1964; 55:463–468.
286. Kruska D. Evidence of decrease in brain size in ranch mink, *Mustela vison* f. *dom.*, during subadult postnatal ontogenesis. Brain. Behav Evol 1993; 41:303–315.
287. Kruska D, Schreiber A. Comparative morphometrical and biochemical-genetic investigations in wild and ranch mink (*Mustela vison*: Carnivora: Mammalia). Acta Theriologica 1999; 44:377–392.
288. Poli MD. Species-specific differences in learning. In: Jerison HJ, Jerison I, eds. Intelligence and evolutionary biology. New York: Springer; 1988:277–297.
289. Pollard JS, Baldock MD, Lewis RFV. Learning rate and use of visual information in five animal species. Aust J Psychol 1971; 23:29–34.
290. Harvey PH. Allometric analysis and brain size. In: Jerison HJ, Jerison I, eds. Intelligence and evolutionary biology. New York: Springer; 1988:199–210.
291. Herre W, Röhrs. Animals in captivity. In: Grzimek B, ed. Grzimek's encyclopedia of mammals. New York: McGraw-Hill 1989.
292. Jerison HJ. Evolution of the brain and intelligence. New York: Academic Press; 1973.
293. Bubenik AB, Bellhouse TJ. Volumetric measurement of brain case cavity. Mammalia 1985; 49:415–420.
294. Apfelbach R, Kruska D. Zur postnatalen Hirnentwicklung beim Frettchen *Mustela putorius* f. *furo* (Mustelidae; Mammalia). Z Säugetierkd 1979; 44:127–131.
295. Kruska D. Vergleichende Untersuchungen an Schädeln von subadulten und adulten Farmnerzen, *Mustela vison* f. *dom.* (Mustelidae; Carnivora). Z Säugetierkd 1979; 44:360–375.
296. Kruska D. The effect of domestication of brain size and composition in the mink (*Mustela vison*). J Zool 1996; 239:645–661.
297. Steffen K, Kruska D, Tiedemann R. Postnatal brain size decrease, visual performance, learning and discrimination ability of juvenile and adult American mink (*Mustela vison*). Mamm Biol 2001; 66:269–280.
298. Kruska D. Domestikationsbedingte Hirgrößenänderungen bei Säugetieren. Z Zool Syst Evol 1980; 18:161–195.
299. Kruska D. Mammalian domestication and its effect on brain structure and behaviour. In: Jerison HJ, Jerison I, ed. Intelligence and evolutionary biology. New York: Springer; 1988:211–250.
300. Schumacher U. Quantitative Untersuchungen an Gehirnen mitteleuropäischer Musteliden. J Hirnforsch 1963; 6:137–163.
301. Lockard RI. The forebrain of the ferret. Lab Anim Sci 1985; 35:216–228.
302. Kruska D. On the evolutionary significance of encephalization in some eutherian mammals: effects of adaptive radiation, domestication and feralization. Brain Behav Evol 2005; 65:73–108.
303. Ashton EH. Some characters of the skulls of the European polecat, the Asiatic polecat and the domestic ferret. Proc Zool Soc Lond 1955; 125:807–809.
304. Yablokov AV. Variability of mammals, revised. Washington DC: Smithsonian Institution; 1974.
305. Korablev PN, Likhotop RI. Asymmetry in the mammalian skull. Vestn Zool 1990; 5:52–58.
306. Bateman JA. Supernumerary incisors in mustelids. Mamm Rev 1970; 1:81–86.
307. Berkovitz BKB. Supernumerary deciduous incisors and the order of eruption of the incisor teeth in the albino ferret. J Zool (London) 1968; 155:445–449.
308. Berkovitz BKB, Silverstone LM. The dentition of the albino ferret. Caries Res 1969; 3:369–376.
309. Glas GH. Numerical variation in the permanent dentition of the polecat, *Mustela putorious* (Linnaeus, 1758), from the Netherlands. Z Säugetierkd 1977; 42:256–259.
310. Ruprecht AL. Supernumerary premolar in *Mustela putorius* Linnaeus. Acta Theriologica 1965; 10.
311. Ruprecht AL. Dental variations in the common polecat in Poland. Acta Theriologica 1978; 23:239–245.
312. Berkovitz BKB. Teeth. New York: Springer; 1989.
313. Miles AEW, Grigson C. Colyer's variation and diseases of the teeth of animals, revised edition. Cambridge: Cambridge University Press; 1990.
314. Glas GH. Over lichaamsmaten en gewichten can de bunzing, *Mustela putorius* Linnaeus, 1758, in Nederland. Lutra 1974; 16:11–19.
315. Lewington JH. Ferret husbandry, medicine and surgery. Oxford: Butterworth-Heinemann; 2000.
316. Lloyd M. Ferrets: health, husbandry and diseases. Oxford: Blackwell Science; 1999.

CHAPTER SIX
Ferret-polecat domestication: genetic, taxonomic and phylogenetic relationships

317. Purcell K, Brown SA. Essentials of ferrets: a guide for practitioners, 2nd edn. Lakewood Colorado: AAHA Press; 1999.
318. Plummer DB. Modern ferretting. Ipswich: Boydell; 1977.
319. Aristotle. Thompson DW. History of Animals. In: 1956 Translated by D'Arcy Wentworth Thompson (Book VI, Part 37: When speaking regarding mice, 'Foxes also hunt them and the wild ferrets in particular destroy them, but they make no way against the prolific qualities of the animal and the rapidity of its breeding'.). Oxford: Clarendon Press; 1965.
320. Pliny the Elder. Natural history, 10 vols. London: Harvard University Press; 1992. Latin text with English translation.
321. Apfelbach R. Wild animal-domesticated animal-experimental animal: Changes in the brain during early ontogeny depend on environmental conditions. Tierärztliche Umsch 1996; 51:157–162.
322. Chivers SM, Einon DF. Effects of early social experience on activity and object investigation in the ferret. Dev Psychobiol 1982; 15:75–80.
323. Einon D. The effects of environmental enrichment in ferrets. In: Smith CP, Taylor V, eds. Environmental enrichment information resources for laboratory animals: 1965–1995: birds, cats, dogs, farm animals, ferrets, rabbits and rodents. AWIC resource series No. 2. Beltsville, MD: US Department of Agriculture; Potters Bar: Universities Federation for Animal Welfare (UFAW); 1995:113–126.
324. Jeppesen LL, Falkenberg H. Effects of play balls on peltbiting, behaviour and level of stress in ranch mink. Scientifur 1990; 14:179–186.
325. Everitt N. Ferrets: their management in health and disease with remarks on their legal status. London: A&C Black; 1897.
326. Birks JDS, Kitchener AC. The distribution and status of the polecat *Mustela putorius* in Britain in the 1990s. In: Birks JDS, Kitchener AC, eds. London: Vincent Wildlife Trust; 1999.
327. Griffiths HI. Mustelids in a modern world: management and conservation aspects of small carnivore : human interactions. In: Griffiths HI, ed. Leiden: Backhuys; 2000.
328. Manlio M, Romina F, Boitani L. Sexual segregation in the activity patterns of European polecats (*Mustela putorius*). J Zool 2003; 261:249–255.
329. Poole TB 1985 Social behaviour in mammals. London: Blackie.
330. Sandell M. The mating tactics and spacing patterns of solitary carnivores. In: Gittleman JL, ed. Carnivore behaviour, ecology and evolution, Vol. 1. Ithaca: Cornell University Press; 1989:164–182.
331. Price EO. The behaviour of domestic animals. In: Cole HH, Garrett WN, eds. Animal agriculture, 2nd edn. San Francisco: WH Freeman; 1980:477–495.
332. Poole TB. Aggressive play in polecats. In: Jewell PA, Loizos C, eds. Play, exploration and territory in mammals. Symposia of the Zoological Society of London. London: Academic Press; 1966:23–44.
333. Poole TB. Aspects of aggressive behaviour in polecats. Z Tierpsychol 1967; 24:350–369.
334. Norbury GL, Norbury DC, Heyward RP. Behavioural responses of two predator species to sudden declines in primary prey. J Wildl Manage 1998; 62:45–58.
335. Norbury GL, Norbury DC, Heyward RP. Space use and denning behaviour of wild ferrets and cats. N Z J Ecol 1998; 22:149–159.
336. Smith GP, Ragg JR, Moller H et al. Diet of feral ferrets (*Mustela furo*) from pastoral habitats in Otago and Southland, New Zealand. N Z J Zool 1995; 22:363–369.
337. Malmkvist J, Hansen SW. Generalization of fear in farm mink, *Mustela vison*, genetically selected for behaviour towards humans. Anim Behav 2002; 64:487–501.
338. Malmkvist J, Herskin MS, Christensen JW. Behavioural responses of farm mink towards familiar and novel food. Behav Processes 2003; 61:123–131.
339. Kusak J, Huber D. Istraživanje radoznalosti mesoždera. Veterinarski Arh 1991; 61:395–409.
340. Petzsch H. Gesellschaftshaltung einer größeren Anzahl von Iltissen (*Putorius putorius* L.) und Frettchen (*Putorius furo* L.) verschiedener Altersstufen. Zool Gart 1955; 21:188–190.
341. Belyaev DK. Destablizing selection as a factor in domestication. J Hered 1979; 70:301–308.
342. Eastment AM, Hughes RN. Reactions of ferret-polecat hybrids to complexity and change. Percept Mot Skills 1968; 26:935–938.
343. Boissy A. Fear and fearfulness in determining behaviour. In: Grandin T, ed. Genetics and the behaviour of domestic animals. San Diego: Academic Press; 1998:67–111.
344. Haskell DG. Experiments and a model examining learning in the area-restricted search behaviour of ferrets (*Mustela putorius furo*). Behav Ecol 1997; 8:448–455.
345. Diener A. Verhaltensanalysen zum Sozialspiel von Iltisfrettchen (*Mustela putorius* f. *furo*). Z Säugetierkd 1985; 67:179–197.
346. Apfelbach A, Wester U. The quantitative effect of visual and tactile stimuli on the prey-catching behaviour of ferrets (*Putorius furo* L.). Behav Processes 1977; 2:187–200.
347. Apfelbach R. Ethologische und neurale aspekte der Nahrungswahl beim Frettchen *Mustela putorius* f. *furo*. Popul Marderertiger Säugetiere 1989; 2:505–514.
348. Aristophanes, Rogers B. Aristophanes, Vol. 3: the Lysistrata, the Thesmophoriazusae, the Ecclesiazusae, the Plutus [edited and translated by Benjamin Bickley Rogers]. Cambridge: Harvard University Press; 1924.
349. Aristophanes, Starkie WJM. Aristophanous Sphekes: the wasps of Aristophanes, with introduction, metrical analysis, critical notes and commentary by W. J. M. Starkie. Amsterdam: AM Hakkert; 1968.
350. Aristophanes, Sommerstein AH. Acharnians. [edited with translation and notes by Alan H. Sommerstein]. Warminster: Aris & Phillips; 1980.
351. Aristophanes, Sommerstein AH. Wasps [edited with translation and notes by Alan H. Sommerstein]. Warminster: Aris & Phillips; 1983.
352. Aristophanes, Sommerstein AH. Peace. [edited with translation and notes by Alan H. Sommerstein]. Warminster: Aris & Phillips; 1985.
353. Aristophanes, Sommerstein AH. Thesmophpriazusae. [edited with translation and notes by Alan H. Sommerstein]. Warminster: Aris & Phillips; 1994.
354. Aristophanes, Sommerstein AH. Ecclesiazusae. [edited with translation and commentary by Alan H. Sommerstein]. Warminster: Aris & Phillips; 1998.
355. Aristotle, Balme DM. History of animals: Books VII–X. [Translated by DM. Balme]. Loeb Classical Library, No. 439. Cambridge: Harvard University Press; 1991.
356. Aristotle, Peck AL. Historia animalium. [Translated by AL. Peck]. Cambridge: Harvard University Press; 1970.
357. Aristotle, Peck AL. History of animals: Aristotle. [with an English translation by A. L. Peck]. Cambridge: Harvard University Press; 1991.
358. Herodotus, Godley AD. Herodotus. [with an English translation by A. D. Godley]. London: William Heinemann; 1938.

359. How WW, Wells J. A commentary of Herodotus, with introduction and appendices. Oxford: Clarendon Press; 1912.
360. Isidore of Seville. Sancti Isidori Hispalensis episcopi opera omnia romæ anno domini mdccxcvii excusa recensente faustino arevalo, qui isidoriana præfationes, notas, collationes, qua antea editas, et codices mss. romanos contulit, nova nunc et accuratiori editone donata pretiosissimisque monumentis aucta. [Migne J-P, ed]. Turnholti, Belgium: Typographi Brepols Editores Pontificii; 1969-1977.
361. Keller JE, Keating LC. Aesop's fables: with a life of Aesop. Lexington: University of Kentucky Press; 1993.
362. Temple O, Temple R. Aesop: the complete fables. New York: Penguin Books; 1998.
363. Theophrastus, Ussher RG. The characters of Theophrastus. London: Macmillan; 1960.
364. Barnett M. Gods and myths of the ancient world: the archaeology and mythology of ancient Egypt, ancient Greece and the Romans. Hertfordshire: Regency House; 1997.
365. Budge EAW. The mummy: chapters on Egyptian funereal archaeology. New York: Biblo & Tannen; 1964.
366. Ikram S. Death and burial in ancient Egypt. Harlow: Longman; 2003.
367. Martin GT. The sacred animal necropolis at North Saqqâra: the southern dependencies of the main temple complex. London: Egypt Exploration Society; 1981.
368. Watterson B. Gods of Ancient Egypt. London: Sutton; 1996.
369. Wilkinson R. The complete Gods and Goddesses of Ancient Egypt. London: Thames & Hudson; 2003.
370. Brewer D. Anubis to Cerberos: dogs of the ancient world. Warminster: Aris & Phillips; 1999.
371. Champdor A. L'Egypte des pharaohs: Saqqara, Abydos, Louqsor, Karnak, Médinet Habou, Edfou, Le Ramesseum, Kom Ombo, Deir el Bahari, Abou Simbel, la Vallée des Rois. Paris: A. Guillot; 1955.
372. Collins BJ. A history of the animal world in the ancient Near East. In: Collins BJ, ed. Boston: Brill Academic Publishers; 2002.
373. Donalson MD. The domestic cat in Roman civilization. Lewiston: Edwin Mellen Press; 1999.
374. Brewer DJ, Redford DB, Redford S. Domestic plants and animals: the Egyptian origins. Warminster: Aris & Phillips; 1994.
375. Reed CA. Animal domestication in the prehistoric Near East. Science 1959; 130:1629–1639.
376. Cansdale GS. All the animals of the Bible lands. Michigan: Zondervan, Grand Rapids; 1970.
377. Moskala J. The laws of clean and unclean animals of Leviticus 11: their nature, theology and rationale (an intertextual study). UMI Dissertation Services, Andrews University, Seventh-Day Adventist Theological Seminary; 1998.
378. Peelman N. The beasts, birds and fish of the Bible. New York: Morehouse-Barlow; 1975.
379. Pinney R. The animals in the Bible: the identity and natural history of all the animals mentioned in the Bible, with a collection of photographs of living species taken in the Holy Land by the author. Philadelphia: Chilton Books; 1964.
380. United Bible Societies. Fauna and flora of the Bible: prepared in cooperation with the Committee on Translations of the United Bible Societies. London: United Bible Societies; 1972.
381. Boessneck J, von den Driesch AA. Roman cat skeleton from Quseir on the Red Sea coast. J Archaeol Sci 1983; 10:205–211.
382. Davies NG. The mastaba of Ptahhetep and Akhethetep at Saqqareh, part I: the chapel of Ptahhetep and the hieroglyphs. Eighth memoir of the Archaeological Survey of Egypt. London: Egypt Exploration Fund; 1900.
383. Davies NG. The mastaba of Ptahhetep and Akhethetep at Saqqareh, part II: the mastaba; the sculptures of Akhethetep. Ninth memoir of the Archaeological Survey of Egypt. London: Egypt Exploration Fund; 1901.
384. Harpur Y. Decoration in Egyptian tombs of the Old Kingdom: studies in orientation and scene content. London: KPI; 1987.
385. Houlihan PF. The animal world of the pharaohs. London: Thames & Hudson; 1996.
386. Macramallah R. Fouilles à Saqqarah. Le mas?aba d'Idout. Imprimerie de l'Institut français d'archéologie orientale, Le Caire; 1935.
387. Murray MA. Saqqara mastabas, part II. London: British School of Archaeology in Egypt; 1937.
388. Newberry PE, Beni Hasan, part I. London: British School of Archaeology in Egypt; 1893.
389. Osborn DJ, Osbornová J. The mammals of ancient Egypt. Warminster: Aris & Phillips; 1998.
390. Boessneck J, von den Driesch A. Studien an subfossilen Tierknochen aus Ägypten. Studien #40, Munich: Münchner Ägyptologische; 1982.
391. Boessneck J. Die Tierwelt des Alten Ägypten. Munich: CH Beck Verlag; 1988.
392. Kurtén B. The carnivora of the Palestine caves. Acta Zool Fenn 1965; 107:1–74.
393. Aihartza JR, Zuberogoitia I, Camacho-Verdejo E et al. Status of carnivores on Biscay (N. Iberian peninsula). Miscellània Zoològica 1999; 22:41–52.
394. Atallah SI. Mammals of the eastern Mediterranean: their ecology, systematics and zoogeographical relationships. Säugetierkundliche Mitt 1977; 25:241–320.
395. Atallah SI. Mammals of the eastern Mediterranean: their ecology, systematics and zoogeographical relationships. Säugetierkundliche Mitt 1978; 26:1–50.
396. Aynard JM. Animals in Mesopotamia. In: Brodrick AH, ed. Animals in archaeology. New York: Praeger; 1972:42–68.
397. Bates PJ, Harrison D. New records of small mammals from Jordan. Bonn Zool Beiträge 1989; 40:223–226.
398. Bodenheimer FS. Animal life in Palestine: an introduction to the problems of animal ecology and zoogeography. Jerusalem: L. Mayer; 1935.
399. Bodenheimer FS. The present taxonomic status of the terrestrial mammals of Palestine. Bull Res Counc Isr 1958; 7B:165–189.
400. Bodenheimer FS. and man in Bible lands. Collection de Travaux de l'Académie Internationale d'Histoire des Sciences n. 10. Leiden: Brill Academic Publishers; 1960.
401. Clarke JE. A preliminary list of Jordan's mammals. Amman: The Royal Society of the Conservation of Nature; 1977.
402. Dobson M. Mammal distributions in the western Mediterranean: the role of human interaction. Mammal Rev 1998; 28:77–88.
403. Haltenorth T, Diller H. A field guide to the mammals of Africa. London: Collins Sons & Co; 1980.
404. Harrison DL, Bates PJ. The mammals of Arabia, 2nd edn. Kent: Harrison Zoological Museum; 1991.
405. Hufnagl E. Libyan mammals. New York: Olander Press; 1972.
406. Kingdon J. The Kingdon field guide to African mammals. London: Academic Press; 1997.
407. Kryštufek B, Petkovski S. New records of mammals from Macedonia (Mammalia). Fragm Balcanica Mus Macidonica Sci Nat 1990; 14:117–127.

CHAPTER SIX
Ferret-polecat domestication: genetic, taxonomic and phylogenetic relationships

408. Lakhdar-Ghazal A, Fartouat JP, Thevenot M. Faune du Maroc: les Mammifères. L'Institut d'Études et de Recherches pour l'Arabisation. Maroc: Rabat; 1975.
409. Panouse JB. Les mammifères du Maroc: primates, carnivores, pinnipedes, artiodactyls. Trav l 'Institut Scientifique Chérifien 1957; 5:1–206.
410. Qumsiyeh MB, Amr ZS, Shafei DM. Status and conservation of carnivores in Jordan. Mammalia 1993; 57:55–62.
411. Qumsiyeh MB. Mammals of the Holy Land. Lubbock: Texas Tech University Press; 1996.
412. Setzer HW. A review of Libyan mammals. J Egypt Public Health Assoc Cairo 1957; 32:41–82.
413. Boessneck J. Die Haustiere in Altägypten. Vereoffentlichungen der Zoologischen Staatssammlung Meunchen III; 1953.
414. El Monaiery AM. Situation of wild mammals in Egypt. Bull Zool Soc Egypt 1955; 12.
415. Flower S 1932 Notes on recent mammals of Egypt, with a list of the species recorded from that kingdom. Proc Zool Soc Lond 1932; 368–450.
416. Hoogstraal HA. Brief review of the contemporary land mammals of Egypt (including Sinai). J Egypt Public Health Assess 1964; 39:205–239.
417. Keimer L. Über zwei Fleischfresser aus der Familie der Mustelidae im Alten und Neuen Ägypten. Mitt dea Dtsch Archèaologischen Instituts 1939; 8:38–41.
418. Osborn DJ, Helmy I. The contemporary land mammals of Egypt (including Sinai). Fieldiana Zool NS 1980; 5:1–579.
419. Russelle T. The fauna of Egyptian deserts. Bull Zool Soc Egypt 1951; 8:5–8.
420. Setzer HW. Mammals of the Anglo-Egyptian Sudan. Proc US Natl Mus 1956; 106:447–587.
421. Setzer HW. The mustelids of Egypt. J Egypt Public Health Assoc Cairo 1958; 33:199–204.
422. Wassif K, Hoogstraal H. The mammals of south Sinai. Egypt. Proceedings of the Egyptian Academy of Science 1953; 9.
423. King C. Immigrant killers. Introduced predators and the conservation of birds in New Zealand. Oxford: Oxford University Press; 1984.
424. Lever C. Naturalized mammals of the world. New York: Longman; 1985.
425. Fox JG. Biology and diseases of the ferret. In: Fox JG, ed. 2nd edn. Baltimore: Williams & Wilkins; 1998.
426. Aubet ME. The Phoenicians and the west: politics, colonies and trade. Cambridge: Cambridge University Press; 1987.
427. Engels D. Classical cats. The rise and fall of the sacred cat. London: Routledge; 2000.
428. Langton B. The Cat in Ancient Egypt. New York: Kegan Paul International; 2000.
429. Malik J. The cat in ancient Egypt. Philadelphia: University of Pennsylvania Press; 1997.
430. Placzek Rev. Dr. The weasel and the cat in ancient times. Trans Soc Biblical Archæology 1893; 9:155–166.
431. Baldwin JA. Notes and speculations on the domestication of the cat in Egypt. Anthropos 1975; 70:428–448.
432. Evelyn-White HG. Hesiod, the Homeric hymns and Homerica, with an English translation. Cambridge: Harvard University Press; 1954.
433. Hine D. The Homeric hymns and the battle of the frogs and mice. [translated by Daryl Hine]. New York: Atheneum; 1972.
434. Butler S. The Iliad of Homer, rendered into English prose for the use of those who cannot read the original. London: AC Fifield; 1914.
435. Lang W, Leaf W, Myers E. The Iliad of Homer [in English prose by Andrew Lang, Walter Leaf and Ernest Myers], revised. New York: Macmillan Press; 1903.
436. Murray AT. The Iliad. [with an English translation by A.T. Murray]. Loeb Classical Library. New York: GP Putnam's Sons; 1924.
437. Pliny the Elder, Bostock J, Riley HT. The natural history: Pliny the Elder. London: Taylor & Francis; 1855.
438. Amigues S. Les belettes de Tartessos. Anthropozoologica 1999; 29:55–64.
439. Plautus, Riley HT. The comedies of Plautus. [translated by Henry Thomas Riley]. London: Bell & Sons; 1912.
440. Morwood J. The pocket Oxford Latin dictionary. Oxford: Oxford University Press; 1994.
441. Ranking J. Historical researches on the wars and sports of the Mongols and Romans: in which elephants and wild beasts were employed or slain and the remarkable local agreement of history with the remains of such animals found in Europe and Siberia. London: Longman, Rees Orme, Brown & Green; 1826.
442. Mason IL, ed. Mongoose. Evolution of domesticated animals. Harlow: Longman; 1984:234–236.
443. Trut LN, Plyusnina IZ, Oskina IN. An experiment on fox domestication and debatable issues of evolution of the dog. Genetika 2004; 40:794–807.
444. Belyaev DK, Ruvinsky AO, Trut LN. Inherited activation inactivation of the star gene in foxes: its bearing on the problem of domestication. J Hered 1981; 72:267–274.
445. Hansen SW. Selection for behavioural traits in farm mink. Appl Anim Behav Sci 1996; 49:137–148.
446. Praslova LS, Trut LN. The effect of the Star gene on the rate of melanoblast migration in embryos of silver foxes (*Vulpes vulpes*). Dokl Akad Nauk 1993; 329:787–790.
447. Trut LNDK. Belyaev's evolutionary concept: ten years later. Genetika 1997; 33:1060–1068.
448. Trut LN. The evolutionary concept of destabilizing selection: Status quo. Z Tierz Zuchtungsbiologie 1998; 115:415–431.
449. Trut LN. Early canid domestication: the farm-fox experiment. Am Sci 1999; 87:160–169.
450. Belyaev DK, Ruvinskii AO, Trut LN. Significance of inherited gene activation inactivation in the domestication of animals. Genetika 1979; 15:2033–2050.
451. Cole L, Shackelford R. White spotting in the fox. Am Nat 1943; 77:289–321.
452. Schaible RH. Developmental genetics of spotting patterns in the mouse. Unpublished PhD Thesis, Iowa State Univerisity; 1963.
453. Tomkins G, Martin D. Hormones and gene expression. Annu Rev Genet 1970; 4:91–106.
454. Bronner-Fraser M. Segregation of cell lineage in the neural crest. Curr Opin Genet Dev 1993; 3:641–647.
455. Dourmishev AL, Dourmishev LA, Schwartz RA et al. Waardenburg syndrome. Int J Dermatol 1999; 38:656–663.
456. Tassabehji M, Read AP, Newton VE et al. Waardenburg's syndrome patients have mutations in the human homologue of the Pax-3 paired bix gene. Nature 1992; 355:535–536.

CHAPTER 7

Ferret handling, hospitalization and diagnostic techniques

'Your ferret will enjoy your company. He may chuckle as you tickle his belly. He will fall asleep in your arms. He will crawl all over you if he has the chance. He will curl up in your hat or coat pocket.'

Mervin F. Roberts, All about Ferrets, 1977

General considerations

Ferrets are owned by a wide variety of people as working animals against wild rabbits and rats. Ferrets are also pet companion animals. Additionally, they are used in laboratory biomedical research. Working ferrets are used to being handled, however a veterinarian should be cautious with them; they can bite but so can dogs and cats. Ferret owners are concerned with their ferrets' welfare and will seek veterinary advice, but only if they think the veterinarian has a positive attitude to ferrets. He should have some knowledge of general ferret matters and as positive an approach to handling ferrets as he has to dogs or cats. It must be remembered that ferrets are domesticated animals and are used to being around humans. Ferrets should be handled gently, remembering that they are seldom still once awake, unless sick, especially as kittens and young adults.

Children can be candidates for nips and bites, as they tend to grab and squeeze things. Ferrets should be kept away from very young children and of course babies, though statistics show that far more children are bitten by dogs than by ferrets. In December 1998, in New Zealand, it was recorded that a ferret strayed from one house, entered another and managed to get into bed with a 2-year-old child. The ferret did bite the child but only when the child had rolled on the ferret.

Ferrets nip as a warning in play but can bite hard into flesh when agitated, alarmed or fighting other ferrets. The bite action is best avoided. Like a terrier, the ferret can hang on tight and be difficult to remove. Ferret kittens are usually nippy but will grow out of it with attention. Nipping, as distinct from biting, is part of the young ferrets' 'play-fight' exercise with their littermates and is seen in all the mustelids. When a kitten nips, it is expecting to be nipped back! To discourage excessive nipping, the kitten is handled and played with as much as possible. If the nips get more persistent, advise ferret owners to give a sharp command 'No!' to alert the ferret to let go, plus perhaps a finger flick under the jaw as a rebuke, with an immediate tender stroking along the ferret's head. With my first ferret, Fred, when he became too rough in play-fight, I would give a sort of whimper and he would immediately stop nipping, lick the spot, then attack again but less fiercely. When playing with a ferret, one can push them away with a hand bunched into a fist when they become nippy. They cannot easily catch hold of your knuckles. Ferrets can nip and also scratch children when they jump up for attention, so care must be taken and they should not be left alone with a youngster who might panic. Ferrets must be supervised when they are with children, as must the children when they are with ferrets.

Ferret/human bonding

The basis of 'bonding' with any pet is frequent handling. Ferrets come to think of humans as part of the 'colony'. There is equal trust. Can you trust a ferret not to savage

CHAPTER SEVEN

Ferret handling, hospitalization and diagnostic techniques

you? At one time when I had a ferret breeding colony, I would open the ferretarium door in the evening and then go and lie on the grass. The garden would be in the evening dark. I would put the bottoms of my trousers in my socks. I would be lying on the grass when I would hear the ferrets rustling around. Hector, a full sable hob, would come along and find me on the grass. He would start at my feet and sniff along my body until he got to my head. I had my hands over my eyes. He would come along sniffing around my face and then find my ear lobe. He would take the lobe in his teeth and just hold, it for a moment – not a bite. Then he would release it and amble towards the family room door wanting to be fed. Now that's ferret/human bonding!

Straying ferrets

Ferrets can get lost like dogs and cats but usually pet ferrets wandering off are excited by new smells. Sometimes they hole up during the day and are active in the evening (like natural polecats). Putting out a small cat basket with bedding from the ferret's home and some food will attract it back and the ferret will be found asleep in the basket the next morning. If a ferret is lost during an evening and does not come back to a call, it might help to just stay put in one place and start digging around, scraping things and looking as if one has found something interesting. The pet ferret might not be able to see you but it can get the human smell and certainly the voice. Nine times out of ten it is driven by curiosity and appears out of the gloom to see what you are doing.

The ferret in the clinic

I used to have a client with a 4-year-old child who came into the clinic with a pet ferret draped happily over his shoulder. When an adult ferret is brought into the veterinary clinic/hospital for examination, remember not to rush the ferret and to handle it gently but firmly; it should be accustomed to handling. Ferrets can be presented in a carrying box (cage), especially if they are hunting ferrets, or, as said, perched on a child's shoulder. They may arrive on a harness with lead.

Hunting ferrets could be excited, unless they are very ill, as they associate the carrying box with something they enjoy; hunting rabbits! Take care in approaching them. Ferreters know their ferrets, so best be guided by them. Let the owner take the ferret out of the box. Try to examine the ferret in as quiet a place as possible, with no barking dogs in the background. They may unnerve the ferret, though on the whole ferrets should be familiar with the smell of dogs and cats around their household. Examine the actions of the ferret once out of the carrying cage.

Healthy ferrets are active ferrets unless sleeping, eating or really sick. Activity will however decline with age but alertness to the surroundings should be there to see as soon as the ferret leaves the carrying basket. (Advise prospective ferret buyers on this point of alertness of the ferret before buying.)

Place the ferret on the examination table, which should be half-covered by a clean towel. Let the ferret sniff around and settle down. It is unlikely to run off like a scared cat but might oblige with a faeces (scat) or urine sample after being confined. Provide a clean plastic scats tray as described in Chapter 3 and, encouraging the ferret, it may produce samples without stress. It also keeps the household pet ferret 'attuned' to the use of the scats tray. The client also observes that you are 'ferret-wise'. Initial examination of urine should show a clear yellow colour. The scats, on a meat diet, should be of a firm elongate dark nature. The type of diet will modify the scats' appearance. These observations are of the healthy ferret, in, e.g. for vaccination. Diarrhoea will be obvious. Constipation is rare with ferrets.

The ferret should have a name! Ask for it and see how the ferret responds to a call. When approaching the ferret, offer a clenched fist, knuckles foremost, as a routine to the ferret before attempting to pick it up. Move slowly! If the ferret is going to bite, it would only get a poor hold on the knuckles. It is more likely to sniff and even lick the knuckles as ferrets like the salt taste of the hand. Again, be careful with hunting ferrets and ask the owner about their temperament. You could be dealing with the equivalent of a Rottweiler! Do not poke fingers at ferrets! Advise ferret owners about children doing the same!

Note the ferret's attitude before attempting to pick it up. If really alarmed by the situation it is in, the ferret might arch its back like a cat and fluff out its tail like a bottle-brush (Fig. 7.1).

Under extreme provocation, the ferret might hiss, attempt to bite, express its musk glands, or all three! Personally, I have never come across this with ferrets but there is always a first time! It is suggested that a spray bottle with a bitter alcohol solution be used for a ferret that did bite to make it let go. In some cases, ferrets get the 'wild-eye' look and will not let go but that is a rare case. In the unfortunate event of really being bitten, plunging the hand and the ferret into a handy bucket of water will do the trick!

At an early stage in the examination, the ferret's rectal temperature should be taken but only if the history and the immediate clinical signs warrant the intrusion. The ferret's temperature can rise marginally due to the stress of the occasion. For examining the skin, place

The ferret in the clinic

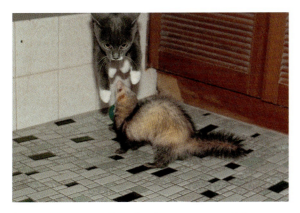

Figure 7.1 Our cat, Mac, has his four paws off the ground when being surprised by ferret, Squeak. *Note:* ferret shows 'bottlebrush' tail.

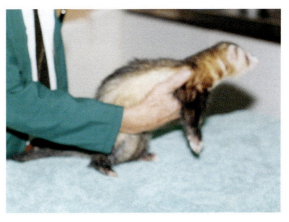

Figure 7.2 Gentle restraint of ferret by raising it off the table, using one hand under its chest. Do not squeeze.

one hand under the chest/abdomen region. The ferret is gently restrained by one hand and the coat checked with the other. There will be a musky smell but there should be no offensive musk gland odour.

The ferret is thus not 'spooked' from being on the examination table. The skin should be pliable to show good hydration. The coat has an 'oily' feel and in fact, a ferret with a good coat easily 'slips' through the hand. The coat of outdoor-living ferrets is usually thicker than that of their indoor-living counterparts, especially in the cold seasons of colder climates than Western Australia. Ferrets have winter and summer moults to some extent. This can be affected by whether the pet ferret is kept indoors all the time under artificial lighting. A thinning of the coat or partial or compete alopecia may indicate an underlying disease problem. Hob ferrets have thinly-haired tails during the mating season and usually regain a full coat later.

With indoor ferrets, the loss of hair over the tail or hindquarters could be the beginning of ferret adrenal disease complex (FADC), which is fairly common in the USA but has also occurred in Australia (Ch. 14). It occurs in sterilized adults, possibly associated with extended photo-periods. An unsterilized jill remaining in heat with a noticeably swollen vulva and complete alopecia could have a potentially fatal post-oestrous anaemia (POA).

Fleas can be common in ferrets, especially those living outside and also in multi-animal households. There may be signs of pruritus with the ferret. Hob ferrets may show scars or bite marks of fighting, especially if they get together in the mating season. Working ferrets can show wounds related to hunting. Skin tumours can occur and mast cell tumours appear to be common in American ferrets (S. Brown, pers. comm. 1991). For further examination, the ferret can be picked up by gently

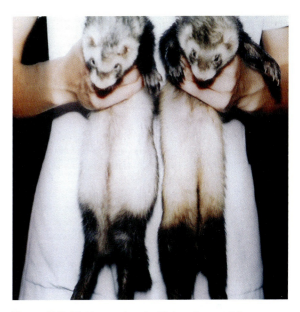

Figure 7.3 Picking up ferret with hand around the upper chest. With these two same-size ferrets, the one on the left as viewed has a enlarged spleen, seen as a noticeable swelling on the left side of the abdomen (see Ch. 13).

lifting with the hand under the chest/abdomen. Do not feel the urge to squeeze tight and be prepared for the ferret to wriggle (Figs 7.2, 7.3).

If the ferret being picked up is relatively heavy or a pregnant jill, it should be supported by a hand under the animal's rump (Fig. 7.4).

Care must be taken with the heavily pregnant jill. It is possible for them to hurt their back especially if they attempt to clamber out of the top of a carrying basket.

CHAPTER SEVEN
Ferret handling, hospitalization and diagnostic techniques

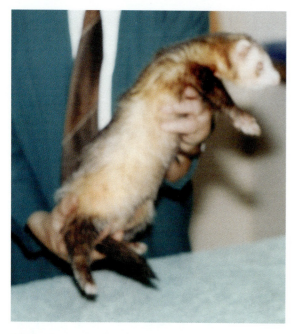

Figure 7.4 Supporting the heavy ferret, especially important with heavily pregnant jills.

A pregnant jill could be examined by ultrasound if available. As an alternative to picking up a ferret for further examination, a small piece of meat can be placed in front of it to take the ferret's attention.

A ferret should tolerate an ear examination using the finest auriscope head. Ear mites (*Otodectes cynotis*) can be common in outdoor and indoor ferrets. Aural cancers of the ear pinnae are not known, even in albino ferrets. A routine ear-swab using a cotton bud moistened with olive oil is a better way to check for ear mites and allows the veterinarian to show the client the moving creatures under the microscope. A positive swab for ear mites and the presence of fleas require overall parasite control to include in-contact dogs and cats.

Working ferrets also pick up 'stick-tight' fleas (*Echidnophaga gallinacea*) from rabbit warrens. These fleas cluster noticeably on the ferret's ears. Ferreters swear that they disappear in a few days but their eggs will be somewhere in the ferret's environment.

While holding the ferret, the feet and nails can be viewed. Ferrets living outside and working ferrets must be checked for the presence of foot mange (*Sarcoptes scabiei*), as this is a dangerous disease in ferrets. If positive, all in-contact dogs must be examined. The ferret's nails are usually kept short in outdoor ferrets but may require clipping, especially in older ferrets. I sometimes get the owner to hold the ferret while clipping the nails. The owner sits down with the ferret on a towel on the lap; the ferret is usually tolerant to the procedure. Alternatively, the nurse can hold the ferret on the table. I find it less stressful for the ferret if they stay with the owner. Naturally, the ferret wriggles!

While considering picking up ferrets never, never, attempt to pick a ferret up by its tail! First, it is painful for the ferret and harms the spinal cord. Second, justifiably annoyed, an agile ferret can climb back up on itself and bury its fangs into your hand in a second! (Find that bucket again...!)

Palpation of the ferret abdomen should be gentle and not rushed. In one US case, a 3-year-old silver mitt castrated hob ferret was examined and an enlarged spleen was noted during a routine examination prior to distemper vaccination.[1] The ferret was given the vaccination s.c. and allowed to rest in the reception room for 30 min as a routine. At home, the ferret was quiet and lethargic and it was put down to a possible stress with the vaccination. It was kept in its cage overnight and found dead in the morning. A post mortem revealed a splenic rupture with the possible cause from the clinical palpation. It can happen.

The nose should be checked for nasal discharge and one must inform the client that ferrets get human influenza and possible 'snuffles' conditions. Any apparent growths on the nose surface could be due to *Cryptococcus neoformans* in outdoor-living ferrets and this is highly dangerous. However, solar-induced nasal cancers are not known, as even white ferrets are mostly nocturnal or house-dwelling. The eyes can be checked for obvious cataracts, which are rare but can affect young and old ferrets. The aetiology of the condition is varied. For a full eye examination, the ferret should be checked in a quiet dark room. Internal eye examinations require patience, possible sedation and use of a mydriatic. To examine the teeth arcade, the ferret can be swung over

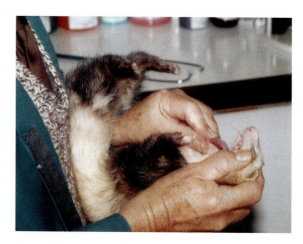

Figure 7.5 Examining the ferret's teeth and mouth.

154

and supported upside down in the crook of the arm or against the body. The lower jaw can be opened with a finger, or if not so bold, with a spatula (Fig. 7.5).

The dental formula has been given in Chapter 2, while details of dentistry and pathology are given in Chapter 21. In the healthy ferret, clean teeth and pink gums should be present but as the ferret ages, tartar builds up on the upper and back premolars and molars. Tooth discolouration may depend on diet. I have found that working ferrets on an all meat/bone diet have good clean teeth. Dental disease with tartar build-up can be dealt with as for cats and dogs under various anaesthetics as in Chapter 16. While examining the mouth, the condition of the tongue and lingual frenulum is checked for the presence of mucoceles, especially in working ferrets, due to fight wounds. Foreign bodies like grass seeds can be a special problem in dry climates.

The external genitalia of the hob and jill can be checked while holding the ferret for teeth examination. The hob testes, penis and baculum (os penis bone) can be palpated for injury, especially in breeding hobs, and for tumours of the testes. Hydroceles, cystic tumours, may be seen in older vasectomized hobs. In the jill, the vulva should be very small, normally hardly noticeable except when swollen in heat. If a jill is in heat, then ask how long the condition has been observed. The jill could pass into post-oestrous anaemia (POA) unless it is prevented by mating, hormonal injection or use of a vasectomized hob. In the spayed jill, a swollen vulva may indicate a retention of some ovarian tissue post-operatively or possibly ferret adrenal disease complex (FADC). I have only seen the alopecia phase of FADC in a sterilized jill without the vulval swelling, as shown in Chapter 14.

To record an obviously sick ferret's temperature, it might be prudent to let the owner hold the ferret on their lap on a towel. Many ferret owners like to assist and with working ferrets, it might be essential that they do. If the ferret is sick, there is usually no trouble, otherwise expect the ferret to wriggle. For the usual vaccinations, there is no point in taking the temperature but this decision must be made on the history and demeanour of the ferret. A plastic digital thermometer with a small bore is preferable to a glass one. The normal body temperature should register 37.5–40°C with stress probably causing the higher value. Ferrets get stressed in situations where more than one ferret is around and involved, such as at ferret shows and ferret racing or 'conveyer belt' vaccination days, which should be banned. If the owner does not hold the ferret, the assisting nurse can do so, with the ferret wrapped in a towel.

The usual auscultation of the heart and lungs may be difficult in an initial examination of an active healthy inquisitive ferret, brought in, e.g. for vaccination. Again,

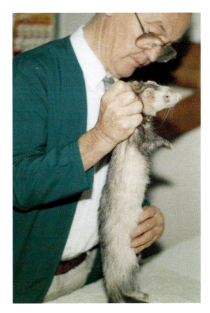

Figure 7.6 'Scruffing' the ferret to palpate internal organs.

a quiet environment without distractions is ideal, so that there is less stress on the ferret, healthy or otherwise. An excited ferret can show an elevated heart rate, usually 180–250 beats per minute, so murmurs are undetected. Pet ferrets in the USA are considered high risks for cardiomyopathy (S. Brown, pers. comm. 1998), therefore take time over a heart check in the older ferret. When checking heart and lungs, the use of a paediatric stethoscope or electronic stethoscope is recommended.

The external lymph nodes and the internal organs can be palpated if the ferret is held gently up with its hind legs on the table. The ferret can also be 'scruffed' and lifted up and the abdomen can be palpated (Fig. 7.6)

In 'scruffing' the ferret is held off the table by using one hand to hold as much skin as possible over the back of the neck starting between the ears. The client should be warned that the ferret is going to be 'scruffed' as they might be alarmed at how their pet is held up.

It is considered that in the 'scruffed' position the ferret can have its ears cleaned, nails clipped, head examined, abdomen palpated, chest auscultated and also be given s.c. or i.m. injections (S. Brown, pers. comm. 1997). *Note*: stroking the abdomen tends to relax the ferret. 'Scruffing' is good for applying ear-drops, when single-handed.

With regard to injecting ferrets, I ask the owner, if willing, to hold the ferret against their body as I inject s.c. I tend to inject the ferret s.c. prone on the examination table and never inject a ferret in the neck, as shown in some books, while 'scruffing'. Some fully grown hunting ferrets might not take lightly to being 'scruffed'! The necks of heavy mature hobs for one thing are less pliable to hold. American veterinarians do not usually treat working ferrets and the pet ferrets they do treat are all sterilized house pets and well-handled. Some breeding jills may be sensitive to 'scruffing' as the hob takes the jill by the neck during mating and a jill may have had a sore neck in the mating season and resent such handling. When 'scruffing' a heavily pregnant jill, I keep her hind legs over the table (Fig. 7.6). While 'scruffing' a ferret, gastric or enteric foreign bodies or bladder stones can be palpated, with experience.

The technique of injecting s.c. a ferret on a towel on the table, is to take it by the scruff and at the moment of injection, press the ferret firmly down just for the second it takes to inject (Fig. 7.7).

The temperament of the ferret at the time, especially working ferrets in countries outside America, must be judged. A sick ferret with abdominal discomfort may allow palpation but if agitated, a twisting motion and attempt to escape may occur. The spleen is one organ most easily palpated on the left side and more so when the ferret is being 'scruffed' or just held with its hind legs still on the table (Fig. 7.2). The ferret spleen may be enlarged naturally in older ferrets but a grossly enlarged spleen with other diagnostic factors may indicate neoplasia and require further investigation. For taking the temperature, the ferret is best wrapped in a towel by the nurse (Fig. 7.8). In the same manner, an injection can be given i.m. into the thigh muscle of the exposed leg.

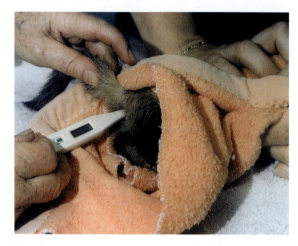

Figure 7.8 Nurse holding ferret for temperature taking. *Note*: the ferret tail is held forward and a white plastic digital thermometer is used.

All ferrets should be weighed during the clinical examination, with kitchen scales or bag and spring scales kept for the purpose. To have the ferret inactive for a moment, unless sick, a small titbit of meat is put on the scale pan. Ferret owners should be encouraged to weigh their ferrets monthly or weekly at home and keep a record to estimate significant gains or losses in weight during the ferret's lifetime.

Taking blood from ferrets

Intravenous blood sampling for laboratory profiles of ferrets is essential but will require practice. The external blood vessels are more prominent in the non-anaesthetized ferret but sometimes sedation or anaesthesia is required for blood sampling. The three main sites for obtaining blood samples are the cephalic and jugular veins and the tail artery. *Note*: when emptying blood from a syringe, Susan Brown advises never to push the blood back out through the needle, as there is a possibility of damaging blood cells.

Cephalic vein technique

This is the normal vein used in the dog and cat but may require use of a sedative in the ferret. With patience, the ferret can be held as you would a cat, with a hand around the ferret's neck, not 'scruffing', with the ferret prone on the table and the nurse holding out the forelimb. Ferrets will wriggle but usually settle down. Wrapping the ferret in a small towel with the foreleg

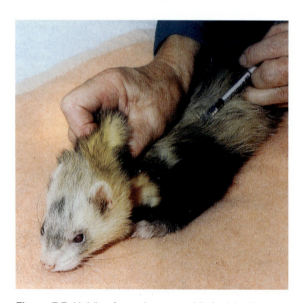

Figure 7.7 Holding ferret down on table for injection.

Taking blood from ferrets

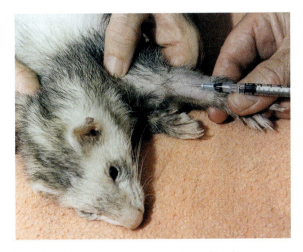

Figure 7.9 Taking blood from the cephalic vein. (Courtesy of John Tingay.)

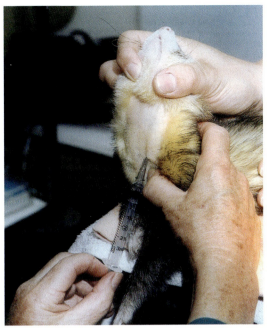

Figure 7.11 Taking blood from the jugular vein. (Courtesy of John Tingay.)

exposed may help. A treat of some kind in front of the ferret might help to distract it. If the ferret is too anxious, use of gas sedation (isoflurane) or ketamine i.m. will aid blood taking. A tourniquet using a miniature alligator clip with a small elastic band is useful. The ferret is held firmly. I prefer to clip the hair. Using a tuberculin syringe with 25 gauge or less needle, it is introduced into the vein and as the blood passes into the syringe the nurse should gently let go of the leg otherwise in short-legged ferrets there might not be enough blood collected. You should get 1 mL for a PVC or blood glucose analysis. It might be quicker to use the 25 gauge needle alone and put on a microtube immediately to collect the blood. In-house analysis is most useful (Fig. 7.9).

For chemotherapy of neoplasia cases, care must be taken in avoiding contamination of the area or person, with dangerous drugs (Fig. 7.10).

Jugular vein technique

This vein is useful as a source of larger amounts of blood, especially for blood transfusion (Fig. 7.11). Using a similar hold to the previous vein, the nurse has to keep a hand around the neck and hold the chin and head up in an extended position with the animal near the end of the table. Thus, the veterinarian can apply pressure at the site of the jugular vein arising from the chest and palpate the vein in the neck in its lateral position. With a thick-necked hob ferret, this can be difficult and the neck should be clipped beforehand It may be advisable to sedate or anaesthetize the ferret but it is possible without. A 22-gauge needle is used and depending on the size of ferret, 15–20 mL can be taken from hobs and perhaps up to 10–12 mL from jills (S. Brown, pers. comm. 1998).

Marini and Fox[2] have described a technique for using the jugular vein by wrapping a conscious ferret in a towel with the ferret's legs secure. The ferret is distracted by Nutri-Cal paste and blood is taken from the jugular vein, which is occluded above and below the bleeding site by digital pressure.

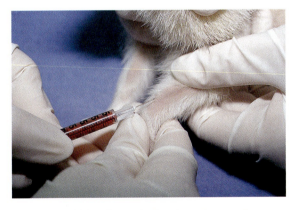

Figure 7.10 Using the cephalic vein under aseptic conditions to administer Doxorubicin chemotherapy for lymphoma (see Ch. 13). (Courtesy of Greg Rich.)

157

CHAPTER SEVEN

Ferret handling, hospitalization and diagnostic techniques

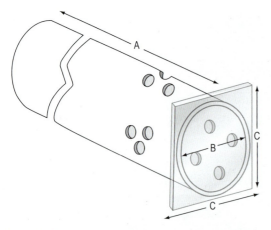

Figure 7.12 Curl restraint device (detail).

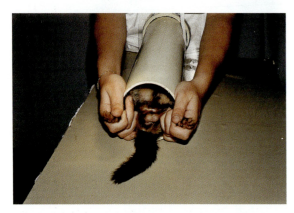

Figure 7.13 The Curl apparatus in use for restraint. *Note* how the nurse holds the ferret's hind legs, which cannot get out of tube.

Caudal artery technique

The technique of bleeding the caudal artery is one used in laboratory situations and requires the use of a Curl restraint device.[3] This is easily made from PVC tubing in two sizes with clear Plexiglas at one end and could be very handy for the practitioner. I made one and used it often (Figs 7.12, 7.13). I used the Curl restraint device for the work I did on cataracts in ferrets (Ch. 12). Figure 7.13 shows how the nurse holds it.

Procedure: The assisting nurse holds the restraint device with the Plexiglas end towards her on a firm surface The ferret is placed at the open end of the tube and usually readily enters (another rabbit warren…?). As the head and thorax are in the tube, the nurse quickly turns the tube over so that the ferret is on its back, holding the ferret by the back legs. The nurse's thumbs are placed on the medial surface of each thigh just below the stifle joint, encircling the thigh with the index finger and thumb and asserting a firm pressure. The ferret wriggles but cannot turn in the tube so there is no danger of nipping and it soon accepts restraint. The veterinarian holds the tail firmly on a firm surface and commences blood collection after first clipping the tail hair and warming the area with a warm soaked cotton ball. Using a 22–25 gauge needle attached to an empty 3 or 6 mL syringe, the needle is inserted into the caudal artery at about a 30° angle to the skin about 2–3 mm caudal to the anus. The needle is advanced until it hits the vertebra and then slowly withdrawn while applying suction pressure on the syringe. It is estimated that 1–3 mL or more blood can be collected by this method.

Note: blood can be taken using the cranial vena cava in a laboratory situation. This method has been adopted by some practitioners (M. Finkler, pers. comm. 2005).

The lateral saphenous vein can be used but restraint in conscious animals is more difficult. However, a quick and simple technique has been suggested for collecting a small volume of blood suitable particularly in insulinoma patients (Ch. 14) where glucose levels must be checked but the ferret not stressed.[4] A lidocaine/prilocaine-based topical anaesthetic cream, a 26 gauge needle, microhaematocrit tubes and a point of care blood glucose analyzer are required. The procedure is to restrain the ferret in lateral recumbency and shave a small area over the lateral saphenous vein. A 1–2 mm strip of lidocaine/prilocaine cream is applied to the area using a cotton bud. After 3–5 min, a 26 gauge needle is inserted into the vein. After a flash of blood appears in the hub of the needle, a microhaematocrit takes the blood to the point of care glucometer to determine the blood glucose concentration.

Note that the systemic absorption in ferrets of topical lidocaine and prilocaine is not known. The 1–2 mm strip used is less than 0.25 mg/kg each of both drugs. It is applied for maximum effect over the target area. This is particularly important in ferrets with known cardiac disease. Remember CNS signs of ataxia, nystagmus, depression and seizures plus nausea and depression are the signs of lidocaine toxicity. Try to avoid pet ferrets getting insulinoma so they will not require blood checking!

The use of intraosseous catheters is described by Lucas (Ch. 20). The use of bone marrow transplant using intraosseous technique has been described by Lennox[5] with a ferret with an undetermined failure of marrow erythropoiesis. Using an intraosseous tibial catheterization of a healthy donor ferret, 2 mL of marrow was extracted and placed in sodium citrate. The marrow was diluted into 5–6 mL of saline and using an intraosseous catheter was infused into the sick ferret. *Note*: epidural administration of morphine gave pain control for both ferrets. The marrow transplant was well received in this interesting case.

Note that further techniques useful for attending to ferrets are given in the ferret emergency chapter, Chapter 20.

The allergy question

There is no doubt that people can be allergic to ferrets as well as cats and dogs. A Japanese survey of 20 symptomatic patients with newly-diagnosed pet allergic asthma includes one with a ferret.[6] The lady had one ferret in-house over 3 years with no other pet. She had a suggestive history of ferret allergy, including bronchial, nasal and ocular symptoms, which improved after removal of the ferret. (*Note*: a specific igE antibody for ferrets and skin test allergen are not commercially available in Japan.) I have always considered the ferret hypoallergic. My wife and son suffered from asthma but we have maintained a collection of pet dogs, cats and ferrets over the years. My ferrets seem to have had a calming not asthma-stimulating influence. Of course, I blame the cat!

Ferret medication considerations

Other than the rabies vaccine and canine distemper vaccine in the USA, there are no medications specifically registered for ferrets. This is an amazing fact, especially in America, where thousands of ferrets are used in biomedical research. Studies on the effects of drugs useful for ferret medicine have been sparse. The few studies that have been conducted have been associated with anaesthetics and analgesics used for ferrets.[7] I have used medicines on ferrets as a straight adaptation from dog or cat use and have presumably been lucky in the drugs; I have not encountered toxicity problems but I do worry about the long-term use of drugs not specified for ferrets.

One particular example of a useful drug is Fipronil (Frontline, Rhone Merieux), which was used in desperation after trying to deal with fleas on a colony of ferrets.[8] However, it has been recorded that this drug is not safe for treating rabbits (Webster, Merial Co., pers. comm. 1999).

Some veterinarians are concerned that vets should make a decision on the use of any drug on ferrets only after consultation with the owner (S. Brown, pers. comm. 1998). There is no doubt that legal concerns may be increasingly in mind for the future regarding the use of current and new drugs on ferrets.

Dog and cat medications are on a body weight basis. For ferrets, being less than 2 kg, a step down calculation from cat values is required but even then the toxicity factor or species reaction can be at the back of one's mind. Ferrets are best given medications by injection, liquid syrups or paste. Use of tablet formulations requires them to be put in solution or suspension and they usually have a bitter taste. I give medications with a pre- and post-dosing of the ferret with a sugar-water solution. It is the only time they get anything too sweet. Oils can be used instead of sugar for drug administration because fat is better for ferrets than sugar and is more easily metabolized. For liquid drugs, the veterinarian needs a stock of insulin or tuberculin syringes for accurate small dosages. A general Ferret Drug Formulary appears in the Appendices.

The ferret expert's hospital

The word 'exotics' still hovers over ferret health. Treatment of pet ferrets, especially in North America, has improved by leaps and bounds. Many USA animal hospitals are all 'exotics' and do not see dogs or cats.

The notes below are given for those vets who may not have had contact with ferret patients and might just be beginning to see a few of the 'critters'. Experienced 'ferret' vets here pass on some valuable information.

Instrumentation and environment

Ideas here are focused on the ferret 'critter' with the help of Susan Brown's and Richard Nye's Midwest Bird and Exotic Animal Hospital, Westchester, Illinois, USA, which I visited in 2002.

Necessary requirements for dealing with such small animals can be listed. It has been said that ferrets should be weighed as routine, so have kitchen scales marked in grams/ounces with basket. Spring scales with a bag are also useful for adults plus a small balance with gram weights for baby ferrets. A small dab of Nutrigel or equivalent on the scales basket will distract a ferret for the time needed to take a reading. Personally, I think that an examination table covered with a clean towel is less threatening to the ferret than a shiny surface.

Basics, which can be added to (with critters in mind!):

Examination room

- Clean towels for handling ferrets. Nail trimmers. Paediatric stethoscope. Styptic powder packed in

CHAPTER SEVEN
Ferret handling, hospitalization and diagnostic techniques

- TB syringe for easy application to nails. Magnifying lens. Mouth speculum
- Auriscope with narrowest examination tube. U/V light
- Curl device for restraining ferrets for blood or genital examination (Fig. 7.12)
- *Plastic* rectal thermometer.

Treatment use

- Catheter tip syringes (35 mL and 60 mL) and curved syringes (≈15 mL) for feeding
- Syringes for injection: 50 unit insulin syringes. 1 mL TB syringes with 25 gauge $^5/_8$ inch needles and 26 gauge $^3/_8$ inch needles
- Syringes for fluid therapy: 35 mL and 60 mL
- Catheters for i.v. 22–25 gauge. The 24–25 gauge catheter is easier to place in the cephalic vein but can use 22 gauge
- For i.o. – 1.5 inch and 2.5 inch 20 gauge and 22 gauge spinal needles
- For urinary: open-end tomcat 20 gauge venocath sleeve; 3 French red rubber tube
- Nasogastric tube 3 French for ferret (Lucas shows placement of tube in Ch. 20)
- i.v. drip sets, paediatric or microdrip (I used ordinary plastic drip sets. Normal gravity sets are *not* recommended)
- Syringe pump: useful for giving small measured amounts of fluid (Razel)
- Sterile empty diluent bottles: used for storing frozen antibiotic formulations and other medicines and for dispensing medicines
- Small incubator
- Nebulizer
- Drugs: a medical list from ferret formularies and texts is required. Arrange for charts showing drug dose relating to body weight. Remember very few drugs are actually approved for ferret use (see Drug Appendix)
- Elizabethan collars 5 or 10 cm
- Heating pads for recovery
- Bleeding ferrets: Use $^3/_4$ to $^3/_8$ inch needles. A $^1/_2$ inch needle is useful for jugular veins in large ferrets. For drawing blood from peripheral veins use no larger than 25 gauge or sometimes 26 gauge. A 22 gauge is useful for jugular bleeding for large volumes of blood for transfusion.

Hospital boarding

- Steel cat cages are adaptable for ferrets as long as the frontage has small diameter wire
- Fibreglass and plastic type cages with clear plastic front doors are useful
- 'Scats' tray and bedding and water source essential for temporarily confined ferret
- Food supply for hospital should be fresh meaty bones (avoid insulinoma)
- Light source should be switched off unless really needed (avoid ferret adrenal disease complex)
- No cooling fans should be directed directly on the ferrets (avoid chills and influenza)
- Temperature control of hospital boarding area should be stable.

Laboratory essentials

- In-house: CBCs, chemical panels, faecal assessment, cytology, Gram stains, urine analysis
- Outside lab: bacterial and fungal cultures, serology for *Cryptococcus* and *Giardia*, etc.
- Hormone assay relating to ferret adrenal disease complex (FADC)
- Cytology and histopathology
- Microtainers with EDTA for CBCs, lithium heparin plasma, separators for chemistries, separators for serology tests
- Haemoccult system. This enables evaluation of occult blood in normal ferrets and ferrets with suspected bleeding[5]
- Mini-tip culturettes and Calgiswabs. Digital scales.

Surgery

- Gas machine delivering halothane, isoflurane, sevoflurane as preferred
- Small face masks, clear plastic is best

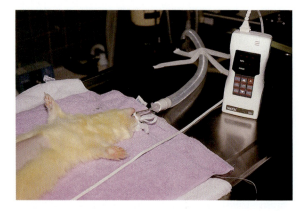

Figure 7.14 Bains pulse oximeter. (Courtesy of Mark Finkler.)

- Endotracheal tubes 2.5–3 mm (non-cuffed)
- Pulse monitor. Ultrasonic Doppler flow detector
- Bains pulse oximeter as seen in Fig. 7.14
- Dental equipment for small animals (see Ch. 21 for dental pathology)
- Ultrasonic scaler e.g. IM3 42-12 (Australia)
- Electrosurgery unit, e.g. Ellman Surgitron, electrodes and bipolar forceps
- Magnifying lens-SurgiTel lupes
- Waterheater blanket (e.g. Thermocare). Safe and warm reusable heat pad
- Masking tape for taping ferret to table. I found Perspex support useful for common operations.

On table surgical materials

- Drapes-VSP surgical drapes 24″ × 24″ clear
- Surgical materials – Size 4-0, 5-0, and 6-0 7-0 PDS, Maxon and nylon. Vicryl
- Haemoclips, small and medium. Disposable skin stapler
- The Satinsky vena cava clamp as used by Avery Bennett (Ch. 18)
- Retractors – Mini-Balfour retractors, Alm retractors, Heiss retractors, elastic retractor system. Eyelid retractors.

Diagnostics

- Radiology equipment should have rare earth screen system and high detail film. (Orthochromic, Dupont)

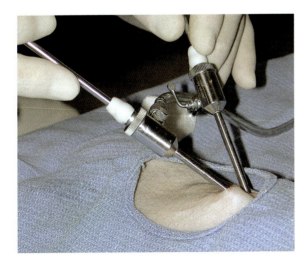

Figure 7.15 Laparoscopy setup. In a multiple puncture technique, note that entry points must be far enough apart for triangulation. (Courtesy of Mike Murray.)

Other choices include mammography film, dental film and non-screen film (Ch. 16)
- Electrocardiography (Ch. 11)
- Echocardiography (Ch. 17)
- Laparoscopy can be carried out on ferrets as a diagnostic tool using mostly equipment used for avians and is described in detail by Murray.[9] Unlike the avian patient, the ferret requires the creation of a pneumoperitoneum (with room air or ideally medical grade CO_2).

Basic laparoscopy equipment

- Single puncture technique: telescope, light cable, light source, 'Insufflator', videocamera, videomonitor, Taylor-sheath/trocar
- Multiple puncture technique: trocar-cannula(s), Veress needle.

Additional hand instruments required

- Palpation probe, clamshell biopsy forceps, punch biopsy forceps, grasping forceps, tru-cut biopsy needle
- The ferret needs to be anaesthetized, intubated and on a ventilator. *Note* that insufflation will have an effect on cardiopulmonary function. A specific 'entry point' must be realized for the organ to be investigated bearing in mind the small nature of the ferret
- Right lateral approach for: liver, gall bladder, pancreas, duodenum, right kidney, right adrenal gland and urinary bladder/prostate
- Ventral midline approach for: liver, gall bladder, pancreas, intestine, spleen, urinary bladder/prostate
- Left lateral approach for: liver, spleen, left kidney, left adrenal gland, urinary bladder/prostate
- The multiple puncture approach has the advantage over the single puncture approach in that an increased range of tissue handling is possible (Fig. 7.15).

For the single puncture technique, the Taylor sheath with its two side ports and single instrument port has the gas source attached to one of the side ports to give insufflation. A 5–10 mm skin incision allows for the Taylor sheath and associated trocar to enter through the body wall after careful blunt and sharp dissection. Once inside the body cavity, insufflation is carried out after the trocar is removed. *Note*: the contralateral side port may be either closed or used to control the intra-abdominal pressure with the aid of a finger pad over the outflow. The instrument port should be kept closed or

CHAPTER SEVEN
Ferret handling, hospitalization and diagnostic techniques

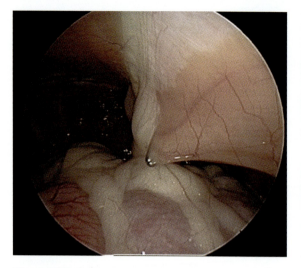

Figure 7.16 A fine mosquito forceps is used to bluntly dissect through the lateral abdominal wall. (Courtesy of Mike Murray.)

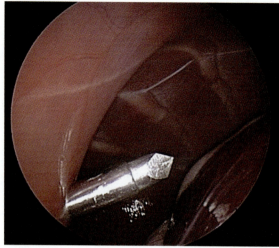

Figure 7.18 Shown is an entry utilizing a traditional trocar/cannula. The sharp point easily punctures abdominal structures. (Courtesy of Mike Murray.)

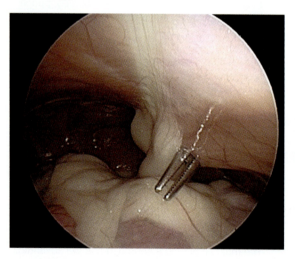

Figure 7.17 Entry of forceps into abdominal cavity produces the defect through which the trocar will be inserted. (Courtesy of Mike Murray.)

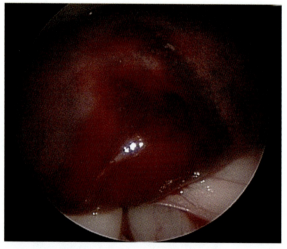

Figure 7.19 In this iatrogenic puncture of the spleen the haemorrhage was self-limiting. (Courtesy of Mike Murray.)

covered by a rubber-sealing bonnet; tissue biopsy can then be taken.

For the multiple puncture technique, with the body cavity distended, the secondary and tertiary ports can be carefully placed.

Entry into the abdomen is indicated by the following views of laparoscopy (Figs 7.16–7.18).

Note: it is important to visualize the secondary equipment as it enters the peritoneal cavity, with no instruments being inserted unless the trocar is visible through the endoscope.

Additional instrument use: Blunt probe, (enhanced visualization) biopsy forceps, (single biopsies) clam-shell forceps, (multiple biopsies), punch-type forceps (for pancreas). Tru-cut biopsy needles (for renal biopsies).

Once the examination is finished, the intra-abdominal pressure is released, the abdominal wall and skin are closed and the ferret allowed to recover. The scope of laparoscopy images can be seen in Figures 7.19–7.30.

Specialized equipment from dog and cat medicine and surgery is serving the pet ferret population.

The ferret expert's hospital

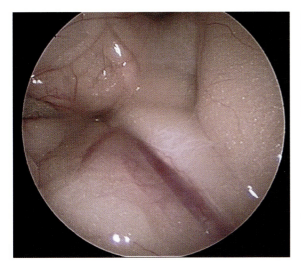

Figure 7.20 Most ferrets are well endowed with abdominal fat, which tends to obscure vision and foul the lens tip. (Courtesy of Mike Murray.)

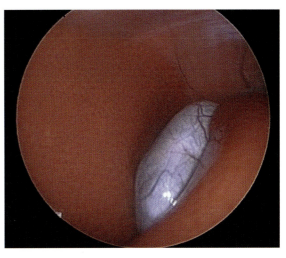

Figure 7.22 The gall bladder is situated between two liver lobes. *Note* the diaphragm in the background. (Courtesy of Mike Murray.)

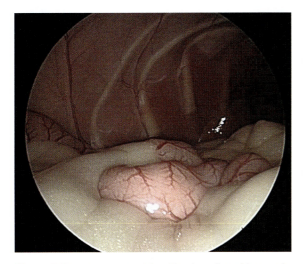

Figure 7.21 Shown is the lateral body wall and loops of small intestine. (Courtesy of Mike Murray.)

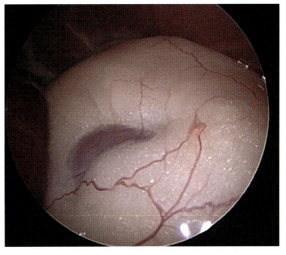

Figure 7.23 The left kidney is embedded in a retroperitoneal fat pad. *Note* the small, accessory adrenal tissue caudolateral to the kidney. (Courtesy of Mike Murray.)

CHAPTER SEVEN
Ferret handling, hospitalization and diagnostic techniques

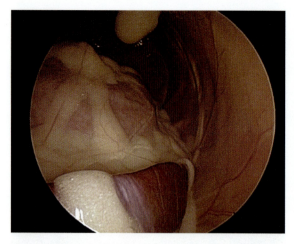

Figure 7.24 A view of the stomach and spleen covered by omentum is seen from the ventral approach. (Courtesy of Mike Murray.)

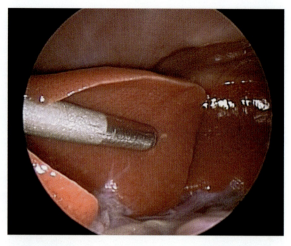

Figure 7.26 A palpation probe is used to reflect the quadrate lobe of the liver. Divisions on the probe are equal to 1 cm. (Courtesy of Mike Murray.)

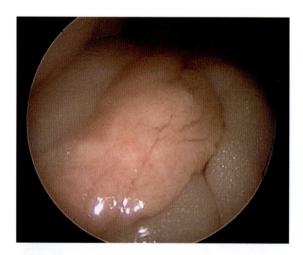

Figure 7.25 This pancreas is grossly normal. (Courtesy of Mike Murray.)

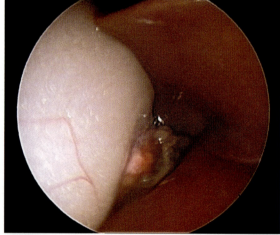

Figure 7.27 Shown is an enlarged right adrenal gland. (Courtesy of Mike Murray.)

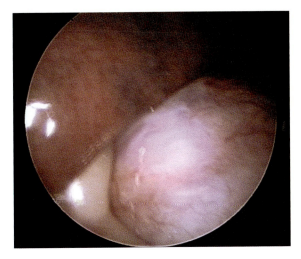

Figure 7.28 A lymphoma was seen in the left kidney. (Courtesy of Mike Murray.)

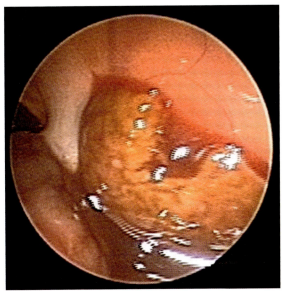

Figure 7.30 A biopsy of the liver seen in Figure 7.29 illustrates a 5 mm clamshell biopsy specimen. The degree of haemorrhage noted here is typical. (Courtesy of Mike Murray.)

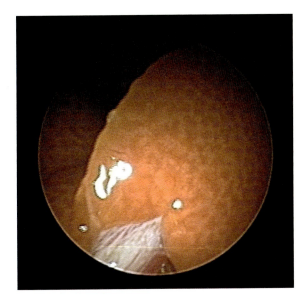

Figure 7.29 Bacterial hepatitis is evident. (Courtesy of Mike Murray.)

References

1. Williams BH. Splenic rupture following palpation in a ferret. Exotic DVM 2001; 3:7–8.
2. Marini RP, Fox JG. Anaesthesia, surgery and biomethodology. In: Fox JG, ed. Biology and diseases of the ferret, 2nd edn. Baltimore: Williams & Wilkins; 1998.
3. Curl JL, Curl JS. Restraint device for serial blood sampling of ferrets. Lab Anim Sci 1985; 35:296–297.
4. Riggs MS, Heatley J, Nevarez J, Mitchell MA. Ferret blood collection: A quick and simple technique. Exotic DVM 2004; 4:6–7.
5. Lennox AM. Working up mystery anemia in ferrets. Exotic DVM 2004; 6:22–26.
6. Shirai T, Matsui T, Suzuki K, Chida K. Effect of pet removal on pet allergic asthma. Chest 2005; 127:1565–1571.
7. Smith DA, Burgmann PM. Drug formulary. In: Hillyer EV, Quesenberry KE, eds. Ferrets, rabbits and rodent. Clinical medicine and surgery Philadelphia: WB Saunders; 1997:392–395.
8. Lewington JH. Frontline for ferrets. Control and therapy series. University of Sydney: Postgraduate Foundation; 1996:189:856.
9. Murray, M. Laparoscopy in the domestic ferret. Exotic DVM 2002; 4:65–69.

Part Two

Medicine

CHAPTERS

8	Viral, bacterial and mycotic diseases	169
9	Ferret gastrointestinal and hepatic diseases by Mark E. Burgess	203
10	Parasitic diseases of ferrets	224
11	Diseases of special concern	258
12	Diseases of the ferret ear, eye and nose	289
13	General neoplasia	318
14	Endocrine diseases	346
15	Managing ferret toxicoses by Jill Richardson	380

CHAPTER 8

Viral, bacterial and mycotic diseases

'Ferrets are susceptible to canine distemper and should be vaccinated yearly against this disease. This is very important because canine distemper is always fatal to ferrets.'

Wendy Winsted, Ferrets, 1981

An overview

Anyone concerned with ferret health will quickly realize that the ferret seems to stand between the dog and cat as regards disease problems, being the third companion animal. Considering viral conditions, ferrets get rabies like other carnivores. They can get canine distemper and many people working ferrets believed they also got feline influenza, in fact ferrets actually get human influenza. All viral infectious diseases in early twentieth century ferret books came under the title of 'the sweats'. With my first ferret, Fred, I gave him both canine distemper and feline enteritis vaccines a week apart to be sure! He showed no ill-effects on using $\frac{1}{6}$ dog/cat dosage.

Added to all other woes, the ferret has been used extensively in biomedical research as a considered good 'model' for the passage of viral and bacterial diseases, besides being used for a variety of experiments on various subjects. Ferrets have been used for the detection of various avian type influenza viruses such as H5N1.[1] Human isolates were fatal to intranasally-inoculated ferrets. Experimentally, ferrets have been found to be susceptible to pseudorabies, poliomyelitis, Newcastle disease, encephalomyelitis and sclerosis.[2]

The Australian 1999 Newcastle disease outbreak in poultry, for instance, was said to be a mutation of the non-virulent Newcastle strain and not an imported virus (Commonwealth Agriculture Department, May statement). With the possible genetic changes of viruses over time and between species, the possibility of new disease patterns arising cannot be discounted. Human influenza was considered in a 1989 review of zoonotic diseases related to ferrets, as being the only disease for which there was a case report concerning transmission from ferret to man. Rabies is still a contentious subject regarding ferrets in the USA even though there has been no infection of man due to ferret bites.[3] Rabies has not been recorded naturally in ferrets in the USA, UK, Europe, Japan, Australia or New Zealand.

There was some concern from American authorities on the rabbit calicivirus possibly mutating between species but, as yet, there has been no proof of the disease being in any other wildlife, or dogs, cats, or ferrets. The horror of human Creutzfeldt–Jacob disease is well known. The possibility of the disease complexes known as transmissible spongiform encephalopathy (TSE) affecting ferrets, from contaminated meat products, is debatable. TSE disease has been seen in farmed mink in the UK.[4]

In Australia, the Hendra virus (HENV) (family Paramyxoviridae, genus Henipavirus) killed horses and two men in 1994. A similar virus, the Nipah virus (NIPV) (genus Henipavirus) was found in pigs in Malaysia in 1999, originally suspected to be Japanese encephalitis (JE), which is spread by mosquitoes.[5] *Note*: ferrets get heartworm disease from mosquitoes (Ch. 10). NIPV was suspected of killing more than 100 people; the symptoms were high fever, aches, eventually coma and death. NIPV, related to but distinct from HENV, is a 'new' megamyxovirus, a genus of the paramyxovirus family. HENV only transmits easily between flying foxes (fruit bats *Pteropus* species) which are the natural hosts to HENV, NIPV and Australian Bat Lyssavirus (ABL).[6] It is

CHAPTER EIGHT
Viral, bacterial and mycotic diseases

considered that a fruit bat first infected pigs with NIPV; however, NIPV seems to be able to transmit easily between pigs and also between pigs and other animals including humans, horses, dogs, goats, and bats.[5]

The position of the ferret in the scheme of things regarding virus infection is still of concern. The 2003 SARS disease complex involving the active coronavirus (an RNA virus)[7] has killed over 700 people in Asia and

Table 8.1 Main infections and parasites in wildlife of European concern regarding veterinary public health

Type	Name	Host	Species frequently mentioned
Virus	African swine fever	Porcine	Wild boar
Virus	Aujeszky disease	Porcine/carnivore	Wild boar/fox
Virus	Avian influenza	Birds	Birds (wild boar?)
Virus	Avian pox	Poultry	Birds
Virus	Classic swine fever	Porcine	Wild boar
Virus	Foot and mouth disease	Ruminants and porcine	Cervid, wild boar
Virus	Hantavirus	Human	Field mice and voles
Virus	Myxomatosis	Rabbit	Wild rabbit
Virus	Newcastle disease	Poultry	Birds
Virus	Rabbit viral haem. disease	Rabbit	Wild rabbit
Virus	Rabies	Mammals	Fox and bats
Bacteria	Anthrax	Mammals	Ungulates
Bacteria	Avian botulism	Ornamental birds	Waterfowl
Bacteria	Avian cholera	Poultry	Birds
Bacteria	Avian tuberculosis	Poultry	Birds
Bacteria	Bovine brucellosis	Bovine	Ungulate
Bacteria	Bovine tuberculosis	Bovine, caprine, human	Cervid, wild boar, badger, carnivore
Bacteria	Leptospirosis	Mammals	Commensal rodents
Bacteria	Listeriosis	Humans	Mammals
Bacteria	Lyme disease	Human	Mammals
Bacteria	Paratuberculosis	Ruminants	Ungulates
Bacteria	Pasteurellosis	Porcine	Mammals
Bacteria	Salmonellosis	Most	Vertebrate
Bacteria	Sheep /goat brucellosis	Ovine and caprine	Ungulate
Bacteria	Swine brucellosis	Porcine	Wild boar, hare
Bacteria	Tularaemia	Hare	Mammals
Rickettsia	Q fever	Ruminants	Terrestrial vertebrate
Protozoa	Leishmaniasis	Human, dog	Wild carnivores?
Protozoa	Toxoplasmosis	Human, cat	Mammals
Cestode	Echinococcosis/ hydatidosis	Human, ovine	Wolf, fox, rodents
Nematode	Trichinellosis	Porcine	Wild boar, fox
Acaria	Mange	Ruminant, equid	Mountain ungulates, fox
Trans enc.	Bovine spond. enc.	Bovine	Zoo animals
Encephalopathy	Encephalopathy	Bovine	Zoo animals

Trans enc., transmissible encephalopathy; Bovine spond. enc., bovine spongiform encephalopathy.
Adapted from Table 1 in Artois et al 2001.[8]

North America and has been traced to cats, raccoons and badgers which are sold in Chinese markets It is thought that the masked palm civet (genetically related to ferrets and cats) transmitted SARS to humans. The SARS coronavirus (SCV) has been shown to infect cats and ferrets and consequently these animals are possible 'models' to test antiviral drugs or vaccine candidates against the disease. The coronavirus can spread fairly well between humans and needs no vector. In a world where air travel is easy it is possible to visualize human to ferret transmission, to pet ferrets, remembering the incubation period in humans can be 2–10 days. In addition, the virus is able to survive outside the body in respiratory secretions or faeces. It is not susceptible to some common household detergents.

Note the ability of the coronavirus to be generally pathogenic in many species is considered to be a result of its RNA make-up. DNA viruses can be accurate reproductions of their own kind, but RNA viruses have errors in replicating (mutation trends) so that the mutation changes are a type of survival mechanism for the virus in adverse conditions, i.e. change from one body to another, animal to man, man to man.[7] The SARS coronavirus in this way shows an ancient similarity to the avian and bovine coronaviruses. Zoonotic virus distributing between the reservoir host (Hr) and the secondary host (Hs), which could in the future be the ferret, has been discussed by Childs.[6]

The control of infectious diseases in Europe and indeed worldwide, in wildlife relates directly or indirectly to those diseases getting to the mustelids, polecats, feral ferrets or even domesticated ferrets.[8] The point is made in Europe that with rabies the dog reservoir is replaced by the red fox (*Vulpes vulpes*) and the bovine form of tuberculosis has been picked up by the Eurasian badger (*Meles meles*). A table of infectious diseases in general

Table 8.2 Comparative viral and bacterial disease susceptibility of the three major carnivores kept as pets; and humans

Disease	Mustelidae	Canidae	Felidae	Humans
Rabies	+	+	+	+
Human influenza	+ fr	–	–	+
Canine distemper	+	+	–	–
Canine hepatitis	–	+	–	–
Canine parvovirus	–	+	–	–
Canine parainfluenza	–	+	–	–
Feline distemper (enteritis)	+ frn	–	+	–
Feline rhinotracheitis	–	–	+	–
Mink viral enteritis	+ frn	–	–	–
Aleutian (parvovirus) disease	+ fmp	–	–	–
Feline chlamydia disease	–	–	+	–
Bordetella bronchiseptica	+	+	–	–
Botulism	+	–	–	+
Leptospirosis	+	+	–	+
Tuberculosis	+	+	+	+

Key to comparative disease susceptibility table:
Mustelidae Domestic ferrets plus mink, otters, badgers, stoats, weasels, etc.
Canidae Domestic dogs plus foxes, dingoes, etc.
Felidae Domestic cats plus tigers, leopards, etc
Human The reader
+ Affects family in question
– Does not affect family in question
fr Indicates that only ferrets get human influenza in the Mustelidae
frn Indicates that only ferrets do *not* get feline enteritis or mink viral enteritis in the Mustelidae (it was thought that feline panleukopenia could replicate when *injected* into a ferret but no clinical signs developed) (Finkler, pers. comm. 2005)
fmp Indicates that both ferrets and mink get Aleutian disease in the Mustelidae

After Dinnes.[45]

CHAPTER EIGHT

Viral, bacterial and mycotic diseases

(Table 8.1) and their hosts is interesting to consider with the fate of the mustelids wild or domestic, in mind. The extent of viral and bacterial infections alone can stimulate thoughts of possible infection of ferrets. In the virus field, the adaptability of any virus to leave its primary host and mutate to invade another species may arise. This may thus threaten all mustelids in the future.

A comparison of disease susceptibility between ferrets, dogs, cats and man is shown in Table 8.2.

Ferret viral diseases

Virus structure is dependant on RNA strands. The taxonomy becomes hard to keep up with as viruses, etc. are broken into groups of nucleic acid 'variations' pathogenic or otherwise. Table 8.3 illustrates the present viruses that could possibly affect ferrets. (Coronaviruses and rotaviruses are discussed further in Chapter 9.)

Rabies

The rabies virus occurs worldwide, with the exception still of Australia, New Zealand, UK, Hawaii, Japan and parts of Scandinavia. These countries do not routinely vaccinate against rabies. Rabies occurs in wild foxes in Europe. A WHO survey, 1977–1998, recorded 464 cases of rabies in wild polecats across Europe. During the rabies surveillance, 48 of the 464 total polecats were said to be rabid ferrets (W. Mueller, WHO/OIE Reference Center for Rabies, Tübingen, Germany, pers. comm. 1998). Dr Mueller was of the opinion however, that the determination of species, whether polecat or ferret, was not always correct. Identification was done by veterinarians not biologists! Ferrets running wild and easily interbreeding with polecats could make identification difficult and it is fairly sure that the 48 rabid ferrets reported were in fact rabid polecats. In a 1998–2004 survey concerning pine marten and other mustelids, Latvia, Lithuania, Poland and Ukraine registered higher number of rabies cases with higher incidence in the targeted pine marten (*Martes martes*). The total rabies cases incidence peaked in 2002 for pine martens and in 2003 for other mustelids (W. Mueller, pers. comm. 2005).

Regarding quarantine, ferrets are not yet allowed to be imported into Australia. In the opinion of the WHO authorities, rabies vaccination for ferrets is not likely to be compulsory in the UK. This might be a safe bet for pet ferrets but it might be different for working ferrets. Rabies is of concern in the USA, where it has been given as the main reason for banning ferrets as pets in California (Ferrets Anonymous, California, pers. comm. 1996). It has been noted experimentally, that ferrets fed rabies-infected mice did not become infected and no serum antibodies were found in the ferret serum, which indicates the bite as the main means of transmission.[3] The mice probably did not get a chance to bite the ferrets!

A Finnish veterinarian in 2004 showed concern that the EU had removed Russia from the list of high-risk countries.[9] Thus Russian owners of dogs, cats and ferrets need not show blood test results. Russians love their pet ferrets and hopefully desire to vaccinate them against rabies. The EU decision was considered political, not scientific and is a worry to Finland. The Baltic States have a problem with sylvatic rabies so the world's guard against rabies cannot be dropped with the advent of more open borders and fast travel. Australia is lucky being an island continent but in respect to rabies the northern islands of Indonesia and New Guinea could be a worry if a dog incubating rabies reached our shores from a fishing boat, etc.

Rabies symptoms: It has been shown experimentally that an incubation period of 28–33 days is possible with death in 4–5 days.[10] The animal shows anxiety and

Table 8.3 Nucleic acid differences of common viruses that may affect ferrets

Viruses	Family	Nucleic acid	Envelope	Size (nm)
Rabies	*Rhabdoviridae*	ssRNA	Yes	70–88 × 130–380
Distemper (CD)	*Paramyxoviridae*	ssRNA	Yes	150–300
Parvovirus (AD)	*Parvoviridae*	ssDNA	No	18–26
Influenza (HI)	*Orthomyxoviridae*	ssRNA	Yes	90–120
Coronavirus (ECE)	*Coronaviridae*	ssRNA	Yes	60–220
Rotavirus	*Reoviridae*	dsRNA	No	80–130
Infectious bovine rhinotracheitis	*Herpesviridae*	dsDNA	Yes	46–48

CD, canine distemper; AD, Aleutian disease; HI, human influenza; ECE, epizootic catarrhal enteritis (Ch. 9); ds, double stranded; ss, single stranded.
After Langlois.[16]

lethargy with possible posterior paralysis.[11] With definite suspicion of infection, e.g. a non-vaccinated ferret and possible exposure to a rabid animal, it must be euthanized and its brain tissue subjected to fluorescent antibody test. The worrying fact to North American pet ferret owners is that if their ferret strayed and was picked up by the local authorities, the ferret, even though vaccinated, might be euthanized directly. A Canadian report study recommended a suspect ferret from a bite situation be kept under observation for 10 days.[12] There is no treatment for rabies bites in animals, though a human survived after being bitten by a rabid bat and given a combination of drugs and an induced coma.[13]

Research on an inactivated rabies vaccine specific for ferrets was carried out.[14] The potential of an immunoperoxidase technique for the diagnosis of general rabies in fresh tissues was found superior to other standard methods e.g. fluorescent antibody test.[15]

The major rabies vaccine for ferrets for the past few years has been IMRAB 3 (Merial) in the USA and Canada. The initial rabies vaccination is a single shot (1 mL) given at 12 weeks of age. The usual yearly boosters apply (Brown, pers. comm. 1999). The vaccine Imrab 3TF (Merial) is used in the USA /Canada, while the latter country also uses Prorab (Intervet Canada).[16]

Rabies vaccination is not carried out in Australia except by the special request of people working in rabies-affected countries like Indonesia. Regarding Australia and New Zealand, rabies would be of extreme concern if introduced and would require a complete re-thinking of our vaccination requirements.

Vaccination site reactions

A technique of giving a vaccination in the ferret neck, between the shoulder blades, was described in the USA, which is higher than I gave injections in dogs, cats or ferrets. It has been known since 1991 that, 3 months to 3 years after FeV or rabies vaccination, cats can get a site tumour, which may be a fibrosarcoma, a malignant fibrous histiocytoma or some sort of mesenchymal tumour. Murray in 1998 demonstrated concern about a ferret vaccine sarcoma in a letter to the AVMA.[17] The damage could be a combination of mechanical trauma and/or reaction to the vaccine material injected. In a 2000 study with dogs and cats, the outcome was a proposal of triennial vaccination at least for cats.[18]

A 2002 assessment of response to commercial vaccines showed that cats differed from mink and ferrets.[19] A total of 24 1-year-old ferrets, 20 4-month-old mink and 20 4-month-old cats were vaccinated with three rabies virus vaccines, two leukaemia virus vaccines, alum adjuvant and saline to see what the local response would be on marked spots of the shaved dorsum area. Injections were given under anaesthesia. Histological findings showed significant differences in the tissue response to the vaccinations between the three species with the cat showing more lymphocytic response to the three rabies vaccines. Production of collagen, fibroblasts and macrophages differed among the three killed aluminium-adjuvant vaccines in the cats but not in the ferrets or mink. In response to the two adjuvanted leukaemia virus vaccines, mink and ferrets produced more binucleate cells. It was considered the response differences in cats were because cats were more likely to get vaccine-associated sarcomas (VAS).

In a retrospective 2003 survey however, ten ferrets were checked and seven were found to have fibrosarcoma development in the areas usually used for vaccination, being the intrascapular aspect of the neck and dorsal aspect of the thorax.[20] Four sample ferrets had been vaccinated with rabies/distemper combinations, two just with rabies, while four had no record of vaccination. The remaining three ferrets each had neoplasia but on the base of the tail, the ventral abdomen and the carpus. The ferret with the ventral abdominal tumour was one vaccinated with rabies/distemper combination. Of the seven, six had definite records of vaccination so the neoplasia were considered to be vaccination site fibrosarcoma or VSF. The tumours were nodular and 10–15 mm wide in the subcutis. The ferrets with VSFs were aged 1–9 years. Follow-up on three ferrets' post-surgical removal of the VSFs showed one tumour recurred after 3 months while the other two ferrets were clear at 8 and 12 months post-operation. The authors of the survey considered the results positive for VSFs in another species besides the cat. There is as yet no proof of a retrovirus involvement in VSFs in the cat or ferret. The location of these tumours at vaccination sites in ferrets suggests that vaccine material may predispose them to reactions.

Lyssavirus of bats in Australia

A human case of Australian Bat Lyssavirus (ABL) (family Rhabdoviridae, genus Lyssavirus) infection has occurred in a person in contact with bats.[21] Tests on dogs and cats that have been inoculated with the rabies-related virus, show that they are susceptible to it, but an epidemic would be unlikely. No work has been done on ferrets. It is considered that domestic animals would be 'dead-end hosts' so there is minimum danger to humans from that source. However, the symptoms of ABL and rabies would be the same. The finding of ABL in two flying foxes[22] in Western Australia illustrates the spread of the disease across the continent. Pet ferrets would only be at risk in the rare chance of them finding an infected carcass.

CHAPTER EIGHT
Viral, bacterial and mycotic diseases

Human influenza (HI)

The ferret is highly susceptible to human influenza and has been important as an experimental model in influenza research since 1935.[3] Ferrets were used to test a potent new Australian-designed drug, GS4104 (Relenza), which has been found to protect them against some of the most dangerous strains, giving hope for similar effects in man.[23] With close contact between people and ferrets, especially in apartment dwellings with closed confined air-conditioning in the USA and other ferret-loving countries, the risk of mutual infection between humans and ferrets has increased, as inhalation is the main means of transmission of 'flu viruses.[3] Ferrets are very susceptible to influenza virus type A.[24] This causes respiratory disease in man, animals and poultry. Influenza with its collection of virulent viruses has been the basis of the fear of a global epidemic.[25]

Clinical signs: Typically, after 48 hours incubation, the ferret has a temperature of 40°C with a moist nose and inappetence. Sneezing occurs and the temperature fluctuates on alternate days as it does with humans. If the ferret continues eating consistently or intermittently, it is a good sign but if a purulent nasal discharge occurs despite medication, the outlook is a possibly fatal pneumonia. That working ferrets can succumb to pneumonia if kept in cold draughty conditions was even pointed out by the writer Nicholas Everitt in 1897.

Treatment is by good nursing, keeping the ferrets in warm and draught-free accommodation, plus broad-spectrum antibiotics for secondary infections. The prognosis is good. Human decongestive room sprays, if available, are useful for ferrets. Interestingly, ferrets can recover within 5 days and will obtain immunity for at least 5 weeks against that particular flu strain.[26] As the nasal sinuses are a particularly vascular area, any permanent cellular damage by persistent infection may lead to a 'snuffles' condition, as described later in this chapter. The human influenza condition must be differentiated from canine distemper.

A neurological syndrome in laboratory ferrets has been recorded where the symptoms were weight loss, high fever, head tremors and ataxia, but recovery occurred with treatment. No infectious agent was isolated but two investigators had succumbed to human 'flu 2 weeks before the ferrets fell sick.[27] (Such neurological symptoms in ferrets living outside, can possibly arise from a meningeal cryptococcosis, see Ch. 12).

H5N1 virus and ferrets

In 1997, the virus H5N1 (a variant of influenza type A) as found in birds caused a human death in Hong Kong and human deaths have occurred since in Vietnam, Cambodia, Thailand and Indonesia.

The lethality of H5N1 has been tested on ferrets from isolates of the virus from humans and poultry.[1] The highly pathogenic H5N1 was found in poultry all over East Asia as from 2004. At the time of writing the H5N1 virus is apparently moving across Europe in migratory birds and infecting domestic poultry in eastern Europe. Vietnamese scientists considered bird flu could mutate to a more dangerous form.

The prevention of any H5N1 epidemic requires a vaccine. Antibodies against both the haemagglutinin (H) and neuraminidase (N), glycoproteins of the virus, are essential to protect against infection and spread, so that any vaccine must contain these proteins. In addition, isolating the H and N genes from a dangerous pandemic virus and altering them to make them user-friendly to humans could produce designer viruses. They can be mixed with another flu virus in the laboratory and used as a vaccine.[25] There is no doubt the ferret continues to play a part in viral experimental research.[28]

Vaccination of ferrets with the usual human influenza vaccine is not usually advised as the disease in ferrets is considered mild. There is wide antigenic variation in the human virus type and the actual immunity conferred is short-lived in ferrets.[29]

Note: swine influenza (SI) virus, another type of influenza virus, affects mice and ferrets and thus could be a problem for working ferrets in country areas near pig farms if an outbreak of SI occurred.[30]

Note: the family Paramyxoviridae includes mumps, Newcastle disease, parainfluenza 1, 2, 3 and 4 plus simian myxovirus SV5 and the morbilliviruses. The morbilliviruses include important pathogens like measles (MV), rinderpest (RPV) and canine distemper (CDV). All morbilliviruses are contagious by air contact.

Canine distemper (CDV)

This is 100% fatal to ferrets and has an incubation period of 7–14 days. Treatment is difficult. In Australia and other countries with ferrets as working animals, the risk comes from contact with foxes that sometimes have dens next to rabbit warrens. The foxes will not disturb the local rabbits but will use them later for training of the fox cubs (Bert Geodes, ferreter, Perth, WA, pers. comm. 1980). The native dingo in Australia is also a possible carrier of distemper. Unfortunately, outback dogs and cross-bred dingoes belonging to aboriginal peoples may not be vaccinated so that the distemper pool may be maintained. Household pet ferrets in Australia and overseas are less likely to contact distemper unless in contact with unvaccinated family dogs bringing in the disease. Thus, overall protection must be advised for dogs and ferrets.

In America, even with blanket vaccination of pet ferrets, a distemper outbreak occurred in a ferret shelter in Westchester country, New York and one case in Chicago, a month apart.[31] Basic education on distemper is still put out by the American Ferret Association. Incidentally, an outbreak of distemper in pet skunks (*Mephitis mephitis*) was recorded in Southern Florida with classic signs (C. MacCullough, pers. comm. 2005). The disease was also seen in Gainesville and Orlando and with cases in Iowa. There was concern that the infection was via pet shops.

Clinical signs: I have seen only one classic canine distemper in the ferret, but have been told of other cases around Australia. The ferret develops anorexia, vomiting, ocular and nasal discharges, which occur after the incubation period, followed by diarrhoea. A characteristic rash develops under the chin and in the inguinal region 10–12 days after exposure. The ocular/nasal discharges become increasingly purulent and as the disease progresses, the foot pads swell up, to become hyperkeratotic. The ferret will die 12–16 days after exposure to the ferret-adapted strain or 21–25 days with the canine strain.[26] The usual progression is for CNS signs with hyperexcitability, excess salivation (which might suggest rabies in some countries) plus muscular tremors, convulsions and eventual death by coma. Classic signs of canine distemper infection in the ferret are shown in Figures 8.1–8.5. Comparative clinical signs of canine distemper and human influenza are illustrated in Table 8.4. The pyrexia of HI fluctuates to high temperatures over days and can be 40°C plus. The CNS signs are seen in the advanced stages of CD but most infected ferrets are euthanized before that point.

Treatment: This is not easy and ferrets usually die of the disease. Some have tried using hyperimmune ferret serum (1.0–1.5 mL i.v., i.o.) from well-vaccinated ferret donors (M. Finkler, pers. comm. 2002). An interesting situation occurred in the USA in 2003.[31] A ferret owned

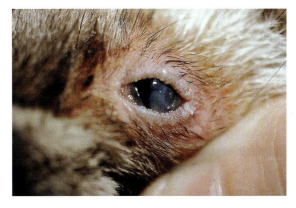

Figure 8.2 Ferret eye discharges. (Courtesy of Dr M. Davidson.)

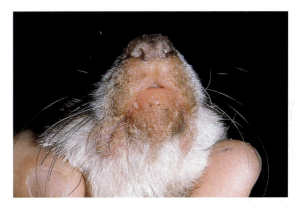

Figure 8.3 Ferret chin rash. (Courtesy of Dr M. Davidson.)

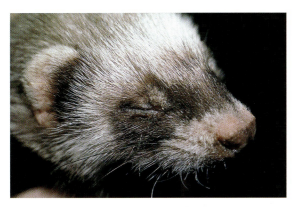

Figure 8.1 Ferret blepharitis. (Courtesy of Dr Michael Davidson, College of Veterinary Medicine, North Carolina State University, Raleigh.)

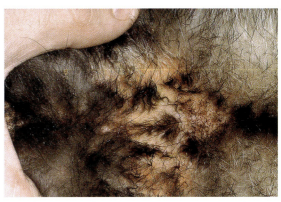

Figure 8.4 Ferret inguinal rash. (Courtesy of Dr M. Davidson.)

CHAPTER EIGHT
Viral, bacterial and mycotic diseases

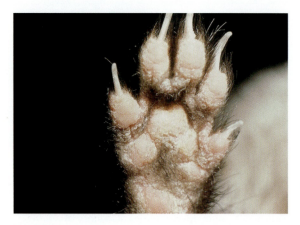

Figure 8.5 Ferret hyperkeratosis of pads. (Courtesy of Dr M. Davidson.)

by a vet hospital manager had sneezing fits and was put on amoxicillin for ferret 'flu. The ferret improved slightly but the manager also had a dog with upper respiratory disease. The dog was a 'rescue' dumped because it had parvovirus and, though nursed through the disease, had not been vaccinated for distemper. The ferret had been vaccinated with Fervac 2 years before but the vaccination was not boosted annually. There was no history of distemper in the hospital but the owner had a large number of raccoons in the front yard where the dog played. (There had been an outbreak of distemper in raccoons on Long Island the previous year.) Both ferret and dog progressed rapidly into classic distemper symptoms. They were vigorously treated against the disease with transfusion, interferon and bovine colostrum for the ferret along with other medications. The dog survived but the ferret succumbed after 5 weeks of treatment.

There is no single vaccine in Australia. Only multivalent vaccines are available, which can be used with care. The vaccines are produced in various mammalian cell lines. Any vaccine produced in ferret cell culture can be fatal to ferrets by actually producing the disease. *Note* that in American native black-footed ferrets, there was an occasion when four ferrets died within 21 days after vaccination with a modified live canine distemper virus vaccine and it was found that there had been insufficient attenuation of the vaccine for the species. The genetic relationship of the black-footed ferret (*Mustela nigripes*) to European ferrets (*M. furo*) remains uncertain, but in the same reference the European ferret has been vaccinated with the vaccine in question without any pathological effects.[32]

Canine distemper vaccination schedules

In the USA, the American Ferret Association has a policy of advising booster vaccinations for canine distemper in healthy ferrets at 8, 11 and 14 weeks of age by s.c. injection.

Vaccines available are:

1. FERVAC D (United Vaccines) modified live virus (MLV) only currently approved ferret vaccine of chick embryo origin.
2. PUREVAX FERRET (Merial) recombinant vaccine, viral-vectored (attached to canarypox virus) able to stimulate both cell-mediated humoral responses to the canine distemper HA and F glycoproteins.

The use of multivalent vaccine for ferrets is not recommended, as it is considered to give a vaccine-induced disease.[33] (However, in Australia we have no option, see below.)

Table 8.4 Canine distemper and human influenza differentiation

Clinical comparative signs	Canine distemper (CD)	Human influenza (HI)
Nasal/ocular discharges	+++	+++
Type of discharges	Severe mucopurulent	Usually mucoserous
Sneezing	+	+++
Coughing	+	+++
Pyrexia	+++	++
Dermatitis	+++	−
Footpad hyperkeratosis	++	−
Central nervous system signs	+	−
Prognosis	F	S

+, May be present; ++, Common; +++, Usual presentation; − Negative. F, fatal; S, self-limiting, can be fatal in neonates or if progressing to pneumonia.
After Rosenthal, with permission.[29]

MLV is a modified virus giving immunity without disease however, it must infect cells to do the job and must survive long enough to stimulate a body immune response. It is suggested that anything which interferes with virus growth prevents enough virus being present to trigger the reaction. The immunity given to the kitten via the mother can interfere with the vaccination and is active for up to 6 weeks or more. This timing of the first vaccination is important.

It has been stated that FERVAC D has some side-effects and fatal reactions.[33] These range from depression with vomiting (sometimes bloody) to bloody diarrhoea, collapse, coma and death. Initial reaction can be pruritus and skin erythema. The ferret can go into shock with pale to gray mucous membranes, a drop in body temperature and a thready pulse. The vaccine reaction can occur anywhere between a few minutes and several hours afterwards, though most occur in the first 20 minutes.

PUREVAX has caused a reaction in a young ferret which had two shots as recommended 2 weeks apart.[34] The ferret slowly declined in health more noticeably after the second injection. It became anorexic with a PCV of 11 (normal 40) but improved on antibiotic, feeding and prednisone in 4 days when the PCV rose to 42. The ferret's appetite resumed and it was suggested by Merial that overstimulation of the ferret immune system had led to a haemolytic anaemia. (As with people, there can be individual reactions to any vaccination.)

It is considered that if rabies and canine distemper vaccinations are given together, any reaction will be from the CD. Both are regularly given together, the reason being that the clients of some practices have to travel long distances for an appointment (S. Brown, pers. comm. 1999).

Greenacre, USA, in a retrospective study into the incidence of an adverse reaction to vaccination with distemper or rabies between 1995 and 2001, found that 14 out of 143 ferrets reacted within 25 minutes.[35] Ten of the ferrets had both vaccinations; three occurred after distemper vaccination alone and one after rabies vaccination alone. They all had a general hyperaemia, mostly on the nose, mucous membranes and footpads. Hypersalivation and vomiting occurred, with five developing dyspnoea; of these, two were cyanotic. Also five had diarrhoea and two of these had haematochezia. One ferret, which reacted to the double vaccination, also had a reaction again the following year with a single rabies vaccine. It should be noted that 9 of the 13 ferrets that had reacted were not supposed to have had any history of previous vaccination but it needs to be remembered that all pet ferrets were derived from Marshall Farms, New York, stock. These ferrets would have been sterilized, descented and vaccinated against canine distemper at 6 weeks of age as were all laboratory ferrets.

Moore et al., USA, also carried out a retrospective study, between 2002 and 2003, on the incidence and risk factors for adverse events associated with distemper and rabies vaccination in ferrets and found the rate very low.[36]

Precaution at vaccinations

It is suggested that ferrets be checked for half an hour after the vaccination for any reaction. In the event of a reaction, the ferret is treated with 0.1 mL of 1:10 000 epinephrine s.c./i.m. for a major reaction, or Dexason SP (1 mg/500 g, i.v./i.m.) or 1 mg diphenhydramine (1 mg/500 g, i.v./i.m.) for minor reactions. *Note*: some American vets routinely pre-treat with 1 mg diphenhydramine before vaccination. Hospital support might be required in severe cases.[33]

Vaccination timing

A check of vaccination timing in a group of kittens would show the level of antibody (titre) dropping with time. Thus, there is a time when the kittens' titre level is dangerously low and the animal is susceptible to infection.

This moment could be as early as 6 weeks in some and as late as 14 weeks in others. Figure 8.6 shows the situation with two ferret kittens.[37] Kitten 1 (white line) has received a high level of passive immunity starting at 25 antibody titre. Kitten 2 (black line) has a lower level of immunity starting at 15. Thus if the titre level 10 is required for infection protection we see kitten 1 becom-

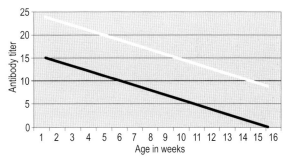

Figure 8.6 Vaccination schedule. The lines represent two different kits. Kit No. 1 (white) received a high level of passive immunity (starting at 25). Kit No. 2 (black), a lower level of immunity (starting at 15). If we assume that a titer of 10 (bold line) is required for protection against infection, then Kit No. 2 becomes susceptible at 6 weeks of age and Kit No. 1 does not become susceptible until 14 weeks of age.

CHAPTER EIGHT
Viral, bacterial and mycotic diseases

ing susceptible at 6 weeks of age and kitten 2 susceptible at 14 weeks of age.

Thus in a population of kittens, if vaccination was given only at 6 week of age or 8 weeks of age there would be part of the population which would not respond to the vaccination and therefore become susceptible to infection. If the first vaccination was at 14 weeks of age many of the kittens would have already lost their immunity. Heiler comments on the problem of assessing titres and what they mean.[38] She points out there are three main methods of measuring antibody levels, being fluorescent molecules technique, haemagglutination inhibition assay and serum neutralization test. In the latter, serum mixed with antibodies is mixed with live virus and is assayed to see how much active virus is still present. The serum goes through dilutions to find out what dilution protects, e.g. titre 1:10 etc. It could be that a titre of 1:32 is effective. Heiler points out that to get the absolute assurance of protection, challenge studies must be done on live animals and that would require sacrificing ferrets in a laborious and costly procedure. She suggests using only approved and proven vaccines and reminds us that the risk of reaction, although very real, cannot be avoided by running a titre. More studies are required on ferret vaccination against canine distemper, which again would require using ferrets.

Galaxy D (Shering Plough Animal Health Co., Omaha, Nebraska) is another commercial USD approved modified live virus chick embryo cell-attenuated vaccine which is used by some but is not labelled for ferrets (M Finkler, pers. comm. 2004). Serological evaluation of the efficacy and safety of live Galaxy D vaccine has been carried out with young ferrets with success.[39]

There has been some research in the USA to indicate that canine distemper vaccine protection might last for up to 3 years. Fort Dodge, Australia has 'Duramune Adult' for dogs for a 3-year vaccination programme (Rapheal, pers. comm. 2005).

Caton has remarked that a statement in *Current Veterinary Therapy XI* pointed out that 'almost without exception there was no immunological requirement for annual vaccination and the immunity to viruses could persist for years or the life of the animal'.[40] This has led to some veterinarians considering annual 'wellness' checks rather than annual vaccinations, however they still agree that some degree of vaccination is needed. Author, Wendy Winstead, at the head of this chapter, was insistent on vaccinations for the deadly canine distemper disease.

Vaccination reactions have been considered previously as anaphylactic shock but Caton points out that ferrets can get lethargy, fever, abdominal tenderness and sore joints. It is also possible that in ferrets with pre-existing health problems, vaccination decreases their immune system and makes them worse. Thus many ferrets with chronic conditions may fail to respond to traditional treatment and homeopathic treatment devotees insist that the vaccination has interfered with the body's ability to heal itself.

Ferrets do not get canine parvovirus, canine adenovirus or canine parainfluenza and thus vaccinations carrying these components are not required for ferrets. At times of virus mutation in the future this might not be the case.

It was considered that multivalent vaccines could cause reactions in ferrets.[33] In Australia and New Zealand, we have only multivalent vaccines and in consultation with the two main vaccine producers, Commonwealth Serum Laboratory Ltd. and Fort Dodge it was established that their multivalent canine vaccines, though not registered for ferrets, can be used.[41,42] Webster's (now Fort Dodge) stated years ago that the global experience with vaccines has been cautious and professional and fitch (ferret pelt production) industries recommended in the past a dose range from one-half to one-sixth of the recommended dog dose. This is despite the fact that the safety and efficiency of these vaccines has been demonstrated at levels five times the fitch dose. Webster's used to have a univalent canine distemper vaccine but it was replaced by a multivalent vaccine so there is probably no chance of getting a single dose vaccine for ferrets yet down under.

However, I have used multivalent vaccines with ferrets with no reaction, providing a recommended dilution technique is used. I originally used Webster's Distemper vaccine at their recommended dose rate of one vial serving six ferrets. Thus using an accurate 1.5 mL sterile water to make up the dog dose, then using a tuberculin syringe for accurate dosing, the individual ferret could be given no more than 0.25 mL s.c. Use of 0.20 mL could be standard. I adapted this procedure with the multivalent vaccines.

I use CSL vaccine 3-1 (Canvac 3) on my own ferrets with no adverse effects. All three living attenuated viruses are produced in continuous cell lines and freeze-dried. I have heard in the past of some deaths in ferrets using 0.5 mL or more of a multivalent vaccine. I have also used the CSL 4-1 at 0.25 mL s.c. with no adverse reaction. Some veterinarians have used the CSL Distemper Hepatitis vaccine. The procedure with CSL Canvac of giving 0.25 mL of a reconstitute vial using 1.5 mL sterile water has been placed in the technical update material for vaccination of ferrets. It is emphasized that there is actually no vaccine currently registered for ferret use in Australia (C. Trumble, Pfizer Animal Health, pers. comm. 2005).

Note. It is considered that canine parvovirus and canine adenovirus are non-pathogenic to ferrets. The canine parvovirus cannot protect against Aleutian disease but I would query if ferrets in some situations are not affected by canine adenovirus, e.g. ferrets boarded in dog kennels.

Whatever multivalent vaccine is used, a whole dog dose is definitely not recommended. Webster's also stated that the effective immunizing dose of vaccines is based on dose titration studies. (In the British Veterinary Codex, 1953, the ferret/fitch dose of an egg-adapted distemper vaccine was $1/1000$th of the dog dose.) Webster's recommended minimal immunizing dose will therefore differ between vaccines of different origins, depending to a large extent on the nature of the virus isolates themselves and the reproduction media and methods employed. It should be recognized therefore that it is the antigenic mass and not the volume *per se* that is important in defining an immunizing dose.

With the multivalent vaccine, it might be prudent to give one dose at 12 weeks of age and then yearly boosters. In the USA, criticism of the yearly booster regime had been stated.[31] It is considered that there is no immunological requirement for the annual re-vaccination. (Only vaccinations involving toxins require boosters.) The AFA recommendations for ferret vaccination still stand as shown previously.

The vaccine-associated sarcoma (VAS)

This has been commented on as relating to rabies and in particular to cats.[20] In the cat, it was found that live vaccines, not attenuated, were associated with VAS. The vaccine aluminium adjuvant was first suspected as an irritant. One veterinarian has quoted vaccine reactions as induced sarcoma, arthralgia (stiffness or pain in the joints), hives, gastrointestinal distress, 'blue eye', autoimmune disease and anaphylaxis in dogs, cats and ferrets.[31]

Annual check-up times

The subject of 'over-servicing' in regard to vaccination programmes has been aired, pointing out that the duration of immunity is a key factor. It is considered, in some quarters, that yearly vaccination has little merit in keeping the antigen titre, of whatever vaccine, up to a protecting level where 3- or 4-yearly boosters would be sufficient and cause less stress on the animal or the pocket of the client. Yearly annual general check-ups should be recommended as a basic procedure whether associated with vaccination or not. It would depend on client compliance but in respect to the ferret-owning clientele, this should be forthcoming in my opinion if they are advised of the need to seek early signs of FADC and insulinoma diseases at the very least.

There have been no trials in Australia to assess if an initial ferret vaccination would suffice for 2 years or more as has been indicated in American literature.[33] At the present time, the vaccination routine is at 6–8 weeks, 12–14 weeks and then a yearly booster of a small accurate dose of a multivalent vaccine as indicated previously. The vaccination incorporates examination, vaccination and certification. Vaccination should be carried out in a *stress-free* environment for the ferret (and vet). That is definitely *not* on ferret show days, ferret-racing days or before ferreting expeditions.

In the UK and Europe, the vaccine Nobivac puppy DP (distemper/parvo) is used only for the distemper fraction. The other vaccine is Delcavac DHPPi (Intervet). This is a combined live vaccine. The distemper fraction again is used from the Onderstepoort strain grown on a Vero cell line. The hepatitis, canine parvovirus, parainfluenza fraction, not really needed, does not appear to harm the ferret. The UK ferrets get a first dose from 12 weeks of age with, note, boosters every 2 years (Oxenham, pers. comm. 1998). In the USA DHPPi is sold as Proguard 5 (i.e. Proguard 7 in combination with Nobivac Leto and Proguard 8 in combination with Nobivac LC0).

Regarding protection of ferrets from canine distemper virus (CDV) a trial was carried out using recombinant pox virus (RPV) vaccines, expressing the H or F gene of the rinderpest virus, which is related to CDV. A single injection of vaccinia virus expressing the H or F genes of RPV was able to protect 60% of 27 ferrets trailed with a challenge from a high dose of CDV.[43] This indicated that RPV antigens expressed by vaccinia virus are able to protect ferrets against a related Morbillivirus and it might lead to a new vaccine for ferrets.

Concern has been raised about other viruses similar to CDV that may affect ferrets. Two strains of Lion (*Panthera leo*) Morbillivirus, Californian and Serengeti types are antigenically related to CDV.[44] (It has been found that ferrets become anorectic at 5–6 days post-intraperitoneal injection of the strains. This leads to ocular nasal discharges at 9–12 days and then deaths from 12–22 days. It is interesting that ferrets vaccinated against mink distemper virus (Onderstepoort strain) are protected against the effects of the two lion strains (Table 8.2).

In Japan, where ferrets from the USA and New Zealand and Europe are the rage, there is no FervacD available, so they have to use multivalent vaccines as in Australia. It appears the vaccines used are Dohy Vac 5 (Krouritsu Shoji Company) and Canine 3 (Kyoto Biken) which are grown on chick embryo. The ferrets are given the full canine dose without any reactions (Yasutsugu Miwa, Tokyo, pers. comm. 2005). This goes against my precise diluting of Canine 3-1 vaccine and worrying about vaccination reactions! It needs more investigation. Of course giving the whole canine dose to one ferret might be wasteful if you could use the vial for four ferrets and get the same protection.

Other ferret diseases

Canine hepatitis is not a disease of ferrets but has been found in mustelids; in skunks. It was postulated that other carnivores may get an asymptomatic infection.[45] Canine parvovirus does not affect ferrets in Australia. A serious overseas disease of ferrets and mink, called Aleutian disease is caused by a different parvovirus. Canine parainfluenza virus does not affect ferrets but another component of the canine cough syndrome does; the bacterium *Bordetella bronchiseptica* in America. Feline distemper (enteritis) does affect mink and other members of the Mustelidae family and may affect ferret kittens. Feline rhinotracheitis does not affect ferrets. However, I have been worried over the years about a 'snuffles' condition in ferrets, which is similar to the rhinitis and sinusitis of cats. Feline chlamydia does not affect ferrets.

Aleutian disease (AD)

This is caused by a parvovirus first discovered in an Aleutian strain of mink on a mink farm (USA) in 1956.

The mink (*Mustela vison*) of primary concern was the gunmetal-coloured Aleutian mink with two autosomal recessive genes for the pelt colour which is called the Chediak–Higashi syndrome.[46] These mink were bred for their remarkable pelt but were highly susceptible to the Aleutian Disease Virus (ADV). In the mink farms in early times, the spleens of distemper-infected mink were used to make an autogenous vaccine to give to other mink and ferrets, which were also farmed. Thus infection passed to ferrets and the ferret ADV would be a mutant of the more virulent mink ADV with the ferret parvovirus showing a feature of sharing a DNA segment like that of the hypervariable capsid region of the mink parvovirus.[11] Initially AD was a chronic wasting disease of mink but only a subclinical problem in fitch ferrets.

There are four strains of AD that affect mink and probably a ferret strain. With mink and ferrets, the severity of the disease depends on the strain of AD but the genetic make-up of the infected animal might also be a factor (M. Oxenham, pers. comm. 1993). Aleutian disease was recorded in ferrets in the USA (1967), then New Zealand (1984), UK (1990), Sweden (1994), Japan (1999), Belgium and the Netherlands (2004).

Differentiation of the AD strains was made possible only by the development of the counter-current immunoelectrophoresis (CIEP) technique in America.

Transfer of AD infection from mink to laboratory or pet ferrets is not explained but AD is highly contagious and an animal handler may have been involved. If laboratory ferrets were taken as pets, the disease could have been dispersed into the relatively high ferret pet population in the USA. In Sweden, there are about 200 mink farms with 80% of mink infected with AD. In 1994, pet and farm ferrets were tested using the CIEP test. Around 150 pet ferrets were tested and found negative. In 1994, ferrets from a farm where they also kept mink were infected with AD. Three ferrets positive for AD were found on the farm, indicating that Swedish ferrets can be infected with the disease, but no pet ferrets were found affected (L. Berndtsson, Fur Animal Dept., National Vet. Institute, pers. comm. 1994).

In New Zealand, where old fitch-farming businesses were active, the possible source of AD infection was originally introduced by breeding stock from the USA. Ferrets have escaped from fitch farms and some farms released their stock into the wild when fitch-farming became unprofitable. Feral ferrets, some possibly from original polecat crosses introduced in the nineteenth century, do occur and there is a policy for trapping them, more out of concern about them killing ground birds and harbouring bovine tuberculosis than AD. If ferret breeders in NZ used captured feral ferrets, which can be quickly domesticated, there might be a possibility of feral ferrets carrying AD bringing the disease to the stock.

In the UK, pet and working ferrets could contract the disease from stray ferrets or polecat contacts, which feral mink might have infected. The latter have been deliberately released by Animal Liberationists and have thrived over time in competition with the native otter. In 1986, an otter death in Norfolk was attributed to possible AD symptoms. Otters can kill and eat mink. Ferrets were interbred with mink on mink farms to increase litter size; thus ferrets are at risk and AD is now endemic in wild mink in the UK. In Russia, European mink have been crossed with ferrets to produce the hybrid Foonoters.[47] There is no AD in that country to date. In Australia, if the import ban on ferrets is lifted and new stock comes in from other countries, they must all be screened for AD.

An excellent account of AD in the UK by Oxenham, with reference to screening, has been done in association with the Wessex Ferret Club (Oxenham, pers. comm. 1993). Basically, AD affects mink and ferrets, but antibodies have been detected in other mustelids. When considering the effects of AD on the body, he

Author's clinical example

To show the difficulty in diagnosis

A sable jill 'Peanut' vaccinated with CSL 3-1 vaccine at 8 and 12 weeks of age developed vestibular disease at 5 months. She was a pet shop ferret and fed Iams food. She was presented with profound weakness on the left front and rear limbs with UMN signs in all four limbs but mostly on the left. She was mentally depressed with reduced appetite. The vestibular signs were on the left side and ear mites were detected bilaterally. The clinical signs suggested a lesion on the left side of the brain stem level of CNVIII. A provisional, broad-range diagnosis was made of parasitic/bacterial otitis being externa, media or possibly interna with a secondary meningitis with a differential of distemper, trauma, toxicity, thiamine deficiency, Aleutian disease and lymphoblastic encephalitis. The jill was treated with Del-Mycin Ear Drops (Delta Labs) on a 5-day course then 10-day break followed by a 5-day course, plus an antibiotic course of clavulanic acid/amoxicillin. A blood check under Domitor sedation proved normal. There were some periods of intermittent improvement over the following weeks but the jill deteriorated, stopped eating and became very weak, losing consciousness. It was euthanized on request. No post mortem was possible.

However, a repeat scenario occurred which is interesting with regard to the wide speculation of causative disease and the possible occurrence of Aleutian disease. A replacement sable hob, Gizmo, from the same pet shop and possibly same breeder, had been vaccinated and fed on Iams kitten food as before and was presented at 7 months of age with vestibular signs similar to the jill. He had a mild right foreleg weakness. Gizmo weighed 1500 g and had ear mites, which were treated this time with intra-aural Ivomectin (0.3 mL repeated 2 weeks later). No other antibiotics were given initially. The treatment removed the mites. He was bright but still weak on the right side. The owner agreed to further antibiotic cover using clavulanic acid/amoxicillin (Pfizer) and enrofloxacin (Baytril). A general weakness occurred with the ferret being immobile and inappetent, with urinary incontinence, so a switch of drugs was made to trimethoprim-sulphamethoxazole for better CNS penetration. A meningitis/encephalitis or brain abscess was suggested or something resembling GME in dogs. Unfortunately, chloramphenicol, another good CNS drug, is not available in New Zealand. In addition, the hob was treated with B vitamin complex for possible thiamine deficiency and was on dexamethasone (0.25 mg/kg s.c.) repeated intermittently every 3 days. There was some improvement in appetite, alertness and less incontinence but this was possibly due to steroid therapy as the hob did continue to decline showing ataxia, weakness and hyperflexion in all limbs. Various suggestions for differential diagnosis were put forward including Aujeszky's disease, toxoplasmosis, canine distemper or a possible parvovirus, the Aleutian disease. The hob had shown no respiratory or skin clinical signs of distemper and had been vaccinated like the previous jill with CSL Canvac 3-1, which was usual in NZ. Eosinophilic gastroenteritis (EG) was even suggested, which is a rare disease in ferrets, dogs and humans and may be an allergic or immunological response to foods. Gizmo was put to sleep at 67 days after the start of problems at 1400 g, immobile and inappent, while Peanut was put down at 47 days.

A full post mortem was done on Gizmo and was interesting as it put Aleutian disease as a possible underlying cause. The morphological diagnosis showed the cerebrum/cerebellum with a moderate lymphocytic meningitis and mild encephalitis. The brain stem had a severe lymphocytic meningoencephalitis and the spinal cord a severe lymphocytic myelitis and meningitis. Celia Hooper (Auckland Animal Health Lab pathologist) commented that the lumbar spinal cord also contained lesions but at this level, they were more severe in the meninges than in the neuropil. The most severe lesions were in the cervical spinal cord and caudal brain stem. No protozoan agents were seen in numerous sections but that does not rule them out. Viruses remained a possibility and though the clinical history and lesions were not typical of CD it could not be ruled out. She stated that Aujeszky disease had not been completely eradicated from New Zealand and could be included in the differential diagnosis but as the inflammation was not suppurative, the negative bacteriology was not surprising. Aleutian disease is certainly a possibility but it is usually more severe in visceral organs and it would be an unusual manifestation to have the most severe lesions in the brain. However, the pancreas, liver, lungs and stomach did contain moderate to severe infiltrations of lymphocytes. The stomach and intestines showed mild to moderate infiltration of eosinophils and plasma cells.

Dr A. Lindsay, Torbay Vet Clinic, Auckland, NZ, pers. comm. 1998.

states that comparisons with diseases of other animals are often mentioned, which include diseases that follow a similar pattern to AD but are in fact quite rare. Examples given are equine infectious anaemia, African swine fever and lymphocytic choroid meningitis of mice.[48] The normal response of an animal to invasion by a virus is to produce specific antibodies that bind that virus and neutralize its effects. If these antibodies do not overcome the virus then the disease progresses. This usually involves the destruction of specific areas of tissue within the body, such as the brain (rabies), liver (canine hepatitis), surface tissue (foot and mouth), etc. What makes AD an unusual type of disease is that mink and ferrets produce massive amounts of immune substances or complexes as a response to the virus, which are deposited in various organs of the body. It is these deposits, which cause the symptoms of AD. Most mink die of kidney dysfunction whilst the symptoms in ferrets are much more variable and in some cases mild to none at all. There has been an interesting study on the effect of repeated live-virus vaccine as a model for vaccine-induced glomerular injury.[49]

Clinical signs

In mink, features of AD were weight loss, lethargy, anorexia, polydipsia, anaemia and melaena with poor pelts.[46] The chronic wasting also leads to infertility, small litter size and stillbirths increase. The Aleutian mink is dramatically affected by the virulent strain of AD while non-Aleutian mink may suffer three classes of infection, the progressive Aleutian strain, persistent non-progressive strain or the nonpersistent, non-progressive strain, which clears in time. It is not known if these conditions relate to ferret infection, which usually show the chronic wasting disease and posterior paresis or paralysis of CNS involvement. In Australia, with a case of posterior paralysis, we would still consider a number of conditions before AD.

Immunology aspects

Although antibodies are produced by the mink and ferret, for some still unknown reason, they do not neutralize the AD virus, hence the persistence of the infection. Another feature of AD is that the virus causes some degree of immunosuppression, so that the ferret is unable to mount a defence against other types of infection. Thus, an AD case surfacing in Australia may be diagnostically masked.

Post mortem signs

AD cases show signs of inflammation in internal organs. In Aleutian mink, the kidneys are small and there is splenomegaly, mesenteric lymphadenopathy, hepatomegaly and bowel haemorrhage.[46] Similar results are seen in ferret post mortems. Kidney sections show glomerulonephritis. The ferret could have respiratory and cardiac disease features in ADV positive cases. With the lungs, consolidation of lobes can occur after an intense coughing illness and results in lung collapse and pleural effusion. CNS involvement can occur some time after the respiratory symptoms giving a posterior paresis leading to an ascending paralysis with effects on bowel and urinary function. The cardiac effects are cardiomyopathy resulting in arteritis showing up at post mortem. The arteritis results from deposition of immune complex substance.

Disease infectivity

With mink, oral or aerosol spread of ADV was likely. The AD can be shown to spread by inoculation of whole blood, serum, faeces, saliva or bone marrow of sick mink. The disease can also pass from mink jills to young with either the progressive or non-progressive subclinical disease, resulting in highly-infected litters. It is not known if this happens with ferrets but oral and aerosol methods are suspected. Infection of kittens from jills is also suspected. It is thus important that strict quarantine measures are taken before accepting in ferrets from AD suspect colonies.

Diagnosis

This can be difficult as demonstrated by the New Zealand example. Other features of the disease besides hind leg lameness are weight loss, which is progressive. Only Gizmo was weighed. Thirst is a sign and sometimes bleeding gums and tarry scats occur plus respiratory symptoms so the signs have a wide spectrum. There can be sudden deaths in stressful situations like ferret shows, etc.

In the UK, a diagnosis of Aleutian disease should ideally be made by:

1. Typical clinical signs.
2. Gammaglobulin levels >20%
3. A positive serological CIEP test (can be used on mink and ferrets).
4. The histopathology picture.
5. Possible electron microscopy with parvovirus particles in bowel lymph gland.

Treatment

There is no treatment possible but hopefully Australia will remain free of such a destructive disease. Affected ferrets must be eliminated from breeding stock. Unfortunately, although AD is caused by a parvovirus it is not the canine parvovirus so that vaccine would not protect. However, in the USA, the ferret AD is considered clinically rare though in some localities 20–30% of ferrets will test positive. In a survey of 500 ferrets in ferret shelters in Illinois, USA, 13% were positive to AD yet only two ferrets developed signs within 3 years (S. Brown, pers. comm. 1997). A prominent USA ferret pathologist reported only 10 cases per year based on submitted PM samples (B. Williams, pers. comm. 1998).

Experimental attempts at treating ferrets with AD have been recorded.[46] Cyclophosphamide in mink was given at 10 mg/kg i.p. 3 times weekly for 13 weeks with a good effect in suppressing host antibody response and deposition of immune complexes in the kidneys, in effect protecting the kidneys at least. *Note* the level of virus growth was not affected by the treatment, which may indicate that direct viral damage to the host is not the cause of classic AD. In ferrets with AD, only fluid therapy is possible to maintain hydration for kidney function and giving nourishment by oral syringe or stomach tube.

Aleutian disease testing in the UK

Accurate diagnosis by blood-testing ferret stock is carried out in the UK and also USA, using the CIEP test (counter-current immuno-electrophoresis test). Infected ferrets (CIEP-positive) are culled. A survey found that not all ferrets in contact with CIEP-positive animals themselves became infected as not all the CIEP-positive ferrets were shedding at the same time.[48] In a 1993 survey, it was found there had been several isolated outbreaks of AD in areas other than central southern England; Berkshire, London, Oxfordshire and Lancashire were affected. The source of infection in ferrets originated from the Wessex area. Evidently, very little ferret screening had been done around the country and only a few positives have been found in areas checked. The routine screening carried out over some years in the Wessex area is shown in Table 8.5. Aleutian disease is a condition to be aware of in ferrets for the twenty-first century with the possible increase of transmission of viral diseases around the world.

The table shows a steady reduction of positive AD until 1992 and then a rise in 1993. The very low incidence in previously-tested ferrets is attributed to the efficient control measures in Wessex and indicates the continuing need for AD screening.

Epidemiology: Oxenham has suggested that wild mink in the UK could be a reservoir of the disease.

A yearly blood test would be required on pet and working ferrets if AD was recorded in Australia. With negative results, ferret breeders would naturally breed with other tested-negative stock and the new stock must be monitored. Cleared ferrets would have to be separated from untested animals. It is known that mink enteritis parvovirus (not AD) can survive outdoors for 5–10 months so this might be the same with mink disease parvovirus (ADV). Cleaning of cages of any suspect ferrets by hot disinfectant washing and drying is to be done. All utensils associated with the ferrets must be cleaned regularly against contamination.

With positive results, the heartache would be whether to keep the ferret/ferrets for the rest of their possible life span. If I had a positive AD case in a ferret colony, the positive would have to be euthanized and the negatives retested at monthly intervals to check the AD clearance. Not a happy prospect for any ferret owner!

In the UK situation of 2005, the small colony of AD-positive ferrets have been maintained for several years. In a letter to the National Ferret Welfare Society, Dr J. Chitty made some interesting points on the status of ferret AD and the future regarding diagnosis (see previous list) and fate of positives. It seems that with the small colony their life span has not shortened and they have died of other diseases. He asserts that a lot the identification of AD disease relates to clinical examination. There are no 'classic' signs of the disease but those listed include hindquarter paresis/paralysis, melaena, lethargy and liver/spleen enlargement. Lymphoma is becoming a common factor of ferret illness. Thus, the cause could be myriad. He has examined seven ferret post mortems with hindquarter paralysis and found six had spinal abscesses and one a spinal haemorrhage. There was no histopathological evidence of AD.

The gammaglobulin level test is useful. However, it is expensive to do and not routine in all laboratories. Moreover, the gammaglobulin levels might also be raised by recent vaccinations, other infective agents or tumours of the antibody-producing white blood cells. There are AD-positive ferrets, which do not have raised gammaglobulins.[50] The CIEP test is little help in these situations as it has been reported that finding the antibody is not synonymous with having the disease. The test is

Table 8.5 Screening tests carried out on Wessex ferrets for Aleutian disease

Year	1990	1991	1992	1993	Totals
No. tested for first time	245	201	242	148	836
No. positive	26 (10.6%)	12 (6.0%)	6 (2.5%)	17 (11.5%)	61 (7.3%)
No. previously tested		154	188	198	540
No. positive		2 (1.3%)	0	2 (1.0%)	4 (0.7%)
Overall total	245	355	430	346	1376
No. positive	26 (10.6%)	14 (3.9%)	6 (1.4%)	19 (5.5%)	65 (4.7%)

M. Oxenham, pers. comm. 1998.

again expensive and not usually done on one sick animal. Ideally, all dead ferrets should have histology examinations, so typical AD lesions may be found and correlated with the preceding clinical signs and testing results. There again typical lesions may be seen without clinical signs,[51] or there may be even no histological changes.[52] It is important that AD diagnosis be accurate to avoid the heartache of destroying a pet ferret.

There is concern for the routine testing of ferrets for AD antibodies. Many ferrets could fluctuate between positive and negative and it may be difficult to decide on these results. Evidently, the main problem appears to be that ferrets do not produce the same level of antibody in response to the AD virus as mink. It has been found experimentally that the rise in gammaglobulin in infected ferrets of 0.5–1 g/dL was lower than that of mink given the same challenge.[53] This shows that the tests for the mink are not sensitive enough to find the smaller rise in ferrets. Thus some ferrets' results could fluctuate with the test. The ideal screening should therefore be very sensitive. The ferrets that are then tested positive are therefore *really* positive. Chitty considers the saliva test less sensitive than the blood test and more difficult to do with the conscious ferret.

Mink produce more antibody than ferrets, which is why the ferret results are so variable. Also with mink, high antibody production is the reason for the severe disease in the species with clumps of antibody and it is the high antibody, not the virus, which causes the damage to small blood vessels, kidneys, heart etc. Thus, the main factor is the mink's highly reactive immune system compared to the ferret. Questions can be asked, if the ferret is not 'hyperactive' in immune response to the virus, will it produce the same disease? Ferrets can get AD but how often and how severely? Should the clinician worry about other diseases such as distemper and lymphoma?

There is also the question of different strains of AD. It was noted in 1982 that when ferrets were inoculated with ferret strains and mink strains of AD, neither produced lesions in the ferrets as severe as those in the mink.[52] So it is seen that current tests do not distinguish between strains of the virus and therefore it may be that some strains are more significant than others.

The question comes back to should AD-positive ferrets be culled? If they are really positive they will go on to infect others and therefore should be culled. But the situation is not clear from the tests to hand. Referring back to the colony of AD-positive ferrets, all but one were very healthy 5 years on from the beginning of the project. The sick ferret was being treated for cardiomyopathy signs. *Note*: none of the AD-positive ferrets in the project had any sign of clinical AD.

Could these ferrets infect others? It was found in 1982 that low levels of virus could be found in the spleens of ferrets 180 days post-infection.[51] No further studies on this point have been made or on virus excretion. Stress and disease cases should be studied on their response to AD.

Is *en masse* testing appropriate? If ferrets do excrete AD and are like the mink, then bringing together many ferrets for testing sessions is not the way to go as it may be a dangerous ideal opportunity for disease spread. It is noted with mink that AD can be aerosol spread and crowding should be avoided.[54]

The situation of UK ferrets with possible positives will be sketchy until there is a more sensitive test. In 1982, using the CIEP test it was found that 42% of 214 healthy ferrets had low levels of antibody.[51] It would be interesting to know how the real situation was with UK ferrets at the present time (J. Chitty, pers. comm. 2005).

European/NZ/Japan AD

Belgium and the Netherlands were previously free of ADV but the disease was brought into Europe apparently by imports of New Zealand ferrets. In early 2004, about 50–100 ferrets were imported from the ferret farm, Southland Ferrets. Other ferrets were imported later from Mystic Farms. The ferrets were beautiful but appeared not to be healthy and several of them died early (H. Moorman, Netherlands, pers. comm. 2005). Post mortems in Holland did not reveal any cause.

In March 2005, a 1-year-old ferret from New Zealand died too early with symptoms of coughing, lethargy, diarrhoea and hind limb weakness. On post mortem, a chronic lymphoplasmacytic inflammation was seen in numerous organs, most prominently in the kidney, liver, spleen, lymph nodes and lungs. Moorman sent tissue to the University of Georgia for testing and Aleutian disease was diagnosed as the cause by the DNA *in situ* hybridization test.

In May 2005, a lot of CIEP tests were performed on ferrets in Holland, 772 ferrets were already tested and 46 showed positive CIEP results. Unfortunately, a Dutch ferret breeder/shelter had given shelter to three New Zealand ferrets in the early months of 2004, until they were euthanized last summer because of a positive CIEP test. *Note*: 33 of 46 ferrets tested positive with the CIEP test were housed at the shelter.

Fortunately, the AD in Holland has not spread very fast but veterinarians and owners are alert to the danger. Several Dutch ferrets were infected mostly because of direct intensive contact or indirect by contaminated cages. The mortality in New Zealand seems much higher than in Dutch ferrets.

Further research on AD in ferret is being carried by Haneke Moorman supported by the Dutch Ferret Foundation 'Stichting de Fret'. The organization paid for samples to be sent to the USA out of widespread concern (Stephenie Bass, pers. comm. 2005).

Japan has an enthusiastic pet ferret ownership with imported ferrets. However, a case of spontaneous Aleutian disease was recorded in 1999.[55] A 3-year-old 1060 g pet jill ferret showed signs of acute dyspnoea and posterior paresis. Though symptomatic treatment was carried out the ferret died 5 days later after becoming comatosed. At post mortem, the body condition appeared good which is a feature of spontaneous AD. There was no hypergammaglobulinaemia in the blood chemistry and histology demonstrated severe inflammatory infiltrates in many organs especially the kidneys. Using PCR products from the kidneys, the gene encoding of the viral capsid was positive for Aleutian disease.

Recently, a survey of 66 ferrets with suspected clinical signs of AD at one private veterinary hospital, between 2003 and 2005, showed the presence of positive results in 23 ferrets using the ELISA test. The origin of the AD ferrets is interesting (Yasutsugu Mawa, pers. comm. 2005). Of 46 ferrets from New Zealand, 19 were ELISA-positive; there were two positives from five Netherlands ferrets and two positives from 15 American ferrets.

This survey does not encourage importation of pet ferrets from some commercial outlets. Where could Australia get clear ferrets from, if importation restrictions were lifted? Russia!

Immune-complex mediated glomerulonephritis (ICGN)

This disease of idiopathic origin of concern to mink farmers[49] is mentioned here as it affects the kidneys, the main target of disease in AD above. A study was carried out as to the effect of repeated vaccination as a possible cause. The vaccines used were against canine distemper, *Pseudomonas aeruginosa* infection, botulism and mink viral enteritis. Canine distemper was given singly to some ferrets and in combination to others. The results did not prove any link between repeated vaccination and ICGN.

However, with the multidosing, there was an increased deposition of immunoglobulin in the kidney glomeruli and this finding deserves further study as vaccines with toxoids, killed bacterial products and inactivated viruses do present a higher antigenic load and are also formulated with adjuvants which are strong immune-stimulating agents. Thus, these vaccine products could more probably result in hyperimmunization and adverse immune-mediated conditions than live virus products. Could the use of multivaccines over a long period have the same effects (see multivalent vaccines reactions earlier)?

Bacterial diseases

Bordetella bronchiseptica

This organism is part of the canine kennel cough (CKC) syndrome and is recognized in the USA as causing disease in ferrets boarded with dogs at a dog kennel or in a veterinary premises.[56] Reference has been made to the problems of boarding ferrets with dogs and cats. In my veterinary hospital, I have experience of a hacking cough of undiagnosed cause in ferrets, which have shared the air with contact dogs in enclosed rooms. It is considered a condition of ferrets in overcrowded conditions and could be of concern in research or breeding establishments where ferrets are kept near dogs (J. Bell, pers. comm. 1999). Vaccination of ferrets for *Bordetella* was carried out by breeding companies, e.g. Marshall Farms, where they also breed dogs. Ferret kittens from Marshall Farms for the pet market are not placed in pet shops till they are 8–10 weeks of age when they are considered safe from kennel cough. Some other commercial breeders sell their kittens to stores at 4–6 weeks but then the kits are not already sterilized at 6 weeks of age as with the growing trend.

Bordetella can cause a thick yellowish nasal discharge and an illness, which can develop into pneumonia. It is prevalent in stressed ferrets, which might well be the case in ferrets boarded with noisy dogs. Only one of my ferrets had shown the cough and this I put down more to the 'snuffles' condition, as related to cats. In many instances, the ferrets are in air contact more with cats than dogs, as the former stay longer in the hospital. Personally, I have never experienced *Bordetella* in ferrets with a severe nasal discharge but usually a unilateral discharge, which has been treated as snuffles. The *Bordetella* pneumonia in ferrets is evidently difficult to treat but the *B. bronchiseptica* isolated from snuffles conditions responds to antibiotics after sensitivity tests on the nasal discharge. However, *Bordetella* can produce a toxin, which will result in convulsions and death and may be confused with a canine distemper diagnosis in ferrets. *Bordetella bronchiseptica* can be avoided by a vaccination 2 weeks before boarding ferrets. It should be boosted on the day of entry for boarding.[56] I have used CSL Canvac BB on my ferrets but have not eliminated unilateral nasal discharge periodically in one ferret, which I consider to be a 'snuffles' case. The vaccine appears safe for ferrets, being a killed product with the dog dose set at one vial. No laboratory trial has been done on ferrets to determine whether a part dose could serve, as with the distemper vaccination. It is important to note that the new intranasal vaccine for *B. bronchiseptica* with canine parainfluenza virus is not suitable for ferrets and could induce the disease.[56]

CHAPTER EIGHT
Viral, bacterial and mycotic diseases

Ferrets can cough for numerous reasons. Considering they are susceptible to lung conditions, it might be prudent to give a coughing ferret an oral antibiotic. I have done so with a ferret living in overnight coughing. It worked. Clavulox palatable drops is a good broad-spectrum standby and one dose may well stop a lot of troubles. I have not regularly vaccinated ferrets in recent years for *Bordetella bronchiseptica*.

'Snuffles': a complex upper respiratory problem

I have compared the cat 'snuffles' to what I call 'snuffles' in ferrets.[57]

Symptoms: With some ferrets, there are sudden paroxysmal bouts of sneezing, with or without nasal discharge. The ferrets have noisy snuffling respiration at times but are not sick. There are a number of differential diagnoses that may apply. In my experience, it has occurred in jills and not hobs. Curiously, with hobs I have had problems with mycotic nasal infections but not in jills (Ch. 12). The finding is purely arbitrary.

At Marshall Farms, New York, it was considered that ferrets' sneezing is related to the human influenza virus (J. Bell, pers. comm. 1997). It could make ferrets sneeze so violently that they fell over, but, like my cases, the ferrets were not actually sick. Bell considered that a *Streptococcus* type C is associated secondarily with the infection. She did say that the sneezing could be due to allergy to the pine and cedar wood chips litter, which we never use. A review of respiratory toxicity of pine and cedar wood bedding has been done.[58] However, Bell used the litter at Marshall Farms for breeding ferrets and also at home with her pet ferrets with no problems. Sneezing as a consequence of pollen allergy with ferrets living outside in a ferretarium, garden or cage situation could be considered.

Marshall Farms used to sell ferrets for influenza research and they were all blood-tested. The pharmaceutical companies required serum from different ferret groups to find a group that had no antibodies. It was evidently difficult to find one, as the people who cared for the ferrets refused to wear masks and there was an infection factor from humans back to ferrets. Again, the ferrets were not sick and the kittens did not even sneeze most of the time. It was concluded that it takes a lot more 'flu virus to affect a ferret than it does a human, which is a comforting thought (J. Bell, pers. comm. 1997).

Diagnosis of 'snuffles'

From the practitioner's point of view, the concern of a snuffles condition is that it may progress to something worse such as pneumonia. The culture of nasal discharge or blood sampling, with bacteriology and sensitivity tests and treatment usually results in 'snuffles' cases being cured. The bacterial picture may be one of certain natural bacteria of the nasal/mouth flora becoming pathogenic to some extent, possibly in a ferret stress situation. Though there is an apparent cure, 'snuffles' can recur. When this happens, it could be that a different bacterium has become dominant and pathogenic in the nasal/mouth flora.

Author's clinical example

'Snuffles' treatment

Two ferrets were involved, jills Tippy and Lucky.[59] A culture of nasal discharge showed similar organisms to those in cats with rhinitis/sinusitis problems. Bacterial flora cultured included those organisms commensal in the nasal cavity, which can become pathogenic in certain circumstances: haemolytic *Escherichia coli*, beta-haemolytic *Streptococcus*, *Staphylococcus aureus*, *Pasteurella multocida*, *Haemophilus* sp., *Bordetella bronchiseptica* and *Pseudomonas aeruginosa*. For both jills, the major bacterial growth was *P. aeruginosa* and the drug sensitivity is shown in Table 8.6. Chloramphenicol at the time (1994) was considered the drug of choice for ferrets but in this case, the *Pseudomonas* was resistant.

Treatment: Tippy was treated successfully with clavulanic acid/amoxicillin (Clavulox palatable drops, Pfizer) and Lucky with doxycycline (Vibravet Paste 100, Pfizer, no longer available in Australia). Of the eight ferret colony members, only Tippy and Lucky showed signs of 'snuffles'. The ferrets respond well to antibiotic, they are not off their food, but there can still be some irritating occasional sneezing bouts without nasal discharge. Possibly, the nasal turbinate membranes are damaged? With another 'snuffles' case, the prominent bacterium was *Pasteurella* sp., sensitive to doxycycline and also to enrofloxacin (Baytril 50 available in injection and oral form)

Table. 8.6 Sensitivity of 'snuffles' organisms in two ferret cases

Antibiotic	Tippy (800 g body weight)	Lucky (980 g body weight)
Tetracycline	R	S
Chloramphenicol	R	R
Doxycycline	R	S
Clavulox	S	R

R, resistant; S, sensitive.

Bacterial diseases

Author's clinical example

The possibility of viral involvement or even sinus problems is shown in the yet to be conclusively diagnosed condition of Teddy of Tasmania. Teddy, born 11 February 2003, is a light sable and arrived in Launceston as an 8-week-old kitten with two brothers and three sisters. He had a slight nose deviation to the right. In this case of possible 'snuffles', the jills were okay but Teddy started sneezing within 3 days of arrival, opposite to what I had found previously.

The ferrets had travelled on a flight from Adelaide to Melbourne and then on to Launceston. On the latter flight, the ferrets shared a compartment with day-old chicks. Quantas do not spray animals in the holds and declared that if there were several animal consignments on board they are kept as far apart as possible. However, in a plane, air circulates and we can all pick up colds!

About 1 month after arriving in Tasmania, Teddy saw a vet. He had been sneezing and coughing for several weeks and became worse 24 hours before the vet visit. He had an increased temperature and was put on Vibravet (doxycycline) 12.5 mg ($\frac{1}{4}$ 50 mg table) b.i.d. for 10 days. On the re-visit, 10 days later, the sneezing had ceased but Teddy was still chesty though sounding better on auscultation. He had however gained weight. He started another course of doxycycline for 8 days.

The owner found out that Blackfoot, one of Teddy's two brothers, had the same clinical signs as Teddy, had been treated with two courses of antibiotic, temporarily improved, but never fully recovered. The other hob, Boofhead, had signs but not as severe and as of March 2005 had no coughs or sneezes for 3 months. *Note*: no other ferrets in contact with Blackfoot or Boofhead developed symptoms.

Teddy had never been vaccinated against canine distemper but received *Bordetella bronchiseptica* vaccination in July 2003 and was sterilized in the August at 1500 g weight. Teddy showed a nasal discharge (Fig. 8.7) and in February 2003, a culture proved negative, only showing normal oral flora. His coughs and sneezes appeared to be coming in cycles, a few days on, a few days off.

In December 2004, Teddy had a bad time coughing and radiographs were done (Fig. 8.8). These were not conclusive. However, Teddy was put on a terbutaline (bronchodilator) syrup and was on Vibravet for 2 months. He was having at least 10 coughing fits a day. In March 2005, he was coughing 2–3 times a day. He was active and eating but his weight was down to 1200 g.

He had two lots of medication, in April and July/August 2005. On examination in August, his heart and lungs were fine. The nasal discharge had some inflammatory cells and lymphocytes and scant bacteria so it was decided to take him off antibiotics for a while. In November 2005, he had been weaned off terbutaline and only coughed occasionally and produced some mucus. With twice daily exercises, he had no problem with clearing his throat and nose. The nasal discharge was the consistency of egg-white. Being off terbutaline his owner noticed 'he has put on weight from 1180 g in August to 1250 g and his body feels firmer, more muscular and he is stronger'.

It would be speculative to put a finger on the direct cause. A slight nasal septum deformation (bent nose), whereby a chronic infection of the fine nasal cartilage might result with a constant discharge, could account for a nasal discharge. The septum damage could be heredity or early trauma. The discharge might have turned pathogenically negative after the intense antibiotic cover earlier. I have always wondered if someone would find a lost *Aelurostrongylus abstrusus* nematode in the ferret, as ferrets do eat snails and slugs (Ch. 10), but not in this case. The virus theories are always hovering in the background, especially when birds are anywhere involved. A RSV association would be interesting to consider. At least Teddy is still active and hopefully a true cause can be discovered of this ongoing case (Christina and Klaus Bernhard, pers. comm. 2003–5).

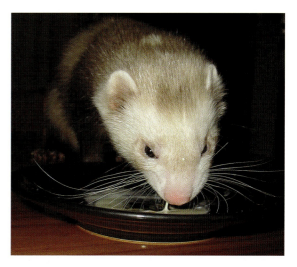

Figure 8.7 Ferret, Teddy, with unilateral nasal discharge and nose bent to the right. (Courtesy of C. Bernhard.)

CHAPTER EIGHT

Viral, bacterial and mycotic diseases

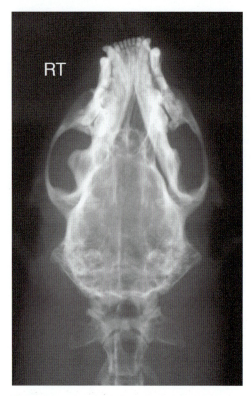

Figure 8.8 Teddy's skull; ventrodorsal. *Note:* deviation to right (compare with Fig. 2.12b). (Courtesy of Dr K. Barrett).

Speculated conditions leading to 'Snuffles':

1. Sinus damage from viral infection such as human influenza or even (?) by feline rhinotracheitis from a passing cat or unvaccinated cat in hospital.
2. Cryptococcosis, a fungal disease that can go quickly to the brain (see Ch. 12).
3. Nasal septum deformation as in the breeding problem 'bent-nose' (Fara Shimbo, Ferret Unity and Registration Organization, Colorado, pers. comm. 1990).
4. Respiratory syncytial virus (RSV) was isolated from chimpanzees in 1956 and is considered a universally important pathogen in infant humans. In the chimpanzees, the disease caused coughing, sneezing and mucopurulent discharge. In humans, it can cause repeated infections throughout life and has been studied as a pathogen for ferrets by Prince and Porter.[60] The virus can cause bronchiolitis and interstitial pneumonia; they were able to replicate the virus in ferret kittens in the nasal tissue but not in the lungs. Although the clinical picture in the kittens showed no nasal discharges or mortality, the post mortem histological sections were consistent with mild rhinitis as seen in human infant infections. It was postulated that RSV could be more pathogenic in the younger animal and decreases in pathogenicity as the animal ages. An unknown mechanism, as the animal ages, acts in the lungs, but not the nose, to depress the pathogenicity of the virus. Thus if ferrets are somehow infected with such a virus from human contact, the nasal passage could harbour an ongoing infection similar to a repeat infection in humans.

Pseudomonas and ferrets

This organism is interesting as a possible pathogen in ferrets. It occurs widely in nature (compare cryptococcosis) and comprises over 140 species. *Pseudomonas aeruginosa* (syn. *pyocynea*) is one of three species pathogenic to man and animals.[61] It is found in soil, water, decaying vegetation and also found on skin, mucous membranes and in faeces. In mink, it causes haemorrhagic pneumonia and is fatal, affecting mink of all ages. It is associated with the stress of autumn moults in laboratory mink. The animals are usually found dead. In the UK, where escaped mink established themselves around rivers, the possibility of this disease of mink affecting other mustelids could be of future concern. In the old fitch farms in New Zealand, ferrets, like mink, would show a bloody nasal discharge and on post mortem signs of haemorrhagic pneumonia in one or more lung lobes. There is no cure but clinically disease-free stock can be vaccinated.[62]

Pseudomonas aeruginosa can become resistant to some antiseptics and disinfectants. In human hospitals it is considered difficult to eradicate the bacterium once it is established so some concern could run parallel with veterinary hospitals in the future.[63] It is found that *P. aeruginosa*, when injected s.c. into rabbits, guinea pigs and mice can produce fever and local abscess formation so its pathogenicity should not be underestimated in small mammals such as ferrets in the right circumstances.[64] Thus ferrets living outside in a garden or ferretarium may be as much at risk as hunting ferrets, which might get the disease in an abscess developing from a bite wound.

Ferret pneumonia

This is a complex and challenging subject; ferret pneumonia can be caused by a number of agents, including viruses, bacteria and parasites, as described in this chapter, plus pathogenic fungi and some internal parasites.

Bacterial pneumonia

The bacterial flora of the nasal cavity and mouth already indicated in relation to 'snuffles' can be implicated in bacterial pneumonia of ferrets. The group of PPLO organisms can feature in lung disease.

Mycoplasma (pleuropneumonia-like organisms: PPLO)

These are part of the normal flora in the respiratory tract of many animals. *Mycoplasma* causes specific diseases in cattle, sheep and goats, fowls and turkeys, mice and rats.[64] It is possible that PPLO are associated with more upper respiratory and pneumonia diseases in ferrets than has been recognized at the moment worldwide, being opportunistic in viral infections. Fox has stated that PPLO are to be found in clinically-normal ferrets as part of the bacterial flora of the mouth and nasal mucosa. This was seen in laboratory-kept ferrets in Japan. In addition, an organism labelled as *Mycoplasma mustelidae* was discovered from the lung tissue of clinically-normal mink kittens in mink farms in Denmark, but has not been recorded widely to date.[65]

The lungs can be invaded by various bacteria as a primary or secondary cause of pneumonia. It has been recorded that *Streptococcus* organisms, e.g. *S. zooepidemicus* along with *Streptococcus* Groups C and G, were implicated in a primary pneumonia as found at post mortem of a ferret after an influenza epidemic in a laboratory ferret colony. *Pseudomonas* infections in 'snuffles' can lead on to pneumonia as suggested earlier. The lungs of ferrets are susceptible to *E. coli* and *Klebsiella* infections along with *Bordetella bronchiseptica* pneumonia, which has been isolated from neonatal ferrets. Thus, there is a wide spectrum of pathogens possibly affecting ferret lungs.

Pneumonia symptoms: It is possible for pneumonia to arise from the nasal infection 'snuffles' with a continuous nasal discharge plus lethargy, pyrexia, anorexia, laboured breathing and increased lung sounds. Chronic cases of pneumonia have cyanotic membranes and cough with sepsis leading to death. A post mortem would show severe lung involvement with suppurative inflammation of all tissues infected.[65]

Diagnosis: This is on clinical signs with radiology and blood check. Examination of tracheal washings is suggested with cats but this might be too stressful for ferrets, especially with severe breathing difficulties. Radiology shows the pattern of alveolar destruction as with other animals. The CBC shows typically elevated total white cells of 20 000 or higher.[66] For differential diagnosis of ferret pneumonia there could be an underlying cardiomyopathy. With outside-living ferrets, there could be heartworm infection, fungal infection, e.g. *Cryptococcus neoformans* or a secondary cancer condition.

Treatment: The use of broad-spectrum antibiotics, good nursing with fluid therapy and possibly forced feeding is the key to success but can be difficult to attain. Chloramphenicol injectable has been a good first choice before sensitivity results are available but resistance is possible as seen with 'snuffles' cases. No oral chloramphenicol is available but the injectable form can be adapted to be given orally. A strong sugar solution is needed, as it is very bitter. Oral trimethoprim-sulfamethoxazole is another useful first-choice antibiotic and synthetic penicillins, like ampicillin.

Chemical-induced pneumonia in ferrets

Chemicals in the air are a major public worry and will also affect ferrets. Aerosol sprays should not be used around ferrets and they should not be left, even for a short while, in underground car parks while their owners go shopping, as they can succumb to petroleum fumes toxicity.

Botulism

Botulism is one of the clostridial infections that can be fatal to ferrets. With ferrets kept outside in a garden, ferretarium or cage, the ferret's tendency to hoard food can be a serious risk to health, especially in hot climates. This is one reason why I decided to feed my ferrets a definite amount of food, initially to eat overnight, so there would be no waste or storing away of food that might spoil the next day.

Free-living indoor ferrets are known to store food in odd places, in and under cupboards, under the fridge, etc. Fortunately, the bacterium is susceptible to antibiotics but the effects on the nervous system of the endotoxin produced by the organism are rapid. Ferrets, like mink, are less resistant to endotoxin effects than are dogs or other carnivores. The type C toxin is highly lethal. *Clostridia* bacteria multiply in decaying carcasses so that working ferrets could be at risk coming across a dead rat or rabbit if they are hungry. Thus ferrets should have some food before working warrens (Bert Geddes, Ferreter, Perth, WA, pers. comm. 1985).

Clinical signs: These occur 18–96 hours after consumption of the botulism toxin, with the ferret showing paralysis, which starts with the hind legs and continues to extend forward for some days. Sensation remains and there is usually no temperature rise. Respiration is shallow with partial paralysis of the intercostals and diaphragm. Salivation, protrusion of the third eyelid, not usually easily seen in ferrets, occurs and finally death results from respiratory failure.

CHAPTER EIGHT

Viral, bacterial and mycotic diseases

Diagnosis: Done on vomitus, scats or suspect stomach contents at post mortem.

Treatment: Must be quick if the disease is suspected. Most cases will die. The ferret is treated with penicillin, vitamin injections and forced feeding. One may get a cure but it takes time. In mink farms, heavy losses can occur with botulism but it is considered that if mink are alive after the 4th day they will get better in 2–3 weeks. Mink can be vaccinated.[62]

Prevention: Vaccination with a *Clostridium botulinum* type C vaccine is done with mink but is impractical with house or garden pet ferrets. Ferreters with numbers of working ferrets might be able to get in with a local sheep farmer to have stock vaccinated with the sheep. Removing excessive food from the ferret is the best method. Ferrets usually sleep during the day, especially in hot climates, (unless working) and should be encouraged to eat late evening or late evening and early morning.

Leptospirosis

Ferreters are aware that using ferrets, in conjunction usually with Jack Russell terriers, to clear out rats and mice in hay sheds, exposes them to rat and mice urine that might contain *Leptospira* organisms. Ferrets have a natural resistance to infection but *L. grippotyphosa* and *L. icterohaemorrhagica* have been isolated from ferrets.[67] In New Zealand, no evidence of leptoviral antigens could be found in a selection of wild weasels, stoats and ferrets. In another survey, a low percentage of stoats in Denmark showed exposure to the bacterium, while weasels and polecats checked were negative. In the UK, however, serological titres for serovars sejroe and Bratislava were detected in weasels.[30] One author does not include leptospirosis in a list of ferret zoonoses.[2]

Clinical signs: The typical findings in the dog include fever, sore muscles, stiffness, weakness, anorexia, depression, vomiting and rapid dehydration. There is possibly bloody diarrhoea, icterus, spontaneous cough and difficulty in breathing. There is polyuria and polydipsia followed later by no urination. Bloody vaginal discharge can be present. Deaths can occur without clinical signs.[68] Relating these symptoms to a possible ferret case shows the wide range of presenting signs. I have known of a ferret with severe jaundice, after definitely eating a mouse. The ferret died even with antibiotic treatment. Unfortunately, no post mortem was possible.

Treatment: Use of penicillin G given i.m. 40 000 IU/kg q.24 h or divide q.12 h until kidney function returns in such cases. Alternatives to penicillin are ampicillin or amoxicillin. Regarding dogs, dihydrostreptomycin is used to eliminate *Leptospira* from the kidney interstitial tissue. (10–15 mg/kg, i.m. q.12 h for 2 weeks). Streptomycin was used if the animal was not in renal failure.[68] Ferrets should not be given any more than 50 mg streptomycin if using the drug at 12-h intervals, as it is toxic in high doses.[26] Now streptomycin is not available on the drug list.

Author's clinical example

Ferret botulism case

A 3-month-old sable hob, Jack, was presented with the insidious onset of paralysis, beginning classically in the hind limbs and moving forwards to involve the forelimbs over a period of 4–5 days (Christmas 1993). He also had green diarrhoea, which was considered later a suspect sign of epizootic catarrhal enteritis (ECE) type disease but not proved. Jack's appetite remained good and he had attempted to play but it became more difficult as time progressed. Clinically, the temperature was normal. Respiration rate had spurts of laboured breathing consistent with respiratory muscle toxicity. Cranial nerve function seemed unaffected but motor reflexes were diminished in both fore and hind limbs. Urine analysis indicated elevated bilirubin levels. Jack unfortunately had a history of food hoarding in the house. Botulism was soon suspected.

Treatment: This consisted of a penicillin injection i.m. and vitamin B$_1$. He was also commenced then on amoxicillin drops (Beechams) at 1 mL twice daily for 10 days, plus he was given a Felobit tablet crushed and concealed in 2 teaspoons of plain yoghurt as a supportive measure. (*Note* the yoghurt might well have helped with the green diarrhoea.) Jack took 3 months to recover with a lot of TLC from his anxious owner.

A follow-up of Jack found that he led a normal life but remained small. A result of being so ill in his growing period? At 5 years of age, Jack started adopting a vague/spaced out stare, remaining standing, but had minor twitching of the whole body. The twitching lasted 15–30 seconds and was intermittent in episodes. He also developed a hind leg weakness. An insulinoma attack might be suggested? However, blood tests were taken with normal results. Fasting blood glucose was taken as well, using another ferret of similar age, colour and sex as a control. The results were normal.

External examinations/palpation found no abnormalities but Jack began to lose weight approximately 2 months after the onset of the vagueness/twitching episodes. He also had some bouts of nausea. Jack continued to deteriorate and after 5 months, he was put to sleep. An exploratory laparotomy had shown no gross abnormalities and a post mortem by a pathologist who had an interest in ferrets found there were certainly no other abnormalities except that one brain hemisphere was a little smaller than the other. Was this some result of the botulism toxicosis in the past?

Val Hucheon, Victoria, Australia, pers. comm. 2005.

I do not feed my animals outside. My ferret Pip, let out into the garden one evening after being fed, then killed a rat and refused to give it up. He would not come in and could have eaten it overnight. The next morning his character changed. He was not his 'weasel' dancing self but somewhat depressed. He did not stop eating however but was more inclined to curl up and sleep. The depression idea panicked me. Was he a leptospirosis case? On the other hand, he could have had a stomachache! He was given amoxicillin 10 mg/kg orally b.i.d. and Animalac to drink as I worried that his depression might be liver function related. He continued for a couple of days to be edgy and non-cooperative. Then he seemed to come out of it, became alert and was taking interest again. Had he been infected by eating the rat? Had my quick intervention with an antibiotic done the trick? I had no blood tests etc. done. I had wondered about vaccination but leptospirosis vaccination is only possible by using a 5-1 vaccine. I might have to consider such vaccination. If ferrets do have a natural resistance to *Leptospira*, could I be worrying for nothing?

Tuberculosis (TB)

Tuberculosis is a serious wasting disease in relation to human health and from this aspect, the presence of *Mycobacterium bovis* etc. in wild and domestic animals is always of concern. Ferrets can get bovine, avian or human strains of tubercle bacillus. In a UK 2002 review, the role of the badger (*Meles meles*) as a reservoir host was discussed.[69] The fox (*Vulpes vulpes*) has been found infected but this was probably due either to its scavenging infected deer carcasses or its habit of occupying abandoned badger setts. In the Mustelidae, negative results were found in a MAFF survey (1996–97) for the stoat (*Mustela erminea*), weasel (*M. nivalis*) and polecat (*M. putorius*) but one positive was found in a mink (*M. vison*) and a second in a stray ferret (*M. furo*).

Mink are feral in the UK having been released from mink farms. The authors note that TB had been found in farmed mink in 1936. Feral ferrets do exist and some have mated with polecats but the density of feral ferrets is nothing to the problem apparently with feral ferrets in New Zealand. It is interesting that six TB cases were found in the domestic cat (*Felis domesticus*).

An otter (*Lutra lutra*) was suspect for TB and again it was surmised that this was because otters had the habit of visiting abandoned badger setts. This could be the reason for an odd feral ferret or polecat cross being infected with TB as they are inquisitive animals. The UK MAFF survey failed to find any native polecats with TB. Tuberculosis infection was found in the mole (*Talpa europaea*) and the brown rat (*Rattus norvegicus*). These are pasture and barn animals so closer to cattle areas.

The question of badger involvement with bovine tuberculosis in the UK and the role of rabbits have been discussed at length.[70–72]

Fox reports on early cases of TB in research facility ferrets in the UK and Europe.[65] The disease was considered rare in the UK.[73] Pet ferret cases of TB were recorded in Germany in 1997 (Henke, G., Berlin, pers. comm. 1999). In the USA, *Mycobacterium avium* was found in a ferret on laparotomy for suspected granulomatous enteritis.[74] A single case of *Mycobacterium microti* was found in a ferret which possibly ate a vole (R. Malik, pers. comm. 2005).

In Norway, a case of *Mycobacterium celatum* (type 3), which affects humans, was found in a 4-year-old male ferret in March 1999.[75] It was noted that there could be a possibility of infection from humans where ferrets were kept as indoor pets. The ferret lost weight and showed coughing over a period of 6 months. It was depressed on examination and showed dyspnoea, dehydration, emaciation and a poor coat. The lungs showed harsh dry sound on auscultation and a radiograph revealed both lungs with multiple disseminated nodular and peribronchial densities. The lung parenchyma looked cystic and the animal was euthanized as the prognosis was grave.

Post mortem results showed an extensive mycobacterial infection with granulomatous inflammations in the lungs and the stomach, with extensive acid-fast bacteria in epithelioid cells and macrophages. Special identification kits were used and the PCR procedure carried out to give a result of *Myobacterium celatum* present as long, slender, sometimes branching bacteria in the ferret tissues.

Person-to-person transmission of non-tuberculous mycobacteria has not been demonstrated, but the ferret did live within a household and would be shedding *Myobacterium celatum* in oral lung excretions and faeces. Thus, the environment would have been contaminated. In humans, immunocompromised patients may show isolates of the bacterium. The pet ferret did not have a history of previous disease so was unlikely to have been immunodeficient. However, in the case of chronic respiratory disease in a ferret, mycobacterial infection is a rare but possible cause.

In Australia, Lucas et al. (2000) recorded two ferrets with *Mycobacterium genavense* infection.[76] This is a new species in the *Mycobacterium avium* complex (MAC) and has been associated with human patients with AIDS and generally as a bird pathogen. The two ferrets were seen by vets regarding eye problems. A 5-year-old castrated sable ferret had hyperplasia of the conjunctiva of the right eye and a peripheral lymphadenomegaly. The second 4-year-old silver jill ferret had a swelling of the conjunctiva of the left eye (Fig. 8.9). The general condition of the two ferrets was unremarkable.

CHAPTER EIGHT

Viral, bacterial and mycotic diseases

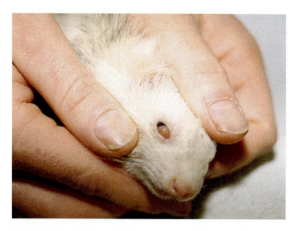

Figure 8.9 Silver jill with swelling of conjunctiva due to *Mycobacterium genavense*. (Courtesy of Dr R. Malik, Post Graduate Foundation in Veterinary Science, University of Sydney.)

The 1200 g male was anaesthetized and smears taken from FNA of the popliteal lymph node, which suggested a mycobacterial infection, i.e. acid-fast bacteria (AFB). The 700 g jill was first treated with antibiotic tetracycline eye ointment with no effect and was later anaesthetized and a section of the swollen conjunctival tissue was taken for histology testing, which proved positive for AFB, with an associated possible mycobacterial rhinitis and cellulitis. Later, biopsy material from both ferrets was RNA tested using the polymerase chain reaction (PCR) and *Myobacterium genavense* was confirmed in both animals.

After examination under anaesthesia for tissue samples, both ferrets recovered and were put on oral medication for the myobacterial infection. The male received 30 mg rifampicin, 12.5 mg clofazimine and 31.25 mg clarithromycin once daily. The antimicrobial agents were well taken in Energel supplement. However, after 3 months, the ferret became inappetent though it was considered cured. It became rapidly worse and had azotaemia, hyperphosphataemia and isosthenuria and was euthanized with suspected renal failure.

The female deteriorated during the days following the biopsy operation. She went on to become depressed, inactive and somewhat aggressive when handled. However, she was given 14 mg rifampicin daily starting 7 days post-biopsy. She did improve and settled down in 4 weeks. At 8 weeks, the medication was stopped but 2 months later, the jill showed a moribund state with an enlarged abdominal mass, which was possibly an ovarian tumour, and died. Unfortunately, a post mortem was not allowed. (I have seen aggressive behaviour in one of my albino jills suffering an ovarian tumour.) Lucas et al. point out that *Myobacterium genavense* is an important avian pathogen but had only twice been reported in companion mammals.

Lunn et al. in Australia (2005) isolated the first cases of pneumonia due to *Mycobacterium abscessus* in two ferrets in the Sydney area.[77] Both ferrets suffered from a chronic pneumonia and were from the same household living indoors but out in the garden for short periods during the day. Both ferrets were on prophylaxis for heartworm (*Dirofilaria immitis*). The two ferrets were presented for examination 6 months apart.

Ferret A was a 560 g 2-year-old sterilized jill with a history of coughing and lethargy for 6 weeks. The ferret had been losing weight as the condition had worsened. The ferret was lean on presentation with increased thoracic breath sounds on both sides. On tracheal palpation, a dry unproductive coughing was initiated. Initially treatment involved doxycycline (5 mg/kg b.i.d.) p.o. (Pfizer Vibravet paste) for 3 weeks, whereby the ferret coughed less and improved over a week. However, the ferret deteriorated in the latter weeks and was represented showing a weight loss to 490 g with more frequent coughing.

A bronchoalveolar lavage (BAL) was decided on to check lung infection. This technique involved the ferret being under isoflurane anaesthesia (Ch. 16). *Note*: butorphanol (0.1 mg/kg s.c.) and midazolam (0.5 mg/kg s.c.) were pre-meds. The ferret was pre-oxygenated with 100% oxygen (flow rate 2 L/min) and then masked down with isoflurane. Next, it was tubed and left on isoflurane at 1.5–2.5%. The ferret breathed spontaneously and radiographs were taken.

The BAL involved allowing the ferret to recover the cough reflex after the isoflurane was discontinued. An open-ended sterile infant feeding tube (3½ French) was passed through the lumen of the endotracheal tube to wedge in the main bronchus. Then 2 mL aliquots of warm saline were injected and immediately aspirated and sent for culture. The ferret recovered well after the ordeal and went home to await culture results. (Diff Quik examination of aspirate showed mucus with numerous inflammatory cells, 91%.)

Blood agar culture aerobically at 25–37°C for 5 days found AFBs which were typed as *Mycobacterium abscessus* by the Queensland Mycobacterium Reference Laboratory. *Myobacterium abscessus* is classified as a rapid growth mycobacterium unlike slow-growing avian species. Quick accurate diagnosis of these dangerous conditions is vital. (Eight other rapid growth mycobacterium (RGM) species exist.) The *M. abscessus* was sensitive to clarithromycin but resistant to many other drugs: enrofloxacin, orbifloxacin, chloramphenicol, doxycycline and the sulfa drugs.

Treatment: The clarithromycin (powder form) was used in oral solution at 150 g/5 mL b.i.d. over 3 months, when the ferret was re-examined and found to be recovering. Body weight was back to 5600 g, so the treatment was stopped as the coughing was becoming rare.

Ferret B was a repeat of Ferret A's condition and underwent the same treatment plus surgery for enlarged spleen and left adrenal gland disease. It had developed alopecia, pruritus and coughing. After surgery, it was placed on prednisolone (1 mg/kg) p.o. daily but its alopecia persisted. It improved on medication and was taken off clarithromycin.

Mycobacterium abscessus is a ubiquitous environmental organism and as dangerous as *Cryptococcus neoformans* (Ch. 12). Being in soil, water and decaying material gives a wide scope for infection of ferrets outside and it can colonize pipes. *Myobacterium abscessus* is saprophytic and infection may be by contamination of wounds, aerosol inhalation, or water. It is apparently more easily treatable than *Cryptococcus neoformans* as long there are effective antibiotics to call on.

The causes predisposing ferrets to develop disseminated mycobacteriosis are not clearly understood, though ferrets digging and 'nosing' soil is a problem. It is known from some epidemiological evidence that ferrets could become infected with a retrovirus capable of inducing a lymphoma but at the moment, there is no evidence that the virus concerned, if it exists, can cause immune deficiency. It can be noted that cryptococcosis, lymphoma and disseminated mycobacteriosis all occur in ferrets so it is theorized that ferrets might have their own immunodeficiency virus. This might indicate cause in the above ferrets with TB and with my two ferrets with cryptococcosis in 1996/97.

In New Zealand, there was concern about feral ferrets being vectors for bovine TB along with possums, deer, pigs, goats, cats and stoats.[78] In May 1994, a report on ferrets, weasels, stoats and cats, tuberculosis in many cases is considered to come from them eating infected carcasses. In one of the TB endemic areas in 1992/93, tuberculosis-positive wild ferrets were found, while ferrets and cats have been incriminated in some cattle breakdowns. The Animal Health Bureau, NZ considered that in a country overrun with rabbits, the ferret prey, ferrets are likely to be the major vector of TB for cattle and deer.[78] The report was concerned about the slow acceptance by veterinary interests of the potential role of other vectors.

It considered that the wide distribution of wild (feral) ferrets and the prevalence of TB in ferrets in some areas highlighted a potential additional vector problem. In the ferrets' defence, they may be important as rabbit calicivirus disease (RCD) vectors. It is known that rabbit calicivirus can survive passage through the dog intestine and can also be transported on external surfaces, so it is thought likely that feral ferrets working burrows move the virus around rabbit areas. As young rabbits are not susceptible to RCD, the use of feral ferrets as a vector for RCD could be important.[79] Thus, the elimination of wild ferrets would increase wild rabbits. There was an opinion that no conclusive proof has been found that ferrets have passed TB on to any other species (Ginkel, M.V. Technical Advisory Officer, MAF New Zealand, pers. comm. 1998).

Further work in New Zealand found that tuberculous possums were the major underlying cause of *Myobacterium bovis* in ferrets.[80] It is also noted that horizontal transmission of *M. bovis* could occur in ferrets in experimental housing conditions.[81] The occurrence of ferret infection with *M. bovis* was found higher by assessing lymph nodes of ferrets carrying the disease but not yet showing symptoms.[82] Thus the feral ferret is a victim of being susceptible, from being let loose in the first place and thus exposed to a terrible disease, TB.

New Zealand fitch farms in their heyday had problems with TB in ferrets due to the eating of infected meat. Therefore, the meat or offal food had to be obtained only from TB-tested cattle. Fitch ferrets were protected from avian TB by bird-proofing the fitch houses and keeping infected poultry and other bird carcasses off the diet. Possibility of the spread of human TB between human and fitch was considered remote.[83] Possum meat, which could be TB-infected, in the fitch diet in some regions of NZ was a concern (Ch. 4). The use of possum meat for feeding working ferrets in the past might be why ferrets were thought to spread TB to cattle.

Mycobacterial disease

Clinical signs: Weakness and wasting with tuberculosis could be confused with Aleutian disease and hind leg weakness with botulism in suspect working or pet ferrets. Bovine mycobacteria cause weight loss, anorexia, lethargy and death. TB-affected farmed mink in the UK and USA show weight loss, emaciation, some abdominal distension, enlarged spleen and lymph nodes and TB is another reason why mink should not be reared near fitch ferrets.[62]

Bovine TB strains tend to be more disseminated around the animal body as infected tubercles while human and avian TB strains provoke local slow-growing tubercular infections. *Note*: because the TB clinical signs in ferrets and mink can at first be vague, there is high zoonotic concern with regard to possible spread to humans as seen in example cases.

Diagnosis: Tubercular lesions are usually found post mortem but they can be picked up by radiography. TB testing of ferrets is possible and has been done

CHAPTER EIGHT
Viral, bacterial and mycotic diseases

experimentally using Freund's complete adjuvant (FCA), which contains killed *Myobacterium tuberculosis*, with a reaction to 10 000 units (200 μg) of tuberculin. However, there are inconsistencies; mink in a colony tested with bovine tuberculin i.d. did not show any delayed hypersensitivity reaction.

Prevention: Farmed ferrets and mink are not treated for bovine TB but culled from farms and breeding establishments. Incidence, if any, is very rare and especially with controlled diets. Bovine TB has been eliminated in Australia. It is said that pet or working ferrets are protected by being on commercially prepared foods. However, these foods themselves could produce possible problems and should be avoided in favour of fresh, infection-clear meats fit for human consumption (Ch. 4).

Listeriosis

Listeriosis has been recorded since 1926 as one of the food-borne diseases and an active animal pathogen.[84] The bacterium is a saprophyte and common in soils. The two pathogenic *Listeria* are *L. monocytogenes* and *L. ivanovii*. Both these agents have groups of genes that facilitate invasion, survival, multiplication and mobility in the intracellular environment. People handling stock can get the disease, people and animals also get it from infected food or feeds. Apart from these contacts, there is no clear evidence of *Listeria* passing between humans and animals or vice versa. In the UK, there appears to be an autumn peak of human listeriosis and a spring peak for animal listeriosis so the two groups do not have a causal relationship. The incubation period between contact with infected food and disease onset can be from 1–90 days. The possibility of serious infection of humans is very low through the food chain. It is important to prevent contamination from the processing environment, which is from raw products or plant and machinery.

This disease can be highly fatal in many animals including ferrets and man, though, as noted above, it had been thought a really mild pathogen. Medical clinicians saw an increase in cases in the 1980s around the world.[84] Fox et al. recorded the presence of *Listeria monocytogenes* in a ferret with adrenal gland disease and cardiomyopathy with concurrent pneumonia and hepatitis. A Russian sable (*Mustela zibellina*) has been shown to carry the organism.[65] *Listeria* is considered a potential risk to ferrets alongside TB and *Salmonella*.[29] Infection can be from soil, which is comparable with cryptococcosis, and clinical signs would be of CNS involvement. Treatment would require very broad-spectrum antibiotics with CNS penetration ability.

Salmonellosis

Food poisoning: a problem of contaminated meat, to be differentiated from botulism. If feeding ferrets natural meat, should it be cooked or uncooked? The latter can be the subject of quick contamination in the Australian climate but it is known for humans to get salmonellosis from market meat products. The Gram-negative facultative anaerobes, *Salmonella newport*, *S. typhimurium* and *S. choleraesuis* have been associated with diseases in ferrets.[3] With ferrets on a meat diet, I have had only one case of salmonellosis, associated with idiopathic otitis interna.[85] The *Salmonella* involved were *S. lavana* in kangaroo meat pet food and *S. muenchen* in butchers' mince. Only one ferret in a colony of 10 was affected. Kangaroo and poultry are considered by some to be high-risk meats for *Salmonella* contamination. Ferreters who are shooters feed their ferrets fresh and frozen culled kangaroo without trouble (A. Geddes, ferreter, Perth, pers. comm. 1998). Some ferret breeders promote feeding day-old chicks. Working ferrets can be fed killed rabbit and will eat the whole carcass including the viscera.

Salmonellosis is considered the most common zoonotic disease in humans, but producing only a gastroenteritis.[86] It is generally known that in most animals *Salmonella* is asymptomatic; these animals can become carriers, including ferrets.

Clinical signs: include vomiting, diarrhoea, fever, inappetence, malaise, abdominal pain and dehydration.

Diagnosis: from the clinical signs and culture of the vomitus or faeces for the Gram-negative pathogen, which can be typed. At post mortem, *Salmonella* is cultured from internal organs.

Epizootology: *Salmonella* disease occurrence is relatively rare in ferrets but has been associated in the past with fitch and mink farms where disease outbreaks could occur from contaminated food. *Salmonella choleraesuis* has been isolated from mink in abortions and ferrets are likewise affected at some times. In a USA survey of laboratory ferrets, various *Salmonella* serotypes were found in the scats, being *S. hadar*, *S. enteritidis*, *S. kentucky* and *S. typhimurium*; the infection was blamed on uncooked meat.[3] A 1965 UK medical microbiology book referring to ferrets advises feeding raw meat and gives no indication of *Salmonella* as a disease of laboratory ferrets.[63] Stress is given as a factor leading to salmonellosis in dogs and cats in overcrowded situations and this could also be said for ferrets. Perhaps in the UK in 1965, laboratory ferrets were not as stressed as they are today? Other possible stresses on ferrets could be unsanitary conditions; in the veterinary hospital, there is conjecture that anaesthetics, surgery and even antibiotics could bring on stress or just the mere change of food/water is said to produce stress in animals and this could be true of both ferrets and mink.

Differential diagnosis: Must include canine distemper, botulism and colibacillosis.

Treatment: Must be by the precise use of the specified antibiotic so that the carrier states can be eliminated plus attention to replacement fluid balance by use of i.v. catheters or s.c. injections.

Colibacillosis

The normal mouth and intestinal flora of the ferret has been recorded.[87] It is known that under some circumstances, organisms can become pathogenic and *Escherichia coli* is one, as seen in 'snuffles'. This gram-negative bacterium is also isolated in acute diarrhoea cases in neonatal ferrets, as it has been picked up in sick puppies and kittens (J. Bell, pers. comm. 1996). The *E. coli* found in the scats does not necessarily point to infection but blood-borne bacteria are highly suspicious. I have seen adult unsterilized unmated jill ferrets, which had developed post-oestrous anaemia (POA), die with a high blood *E. coli*.[57] Ferret kittens may be born to jills, which begin an endometritis for some reason, and the kittens are at risk of a coliform infection. This is seen in aging jills. Thus, jills with poor nutrition and colostrum deficiency can produce sickly kittens and all factors of poor husbandry can play a part.

Treatment: Sick ferrets with colibacillosis showing acute enteritis and septicaemia should have rehydration fluids, good nutrition and warmth plus a suitable broad-spectrum antibiotic based on bacterial culture. Toxicity to some drugs may be higher in ferrets than dogs and cats, e.g. doxycycline (Vibravet Paste, Pfizer) is a fluoroquinolone, which should not be used in young kittens as it causes cartilage damage.

Prognosis: With young ferrets it is guarded, though the possibility of zoonosis between the kittens and ferret owner is unlikely compared with salmonellosis. However, young children who are fascinated by young ferret kittens should be kept well away and any immunosuppressed people should avoid contact with them. Standard hygiene procedures should apply after handling sick ferrets.

Note the condition of haemolytic uraemia syndrome involving *Escherichia coli* has been studied.[88] Fifteen strains of beta-haemolytic *E. coli*, from diarrhoea and diseased tissues of infected ferrets, were found positive in specific PCR assays showing the presence of the candidate virulence factor strains CNF1, hlyA and pap1. The authors suggested s further study of the bacterial strains. *Note*: the gastrointestinal 'wasting' diseases are discussed in detail by Burgess in Chapter 9.

Anaerobic bacterial diseases

Anaerobic bacteria are of interest when considering ferrets found in unhygienic conditions and possibly working ferrets which have been involved in fights but have not had wounds immediately attended to, as with ferreters going bush. They should be of historical interest only but are worth looking out for with regard to working ferrets. A number of species of non-sporing anaerobic Gram-negative rod-like bacteria inhabit the oral cavity, upper respiratory tract, intestinal tract, and genital tract in man and animals.[89] Some of these organisms have been isolated in inflammatory processes, particularly accompanied by necrosis and ulceration. Many of these bacteria have been overlooked in bacteriological diagnosis because they grow only under strict anaerobic conditions and need special growth media for isolation.

Examples: Fusiformis species (now *Dichelobacter nodosus*); *Bacteroides* species (*Bacteroides fragilis*)

Cultures of these organisms have a characteristic foetid odour and they grow only with difficulty from serum, blood and tissue in anaerobic conditions with excess CO_2. These two anaerobic species are however obligate parasites of man and animals and may under certain conditions become pathogenic and invade tissues. Usually the anaerobic bacteria are found mixed with other organisms, e.g. *E. coli*, and it is difficult to know if they are invaders.

Fusiformis

Fusiformis infection used to occur in ferrets in unsanitary conditions and was called 'footrot' by ferreters as it is a disease akin to footrot in sheep.

Symptoms: The ferret develops raw sore necrotic feet pads with progressive tissue destruction. The infection should rarely, if ever, be observed now, except in cases of ferret neglect in wet muddy areas. It has been known in the past in Australia and the UK. *Note*: nowadays it would be a case for the RSPCA. Footrot should not be confused with mange in ferrets, as some ferreters are prone to call mange footrot, which it is not. Ferret mange (from sarcoptic scabies mite) should be called foot mange as it develops basically from the feet and thus the confusion with footrot.

Treatment: by isolation of affected ferrets in dry conditions and treating with sheep footrot preparation spray.

CHAPTER EIGHT
Viral, bacterial and mycotic diseases

Bacteroides

These types of infections I have seen in swollen lesions in the groin of a working ferret, which had a history of fighting. When the lesion was excised under G/A, it revealed a terrible-smelling pus-filled gland, which had to be completely excised. The foetid pus was produced by a heavy growth of a mixture of *Bacteroides* and *E. coli* found on laboratory culture.

Treatment: This is by daily chloramphenicol injections with the wound left open to drain and flushed daily with hydrogen peroxide. The treatment takes over 2 weeks to resolve the wound. *Note* that some *Bacteroides* infections are drug-resistant and can lead to deaths in ferrets.

Streptococcus/Staphylococcus infections

Streptococcus and *Staphylococcus* bacteria, along with *E. coli*, affect pet ferrets similarly to fitch ferrets and mink.[90] *Streptococcus* infections occur in kittens where the jill has sustained a milk-borne infection due to unhygienic conditions. *Staphylococcus* infections are associated with mastitis, acute and chronic, in the lactating jill and will be the major cause of deaths of the litter and even the jill if not treated promptly.[91] Working ferrets, especially hobs, if fighting during the mating season, can sustain *Staphylococcus*-infected wound abscesses (Fig. 8.10). Therefore, hobs should be kept separate during this time. Working ferrets have the chance of being bitten by feral cats or kicked by buck rabbits. Requires drainage under G/A.

A dental abscess at the root of a broken tooth was seen in one ferret as a swelling on the side of the face

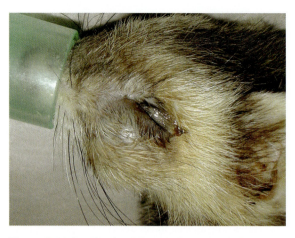

Figure 8.11 Swollen ferret face from canine root abscess. (Courtesy of William Lewis, The Wylie Veterinary Centre, Essex, UK.)

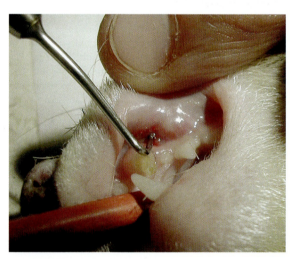

Figure 8.12 View of broken canine tooth of upper jaw. (Courtesy of William Lewis.)

below the eye (Fig. 8.11). With the animal under gaseous G/A and tubed, inspection of the broken tooth showed pus from the infected gum (Fig. 8.12). With the broken tooth removed, an awl was passed upwards from the mouth to open up the root abscess which was drained as shown in Figure 8.13. With the flushing of the wound, healing was commenced under antibiotic cover. Laboratory ferrets can sustain abscesses from sharp objects in cages and breeding colonies should be monitored for males fighting near the mating season.[92]

Staphylococcus infections can occur in the ferret mouth due to bone spicules, where the ferret's powerful bite forces a spicule deep into the tissues. It can

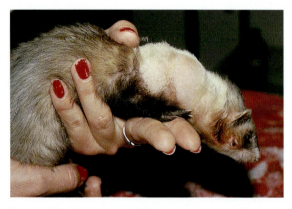

Figure 8.10 My hob ferret, Sammy, after being bitten. *Note* the swelling on dorsal part of neck – soft abscess, opened under G/A and drained.

Mycotic diseases of ferrets

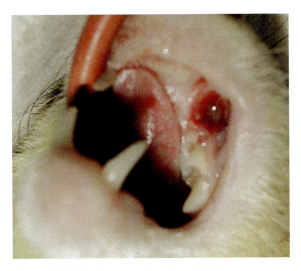

Figure 8.13 Tooth removed and pus draining. (Courtesy of William Lewis.)

result in a submandibular swelling and mucocele of the sublingual tissues.[57] Sublingual mucoceles are tight fluid-filled cavities on the ranula of the tongue (see Fig. 2.16). Mucoceles can also occur in the salivary glands if damaged by sharp objects such as penetrating grass seed awns.

Treatment: By a general anaesthetic, incision of the mucocele and antibiotic cover. Once incised and cut, the surface is dressed with a swab of dilute iodine to kill the surface cells. Salivary gland mucoceles require incision and possible removal of the salivary gland by delicate surgery. The positions of the five salivary glands are shown in Figure 2.14.

Grass seed abscesses

In Western Australia and many countries with hot dry summers, ferrets living outside or working ferrets face the problem of grass seed awns penetrating the skin. Hob ferrets can get suppurative wounds in the groin and penis sheath due to grass awn penetration, when working in the bush or simply urine-marking their territory, by moving along the ground, pressing their groin area down, urinating and chattering as they go. *Staphylococcus* abscesses are the result. For this reason ferrets should not be bedded down or play in hay in large sheds or ferret courts. Straw is better.

Treatment: An abscess requires vigorous attention with surgical drainage and flushing the wound plus essential broad-spectrum antibiotic cover. Liquid or paste drugs are preferred and are easily administered; the owner should be encouraged to give a complete course to prevent development of drug resistance.

With reference to possible antibiotic resistance, the presence of vancomycin resistant enterococci (VRE) has been found in New Zealand food animals.[93] Nearly 90% of VRE isolates were recovered from broilers and this has happened in Australia. The possibility of drug resistant microbes affecting ferrets fed on chicken produce could then happen?

Mycotic diseases of ferrets

Skin pathogens: Skin mycotic diseases affecting ferrets are uncommon.

Ringworm: The common fungal invader of dogs, cats and ferrets. Includes *Microsporum canis* and *Trichophyton mentagrophytes*. I have never come across ringworm. It would be a zoonosis problem, as with cats, especially with small children. There is a record of a ferret colony which did get infected from a cat as did some mink, where cats were allowed to sleep in bedding stored for the mink.[94] Ryland also recorded *Microsporum canis* in young ferrets possibly infected by cats.[26] Spread of disease is by contact between animals or with contaminated areas of bedding and thus housed ferrets in colonies are at risk.

Animal attendants could be infected and the zoonosis aspect of skin fungi is well known. Attention to separating infected ferrets ands strict hygiene is required.

Clinical signs: Classic ringworm lesions, with young animals to be most at risk. The circular areas of alopecia and inflammation can occur anywhere on the body. The skin becomes thickened, itchy and then scaly.

Diagnosis: Usually by the Wood's lamp technique and checking hairs microscopically for the characteristic arthrospores.

Treatment: Any infected ferrets can be treated with griseofulvin at 25 mg/kg by mouth but the disease can be self-limiting.

Mucormycosis

Seen in New Zealand fitch farm ferrets, the fungus *Absidia corymbifera* (syn. *ramosa*) was commonly found in association with *Otodectes cynotis*. It is not normally present in ferret ears though it is widespread in the environment like other fungi.[95] The avoidance of mouldy litter is advised. Strict cage disinfection was standard practice in fitch farms.

Clinical signs: Ear scratching is the classic sign of ear mite and along with it fungal infection found in the brown earwax. In severe cases, the ferret may be depressed and lethargic. A torticollis is seen as associated with inner ear infections (Ch. 12). There is a loss of balance, circling, even prostration, with the affected ear turned down towards the body (see Fig. 12.5). The disease can lead to damage to the petrous temporal bone showing granulomatous inflammation and necrosis with a following granulomatous meningoencephalitis. In extreme infection the temporal and pyriform lobes of the cerebrum show lesions, which may appear on the cerebellum and brainstem areas.[94]

Diagnosis: By finding the ear mites associated with the fungi in external auditory wax. The fungus can be extracted from the regional lymph nodes and demonstrated on tissue section.

Treatment: Requires the immediate removal of the ear mites and ear cleaning. The question of antibiotic use on the fungus is questionable in itself as the antibiotic might predispose the ferrets to getting a secondary fungal infection. Possibly prevention is better than cure in this condition and keeping ears clear of mites is the right way to go.

Malassezia infection

Malassezia is becoming responsible for increasing incidence of dermatitis especially in dogs. The most common yeast is opportunistic in skin and ear infections to cause extreme pruritis.[96] *Malassezia pachydermatis* is the most common of seven species of the yeast and isolated especially from the dog and less so from the cat. *Note*: it is on the skin, in anal sacs and in mucus of healthy cats who also may have *M. sympodialis* and *M. globosa*. Dogs and cats can be companions in a household situation along with pet ferrets.

Malassezia species have been associated with ferrets in the UK.[97] In a colony of 50 ferrets, eight developed crusting and necrosis of the ear pinnae. The disease spread to another six ferrets with all ferrets having *Otodectes* sp. infection. It was considered that *M. pachydermatis* was acting as an opportunistic pathogen. An ear infection is liable to spread to the face. With the infected ferrets, treatment with topical betamethasone, neomycin and monosulfiram failed and the ear pinnae had to be ablated. Histologically the involved epidermis had inflammatory cells and yeast beneath the corneum but no acanthosis. However, large areas of necrosis and haemorrhage were seen.

Diagnosis: Again earwax material will show *Malassezia* yeast cells on microscope inspection. The cells measure 3–8 μm in diameter; they are round or oval and usually in clusters.

Treatment: With the UK ferrets, oral ketoconazole at 5–10 mg/kg b.i.d. and topical application of miconazole, polymyxin and prednisolone were used, giving an improvement in 5 days. All in-contact ferrets were treated. *Note*, it is again important to remove the ear mite infestation (Ch. 12).

Fox lists fungi causing systemic infections in the ferret: (1) *Blastomyces dermatidis*, (2) *Coccidioides immitis*, (3) *Histoplasma capsulatum* and (4) *Pneumocystis carinii*.[94] The first three organisms are widespread soil contaminants like *Cryptococcus bacillisporus* while the fourth was considered a protozoan but now is classified as a fungus. The difficulty in the treatment of these dangerous fungal infections can be considered.

Blastomycosis

This is a primary condition caused by *Blastomyces dermatidis*, with a chronic granulomatous invasion of the lung tissue and possible skin lesions. A clinical example of ferret infestation was seen in the 1980s along with cases in dogs and humans in that period.[94] The disease incidence is sporadic, from the soil and possibly by inhalation of conidia in dust. There is apparently no animal/animal or animal/human transmission. It has not been recorded in Australia or NZ but in the USA, Canada, Africa and rarely in Central America. Ferrets housed outdoors may be at higher risk.

Clinical signs: Ferrets develop a chronic granulomatous mycosis in the lungs, giving signs of cough and sneezing. A cutaneous blastomycosis gives ulcerative swellings, which spread slowly over the skin. The footpads can have ulcerative swellings.

PM signs: In the US case, a reticulonodular interstitial pneumonia was seen. The lung had focal consolidation and pleural fluid. There was a bilateral diffuse granulomatous pneumonia and pleuritis, a meningoencephalitis and an enlarged spleen.

Diagnosis: It could be another cause of chronic respiratory disease in ferrets and the yeast organisms can be extracted from skin or lung aspirate. Tissue imprints will show budding yeasts. It is noted that as with the dog infection, characteristic 'snowstorm' interstitial changes can be seen. Circulating antibody titre to the organism can be shown by agar immunodiffusion test.

Treatment: In dogs is by amphotericin B (AB) and ketoconazole (KTZ). This can be more difficult in the ferret as the AB must be given i.v. The dosage of AB (0.5 mg in 1 mL 5% dextrose) for the US ferret was 0.8 mg AB/kg. In addition, 5 mg KTZ was given p.o. The BUN was monitored and fluids given s.c. However, the AB caused anorexia, pyrexia and azotaemia so the AB dose was reduced to 0.25 mL (0.4 mg/kg) and checked by the BUN levels. The ferret showed a resolution of the forepad ulcer and regression of primary lesions. It became difficult to give the AB by i.v. injection so that only the KTZ was continued s.c. every other day. Two weeks after the s.c. treatment began the ferret relapsed and was euthanized. It is not easy to treat ferrets with some diseases and especially over long periods where the actual drugs used may have a cumulative toxicity factor.

Coccidioidomycosis

The fungal pathogen in this case is *Coccidioides immitis*, found particularly in low-lying sandy alkaline soils in the USA. Interestingly, it likes a high temperature environment.[94] The mycelium of the fungus produces arthrospores, which can become airborne and infective.

This disease has been recorded in ferrets in the USA. One ferret (18-month-old male) showed signs over 3 weeks of lethargy and weight loss. It had lost 36% of weight over 6 months. At presentation, it was said to have been coughing for 3 days and showed moderate pharyngeal hyperaemia. Blood check and temperature were normal.

Treatment: The ferret was given 25 mg tetracycline t.i.d. for 7 days but after 2 weeks, the cough had worsened and the submandibular glands were enlarged. Radiographs showed increased lung interstitial pattern in the cranial lobes. The treatment was changed to oral amoxicillin at 12.5 mg b.i.d. for 10 days. No improvement occurred after addition of 1.25 mg prednisolone daily for 16 days.

Coccidioidomycosis test was at first negative and then, 1 year later, when the ferret was seen with more weight loss, the test was positive. The ferret then was lethargic, weak was still losing weight and showed an abdominal mass plus lame right front leg. The scats were bloody. The WBC count was at a stress level of 24 000/μL. As coccidioidomycosis was diagnosed, the ferret was given 10 mg KTZ b.i.d. but with no improvement, so the ferret was euthanized 6 weeks after treatment began. No post mortem was possible.

Another US ferret became sick 2 days before presentation. It had been a pet shop ferret and when clinically examined was anorectic and lethargic with radiographs showing two radiodense areas of the mediastinum and caudal right lung lobe. A tracheal wash was attempted under G/A but the ferret died. However, a post mortem showed *Coccidioides* organisms in the lungs and lymph nodes.

Yet another US ferret was presented with a draining wound on the left stifle and showed symptoms of nasal discharge, weight loss and dehydration.

Treatment: 2 mg gentamycin was given to the ferret and the owner told to give oral amoxicillin plus oral vitamin B complex for 7 days. The wound was to be cleaned with peroxide daily. When checked 3 weeks later, the tibiotarsal region showed a swollen draining tract from which a smear was made revealing bacteria and neutrophils. Gentamycin was tried again for 4 days without success. Then amikacin sulphate was used at 6 mg/kg b.i.d. s.c. with an improvement shown so that the dosage was upped to 6 mg/lb once daily. After initial response, the draining swollen area recurred. Radiographs revealed a swollen radiodense area of the right radius. The ferret was euthanized 2 days later as there was no recovery progress. On examination of the draining tract, the area of the muscle and soft tissue of the right corpus and right and left tarsus were involved and from the right tarsus area. *Coccidioides* species were lifted for microscopy. No post mortem was possible.

It is noted that inhaled arthrospores of *C. immitis* can produce respiratory signs in 1–3 weeks in the dog and man.

Diagnosis: The diffuse interstitial pattern of infected lungs may be an indication of this disease on X-ray. Swelling of the mediastinal lymph nodes may be another clue. The disease can spread from the lungs to affect bone and joints, as seen in the last ferret case, and also any abdominal organs, the heart and CNS and even the male testicles. Osteomyelitis may be present on X-ray. Actual confirmation of *C. immitis* is by cytology or biopsy examination of tissues.

Treatment: This disease requires long-term treatment with ketoconazole (KTZ) being used in dogs and cat. The dose indicated for ferrets is 20 mg/kg b.i.d. In my opinion, as with cryptococcosis treatment, KTZ may be likely to be hepatotoxic to the ferret long before it has completely killed the pathogen it is aimed at. Having said that, prognosis of the disease in humans is good even without treatment, but guarded in dogs. There is not enough clinical data on ferret prognosis but it is possibly guarded too as it still is with cryptococcosis.

Histoplasmosis

This pathogenic organism is *Histoplasma capsulatum*, which is not contagious but is infectious.[94] This disease is said to infect by the respiratory route and a case was seen in a working ferret in the USA. Ferreting is not common now in the USA but the ferret involved was used to hunt rats and rabbits. It lived on dog food, table scraps and rabbit heads and this diet could be compared with the nutrition ideas in Chapter 4. The disease usually affects dogs, so that might be a connection with working ferrets. In the USA, it has been seen in the central continental area where *H. capsulatum* is found in the soil.

The symptoms were severe abdominal pain, enlarged spleen and subnormal temperature. In another ferret, subcutaneous nodules were noted in the skin. Again, this disease would have to be differentiated from cryptococcosis. In ferrets, the disease may run the same course as with dogs, showing pneumonia, ascites and

CHAPTER EIGHT
Viral, bacterial and mycotic diseases

lymphadenopathy with a positive diagnosis being made from fungal culture and/or biopsy.

Pneumocystis carinii

This organism is interesting as it was considered to be a protozoan. It has been re-classified on the homology of the parasite's basic genes with those found in fungi. The parasite can infect ferrets, rats, mice and even man. The *P. carinii* from these hosts appear morphologically similar but there are antigenic and genetic differences.[94] It is considered that further study of *P. carinii* as a zoonotic organism is required. The parasite is said to inhabit the lungs as a commensal in laboratory and some domestic animals including ferrets. It apparently affects immunocompromised animals under drug treatment or with some disease.

Pneumocystis carinii pneumonia in ferrets

The ferret has been used as a laboratory study of the disease while being under long-term cortisone medication (cortisone acetate 10–20 mg/kg s.c. for 9–10 weeks). The organism was found in all 11 ferrets under trial and caused disease in six animals, and should be considered as a possible disease problem with ferrets under long-term steroid therapy.

Ferrets are resistant to losing body weight, as are humans, when under corticosteroid therapy. Pneumocystic pneumonia can occur with ferrets undergoing long-term steroid treatment Also, it should be noted that in adrenal gland neoplasm, where the blood cortisone levels will be high, *P. carinii* might be present in sick animals (Ch. 14). Diagnosis would be by finding trophozoites by a bronchoalveolar lavage. Treatment is by using oral trimethoprim–sulfamethoxazole, in any infected ferrets, as with rats and humans. Histology showed interstitial pneumonia, focal mononuclear cell infiltrates and many cysts and trophozoites under GMS and Giemsa stains.

References

1. Govorkova EA, Rehg JE, Krauss S et al. Lethality to ferrets of H5N1 influenza viruses isolated from humans and poultry in 2004. J Virol 2005; 79:2191–2198.
2. Andrew PLR, Illman O. (1997) The Ferret. In: Poole T, ed. UFAW handbook on care and management of laboratory animals. UK: University Federation for Animal Welfare; 1997:436–455.
3. Marini RP, Adkins D, Fox JG. Proven or potential zoonotic diseases of ferrets. J Am Vet Med Assoc 1989; 195:990–994.
4. Associated Press editorial. The horrors of mad cow disease. The big weekend, The West Australian 1998; 6 June:2.
5. Anon. Exotic Animal Diseases Bulletin. Aust Vet J 1999; 77:474–475.
6. Childs JE. Zoonotic viruses of wildlife: hither from yon. Arch Virol 2004(suppl); 18:1–11.
7. Hood J. SARS sensationalized or serious threat? The Veterinarian 2003; May:20–21.
8. Artois M, Delahay R, Guberti V, Cheeseman C. Control of infectious diseases of wildlife in Europe. Vet J 2001; 162:141–152.
9. Koppine J. Letter from Europe. Aust Vet J 2004; 82:664.
10. Niezgoda M, Briggs DJ, Shadduck J et al. Pathogenesis of experimentally-induced rabies in domestic ferrets. Am J Vet Res 1997; 58:1327–1331.
11. Fox JG, Person RC, Gorham JR. Viral diseases. In: Fox JG, ed. Biology and diseases of the ferret, 2nd edn. Baltimore: Williams and Wilkins; 1998:355–375.
12. Gustafson B. Rabies studies in Canada. Am Ferret Rep 2002; 12:3.
13. Associated Press. Rabies survivor goes home. The West Australian 2005; 3 January:29.
14. Rupprecht CE. Evaluation of an inactivated rabies vaccine in domesticated ferrets. J Am Vet Med Ass 1990; 196:1614–1616.
15. Arslan A, Saglam YS, Temur A. Detection of rabies viral antigens in non-autolysed and autolysed tissues by using an immunoperoxidase technique. Vet Rec 2004; 155:550–552.
16. Langlois I. Viral diseases of ferrets. Vet Clin North Am Exot Anim Pract 2005; 8:139–160.
17. Murray J. Vaccine injection-site sarcoma in a ferret (letter). Am Vet Med Assoc 1998; 213:955.
18. Newby J. The needle and the damage done? The Veterinarian 2000; September:6–9.
19. Eggers CE, Dubielzig RR, Schultz D. Cats differ from mink and ferrets in their response to commercial vaccines: a histological comparison of early vaccine reactions. Vet Path 2002; 39:216–227.
20. Munday JS, Steadman NL, Richey LJ. Histology and immunohistochemistry of seven ferret vaccination-site fibrosarcomas. Vet Pathol 2003; 40:288–293.
21. Australian Veterinary Association. AVA Information Sheet, Issue No.1; 1996:11 November.
22. Hood, J. Lyssavirus hits WA flying foxes. The Veterinarian 2001; August:1–4.
23. O'Neill G. Flu 'penicillin' to face human test. Australia; The Age 1993; 24 April:21.
24. Wilcox G. Personal notes on virus taxonomy. School of Veterinary and Biomedical Sciences. Perth: Murdoch University; 2005.
25. Alhouse P, Tomlin S. Avian flu: Are we ready? Nature 2005; 435:399–740.
26. Ryland LM, Bernard SL, Gorman JR. A clinical guide to the pet ferret. USA; Compend Contin Edu Small Anim Pract 1993; 5:25.
27. Niemi SM, Newcomer CE, Fox JG. Neurological syndrome in the ferret (*Mustela putorius furo*). Vet Record 1984; 11:455–456.
28. von Messling V, Springfield C, Devaux P, Cattaneo R. A ferret model of canine distemper virus virulence and immunosuppression. J Virol 2003; 77:12579–12591.
29. Rosenthal KL. Respiratory diseases. In: Hillyer EV, Quesenberry KE, eds. Ferrets, rabbits and rodents: Clinical medicine and surgery. Philadelphia: W.B. Saunders; 1997:77–84.
30. Cruikshank R. Swine fever virus. In: Baron S, ed. Medical Microbiology, 2nd edn. Edinburgh: Churchill Livingstone; 1965:455–456.

31. Grey CA. Annual vaccines. Am Ferret Report 2003; 13:3.
32. Carpenter JW, Appel MJ, G. Erickson RC et al. Fatal vaccine-induced canine distemper virus infection in black-footed ferrets. J Am Vet Med Assoc 1976; 196:961–964.
33. Finkler M. Practical ferret medicine and surgery for the private practitioner. Roanoak: Roanoak Animal Hospital; 1999.
34. Owens D. Purevax distemper vaccine reaction. The F.A.I.R. Report 2004; XII:Issue 3.
35. Greenacre CB. Incidence of adverse events on ferret vaccination with distemper or rabies vaccine:143 cases (1995–2001). J Am Vet Med Assoc 2003; 223:663–665.
36. Moore GE, Glickman NW, Ward MP et al. Incidence and risk factors for adverse events associated with distemper and rabies vaccine administration in ferrets. J Am Vet Med Assoc 2005; 226:909–12.
37. Gandolf R. Distemper vaccines. Medical News. Am Ferret Report 2004; 14(3):6.
38. Heiler R. Antibody titers and what they mean. Immunology 101, Part 3. Am Ferret Report 2005; 15:13–14.
39. Wimsatt J, Jay MT, Innes KE et al. Serological evaluation, efficacy and safety of a commercial modified-live canine distemper vaccine in domestic ferrets. Am J Vet Res 2001; 62:736–740.
40. Catton K. Rethinking annual vaccinations. Medical News. Am Ferret Report 2002; 12:16.
41. Lewington JH. Vaccination of ferrets. Control and Therapy Series. University of Sydney: Postgraduate Foundation 1992; 164:396.
42. Smith H, Lindsay M, Reed G. Vaccination of ferrets. Control and Therapy Series. University of Sydney: Postgraduate Foundation 1992; 165:413–414.
43. Jones L, Terorio E, Gorham, J et al. Protective vaccination of ferrets against canine distemper with recombinant pox virus vaccine expressing the H or F genes in rinderpest virus. Aust J Vet Res 1997; 58:590–592.
44. Evermann JE, Leathers CW, Gorman JR et al. Pathogenesis of two strains of lion (*Panthera leo*) Morbillivirus in ferrets (*Mustela putorius furo*). Vet Path 2001; 38:311–316.
45. Dinnes MR. Table 2. In: Kirk R, ed. Current veterinary therapy, VII edn. Philadelphia; W. B. Saunders; 1980:711.
46. McCrackin Stevenson MA, Gates L. Aleutian mink disease parvovirus: implication for companion ferrets. Compend Contin Edu Small Anim Pract 2001; 23:178–185.
47. Heozov M. Intermustelidae hybrids. International Ferret Newsletter 2004; Nov/Dec:11–20.
48. Oxenham MB. Aleutian disease in the ferret: A review. Wessex Ferret Club Magazine 1993: May.
49. Newman SJ, Johnson R, Sears W, Wilcock B. Investigation of repeated vaccination as a possible cause of glomerular disease in mink. Can J Vet Res 2002; 66:158–164.
50. Besch-Wiliford CL, Biology and medicine of the ferret. Vet Clin N Am Small Anim Pract 17:1155–83.
51. Porter HG, Porter DD, Larsen AE. Aleutian disease in ferrets. Infect Immunol 1982; 36:379–86.
52. Lloyd M. Ferrets: Health, husbandry and diseases. Oxford: Blackwell; 1999.
53. Porter DD, Larsen AE, Porter HG. Aleutian disease of mink. Adv Immunol 1980; 29:261–86.
54. de Geus B, van Eck J, van de Louw A. Transmission of Aleutian disease virus by air. Scientifur 1996; 20:350–54.
55. Une Y, Wakimoto Y, Nakano Y, Konishi M, Nomura Y. Spontaneous Aleutian disease in a ferret. J Vet Med Sci 2000; 62:53–55.
56. Bell J. The pet ferret owners manual. New York: Christopher Maggio Studio Publishers; 1995.
57. Lewington JH. Ferrets: a compendium. Vade Mecum series C No 10. Sydney University: Postgraduate Foundation; 1988.
58. Johnson J. Respiratory toxicity of cedar and pine wood: a review of the biomedical literature from 1986 through 1995. Online. Available: www.trifl.org/cedar shtml; 1995.
59. Lewington JH. *Pseudomonas* and ferret 'snuffles' disease. Control and Therapy series. University of Sydney: Postgraduate Foundation 1994; 181:728.
60. Prince GA, Porter DD. The pathogenesis of respiratory syncytial virus infection in infant ferrets. Am J Path 1976; 82:339–352.
61. Carter CR, ed. *Pseudomonas*. In: Essentials of veterinary bacteriology and mycology, 3rd edn. Philadelphia: Lea and Febiger; 1986:156–159.
62. Fraser CM, ed. Husbandry and diseases of mink management. In: The Merck Veterinary Manual, 7th edn. Rahway: Merck; 1999:1050–1056.
63. Cruickshank R. *Pseudomonas: Loefflerella*. In: Cruickshank R, Duguid JP, Marmion BP, Swain RHA, eds. Medical Microbiology, 12th edn. New York; Churchill Livingstone; 1975:341–344.
64. Soltys MA. Bacteria and fungi pathogenic to man and animals. London: Baillière Tindall; 1963.
65. Fox JG, ed. Bacterial and mycoplasmal diseases. In: Biology and diseases of the ferret, Baltimore: Williams and Wilkins; 1998:321–354.
66. Jenkins JR, Brown SA. Practitioners' guide to rabbits and ferrets. Lakewood: American Animal Hospital Association; 1993:43–93.
67. Oxenham M. Ferrets. In: Beynon PH, Cooper JE, eds. Manual of exotic pets. Brit Small Anim Vet Assoc 1991:97–110.
68. McDonough PL. Leptospirosis. In: Tilly PL, Smith FWK Jr, eds. Five-minute veterinary consult canine and feline. Baltimore: Williams and Wilkins; 1997:768–769.
69. Delahay RJ, De Leeuw AN, Barlow AM, Clifton-Hadley RS, Cheeseman CL. The status of *Mycobacterium bovis* infections in UK wild mammals: a review. Vet J 2002; 164:90–105.
70. Hutchings MR, Harris S. Effects of farm management practice on cattle grazing behaviour and the potential for transmission of bovine tuberculosis from badgers to cattle. Vet J 1997; 153:149–162.
71. Daniels MJ, Lees JD, Hutchings MR, Greig A. The ranging behaviour and habit use of rabbits on farmland and their potential role on the epidemiology of paratuberculosis. Vet J 2003; 165:248–257.
72. Hancox M. Flying kites: the great badger and bovine TB debate. Biologist 1995; 42:159–161.
73. Porter V, Brown N. The complete book of ferrets. Bedford: D&M Publications; 1997.
74. Schultheiss PC, Dolgin OW. Granulomatous enteritis caused by *Mycobacterium avis* in a ferret. Am Vet Med Assoc 1994; 20:1217–1218.
75. Valheim M, Storset AK, Aleksersen M, Brun-Hansen H. Disseminated *Mycobacterium celatum* (type 3) infection in the domestic ferret (*Mustela putorius furo*) Vet Pathol 2001; 38:460–463.
76. Lucas J, Lucas A, Furber H et al. *Mycobacterium genavense* infection in two aged ferrets with conjunctival lesions. Aust Vet J 2000; 78:685–689.
77. Lunn JA, Martin P, Zaki S, Malik R. Pneumonia due to *Mycobacterium abscessus* in two domestic ferrets (*Mustelo putorius furo*). Aust Vet J 2005; 83:542–545.
78. Parliamentary Commissioner for the Environment. Possum management in New Zealand. Wellington: Parliamentary Commissioner for the Environment; 1994.

79. Williams JM. Possible implication of rabbit calicivirus disease (RCD) In: RSNZ, eds. Workshop on ferrets as vectors of tuberculosis and threat to conservation. Wellington: The Royal Society of New Zealand; 1996.
80. Caley P. Broad scale possum and ferret correlates of macroscopic *Mycobacterium bovis* infection in feral ferret populations. NZ Vet J 1998; 46:157–162.
81. Qureshi T, Labes RE, Lambeth M, Griffin JF, Mackintosh CG. Transmission of *Mycobacterium bovis* from experimentally infected ferrets to non-infected ferrets (*Mustela furo*). NZ Vet J 2000; 48:99–104.
82. deLisle GW. Surveillance of wild life for *Mycobacterium bovis* using culture of pooled tissue samples from ferret (*Mustela furo*) NZ Vet J 2004; 53:14–18.
83. Wallace DN. Fur farming fitch diseases in farm production and practice. Wellington: Ministry of Agriculture and Fisheries; 1983.
84. McLauchlin J. Animal and human listeriosis: a shared problem? Vet J 1997; 153:3–5.
85. Lewington JH. Idiopathic otitis interna of the ferret. Control and Therapy Series. University of Sydney: Postgraduate Foundation 1989; 151:183–184.
86. Loan MG. Risk of pet ownership: The family practitioner's viewpoint. Vet Clin North Am Small Anim Pract 1987; 17:17–25.
87. Smith ME. Normal mouth and intestinal flora of the ferret (*Mustela furo*). Nature 1980; 173:1048.
88. Marini RP, Taylor NS, Liang AY et al. Characterization of hemolytic *Escherichia coli* strains in ferrets: recognition of candidate virulence factor CNF1. J Clin Microbiol 2004; 42:5904–5908.
89. Soylts MA. Bacteria and fungi pathogenic to man and animals. London: Baillière Tindall; 1963.
90. Gorman JR, Hagen KW, Farrell RK. Mink: diseases and parasites. Agricultural handbook. USA Department of Agriculture; 1972:175.
91. Bell J. Infectious diseases of ferrets. Proc North Am Vet Conf 1993:721–23.
92. Fox JG, Anderson LC, Loew FM, Quimby FW. Laboratory animal medicine, 2nd edn. San Diego: Academic Press; 2002:483–517.
93. Hood J. VRE found in New Zealand food animals. The Veterinarian 2003; June:1.
94. Fox JG. Mycotic diseases in biology and diseases of the ferret, 2nd edn. Baltimore: Williams & Wilkins; 1998:393–403.
95. Animal health division. Mycotic diseases surveillance, New Zealand. Ministry of Agriculture and Fisheries 1984; 1:5–6.
96. Matousek JL, Campbell KL. *Malassezia* dermatitis. Compend Contin Edu Small Anim Pract 2002; 24:224–231.
97. Dinsdale JR, Rest JR. Yeast infection in ferrets (letter). Vet Rec 1995; 16:647.

CHAPTER 9

Ferret gastrointestinal and hepatic diseases

Mark E. Burgess

'Whenever you find yourself on the side of the majority, it is time to pause and reflect.'

Mark Twain

Introduction

The ferret gastrointestinal (GI) tract is short and fairly simple, typical of a carnivore digestive system. It comprises a simple stomach, duodenum, 'jejunoileum' (jejunum and ileum are indistinguishable), and colon. Ferrets lack a caecum or ileocolic junction. The normal gastrointestinal transit time is rapid, varying from 148 to 219 min.[1]

The ferret gut is also extremely reactive and commonly demonstrates a strong inflammatory response from a variety of aetiologies. Chronic gastroenteritis is common, and in the author's experience often results in clinical disease, or in alterations of gut function, such as delayed gastric emptying and greatly slowed gastrointestinal transit times.

Our understanding of the pathophysiology of the common gastroenteropathies in ferrets is incomplete. Two factors have slowed our recognition and understanding of ferret gut pathology. First, many ferrets with chronic gastroenteritis demonstrate only subtle signs of illness which are often overlooked. Second, there are commonly held misconceptions regarding ferret gastroenteric disease, which persist despite considerable histopathologic evidence which should force us to rethink some of the current views of the ferret gut. This chapter is an attempt to present ferret gastrointestinal (and hepatic) diseases in a logical and practical format, emphasizing those diseases with high clinical relevance, and de-emphasizing some diseases which have received much attention to date but which may be clinically less important.

Overview of gastrointestinal disease (cranial to caudal)

- Oral ulcers
- Megaoesophagus
- Gastric foreign bodies and trichobezoars
- Gastric ulcers
- *Helicobacter* gastritis
- Inflammatory bowel disease
- Intestinal foreign bodies
- *Coccidia*
- Coronavirus enteritis (ECE)
- Eosinophilic granulomatous disease
- Bacterial overgrowth/enteritis
- Enterotoxaemia
- Aleutian disease virus
- Neoplasia: lymphoma, pancreatic adenocarcinoma, etc.
- Proliferative bowel disease
- Proctitis.

Overview of GI disease based on clinical incidence

Diseases with high clinical incidence:

- Oral ulcers
- Gastric and intestinal foreign bodies, trichobezoars
- Coronavirus enteritis (ECE)

- Inflammatory bowel disease
- Bacterial overgrowth/enteritis
- Gastric ulcers.

Diseases with moderate clinical incidence:

- Proctitis
- Neoplasia
- *Helicobacter* gastritis.

Diseases with low clinical incidence:

- Megaoesophagus
- Aleutian disease virus (causing GI signs)
- Enterotoxaemia
- Proliferative bowel disease
- Coccidiosis
- Eosinophilic granulomatous disease.

Overview of hepatic diseases

- Lymphocytic hepatitis
- Suppurative hepatitis
- Hepatic lipidosis
- Vacuolar hepatopathy
- End stage liver disease (cirrhosis)
- Biliary cysts
- Metastatic neoplasms
- Primary hepatic neoplasms.

Clinical findings associated with various gastrointestinal disorders

- *Nausea* (bruxism, pawing at mouth, salivation, vomition): gastric foreign body, trichobezoar, gastric ulcer, inflammatory bowel disease, bacterial overgrowth and/or enteritis, coronavirus enteritis (first 48 h), intestinal foreign body, intestinal lymphoma, *Helicobacter* gastritis. Eosinophilic granulomatous disease (uncommon) and proliferative bowel disease (rare) may produce nausea
- *Regurgitation* (ejection of food within 5 min postprandial, with minimal nausea; patient often eats after regurgitating): megaoesophagus
- *Anorexia*: nearly any gut lesion may produce this sign
- *Diarrhoea* (greenish, or brown, or mucoid, or loose 'birdseed' stools): bacterial overgrowth and/or enteritis (often greenish, often mucoid), coronavirus enteritis (bright green, may fade to brown with antibiotic therapy), inflammatory bowel disease (greenish to brown, mucoid to birdseed). *Note*: bacterial enteropathies may occur secondary to sudden diet changes, dietary indiscretion, or secondary to nearly any other intestinal lesion, such as inflammatory bowel disease, coronavirus enteritis, or intestinal lymphoma. Uncommon diseases that may produce diarrhoea include eosinophilic granulomatous disease and proliferative bowel disease
- *Weight loss/muscle wasting* despite good appetite: inflammatory bowel disease, bacterial overgrowth/enteritis, coronavirus enteritis, intestinal lymphoma. Eosinophilic granulomatous disease (uncommon) and proliferative bowel disease (rare) may cause wasting
- *High fever*: acute bacterial enteritis and/or hepatitis (often secondary to underlying gut pathology), septicaemia (secondary to severe gastroenteritis), acute coronavirus enteritis or perforated gastrointestinal ulcer with septic peritonitis
- *Melaena* (acute or chronic): gastric or duodenal ulcers, gastric foreign body, inflammatory bowel disease, *Helicobacter* gastritis, gastrointestinal lymphoma
- *Proctitis* (red, swollen anal mucosa): secondary to any chronic enteropathy, especially with chronic diarrhoea; e.g. inflammatory bowel disease, coronavirus enteritis, bacterial overgrowth
- *Palpable thickened bowel*: intestinal lymphoma, eosinophilic granulomatous disease (uncommon), proliferative bowel disease (rare)
- *Palpable mesenteric lymphadenopathy*: intestinal lymphoma, inflammatory bowel disease, eosinophilic granulomatous disease (uncommon), proliferative bowel disease (rare)
- *Tenesmus*: inflammatory bowel disease with colitis, bacterial overgrowth/enteritis, intestinal lymphoma, eosinophilic granulomatous disease (uncommon), proliferative bowel disease (rare)
- *Rectal prolapse*: (a) Mild: inflammatory bowel disease, bacterial enteritis/colitis, intestinal lymphoma, eosinophilic granulomatous disease (uncommon). (b) Severe: proliferative bowel disease (rare), or other severe colonic pathology, e.g. severe colitis, intestinal lymphoma (all rarely cause severe prolapse)
- *Leukocytosis*: may be seen with most gut pathology, especially if secondary bacterial overgrowth or enteritis occurs
- *Eosinophilia*: inflammatory bowel disease (occasionally); eosinophilic granulomatous disease (uncommon disease, but eosinophilia is common with this disease)

- *Neutrophilia*: bacterial overgrowth and/or enteritis, often secondary to underlying gut pathology such as inflammatory bowel disease, coronavirus enteritis, intestinal lymphoma, eosinophilic granulomatous disease. Intestinal foreign bodies may also produce neutrophilia, especially with bowel necrosis and/or rupture
- *Lymphocytosis*: inflammatory bowel disease, intestinal lymphoma, possibly *Helicobacter* (uncommon).

Gastrointestinal diseases (cranial to caudal)

Oral ulcers

Oral ulcers commonly occur on the palate secondary to self mutilation (pawing at the mouth with the forepaws). These are usually circumscribed, shallow oval to round red ulcers on the palate (cranial or caudal), 3–10 mm in diameter. Pawing at the mouth is common in ferrets with gastrointestinal disease causing nausea or abdominal pain; it is also common with administration of foul tasting medication, e.g. metronidazole.

Treatment includes identifying and correcting the underlying cause (e.g. gut lesions, medications) and trimming the front toenails short. Sucralfate (Carafate) suspension 100–125 mg orally may adhere to the ulcer; oral antibiotics may be used to minimize secondary infection.

Prevent iatrogenically induced ulcers by restraining the ferret during and after medicating; administer a sweet liquid such as a sugary syrup immediately before and after giving a foul or bitter tasting drug.

Megaoesophagus

An infrequent disease in ferrets, its etiology is poorly understood in many cases.[2,3] It appears to be an acquired, not congenital condition. We have histopathologically linked some cases to underlying gastritis with associated gastric acid reflux and oesophagitis.[4]

Signs include distress while eating, choking/coughing, extending the neck postprandially, and regurgitation within 5–10 min (or sooner) postprandial. Neck palpation sometimes reveals fluid and gas distension of the proximal oesophagus, on the left side of the neck just caudal to the head. Radiographs may show retained air or food in the oesophagus. Radiographic diagnosis is enhanced by administering a barium swallow mixed with food, followed by an immediate radiograph; findings typically are a dilated cervical and thoracic oesophagus with retained food and barium (Ch. 16).

Treatment may be unrewarding if oesophagitis is not involved. Cisapride dosed at 0.5 mg/kg p.o. b.i.d. has produced minimal benefit in our patients. For cases with reflux oesophagitis, total resolution of signs can sometimes be achieved via administration of acid blockers such as ranitidine (Zantac) or famotidine (Pepcid). We have had more experience using ranitidine; our usual dose is 3.5 mg/kg p.o. b.i.d. for several weeks, possibly long term. Sucralfate (Carafate) suspension may be administered at 100–125 mg per ferret p.o. b.i.d./t.i.d.; this may adhere to both gastric and oesophageal ulcerations and aid healing. Metoclopramide (Reglan) may be used to encourage gastric emptying and reduce reflux; typical dosing is 0.5–1.0 mg/kg p.o. b.i.d.

Feed liquefied food such as Hill's a/d gruel; elevate the front of the ferret's body while eating (one may place food on an elevated platform). Patients with reflux oesophagitis that respond well to acid blockers may eventually be returned to a normal diet. Underlying gut pathology should be identified and addressed when the patient is stabilized. Rarely reflux oesophagitis may lead to distal oesophageal stricture; prognosis in these patients is grave.

Gastric foreign bodies and trichobezoars

These are seen in any age animal. Ingested rubber materials and trichobezoars are common. Affected ferrets are often asymptomatic; signs can include vomition, anorexia, melaena, lethargy, weight loss, bruxism or pawing at the mouth. Subclinical cases may still develop gastritis (see Inflammatory bowel disease comments).

Palpation may discern the foreign body, but clinicians may find that the stomach rests too far cranially (between the ribs) for easy palpation. Radiographs with a barium swallow may or may not visualize the object; even trichobezoars often fail to retain barium due to their smooth dense composition and mucus-coated surface (Ch. 16). An air contrast gastrogram may aid visualization. Serum chemistries may show elevated lipase (over 500 IU/L at commercial veterinary diagnostic laboratories,[5,6] or over 1000 IU/L using an in house IDEXX VetTest® machine[7] – see Inflammatory bowel disease discussion), as well as elevated globulin (over 3.0 g/dL).[8]

Prevent foreign bodies by severely restricting access to ingestible items, especially those with a soft rubbery texture. Prevent trichobezoars by brushing moulting animals, and using a feline hairball laxative in moulting animals and other animals deemed to be at risk (such as cage mates who groom the moulting ferret, or ferrets with a prior history of trichobezoars). Ferrets with

CHAPTER NINE
Ferret gastrointestinal and hepatic diseases

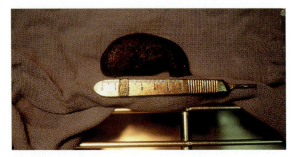

Figure 9.1 An unusually large trichobezoar which filled the stomach of the affected ferret.

significant gastritis may exhibit reduced gastric motility and a potentially higher risk for hair retention (see Inflammatory bowel disease).

Treatment of gastric foreign bodies and trichobezoars is usually via gastrotomy; endoscopic removal is possible with smaller objects. The small bowel does not allow passage of any but the smallest objects, so removal is usually required. Trichobezoars in ferrets are usually too dense and firm to dissolve with medications, and too large to pass though the bowel even with lubricants. Figure 9.1 shows an unusually large trichobezoar which filled the stomach of the affected ferret. A gastrotomy or enterotomy in this species may be treated with 7 days of postoperative antibiotics, such as enrofloxacin 5 mg/kg p.o. b.i.d. plus amoxicillin 10 mg/kg p.o. b.i.d.

Gastric palpation is recommended during any laparotomy procedure; incidental gastric foreign bodies are common findings and should be removed when detected (Ch. 18).

Gastric ulcers

Ferrets have been described as being prone to gastric ulcers secondary to various factors,[9] including azotaemia, ulcerogenic drugs, foreign bodies, and *Helicobacter* overgrowth.[10,11,12] Many of our patients with ulcers have concurrent generalized gastroenteritis (inflammatory bowel disease). Signs may include melaena (tarry stools), anorexia, vomition, bruxism and weight loss. In extreme cases, gastric or duodenal ulcers can rupture a blood vessel and cause severe prolonged bleeding, leading to anaemia or shock. Severe ulcers can occasionally perforate the gut, leading to septic peritonitis and death if not corrected. Figure 9.2 shows a necropsy gastric specimen with numerous severe ulcerations.

Any patient with signs of GI ulcers should ideally have a blood profile evaluated, and if evidence of chronic gut inflammation is present (e.g. elevated serum lipase or globulin), gut biopsies should be recommended when the patient is stable. Any unrecognized foreign bodies would also be detected during a biopsy procedure (Ch. 18). Histopathology is typically required to definitively identify an underlying gut disorder, such as inflammatory bowel disease, *Helicobacter* gastritis, lymphoma, etc.

More conservative treatment would include an acid blocker such as ranitidine (Zantac), famotidine (Pepcid), or omeprazole (Prilosec). See *Helicobacter* gastritis for drug doses. In addition, sucralfate (Carafate) may be used to aid ulcer healing, at 100–125 mg/ferret p.o. b.i.d./t.i.d. for 5–7 days or until signs resolve. Ideally give sucralfate on an empty stomach (no food or other drugs present). Sucralfate may bind to food or other medications, reducing its binding to ulcerated mucosa, and reducing absorption of other medications. Trial therapy for *Helicobacter* infection could be initiated (see *Helicobacter* gastritis). Alternatively, enrofloxacin 5–10 mg/kg p.o. b.i.d. plus amoxicillin 10–20 mg/kg

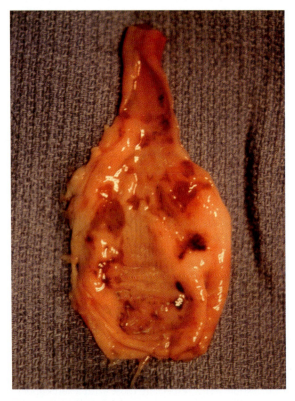

Figure 9.2 A necropsy specimen of stomach and proximal duodenum, showing severe gastric ulcerations. This patient died from blood loss associated with haemorrhage from the ulcers. *Helicobacter* was not detected histopathologically.

p.o. b.i.d. can be used to control a bacterial overgrowth or enteritis in the small bowel (in the event that melaena is arising from hemorrhagic enteritis and not a focal ulcer).

Helicobacter gastritis

Helicobacter mustelae is a spirilliform bacterium that lives in the stomach (primarily the pyloric region) and first 1 cm of the duodenum in the ferret. Research models have promoted *Helicobacter* as a significant gastric pathogen in the domestic ferret, based on its ability to produce lesions in controlled research settings.[10,11,12,13,14] These studies have shown that *Helicobacter* is common in the ferret stomach and may be nearly ubiquitous in the domestic ferret population, at least in the USA. Typically, when an organism is so universally distributed in a host population, it is well host-adapted and tends to behave as 'normal flora' in most situations. Our clinical experience supports this; *Helicobacter* appears to have low pathogenicity in most of our ferret patients; in some cases, it may produce a mild to severe lymphoplasmacytic gastritis. Prior authors noted clinical disease occurring mostly in 3–5-month-old stressed ferrets.[15] However, this organism is now often assumed to be responsible for gastritis, gastric ulcers, or other gastrointestinal lesions in both young and old ferrets. Often the diagnosis is unconfirmed and response to antibiotic treatment is interpreted as confirmation of the disease. There are, however, multiple gastrointestinal disorders that show clinical improvement with antibiotic therapy (due to resolution of secondary bacterial overgrowth in the gut); response to treatment is non-specific and does not verify a specific aetiologic agent. *Helicobacter* has been claimed to cause diarrhoea with progressive wasting,[15] which are signs one would not expect even with gastric pathology; every case we have seen has had concurrent enteric disease (separate from *Helicobacter*) which was producing these clinical signs. Chronic blood loss due to severe gastric ulceration might, in severe cases, be able to produce wasting disease.

Faecal cultures, rapid urease testing of gut tissue samples, PCR (polymerase chain reaction) testing of faeces or biopsy samples, urea breath testing, stool antigen testing, and serum antibody testing can all identify a *Helicobacter* carrier.[16] However, as most ferrets are thought to be carriers, such testing is probably not useful, unless as an assessment of post-treatment eradication of the bacteria. Gastric (and intestinal) histopathology is needed to confirm a causal relationship between infection and the presence of gut lesions. Visualization of the bacteria is maximized using a silver stain (Warthin–Starry stain).

The difficulties inherent in applying laboratory research models to everyday clinical cases are numerous. The original studies promoting *Helicobacter* as a ferret pathogen involved small numbers of animals and lacked histopathologic examination of the gut, other than the stomach and proximal 1–2 cm of the duodenum where *Helicobacter* could be expected to colonize.[10,11,12] Concurrent enteritis or generalized gastroenteritis would not have been detected. Some studies utilized ferrets from a large breeder facility known to have coronavirus enteritis in its ferret population[12,17]; this virus causes lymphoplasmacytic inflammation of the ferret gut.[18] Whether concurrent coronavirus infection would influence histopathologic findings in those *Helicobacter* studies is unknown. In a study utilizing combination drug therapy to eliminate ferret *Helicobacter* infection,[17] bacterial eradication was proven successful, but the level of gastritis did not improve in five out of six ferrets. This is in contrast to human research with *Helicobacter pylori* which demonstrated that bacterial elimination produced resolution of gastritis.[19] Such results should make us question whether *Helicobacter* was the only inciting agent of the gastritis in those research cases. Perhaps a *Helicobacter*-induced gastritis might persist awhile after bacterial elimination, as can sometimes occur with humans; or perhaps other factors were inciting the inflammatory response. Some reports state that *Helicobacter* infection in ferrets is associated with chronic gastritis that increases in severity over time.[14] Whether this occurs in non-stressed house ferrets in normal clinical situations is less certain. Review of another study suggests only mild pathology induced by experimental infection: all four ferrets had *Helicobacter* colonization of the gastric fundus and antrum, but the fundal mucosa showed negligible changes, and the antral mucosa showed only mild inflammation in three ferrets (the fourth remaining normal). The severity of the lesions did not increase during the 6-month interval of the study.[10]

Helicobacter has been shown to occasionally incite development of lymphoma in the gastric mucosa (in the mucosa associated lymphatic tissue, i.e. 'MALT' lymphoma).[13] It should be noted that other forms of gastroenteritis can commonly lead to lymphoma, occasionally in the gastroenteric mucosa, but more often in the mesenteric lymph nodes associated with the gut;[8] see Inflammatory bowel disease.

Histopathologic examination of hundreds of ferret gastrointestinal biopsies has shown that in the author's pet ferret patients, *Helicobacter* does not appear to be the primary aetiologic agent for most gastroenteric lesions observed.[4,8] On pyloric-region gastric biopsy and histopathology (with silver staining) we can find the bacteria in less than 50% of ferrets with confirmed gastritis; only a small percentage of these have heavy numbers of bacteria present. In most cases, the bacteria seem to be an incidental finding or at most a partial contributor to the inflammatory lesions. When the stomach is biopsied 2–3 cm proximal to the pylorus, we find *Helicobacter* only about 4% of the time, with only about 2% of cases having a large number of bacteria present – yet biopsies taken in this region reveal significant gastritis also. This is in contrast to the claims made in the original research studies of *Helicobacter mustelae*, wherein the researchers proposed a causal link between the bacteria and inflammatory lesions due to visualizing a close geographic association of the bacteria to the observed lesions.[11,12]

In the author's experience, most ferrets with gastritis also have enteritis which equals or exceeds the gastric lesions in severity. In a recent sampling of 115 recent gut biopsy cases, only 34 cases (29.5%) had pyloric gastritis which was more severe than the enteritis; of these, only 22 (19%) had detectable *Helicobacter* on pyloric area biopsy. By contrast, 81 cases (70%) had enteritis which equalled or exceeded the gastritis in severity – in 53 cases (46%) the enteritis was much more severe than the gastritis on biopsy. *Helicobacter* should not produce these enteric lesions; in hundreds of enteric biopsy samples (silver-stained), we have never detected *Helicobacter*-like organisms in mid-duodenal or jejunal biopsies, nearly all with enteritis present. Detection of *Helicobacter*-like organisms in intestinal fluid contents or the bowel lumen is to be expected; the organism must pass through the gut and out of the body if it is to infect additional hosts. But no causal link between this bacterium and active enteritis can be concluded, when the organism cannot be detected in any biopsies of intestinal mucosa.

One study noted antigastric autoantibodies in ferrets infected with *Helicobacter*; this might explain persistence of gastritis after bacterial eradication.[20] However, those antibodies reacted with parietal cells from the gastric mucosa, but not with duodenal or colonic mucosa, so even an immune-mediated response triggered by *Helicobacter* would not appear likely to induce enteritis. In conclusion, most ferrets with gastric disease have a more generalized gastroenteritis, with *Helicobacter* present either incidentally or as a partial contributor to the gastric lesions. Only a small percent of cases (1.7%) showed heavy *Helicobacter* growth in the gastric mucosa with a significant gastritis and minimal enteritis; these cases may be examples of primary *Helicobacter* gastritis. Based on these data, it is evident that although the bacteria may be pathogenic in certain situations, *Helicobacter*-induced pathology is probably far less common in the ferret than is currently assumed, and the bacteria are blamed for many lesions which in reality are being induced by unrelated pathology.

Signs of *Helicobacter* gastritis would include nausea, anorexia, vomiting, melaena, or bruxism; these signs all are typical of gastritis. *Helicobacter* would *not* be expected to directly produce signs of enteritis such as chronic diarrhoea without melaena, mucoid stools, greenish stools, or weight loss despite good appetite (unless from chronic vomition, or chronic heavy blood loss). Diagnosis ideally should be confirmed with surgical biopsy (not endoscopy); this allows for histopathologic sampling both of the pyloric stomach and small bowel, as well as mesenteric lymph nodes (to assess for cellular or architectural atypia and risk of lymphoma development). (See Inflammatory bowel disease discussion regarding lymph node histopathology.) If gastritis with *Helicobacter* in the lesions is confirmed via biopsy, or if the clinician elects presumptive treatment to eliminate possible infection, then several treatment protocols are available. In the past, metronidazole at 20 mg/kg p.o. b.i.d./t.i.d. plus amoxicillin at 10 mg/kg p.o. b.i.d./t.i.d. for 14 days or longer was said to eliminate infection.[14] More recent protocols have increased dosing, frequency and duration of therapy due to apparent antibiotic resistance developing.[13] Addition of bismuth subsalicylate (Pepto-Bismol) 0.5 cc p.o. b.i.d. may enhance treatment effectiveness, as bismuth compounds may aid bacterial elimination.[17] One may add acid blockers such as ranitidine (Zantac) at 3.5 mg/kg p.o. b.i.d., or famotidine (Pepcid) at 0.25–0.5 mg/kg p.o. s.i.d., or possibly omeprazole (Prilosec) at 0.7 mg/kg p.o. s.i.d. Human studies have demonstrated that acid blockers can enhance bacterial elimination.[21,22,23]

Metronidazole and bismuth subsalicylate are both distasteful to ferrets. Omeprazole is supplied as capsules containing numerous slow release granules, so is more difficult to dose in small patients; in our initial use with higher doses of this drug (4 mg/kg p.o. s.i.d.) some patients exhibited malaise and anorexia not seen with other acid blocking drugs. *Note*: when dosing this drug, one must open the capsule and count out individual granules to achieve an accurate dose.

Another protocol uses clarithromycin at 25 mg/kg p.o. b.i.d. for 14 days, combined with ranitidine bismuth citrate (not available in the USA).[17] Alternatively, clarithromycin may be combined with amoxicillin (10–40 mg/kg p.o. b.i.d./t.i.d.) and ranitidine (3.5 mg/kg p.o. b.i.d.) for 14–28 days. Pepto-Bismol can be added to this combination. A recent published human protocol used clarithromycin plus amoxicillin plus omeprazole (at human doses) and showed elimination of infection.[21] Drug resistance can easily develop with all these protocols; some human protocols now use metronidazole in place of clarithromycin due to antibiotic resistance.[22,23] One human study showed that concurrent use of sucralfate with combination antibiotic therapy enhanced efficacy similar to using proton pump inhibitors; the sucralfate bound the antibiotics and the bacteria at the mucosal surface, enhancing bacterial clearance.[24] The author's current preference is to use drug combinations that are palatable, increasing owner and pet compliance; a fairly palatable combination is clarithromycin, amoxicillin, sucralfate and ranitidine; the first three are given together, and the ranitidine is given at least 1 hour apart to allow proper absorption from the gut without binding to the sucralfate. Famotidine would be a good alternative to ranitidine.

We have noted occasional persistence of *Helicobacter* in the ferret gut when using the above treatment protocols. This could be due to drug resistance or inconsistent drug administration, but also may be related to re-infection from the pet's own faeces or from other ferrets in contact with the treated patient. Ideally, all contact ferrets should be treated for *Helicobacter* simultaneously to maximize potential for total elimination of the organism. Their cage environment and litter boxes should be disinfected regularly during the treatment course.

If gastric ulcers are suspected due to presence of melaena, bruxism, or severe nausea, then sucralfate (Carafate) suspension may be used at 100–125 mg per ferret p.o. b.i.d./t.i.d. until signs resolve.

Inflammatory bowel disease (lymphoplasmacytic gastroenteritis)

This is an idiopathic chronic inflammation of the gastrointestinal tract, usually involving both stomach and small bowel (duodenum and jejunum). The ileum and colon are likely involved in many cases as well, based on clinical signs of colitis and proctitis; however, these sites are usually not sampled histopathologically except on necropsy. It is usually seen in ferrets over 1 year old; most commonly over 2 years old. This is one of the most common significant disease syndromes in pet ferrets today (in the USA), certainly as common as adrenal tumours or insulinomas. It is also the most underdiagnosed disease in ferrets, being virtually unrecognized until fairly recently.[8]

The inflammation of the gut mucosa and lamina propria is primarily lymphoplasmacytic, especially in the stomach, but often has a lesser eosinophilic component (mostly in the bowel). Of 115 recent intestinal biopsy cases, 35 cases (30.4%) demonstrated lymphoplasmacytic enteritis; 77 cases (66.9%) had both lymphoplasmacytic and eosinophilic infiltrates; 3 cases (2.6%) had purely eosinophilic enteritis. Of 120 recent gastric biopsy cases, 106 (88.3%) demonstrated lymphoplasmacytic gastritis; 14 cases (11.7%) had both lymphoplasmacytic and eosinophilic infiltrates; no cases had a purely eosinophilic gastritis.

Inflammatory bowel disease (IBD) cases with an eosinophilic component to the gut inflammation must be distinguished from a less common disease, eosinophilic granulomatous disease (also called eosinophilic gastroenteritis – a bit of a misnomer). This is a multi-organ disease involving eosinophilic infiltrates and granulomas of lymphatics and multiple tissues; it does involve the gut as well, but the condition is not a gut mucosa-oriented inflammatory disease and therefore is not a form of true 'inflammatory bowel disease'. In our IBD cases, the inflammatory response primarily involves the gut mucosa and lamina propria.

Possible inciting factors for inflammatory bowel disease could include food hypersensitivity, carbohydrate overload, bacterial overgrowth, gastric foreign bodies, bacterial or viral infection, toxins, aberrant immune response, etc. *Helicobacter* infection can sometimes produce a lymphocytic gastritis; coronavirus infection produces a lymphocytic enteritis. Prolonged or extravagant immune response to these infectious agents might result in chronic gastritis or enteritis that persists even when the inciting organism is eliminated.

IBD is often non-symptomatic until very advanced. Signs may be subtle, and may include a lack of proper musculature (protein malabsorption), weight loss, sporadic diarrhoea, melaena (with gastritis), bruxism due to nausea, or vomiting. Signs may be mild and chronic, or acute and severe. Acute diarrhoea (often greenish) and malaise may occur with secondary bacterial overgrowth/bacterial enteritis. Acute melaena, nausea and anorexia may occur with gastric ulceration. Acute suppurative hepatitis may be seen, producing fever, leukocytosis, occasionally icterus, and severe malaise. Figure 9.3 shows a typical IBD stool, with a mixture of greenish stool (likely due to bacterial overgrowth) and melaena (due to gastric or duodenal ulceration).

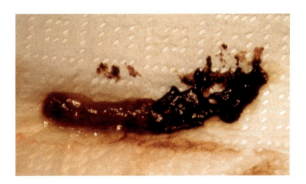

Figure 9.3 Stool from a patient with inflammatory bowel disease. The sample demonstrates green mucoid characteristics in one portion, typical of bacterial enteritis/bacterial overgrowth. The other portion of the stool demonstrates melaena suggestive of gastric or intestinal ulceration.

CHAPTER NINE
Ferret gastrointestinal and hepatic diseases

Often IBD is detected when patients are presented for concurrent disease (e.g. adrenal or islet cell tumours), and a thorough history, physical exam and blood profile show evidence of gut disease.

Preliminary diagnosis (i.e. high index of suspicion) can usually be made via a comprehensive blood profile and clinical signs (if present). Essential tests for evaluating gut disease include a complete blood count (CBC) test, plus serum lipase, globulin, alanine aminotransferase (ALT), and gamma-glutamyltranspeptidase (GGT). Other recommended tests in any comprehensive ferret profile include glucose, blood urea nitrogen (BUN) and creatinine kinase (CK), amylase, bilirubin, albumin, calcium, phosphorous, aspartate transaminase (AST) and alkaline phosphatase.

At our practice, comparison of serum chemistry values with gut histopathology on hundreds of cases has revealed some correlations. Elevation of lipase over 500 IU/L at commercial US veterinary laboratories,[5,6] or over 1000 IU/L using an in house IDEXX VetTest® machine[7] is consistent with gastritis or gastroenteritis in ferrets. In the author's experience, clinical pancreatitis is rare in ferrets, and produces serum elevations of both amylase and lipase. Gastric lipase seems to be the main component of most serum lipase elevations in ferrets, and amylase remains low (<100 IU/L).[8] Serum lipase elevations of gastroenteric origin have been documented in dogs and cats.[25,26,27,28]

Elevated serum globulin levels suggest inflammatory response; most confirmed IBD cases have high serum globulin levels, between 3.0 and 5.5 g/dL.[8] Serum globulins higher than 6.0 g/dL can be seen with very severe IBD, but Aleutian disease virus must be considered as a differential diagnosis whenever serum globulins approach 6.0 g/dL or above. ALT and GGT may be elevated due to secondary lymphocytic hepatitis or less commonly suppurative hepatitis (see Hepatic diseases). CBC findings are variable. A leukocytosis may be present, with a relative or absolute lymphocytosis. In other cases, a neutrophilia may be seen, suggestive of secondary bacterial infection in the gut or liver. Because chronic gastroenteritis is common, insidious and potentially fatal, annual comprehensive CBC and chemistry profiles should be recommended on all ferrets over 3 years old.

If many cases are subclinical or have only subtle signs, why diagnose and treat IBD aggressively? Because sequelae may be severe and fatal, even though the patient tolerates the underlying gastroenteritis for months or years. Sequelae include:

1. Chronic stomach or intestinal damage leads to fibrosis, bleeding ulcers, spontaneous gastric or intestinal rupture, intestinal villous atrophy and malabsorption, and/or progressive weight loss.
2. Secondary bacterial overgrowth or enteritis can produce severe illness including diarrhoea, vomition, anorexia, weight loss and sepsis.
3. Altered gastric motility may predispose to gastric acid reflux and oesophagitis, leading eventually to megaoesophagus.[4] Gastric motility alterations may also predispose to trichobezoar formation, although this connection is less easy to demonstrate.
4. Chronic malabsorption and protein deficiency can lead to muscle wasting. In theory, the cardiac muscle may be affected as well as skeletal muscles, with multiple amino acid deficiencies possibly leading to cardiomyopathy.
5. Lymphocytic enteritis can lead to ascending portal lymphocytic hepatitis; occasionally this leads to secondary bacterial infection and suppurative hepatitis.[8] Occasionally, chronic hepatitis may end in cirrhosis.
6. The most severe sequel to chronic gastroenteritis is lymphoma; this arises typically in the mesenteric nodes which have become severely hyperplastic in response to chronic gut inflammation.[8] Less often lymphoma can arise in the mucosa of the stomach or bowel. In the author's experience, undiagnosed chronic gastroenteritis is the most common trigger for lymphoma development in the pet ferret, in particular lymphomas arising in the mesenteric nodes (Ch. 13). Chronic gastroenteritis has been linked to increased risk of lymphoma development in other species as well.[29,30,31,32]

Figure 9.4 is a schematic of lesions, which may occur in various organ systems as sequelae to chronic gastroenteritis. The sequential events in the various pathways lead to end-result lesions which may be detected clinically; these lesions are shown in darker highlighted boxes. Those with question marks have a hypothesized causal association with gastroenteritis but have not been conclusively linked at this time.

Confirmation of diagnosis of IBD should be ideally done via histopathology. Gut biopsies should be obtained of the pyloric stomach, mid-duodenum, and mid-jejunum. The pyloric area biopsy should be just proximal to the pylorus itself, toward the lesser curvature of the stomach. Bowel biopsies should be on the antimesenteric border. Full thickness biopsies should be obtained ideally. A 5–7 mm wedge is easily taken for gastric biopsies; intestinal biopsies are typically only 2–3 mm long. A reversed scalpel blade is used to nick the antimesenteric surface of the bowel; the tissue everts with gentle digital pressure, allowing trimming of tissue off one margin with curved Metzenbaum scissors. Closures with 5-0 monofilament such as PDS or Maxon in simple interrupted pattern work well; gentle technique is impor-

Gastrointestinal diseases (cranial to caudal)

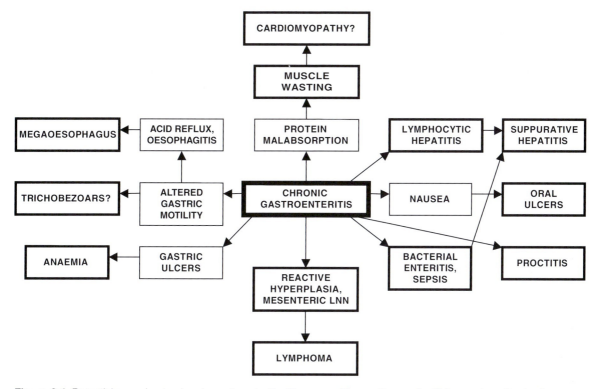

Figure 9.4 Potential sequelae to chronic gastroenteritis. Diseases with question marks (?) have a hypothesized causative association with gastroenteritis but have not been conclusively linked at this time. LNN, lymph node neoplasm.

tant to minimize tissue tearing with the small gauge suture. Gastric closure can be two layer (Ch. 18). Postoperative antibiotics are indicated whenever the gut is entered; e.g. enrofloxacin at 5 mg/kg p.o. b.i.d. plus amoxicillin at 10 mg/kg p.o. b.i.d. for 7 days postoperatively, or longer if the patient has evidence of bacterial disease.

Lymph node biopsies should be taken if any mesenteric nodes are visible. The most commonly enlarged and easily visualized are the gastric lymph nodes located in the fat near the lesser gastric curvature, and the duodenal (peripancreatic) node located just caudal to the pylorus. Figure 9.5 shows a grossly enlarged duodenal lymph node at the proximal end of the duodenum near the pylorus; a very large gastric lymph node is also visible in the fat near the lesser curvature of the stomach. Reactive lymph nodes in ferrets, unlike those of dogs and cats, demonstrate a gradation of pathology, which may be difficult to interpret: they may progress from mild to severe hyperplasia, then exhibit considerable cellular and/or architectural atypia, prior to transformation into lymphoma. A pathologist accustomed to interpreting canine and feline lymph node biopsies may mistakenly diagnose lymphoma in ferrets when the

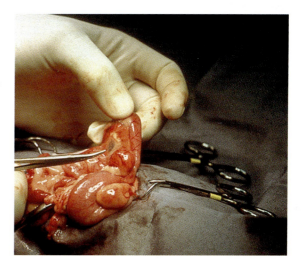

Figure 9.5 Severe enlargement of duodenal (peripancreatic) and gastric lymph nodes. The duodenum is held elevated, with forceps pointing toward the duodenal node adjacent to the pylorus. The stomach sits in the foreground, with a large gastric lymph node visible in the fat adjacent to the lesser gastric curvature.

CHAPTER NINE
Ferret gastrointestinal and hepatic diseases

nodes are only hyperplastic or preneoplastic. Therefore, pathologists not familiar with the histologic appearance of ferret lymph nodes should interpret nodal changes conservatively. Lymphoma should be suspected when histologic exam reveals obliteration of nodal architecture, and when gross exam of the patient reveals very large firm mesenteric or peripheral lymph nodes. Hyperplastic nodes, even when fairly large (over 1 cm diameter) are usually soft, and often oedematous; they may rupture when handled and drain serous fluid. Neoplastic nodes tend to be firm and solid even when sectioned. Ideally biopsy an entire node, as wedge biopsies may not represent the complete nodal architecture or cell population especially if the wedge sample enters a lymphoid follicle. Patients with cellular or architectural atypia in the nodes (which signify a potential for future transformation to lymphoma) warrant aggressive treatment. Figure 9.6 is a (ventral aspect) diagram of gut and lymph node biopsy sites in the ferret. If serum ALT or GGT elevations were noted, the liver should be biopsied as well; the tip of a lobe (such as the quadrate lobe) may be easily biopsied via suture ligation.

Biopsies should be read by a pathologist experienced in interpreting ferret gut histopathology. The author's samples are read by Dr Mike Garner.[a] The gut and lymph node lesions are identified, and graded as mild, moderate or severe, and any atypia is noted. Possible contributors to gut inflammation, such as *Helicobacter* or cryptosporidia are also noted when detected.

Treatment is aimed at eliminating possible underlying causes of gut inflammation and suppressing the inflammatory response. The long-term goals are suppressing the disease, thereby minimizing further tissue damage, allowing healing of gut mucosa, rebuilding the body's muscle mass, and preventing development of lymphoma. Initial therapy may include controlling existing sequelae such as gastric ulcers or bacterial overgrowth/enteritis; some patients present in poor condition and require aggressive supportive therapy prior to any surgical biopsy. Patients with signs suggestive of bacterial enteritis (diarrhoea, mucoid stools, green stools, bruxism, anorexia, thin body condition) may be treated initially with enrofloxacin at 5 mg/kg p.o. b.i.d. for 14 days plus amoxicillin at 10–20 mg/kg p.o. b.i.d. for 14 days; treatment may be extended if signs recur when medication is withdrawn. Force feeding with Hill's a/d diet, occasionally with added high calorie supplements such as Nutrical (EVSCO, USA), Ferretvite (8 in 1 Pet Products, USA) or human Ensure (Abbott Laboratories, USA), may help stabilize underweight weak patients. If gastroduodenal ulcers are suspected, they should be treated accordingly (see Gastric ulcers). Antiemetics such as metoclopramide (0.5–1.0 mg/kg p.o. or s.q. s.i.d./b.i.d.) may be useful if the patient appears nauseated when fed.

Ideally, long-term treatment should be based on gut histopathology. Treatment may begin once post-surgical healing is complete, usually 10–14 days postoperatively. If gastric biopsies reveal a significant *Helicobacter* presence coupled with lymphocytic gastritis, treatment to eliminate this organism should be initiated (see *Helicobacter* gastritis). Alternatively, as most ferrets carry *Helicobacter* in their gastric mucosa, one may decide to treat every gastritis patient presumptively, although *Helicobacter* may not be a significant contributor to gastritis in many patients. Presumptive treatment for *Helicobacter* should be performed in any patient who did not undergo gut biopsy as part of the diagnostic workup.

After *Helicobacter* treatment (if performed) is completed, long-term anti-inflammatory therapy should begin. Our drug of choice is azathioprine (Imuran); long experience with this drug in ferrets has shown it to be superior to corticosteroids in several respects. Corticosteroids used at immunosuppressive doses in ferrets will eventually produce unwanted side-effects, including loss of body condition (muscle wasting, fat deposition and 'pot belly'), hair thinning, increased risk of gastric ulceration, and hepatopathies. Patients with pre-existing hepatic pathology such as lymphocytic hepatitis or vacuolar hepatopathy (from concurrent adrenal endocrinopathy) seem particularly prone to prednisone-induced hepatopathies. These patients will sometimes demonstrate clinical malaise and severe elevation of serum hepatic enzymes (ALT, GGT) after even brief dosing with

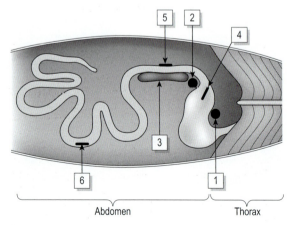

Figure 9.6 Gastrointestinal and mesenteric lymph node biopsy sites. **1.** Gastric lymph node; **2.** Duodenal lymph node; **3.** Right lobe of pancreas; **4.** Gastric biopsy site; **5.** Duodenal biopsy site; **6.** Jejunal biopsy site.

[a] Dr Mike Garner, Northwest ZooPath, Snohomish, Washington, USA. Tel: 1-360-794-0630; e-mail: zoopath@aol.com

corticosteroids. None of these sequelae are commonly seen with azathioprine, and bone marrow suppression or immune insufficiency are rare at the doses recommended. Azathioprine is easily compounded into a 5 mg/mL suspension which is pleasant tasting and stable for months. The azathioprine dosing protocol varies depending on the severity of the lesions being treated. Patients with gastroenteritis classified as mild or moderate may be placed on azathioprine dosed at 0.9 mg/kg p.o. q. 48 h. (This conservative dose regimen is also used if the patient did not undergo gut biopsy and is being treated presumptively based on history, clinical signs and CBC/serum chemistry findings.) The dosing frequency may be increased to 0.9 mg/kg p.o. s.i.d. in patients with severe or refractory clinical signs. Patients with gastroenteritis classified as severe, or who have lymphoid atypia present in gut mucosa or lymph node biopsies, should be placed on daily azathioprine dosing immediately. Cellular or architectural atypia in the nodes suggest potential for future transformation to lymphoma and always should be treated aggressively.

If prednisone is used instead of azathioprine, the dose is typically 2 mg/kg p.o. s.i.d.; concurrent use of corticosteroids with azathioprine may increase the risk of drug side effects and is not usually recommended.

Response to azathioprine is gradual, and 6 to 12 weeks may be needed for suppression of inflammation, healing of gut mucosa, resolution of clinical signs, and improvement in overall body condition. Rarely bone marrow suppression may be seen at s.i.d. dosing, usually manifesting as neutropenia. One patient demonstrated a gradual non-regenerative anaemia which improved when the azathioprine dose was reduced. Ideally perform a CBC within 3–4 weeks of starting therapy, then every 2–3 months thereafter. Patients who are stable on initial evaluations may be checked less frequently long term. Serum chemistries should be checked after 3–4 weeks on therapy, then every few months thereafter; the primary tests of concern are the serum lipase and globulin levels which may reflect the severity of the gut inflammation and hepatic enzymes (ALT and GGT), especially if hepatitis has been documented previously.

A small percentage of patients may not demonstrate adequate improvement in clinical appearance or in CBC/serum chemistry parameters on the above azathioprine doses. If no leukopenia is noted, the dose may gradually be increased to effect in these patients. Response to each dosage increase should be evaluated for 6–8 weeks prior to additional increases; re-check the CBC and serum chemistries 4–6 weeks after any dose increase to assess response and drug tolerance.

Dietary management is also recommended if the ferret will eat alternate diets. Several approaches may be taken:

1. *Allergen avoidance-hydrolyzed diets* such as Hills Z/D feline, or other strictly formulated feline select protein diets that avoid common protein sources (meats and grains), may allow reduction of gut inflammation if an underlying food hypersensitivity exists. An 8–10-week strict feeding trial is recommended. Some of our patients have shown clinical improvement (better stools, weight gain) on such diets, but whether this was due to allergen avoidance or simply better digestion of a particular formulation is uncertain. Many ferrets fail to show clinical improvement on these diets.

2. *Carbohydrate reduction*: Some carnivores are known to have trouble with chronic diarrhoea and digestive disturbances when fed dry kibble diets, whereas canned formulas produce fewer problems. The difference is thought to be the higher carbohydrate content of dry foods; starch is added to help form a more cohesive kibble. More recently, some low carbohydrate dry foods have been produced, such as Purina DM feline diet, Hills MD feline, and Pretty Pets Natural Gold diet for ferrets. These tend to have very high protein content and significantly reduced carbohydrate content, in theory ideal for ferrets. Some of our patients who fail to improve on allergen avoidance formulas have instead shown improvement on low carbohydrate formulas.

3. *Increased dietary fibre*: Some patients with chronic diarrhoea and bacterial overgrowth show clinical improvement when a high fibre formula such as Hill's W/D feline is added to the diet, either as part of a mix or as the exclusive diet. Despite the lower fat content, some patients actually gain weight due to improved gut function.

Despite dietary management, elimination of contributing factors such as *Helicobacter* or foreign bodies, and use of anti-inflammatory medications, IBD tends to be a long-term disease which remains active but suppressed with treatment. Therefore, chronic medication and monitoring are usually necessary. Resolution of clinical signs does not indicate a cure; only about half of our IBD patients had recognizable clinical signs *prior* to treatment, and were detected initially via evaluation of serum chemistries. With early detection, proper work-up and treatment, lymphocytic gastroenteritis can be controlled and severe sequelae avoided in most patients. With good control, we can minimize chronic wasting and loss of body condition, and reduce risk of mesenteric lymphoma. As a result, we see more ferrets living past the age of 8 years than ever before.

Intestinal foreign bodies

These are typically ingested pieces of soft rubbery material which ferrets are prone to chew and swallow; small trichobezoars can also occasionally leave the stomach and become lodged in the small bowel, usually the duodenum or proximal jejunum.

Signs are usually acute and severe, and may include bruxism, anorexia, vomiting, lethargy, weakness, fever or hypothermia, gastric distension and shock. If the object is slowly moving, signs may be less severe; the patient may be even be drinking or eating minimal amounts.

Careful palpation often reveals a firm movable abdominal mass effect. Radiographs often show a gas pattern in the stomach and proximal bowel with moderate distension; rarely a radio-dense foreign body such as a fruit pit may be seen; more often the object is radiolucent material such as soft rubber (Ch. 16). Barium may reveal a flow obstruction, but often does not outline the foreign body. Treatment is via enterotomy; use postoperative antibiotics for 7–14 days; enrofloxacin + amoxicillin is a good combination. Bowel resection and anastomosis is occasionally indicated if the obstructed bowel segment appears non-viable (Ch. 18).

Coccidia

No gastrointestinal parasite is very common in ferrets in the USA, but coccidiosis is occasionally seen, usually in stressed juvenile ferrets. Suspect concurrent disease with immune suppression if coccidiosis is detected in an adult ferret. Signs, when present, may include diarrhoea, tenesmus, mildly prolapsed rectal mucosa, and in severe cases, dehydration or weight loss. Diagnosis is via faecal flotation; treat with oral sulfonamides for 3 weeks. Albon (sulfadimethoxine) is effective; administer at 50 mg/kg p.o. s.i.d. on day 1, then 25 mg/kg p.o. s.i.d. for 14–20 days. Trimethoprim-sulfa is an alternate therapy, used at 30 mg/kg p.o. s.i.d./b.i.d. for 14–21 days (see Ch. 10).

Coronavirus enteritis (ECE)

This is a relatively new viral disease appearing first in the Eastern USA over a decade ago[18]; it rapidly spread across the USA, possibly as a result of large scale breeder facilities producing infected ferrets. It has been named epizootic catarrhal enteritis (ECE).

This virus is highly contagious via contact with infected ferrets, or their faeces or fomites. Coronaviruses may persist in the environment for considerable intervals (weeks or longer) under the right conditions. Disinfectants easily kill the virus.

This infection is unusual in 2 respects: (1) The younger the host is at time of infection, the fewer clinical signs are generally seen. (2) The ferret carries the virus long after clinical signs have resolved, and remains contagious to other ferrets for up to 6 months, perhaps longer.

Ferrets under 4 months old at time of infection often show no clinical signs. Ferrets 5–18 months old usually show mild to moderate signs, with severity gradually increasing with increased host age. Ferrets over 4–5 years old have the greatest risk of becoming severely ill when infected. However, the virulence of this virus appears to have been greatly reduced since the early years of viral spread across the USA. Whereas ferrets in the early 1990s often became severely ill (and many older ferrets died due to severe intestinal damage and nutrient malabsorption), death from ECE is uncommon now even in older ferrets, if adequate treatment is provided.

Onset of signs usually occurs within 48–96 h of exposure. Vomition is often seen in the first 48–72 h of illness, usually ceasing thereafter. Greenish mucoid to watery diarrhoea is the most common clinical sign, with rapid weight loss being seen in more severe cases. Milder cases may show little weight loss; diarrhoea is sometimes brown rather than green. Occasional cases may have melaena due to gastric or intestinal ulceration. Weight loss in severe cases may be extreme within the first 7–10 days of the illness even if the ferret is eating well. This is due to severe damage to enteric mucosa, with nutrient malabsorption and possibly protein-losing enteropathy contributing to the wasting disease.

Ferrets are not overly prone to hepatic lipidosis, but the rapidity of weight loss with this disease can sometimes produce significant lipidosis, especially in ferrets who were initially heavy. The gut inflammation can also predispose to ascending biliary or portal hepatitis, potentially impacting hepatic function.

No diagnostic serology is available; suspect ECE based on clinical signs of (usually) greenish diarrhoea with rapid onset, *plus* history of recent exposure to a new ferret. (This exposure could include the owner handling a baby ferret at a pet store.) The index of suspicion is higher if multiple ferrets are showing signs concurrently. Routine blood profiles may show mild lymphocytosis, as the inflammatory response in the intestine is primarily lymphoplasmacytic. However, secondary bacterial infection may induce a neutrophilia, or the leukocyte counts may be normal, so CBC changes are not diagnostic. Serum chemistry testing may reveal elevation of serum lipase or globulin due to gut inflammation (see Inflammatory bowel disease discussion), and elevated ALT or GGT if ascending lymphocytic hepatitis or hepatic lipidosis is present. Serum CK and AST tests may be elevated if muscle damage is present due to wasting disease. Hypoalbuminaemia may be seen with severe wasting illness. A more definitive diagnosis can be made via histopathologic examination of intestinal biopsies (usually post mortem). Immunohistochemistry testing of the gut mucosa for coronavirus can be performed.

Treatment is mainly supportive. Antibiotics may reduce secondary bacterial enteritis and improve clinical signs, reducing nausea and diarrhoea. Often the stool becomes less green with antibiotic usage. Metronidazole in particular seems to improve stool color and consistency, possibly due in part to its anti-inflammatory effects – the usual dosage is 20 mg/kg p.o. b.i.d. Enrofloxacin (5 mg/kg p.o. b.i.d.) plus amoxicillin (10–20 mg/kg p.o. b.i.d.) also can produce clinical improvement and is more palatable.

Severe malabsorption cases may show progressive wasting despite aggressive feeding, and may need extensive supportive care including total parenteral nutrition (Ch. 20). However, this is a rare scenario in the past 6 years as the most virulent viral strains seem to have vanished, likely due to selective pressures favoring milder strains which allow host survival and prolonged viral shedding.

No vaccines are available. Prevention is via avoidance; owners of older ferrets should exercise caution when handling unknown ferrets, especially juveniles. There is risk when purchasing a new young ferret as a companion for an older pet, especially if the ferret came from a large scale breeder facility in the USA. When handling such animals in hospital, proper isolation and disinfection techniques should be utilized to minimize contagion to other patients.

Eosinophilic granulomatous disease ('eosinophilic gastroenteritis')

This is an uncommon disease of unknown etiology.[33,34,35] It is characterized by eosinophilic infiltrates and granulomas involving the abdominal lymphatics and multiple organs. The intestines are usually involved when cases are recognized, but the inflammatory process does not appear to originate in the gut mucosa; it is more an eosinophilic lymphangitis. Thus, this is not a form of true 'inflammatory bowel disease', and the term 'eosinophilic gastroenteritis' is misleading.

Potential aetiologies could include allergic or parasitic disease; no parasites have been shown to be linked to this syndrome. Clinical signs, when present, can include diarrhoea of variable appearance, anorexia, weight loss, vomiting or lethargy. Severe cases may exhibit grossly bright red, thickened small bowel loops, some with clear cystic structures on the serosal surfaces (lymphangiectasia). This disease can be severe and can produce more profound gross lesions than with most

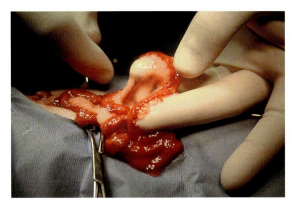

Figure 9.7 Eosinophilic granulomatous disease. In this advanced case, the intestinal loops are diffusely bright red, with clear vesicles (lymphangiectasia) present on the serosal surfaces.

inflammatory bowel disease (IBD) cases (Fig. 9.7). Early cases can be subclinical as with IBD.

Diagnosis follows the same clinical and CBC/serum chemistry parameters as with IBD; occasionally an absolute and relative eosinophilia may be seen. Gut and lymph node biopsy is needed to confirm diagnosis, and to differentiate this disease from IBD which often has an eosinophilic component. Eosinophilic granulomatous disease is uncommon and should not rate a high index of suspicion unless severe eosinophilia is present or grossly red thickened bowels are noted surgically. Intestinal lymphoma may also produce diffusely thickened red bowel segments on occasion.

Treat as with IBD; try to use a select protein diet if possible. This disease may be more difficult to manage than IBD but usually responds to anti-inflammatory treatment (azathioprine at 0.9 mg/kg p.o. s.i.d. long term).

Bacterial overgrowth/bacterial enteritis

Bacterial overgrowth and/or enteritis appear to be common in ferrets, usually secondary to underlying gut pathology such as inflammatory bowel disease or coronavirus enteritis. Other possible inciting factors could include dietary indiscretion, diet changes, coccidiosis, intestinal neoplasia, debility and foreign body ingestion.

Signs usually include diarrhoea (often greenish); more severe cases may demonstrate bruxism, anorexia, weight loss and occasionally vomition. Signs may be mild and sporadic; episodes are typically acute but may be weeks or months apart. Repeated episodes (if unrelated to diet changes or dietary indiscretion) strongly suggest underlying gut pathology.

Treat with broad spectrum antibiotics; enrofloxacin 5 mg/kg p.o. b.i.d. + amoxicillin 10–20 mg/kg p.o. b.i.d.

for 10–14 days usually works well. Metronidazole may also be used at 20 mg/kg p.o. b.i.d.

Enterotoxaemia

Bacterial enterotoxaemia is an uncommon but potentially deadly sequel to severe gastrointestinal disease and disruption of normal gut flora, such as can occur with inflammatory bowel disease, bacterial overgrowth, coronavirus enteritis, etc. Weak debilitated animals may be more prone, but incidence of enterotoxaemia is always low. The responsible organism is probably a *Clostridium* species.

Signs include diarrhoea, depression, hypothermia, shock and death. Enterotoxaemia may be suspected in a patient who has gastrointestinal disease and initially seems stable, then suddenly destabilizes, is very weak and is hypothermic. Differential diagnoses could include septicaemia, or septic peritonitis due to a perforated ulcer, or acute heavy gut bleeding due to ulceration, etc.

Treatment must be rapid and aggressive. Give broad spectrum antibiotic therapy which targets anaerobic infections well (such as metronidazole 20 mg/kg b.i.d. and amoxicillin 10–20 mg/kg b.i.d.). Toxin binding agents such as activated charcoal may be of benefit. Warmed i.v. fluids and supportive care are indicated (Ch. 20).

Mortality may be high with enterotoxaemia. Prevention is the better approach to this problem; use broad spectrum antibiotics such as enrofloxacin plus amoxicillin with any patient demonstrating significant signs of GI disease. Initiate supportive care if progressive weight loss is noted, before the patient is debilitated. Necropsy reveals large areas of small bowel which are dark red to black in color; otherwise findings are unremarkable (Fig. 9.8).

Aleutian disease virus

This is a chronic parvoviral disease of ferrets which may be subclinical or may on occasion produce clinical signs and hypergammaglobulinaemia. The virus can damage multiple organ systems, including kidneys, eyes, lungs and brain.[4] (See also discussion in Ch. 8.) This disease is mentioned here because wasting disease and diarrhoea with melaena have been reported in severe cases.[36] In the author's experience, ferrets with significant clinical Aleutian disease usually demonstrate an elevation in total serum globulin, occasionally as high as 14.0 g/dL. Other causes of chronic inflammation such as inflammatory bowel disease may also elevate serum globulin levels. However, total serum globulin levels in excess of 6.0 g/dL tend to be highly suspicious for Aleutian disease viral infection, as other inflammatory diseases usually produce lesser elevations.[8] Aleutian disease virus should be suspected when high serum globulin levels and chronic wasting disease or malaise are noted. Renal disease, mild respiratory distress due to viral pneumonia, ocular lesions such as uveitis, or CNS signs may also be present with this disease. Until recently, serologic confirmation of viral infection was available using counter-immunoelectrophoresis (United Vaccine Lab, USA). This laboratory no longer offers Aleutian virus testing, but the test is now available through the Blue Cross Animal Hospital, which has obtained United Vaccine Lab's reagents. (Serum samples should be addressed to Blue Cross Animal Hospital, c/o Dr Blau/CEP testing, 401 North Miller Avenue, Burley, Idaho, USA 83318.) Although serology can detect a viral carrier, causal linking of viral infection to gut lesions would require histopathology. Histologic findings would typically be a primarily plasmacytic inflammatory infiltrate in the gut tissues.[4] Treatment is primarily supportive care and anti-inflammatory medication; azathioprine dosed at 0.9 mg/kg p.o. s.i.d. has reduced serum globulin levels and reduced severity of signs in some of the author's patients. Broad spectrum antibiotics such as enrofloxacin 5 mg/kg p.o. b.i.d. plus amoxicillin 10 mg/kg p.o. b.i.d. may reduce severity of diarrhoea and malaise by reducing secondary bacterial overgrowth or enteritis. This is an uncommon primary cause of gastrointestinal disease in the ferret in the author's experience, and should have a low index of suspicion when evaluating most ferrets with gastrointestinal signs.

Neoplasia

Lymphoma is the most common gastrointestinal neoplasm encountered, likely due in many cases to chronic unrecognized inflammatory disease of the gut, such as caused by inflammatory bowel disease, *Helicobacter* gastritis, food hypersensitivity, or other factors. Lymphoma often appears to arise in the mesenteric lymph nodes first, but also can arise in the gut mucosa, or metastasize there from other locations. Signs vary depending on the location and extent of the lesions (Ch. 13). Often gradual weight loss and/or palpable abdominal masses are noted. Discrete masses involving the gut can lead to

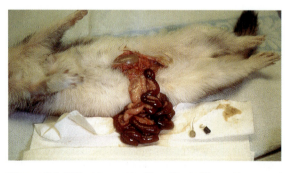

Figure 9.8 Enterotoxaemia. The affected bowel loops are dark red to black, typical of Clostridial enterotoxaemia. This necropsy was performed immediately post mortem.

bowel obstruction. Intestinal lymphoma can also cause diffusely thickened red bowels that resemble those seen with eosinophilic granulomatous disease. The red thickened lesions can be localized to small segments of bowel or involve the entire gut from duodenum to rectum. Diffuse infiltration of the bowel or stomach wall can lead to spontaneous perforation of the gut and septic peritonitis. The CBC may be unremarkable; lymphocytic leukaemia occurs only in a small percentage of cases. Serum chemistry tests may reveal elevated lipase and globulins suggestive of chronic gut inflammation; CK may be elevated with weight loss and muscle wasting. ALT may be elevated if neoplasia involves the liver.

Treatment of lymphomas is via chemotherapy; protocols vary from simple and inexpensive (e.g. prednisone alone), to moderately aggressive and moderately effective (e.g. Tufts University protocol), to the most aggressive and probably most effective (e.g. University of Wisconsin protocol). Response to treatment may be more rewarding with high grade lymphomas (Ch. 13).

Other neoplasia involving the gut is occasionally seen, such as pancreatic (exocrine) adenocarcinoma or primary bowel cancer. Signs vary depending on the location and extent of lesions, as with lymphoma. Prognosis for cure is poor with most of these neoplasms unless the lesion is localized and resectable (Ch. 13).

Proliferative bowel disease (proliferative ileitis)

This rather rare condition is caused by an intracellular bacterium, *Lawsonia intracellularis*.[37] The disease is characterized by inflammation and thickening of the ileum and/or colon (which often become palpable) and by diarrhoea of variable appearance and severe wasting. Unlike coronavirus, this disease affects mostly young ferrets younger than 1.5 years old, and does not respond to supportive care alone. Also, this disease targets the lower bowel, and can produce severe tenesmus and rectal prolapse.

Treatment is with chloramphenicol at 50 mg/kg p.o. b.i.d. for at least 2 weeks, longer in severe or chronic cases. Other antibiotics appear to be less effective.[37]

This illness appears to be rare, at least in the Western USA, and the author has not seen a confirmed case in nearly 20 years of clinical practice involving ferrets. The author's pathologist Dr Mike Garner (see p. 212) reads histopathology samples from across the USA and has only seen one case of this disease. Most enteric disease (with diarrhoea) which the author sees in ferrets responds clinically to amoxicillin combined with enrofloxacin or metronidazole, plus addressing any underlying gut disease. Thus proliferative bowel disease should have a very low index of suspicion, unless a palpably firm thickened lower bowel segment is noted or severe rectal prolapse is seen. Even with those clinical findings, intestinal lymphoma would be a more likely diagnosis than proliferative bowel disease in the author's experience.

Proctitis

This condition is occasionally seen, and appears as a grossly red, swollen and sometimes protruding anus. Severe cases may appear to have rectal mucosa prolapsing moderately. Tenesmus and pain on defecation are often noted.

Proctitis is seen most commonly concurrent with other gut pathology, such as inflammatory bowel disease, bacterial enteritis, or other disease that produces chronic diarrhoea or colitis. In these cases, proctitis could result from soiling and irritation of anal tissues due to chronic diarrhoea, or could represent a direct extension of an inflammatory process involving the rectal mucosa.

Initial treatment involves topical anti-inflammatory medication; one of the more effective is Anusol-HC (human haemorrhoid cream with hydrocortisone). Alternatively, an antibiotic + cortisone combination cream may be useful. Some cases respond better when oral enrofloxacin is used concurrently, suggesting a bacterial component to the proctitis. This condition may recur; long-term management should include evaluation for (and treatment of) any other gastrointestinal pathology present.

In rare cases of true rectal prolapse, the tissue should be replaced in situ and a 3-0 nylon purse string suture applied to prevent recurrence of the prolapse; the suture should be maintained for 14–21 days minimum provided that the patient tolerates the sutures well and can defecate normally.

Hepatic diseases

Hepatic pathology is common in ferrets and is often subclinical. The most common diseases encountered are hepatitis (usually ascending portal inflammation secondary to gastroenteritis), vacuolar hepatopathy (secondary to adrenal hormonal dyscrasias or cortisone administration), or a combination of both of these processes. Less commonly, neoplasia or other pathology may be seen. Serum chemistry evaluation is a useful tool in detecting hepatic pathology and in monitoring response to treatment. Histopathology is often required for definitive diagnosis and grading of lesions.

Lymphocytic hepatitis

This is very common in pet ferrets and is often unrecognized as it is usually subclinical. Lymphocytic hepatitis usually occurs secondary to gut disease, e.g. inflammatory bowel disease or other causes of chronic gut inflammation such as coronavirus.[8] A published report identified spirilliform bacteria resembling *Helicobacter* in hepatic biopsies of several ferrets with cholangiohepatitis,[38] but none of our cases have yielded similar findings.

The inflammation is typically a lymphocytic portal hepatitis, suggesting an ascending inflammatory process from the gut. Biliary inflammation is often noted.

Most cases are diagnosed incidentally when a blood profile is run; most patients are over 1.5 years old when diagnosed. Signs, if present, may include lethargy, anorexia, weight loss, bruxism, diarrhoea or vomition. Many of these signs could be due to gut disease which is often present. Preliminary diagnosis (i.e. high index of suspicion) is made via serum chemistry analysis. Lymphocytic hepatitis usually produces moderately elevated serum ALT (200–500 IU/L) and often GGT. Concurrent vacuolar hepatopathy from adrenal endocrinopathies may elevate the ALT further. Concurrent gut inflammation may produce elevated serum lipase and/or globulin levels. Most cases of lymphocytic hepatitis do not show elevation of serum AST, alkaline phosphatase or bilirubin. These are insensitive tests for hepatic disease in ferrets and typically elevate only with severe hepatic lesions such as suppurative hepatitis or neoplasia. AST is also a non-specific test and elevates readily with muscle damage, including wasting due to severe weight loss. Check for elevated CK if the serum AST exceeds the ALT, because even with severe liver disease ALT always elevates faster and more dramatically.

Interpreting serum chemistries:

- ALT = 200–700 IU/L: Mild to severe lymphocytic hepatitis, or mild to moderate suppurative hepatitis, or vacuolar hepatopathy, or occasionally lipidosis
- ALT = over 1000 IU/L: Severe suppurative hepatitis, or neoplasia
- GGT – over 10 IU/L: Ascending biliary inflammation and/or stasis suggested
- AST elevation only is seen in severe hepatic disease or muscle wasting
- Alkaline phosphatase elevation suggests severe biliary pathology and/or obstruction, such as with severe suppurative hepatitis or neoplasia
- Bilirubin elevation (over 0.9 mg/dL) suggests severe suppurative or neoplastic hepatic disease, or haemolysis. However, ferrets clear bilirubin very efficiently via the kidneys; urinalysis often reveals bilirubinuria with normal serum bilirubin concentrations.

Confirmation of diagnosis is via liver biopsy, ideally via laparotomy. Ultrasound-guided biopsy may be performed; avoid needle aspirates as they often are not diagnostic (Ch. 17). Most cases warrant gut biopsies as hepatitis in ferrets usually is secondary to chronic gastroenteritis; include the mesenteric lymph nodes (see Inflammatory bowel disease). Suture ligature of a lobe tip is an easy biopsy technique, if no focal hepatic lesions are noted.

Treatment is similar to that for inflammatory bowel disease. Azathioprine dosed at 0.9 mg/kg every 1–2 days p.o. is recommended long term; monitor progress via evaluation of serum ALT and GGT regularly (and lipase/globulin, if these are elevated due to gastroenteritis). Also evaluate the CBC 4 weeks after initiating therapy, then every 3–4 months thereafter while using azathioprine. Human studies have shown that azathioprine combined with low dose prednisone controlled inflammation as well as high dose prednisone alone. Some anecdotal reports in canine chronic active hepatitis indicated improved results when azathioprine was used with prednisone, as opposed to prednisone alone.[39] In ferrets, prednisone can exacerbate hepatic pathology in some cases and is not recommended. Some ferrets with pre-existing hepatopathies may demonstrate severe elevations in serum ALT levels soon after prednisone dosing begins, often with profound clinical malaise.[4]

Cases with severe or refractory elevations of ALT or GGT may benefit from addition of ursodiol (Actigall) at 15 mg/kg p.o. s.i.d. to reduce biliary stasis via thinning of biliary secretions; it also has anti-inflammatory effects. S-adenosylmethionine (SAMe) may be of benefit in some cases also – it reportedly has antioxidant and cell membrane-protective properties. The typical dose is 20 mg/kg per day for dogs; we have not evaluated its use in ferrets at this time. Silymarin (milk thistle) is a flavinolignan mixture with purported antioxidant properties. Its efficacy in treating liver disease in humans, dogs, cats and ferrets has not been demonstrated adequately.

Control of ferret hepatitis usually requires recognition and control of any concurrent gut pathology such as inflammatory bowel disease; control of gastroenteritis often resolves the hepatitis. Untreated lymphocytic hepatitis may lead to episodes of acute suppurative cholangiohepatitis, cirrhosis or possibly neoplasia.[4,40]

Suppurative hepatitis

This form of hepatitis is far less common than lymphocytic hepatitis, but is more recognizable due to its often profound clinical signs. Mild cases may be subclinical, but severe cases can be acute and dramatic. There is probably underlying lymphocytic gastroenteritis present in most cases, leading to intestinal bacterial overgrowth, ascending biliary inflammation, and lymphocytic hepatitis, all of which predispose the patient to bacterial cholangiohepatitis. In a few cases, liver biopsies reveal neutrophilic infiltration patterns suggestive of bloodborne sepsis, but most are portal hepatitis typical of ascending disease from the GI tract.[4]

Acute severe cholangiohepatitis produces significant clinical signs: lethargy, anorexia, fever, vomition or diarrhoea may all occur, as well as icterus. Normal ferrets may have a slight yellowish cast to the skin due to sebaceous secretions, and icterus may be subtle and overlooked. The nose, ears and oral cavity are good locations for visualizing icterus, as is the serum (Fig. 9.9). Urine may be vivid deep yellow or greenish tinged with bilirubinuria.

Subclinical cases are discovered via serum chemistry analysis; usually serum ALT and GGT are the best indicators of ferret hepatopathy and are likely to elevate even with milder cases (see lymphocytic hepatitis for discussion of serum chemistry evaluation). Severe cases may demonstrate ALT levels well over 1000 IU/L, with lesser elevations of GGT, AST and even alkaline phosphatase. Serum bilirubin may be elevated. Ferrets clear bilirubin efficiently via the kidneys, which may lead to bilirubinuria with fairly normal serum bilirubin levels. The CBC may reveal leukocytosis with neutrophilia in some cases.

Definitive diagnosis is via histopathology; in milder cases, this is the only way to differentiate this condition from the more common lymphocytic hepatitis. Severe cases with large chemistry elevations should create immediate suspicion of suppurative disease, and broad spectrum antibiotic therapy should begin. An effective combination is enrofloxacin at 5–10 mg/kg p.o. b.i.d. + amoxicillin at 10–20 mg/kg p.o. b.i.d. for at least 14 days. Supportive care (fluids, force feeding, control of diarrhoea or nausea, etc.) should be given as needed. Serum chemistries and clinical appearance often improve dramatically within 3–5 days, and the patient may appear clinically normal at the end of therapy. Serum chemistries should be evaluated after 14 days even if recovery appears complete. Mild persistent ALT or GGT elevations suggest underlying pathology such as lymphocytic hepatitis; elevated serum lipase and/or globulin levels may also suggest underlying gut pathology such as inflammatory bowel disease. Suppurative hepatitis is usually secondary to another disease process; this should be investigated and addressed in order for long-term management of the patient to be successful (i.e. hepatic and gastrointestinal biopsies may be indicated).

Vacuolar hepatopathy

This is a histopathologic diagnosis, wherein increased vacuolization of hepatocytes is observed. The typical cause is endocrinopathy, such as caused by adrenal tumours with elevation of sex hormones such as estradiol. Corticosteroid administration may also produce this condition.

Most cases are subclinical, but might be suspected when mild to moderate persistent serum elevations of ALT (and sometimes GGT) are seen in a patient with adrenal disease. The main differential diagnosis is lymphocytic hepatitis; only hepatic biopsy can differentiate the two conditions. Clinical signs tend to be mild and nonspecific, e.g. malaise, mild anorexia, or lethargy.

This condition usually produces minimal to mild ALT elevations (200–350 IU/L). However, cases with concurrent lymphocytic hepatitis and vacuolar hepatopathy may demonstrate persistent serum ALT levels as high as 400–550 IU/L, with minimal clinical signs and no apparent progression of disease for long periods.

Treatment includes elimination of underlying causes, i.e. adrenal disease or prednisone administration. Other therapies when clinical signs are present may include ursodiol (Actigall) at 15 mg/kg p.o. s.i.d., anti-nausea medications and general supportive care.

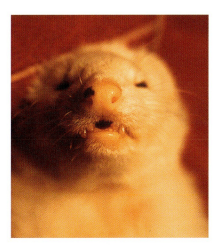

Figure 9.9 Icterus in a ferret with suppurative hepatitis. *Note* the yellow nose and lips. Icterus is often subtle and overlooked in ferrets.

Hepatic lipidosis

Ferrets are not overly prone to severe lipidosis, but certain situations may predispose a patient to this disease. The most common would be a heavy older ferret who loses weight suddenly, such as from infection with coronavirus enteritis. Other hepatic disease such as lymphocytic hepatitis may compromise hepatic function and predispose to lipidosis in the face of weight loss. Steroid usage, endocrine dyscrasias and other factors may also influence the incidence of this disease.

The clinical presentation is variable. Many cases of lipidosis are subclinical, and presenting signs are often related to whatever disease process precipitated the initial weight loss (e.g. coronavirus enteritis, suppurative hepatitis, neoplasia, sepsis, etc.). Only in severe cases is the liver grossly enlarged enough to identify via palpation. Serum chemistries may be normal or may show mild elevation of ALT and GGT similar to lymphocytic hepatitis (see Lymphocytic hepatitis for discussion of serum chemistry evaluation). Radiographs or ultrasound may detect hepatomegaly (Chs 16, 17).

Diagnosis is via surgical inspection and/or biopsy. A transdermal biopsy may be performed if no surgery is elected. Grossly the liver appears pale brown to yellowish, and the lobes tend to be swollen and rounded.

Treatment includes controlling concurrent diseases (especially those causing weight loss), maximizing caloric intake, and minimizing liver pathology. If the patient is eating, supplement the normal diet with Hill's a/d canned food and a high calorie supplement such as Ferretvite, Nutrical, human Ensure, etc. to add calories. Anorexic animals can be force fed a/d and Nutrical unless vomiting. Broad spectrum antibiotics are safe and may inhibit GI bacterial overgrowth or low-grade suppurative hepatitis; a good combination is enrofloxacin at 5 mg/kg p.o. b.i.d. + amoxicillin at 10 mg/kg p.o. b.i.d. Ursodiol (Actigall) may be used to reduce biliary stasis, dosed at 15 mg/kg p.o. s.i.d. Prognosis is good with most ferret lipidosis patients, provided that the underlying cause of the lipidosis is identified and resolved.

End stage liver disease (cirrhosis)

This uncommon condition is the end result of chronic damage to the liver, most likely due to undiagnosed chronic hepatitis. At this stage, the liver is close to failing, and patients may present with either acute or chronic lethargy, nausea, vomition, diarrhoea, anorexia, icterus and weight loss. Patients who seem to become ill acutely may have acute bacterial hepatitis. The prognosis is poor once cirrhosis is confirmed.

Serum chemistries are compatible with liver damage *and* loss of function. Serum ALT and GGT may be mildly to markedly elevated and bilirubin is usually elevated also. AST and even alkaline phosphatase may elevate. Serum bile acids may be elevated as well. Lipase and globulin levels may be high with concurrent gut pathology (see Lymphocytic hepatitis and Inflammatory bowel disease for discussion of serum chemistry evaluation of hepatic and gut parameters, respectively).

A definitive diagnosis is made via biopsy. Ultrasound may detect changes in size and consistency of the liver suggestive of cirrhosis (Ch. 17). If biopsy is surgical, preoperative supportive care may be needed to strengthen and stabilize the patient prior to surgery. Antibiotics may produce significant improvement in signs and serum chemistries in some cases. Grossly, the liver appears small, firm, and irregular, sometimes with nodular regeneration visible. Histopathology shows bridging fibrosis with areas of regeneration, but overall loss of healthy hepatocytes. Underlying lymphocytic or neutrophilic inflammation may be noted.

The long-term prognosis is poor. Patients may be maintained on a high calorie low protein diet such as Hill's k/d feline; if needed one can mix in Hill's a/d diet or high calorie supplements such as Nutrical to improve palatability. Long term antibiotic therapy may be indicated, especially if histopathology revealed a suppurative component or the patient shows initial improvement on antibiotics. Long-term enrofloxacin dosed at 5 mg/kg p.o. s.i.d. may be enough to prevent re-infection. Ursodiol dosed at 15 mg/kg p.o. s.i.d. may also be used long term.

Biliary cysts and cystadenomas

These are histologically benign cystic structures located in one or more hepatic lobes; they are variable from small and focal to large and numerous. Dr Mike Garner (see p. 212) at Northwest ZooPath notes that they are common in both domestic and black-footed ferrets. Cystadenomas are benign but may be progressive in development; in extreme cases, the cystic masses may replace large portions of hepatic parenchyma in multiple lobes. In theory, if these lesions become extensive they could result in loss of hepatic function. However, few have resulted in clinical hepatopathy in the author's experience, and most often, the cystic masses were an incidental finding during a laparotomy. Large cysts may be palpable as soft masses in the cranial abdomen or may be visible on radiographs; smaller lesions may be detected via ultrasound (Chs 16, 17). No serum elevations of hepatic enzymes are usually seen; mild to moderate increases in ALT and GGT occasionally occur. Treatment (if elected) is surgical removal; in severe cases, the lesions may recur. Figure 9.10 shows moderately large biliary cysts in a necropsy specimen.

Hepatic neoplasia

Primary or metastatic neoplasms are occasionally seen in the ferret liver (Ch. 13). These are difficult to suspect unless detected via palpation, radiographs or ultrasound

Gastrointestinal diseases (cranial to caudal)

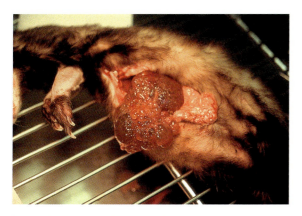

Figure 9.10 Large biliary cysts in a ferret; these were incidental findings and not the cause of death.

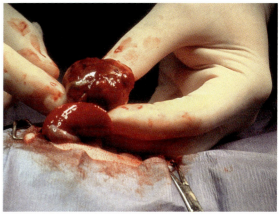

Figure 9.12 Hepatoma in a liver lobe; the single mass is elevated, showing the normal liver lobe it is attached to (below the mass).

(Chs 16, 17). Clinical and serum chemistry findings resemble those seen with hepatitis. Neoplasia in the liver may also be suspected whenever severe elevations are seen in key serum chemistries, in particular ALT and GGT, and sometimes AST, alkaline phosphatase, or bilirubin. The main differential diagnosis is suppurative hepatitis (see Lymphocytic hepatitis for discussion of serum chemistry interpretation). The most common tumours seen in ferret livers are metastatic masses from other sites, mainly adrenal cortical adenocarcinomas and lymphomas. Both of these neoplasms tend to produce pale multiple masses when they involve the liver; some right adrenal tumours invade the caudate liver lobe locally without general metastasis (Fig. 9.11).

Primary hepatic masses are less common. They tend to be darker in colour, resembling the colour of normal liver to some extent. Several types are seen. *Helicobacter*-like organisms were reported associated with hepatitis and hepatic neoplasia in one study,[38] but none of our cases in the past 18 years have had similar findings.

Hepatomas are benign hepatocellular neoplasms which can produce clinical disease, either via damage to hepatic tissue and function, or possibly via inducing hypoglycemia. Hepatic neoplasms have been shown to be capable of inducing hypoglycemia in other species.[41,42,43] Clinical signs may include lethargy, salivation, weight loss, anorexia, bright orange-yellow or greenish urine (bilirubinuria), and icterus. Serum chemistries in an example case showed ALT = 1050 IU/L, AST normal, GGT = 37 IU/L, alkaline phosphatase normal, globulin = 3.6 g/dL and glucose = 38 mg/dL. Insulinoma is an obvious differential diagnosis for the hypoglycaemic component. Surgical findings are typically a single dark irregular liver-coloured mass involving one lobe, usually resectable (Fig. 9.12). Treatment is via excision; the prognosis is good.

Hepatocellular adenocarcinoma is a malignant aggressive neoplasm which may involve one or more lobes and may metastasize. Serum chemistries in a sample case showed ALT = 4035 IU/L, AST = 596 IU/L, GGT = 102 IU/L, alkaline phosphatase normal, lipase = 605 IU/L, globulin = 3.1 g/dL and glucose = 53 mg/dL. Treatment is via surgical resection if possible. Gross findings are one to many dark irregular liver-coloured masses involving one or more liver lobes, with visible metastasis sometimes seen. Solitary masses may be excised; with more aggressive lesions debulking the tumour mass might slow the clinical progression for a time. The prognosis is poor if the lesions are not detected early.

Biliary adenocarcinoma is occasionally seen. Findings and aggressive behaviour are similar to those of hepatocellular adenocarcinoma; treatment and prognosis are similar as well.

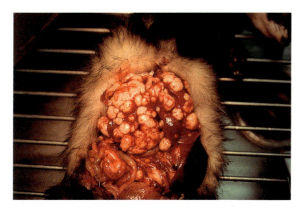

Figure 9.11 Metastatic adrenal cortical carcinomas in the liver of a ferret.

References

1. Evans HE, An NQ. Anatomy of the ferret. In: Fox JG, ed. Biology and diseases of the domestic ferret, 2nd edn. Baltimore: Williams and Wilkins; 1998:19–69.
2. Harris CA, Andrews GA. Megaoesophagus in a domestic ferret. Lab Anim Sci 1993; 43:506–508.
3. Blanco MC, Fox JG, Rosenthal K, et al. Megaoesophagus in nine ferrets. J Am Vet Med Assoc 1994; 205:444–447.
4. Burgess M, Garner M. Unpublished clinical and histopathologic data from clinical cases, 1995–2005.
5. IDEXX Veterinary Laboratories, Portland, Oregon, USA.
6. Antech Veterinary Laboratories, Portland, Oregon, USA.
7. Vet Test Chemistry Analyzer, IDEXX Laboratories, USA.
8. Burgess M, Garner M. Clinical aspects of inflammatory bowel disease in ferrets. Exotic DVM 2002; 4:29–34.
9. Hoefer, HL. Gastritis and ulceration. In: Hillyer EB, Carpenter JW, eds. Ferrets, rabbits and rodents: Clinical medicine and surgery, 2nd edn. Philadelphia: WB Saunders; 2004:26–28.
10. Fox JG, Otto G, Taylor NS, et al. *Helicobacter mustelae*-induced gastritis and elevated gastric pH in the ferret (*Mustela putorius furo*). Infect Immun 1991; 59:1875–1880.
11. Fox JG, Otto G, Murphy JC, et al. Gastric colonization of the ferret with *Helicobacter* species: natural and experimental infections. Rev Infect Dis 1991; 13:671–680.
12. Fox JG, Correa P, Taylor N, et al. *Helicobacter mustelae*-associated gastritis in ferrets. Gastroenterology 1990; 99:352–361.
13. Erdman SE, Correa P, Coleman LA, et al. *Helicobacter mustelae*-associated gastric MALT lymphoma in ferrets. Am J Pathol 1997; 151:273–280.
14. Fox JG, Marini RP. *Helicobacter mustelae* infection in ferrets: pathogenesis, epizootiology, diagnosis, and treatment. Semin Avian Exotic Pet Med 2001; 10:36–44.
15. Bell JA. *Helicobacter mustelae* gastritis. In: Hillyer EB, Carpenter JW, eds. Ferrets, rabbits and rodents: Clinical medicine and surgery, 2nd edn. Philadelphia: WB Saunders; 2004:33–34,37.
16. Flatland B. *Helicobacter* infection in humans and animals. Compend Contin Edu Small Anim Pract 2002; 24:688–696.
17. Marini RP, Fox JG, Taylor NS, et al. Ranitidine bismuth citrate and clarithromycin, alone or in combination, for eradication of *Helicobacter mustelae* infection in ferrets. Am J Vet Res 1999; 60:1280–1286.
18. Williams BH, Kiupel M, West KH, et al. Coronavirus-associated epizootic catarrhal enteritis in ferrets. J Am Vet Med Assoc 2000; 217:526–530.
19. Parsonnet J. The epidemiology of C. *pylori*. In: Blaser MJ, ed. *Campylobacter pylori* in gastritis and peptic ulcer disease. New York: Igaku-Shoin; 1989:51–60.
20. Ó Cróinin T, Clyne M, Appelmelk BJ, et al. Antigastric autoantibodies in ferrets naturally infected with *Helicobacter mustelae*. Infect Immun 2001; 69:2708–2713.
21. Zhonghua Yi. Effects of different triple therapies on duodenal ulcer-associated *Helicobacter pylori* infection and a one year follow up study. Xue Za Zhi 2004; 84:1161–1165.
22. Calvet X, Montserrat A, Guell M, et al. Raniditine bismuth citrate, tetracycline and metronidazole followed by triple therapy as alternative strategy for *Helicobacter pylori* treatment: a pilot study. Eur J Gastroenterol Hepatol 2004; 16:987–990.
23. Kato S, Konno M, Maisawa S, et al. Results of triple eradication therapy in Japanese children: a retrospective multicenter study. J Gastroenterol 2004; 39:838–843.
24. Watanabe K, Murakami K, Sato R, et al. Effect of sucralfate on antibiotic therapy for *Helicobacter pylori* infection in mice. Antimicrob Agents Chemother 2004; 48:4582–4588.
25. Strombeck DR, Guilford WG. Plasma lipase. In: Strombeck DR, Guilford WG, eds. Small Animal Gastroenterology. Davis, CA: Stonegate Publishing; 1990:445.
26. Carriere F, Laugier R, Barrowman JA, et al. Gastric and pancreatic lipase levels during a test meal in dogs. Scand J Gastroenterol 1993; 28:443–454.
27. Carriere F, Rogalska E, Cudrey C, et al. In vivo and in vitro studies on the stereoselective hydrolysis of tri- and diglycerides by gastric and pancreatic lipases. Bioorg Med Chem 1997; 5:429–435.
28. Burrows CF. Secretion and localization of dog gastric lipase: viewpoint. Alpo Viewpoints in Vet Med 1993; 3:1.
29. Charlotte F, Sriha B, Mansour G, et al. An unusual case associating ileal Crohn's disease and diffuse large B-cell lymphoma of an adjacent mesenteric lymph node. Arch Pathol Lab Med 1998; 122:559–561.
30. Woodley HE, Spencer JA, MacLennan KA. Small-bowel lymphoma complicating long-standing Crohn's disease. AJR Am J Roentgenol 1997; 169:1462–1463.
31. Greenstein AJ, Mullin GE, Strauchen JA, et al. Lymphoma in inflammatory bowel disease. Cancer 1992; 69:1119–1123.
32. Wasmer ML, Willard MD, Helman RG, et al. Food intolerance mimicking alimentary lymphosarcoma. J Am Anim Hosp Assoc 1995; 31:463–466.
33. Fazakas S. Eosinophilic gastroenteritis in a domestic ferret. Can Vet J 2000; 41:707–709.
34. Palley LS, Fox JG. Eosinophilic gastroenteritis in the ferret. In: Kirk RW, Bonagura JD, eds. Kirk's current veterinary therapy XI: Small animal practice. Philadelphia: WB Saunders; 1992:1182–1184.
35. Fox JG, Palley LS, Rose R. Eosinophilic gastroenteritis with Splendore-Hoeppli material in the ferret (*Mustela putorius furo*). Vet Pathol 1992; 29:21–26.
36. Morrisey JK. Aleutian disease. In: Hillyer EB, Carpenter JW, eds. Ferrets, rabbits and rodents: Clinical medicine and surgery, 2nd edn. Philadelphia: WB Saunders; 2004:66–68.
37. Bell JA. Proliferative bowel disease. In: Hillyer EB, Carpenter JW, eds. Ferrets, rabbits and rodents: Clinical medicine and surgery, 2nd edn. Philadelphia: WB Saunders; 2004:34–37.
38. Garcia A, Erdman SE, Xu S, et al. Hepatobiliary inflammation, neoplasia, and argyrophilic bacteria in a ferret colony. Vet Pathol 2002; 39:173–179.
39. Richter, Keith DVM, DACVIM. Selected canine hepatopathies. Continuing education lecture, Portland, Oregon, 2004.

40. Yano Y, Yoon S, Seo Y, et al. A case of well-differentiated hepatocellular carcinoma arising in primary biliary cirrhosis. Kobe J Med Sci 2003; 49:39–43.
41. Tietge UJ, Schofl C, Ocran KW, et al. Hepatoma with severe non-islet cell tumour hypoglycemia. Am J Gastroenterol 1998; 93:997–1000.
42. Yamaguchi M, Kamimura S, Takada J, et al. Case report: Insulin-like growth factor II expression in hepatocellular carcinoma with alcoholic liver fibrosis accompanied by hypoglycemia. J Gastroenterol Hepatol 1998; 13:47–51.
43. van Wijngaarden P, Janssen JA, de Man RA. Hepatocellular carcinoma complicated by non-islet cell tumour hypoglycemia. Ned Tijdschr Geneeskd 2002; 146:859–862.

CHAPTER 10

Parasitic diseases of ferrets

'Practically all wild mammals, even healthy ones, carry at least a few parasites, internal and/or external.'

Carolyn King, The Natural History of Weasels and Stoats, 1989

Let us see if this relates to ferrets remembering there is always a risk of new or exotic parasites somehow getting into other countries. The various life cycles are of interest where pet ferrets are in close contact with dogs and cats and when an intermediate host is involved which might attract a ferret to eat it.

Ferret internal parasites

Ferrets can be infected with internal parasites of the dog, cat or other mustelids such as mink, and this should be considered at clinical examination. Unlike American pet ferrets, those in other countries often live largely outdoors and can be used for hunting, so the risk of infection could be increased in these circumstances.

Important protozoan diseases

Parasite taxonomy is changing with the availability of DNA sequencing. At present, the protozoan parasite species considered below are of interest and occur in the text below. The general classification headings have been made with the help of Russell Hobbs, parasitologist, Murdoch University Veterinary School. The chapter gives a general account of disease-producing species with reference to the ferret taking part as a possible secondary host, as indicated in the life cycle diagrams.

Phylum Sarcomastigophora
    Subphylum Mastigophora
        Class Zoomastigophorea
            Order Kinetoplastida
                Family Trypanosomatidae
                      Genus *Leishmania*
            Order Diplomonadida
                Family Hexamitidae
                      Genus *Giardia*
Phylum Apicomplexa
    Class Sporozoasida
        Subclass Coccidiasina
            Order Eucoccidiorida
                Suborder Adeleorina
                      Family Hepatozoide
                          Genus *Hepatozoon*
                Suborder Eimeriorina
                      Family Eimeriidae
                          Genus *Eimeria*
                          Genus *Isospora*
                      Family Sarcocystidae
                          Genus *Sarcocystis*
                          Genus *Toxoplasma*
                          Genus *Neospora*
                      Family Cryptosporidiidae
                          Genus *Cryptosporidium*

Toxoplasmosis

All carnivores are susceptible to this disease and the ferret could possibly act as an intermediate host to

Important protozoan diseases

Toxoplasma gondii, one of the most ubiquitous parasites known. It is an intracellular parasite. Serological studies in the USA found at least 30% of cats and humans have been exposed to the parasite.[1] It has been found, on histology, in experimental ferrets used for distemper research. It has also been obtained from one ferret and two ferret-polecat hybrids via in vivo passage of brain tissue in mice.[2] It should be noted that the mustelid *Toxoplasma* are morphologically, biologically and serologically indistinguishable from those isolated from rabbits in the UK.[2]

Deaths of neonate ferrets have been a problem in fitch farms in the USA. The deaths are without clinical signs and post mortem findings show extensive necrotic areas in the lungs, heart and liver along with *Toxoplasma*-like organisms. Deaths and the presence of *Toxoplasma* in 1-day-old ferret kittens indicate a congenital infection.[2]

A congenital *Toxoplasma*-like disease was found in New Zealand on a fitch farm where 30% of 750 neonatal kittens died without observed clinical signs. The main diet had been frozen sheep meat. About 1 month prior to mating, the jills who bore these kittens had gone into an unusual period of anorexia. On post mortem of the kittens, multifocal necrotic areas associated with *Toxoplasma*-like organisms were found in the liver, lungs and heart, which indicated toxoplasmosis. The surviving kittens from the affected litters showed stunted growth and no signs of *Toxoplasma* by histological or serological examination; neither could the infection be shown by injection of infected material into mice. Because of these facts, a congenital acute disease was thought likely.[3]

Between 1992 and 1999 an epizootic outbreak of the disease occurred in 22 adults and 30 kits of captive *Mustela nigripes* (endangered black-footed ferrets, BFF) in the USA.[4] These animals appear to be highly susceptible to acute and chronic toxoplasmosis. The clinical signs included anorexia, lethargy, corneal oedema and ataxia. High antibody titers to *Toxoplasma gondii* were found in ten individuals and those that died showed *T. gondii*-like organisms in many organs. It was considered that frozen uncooked rabbit was the source of

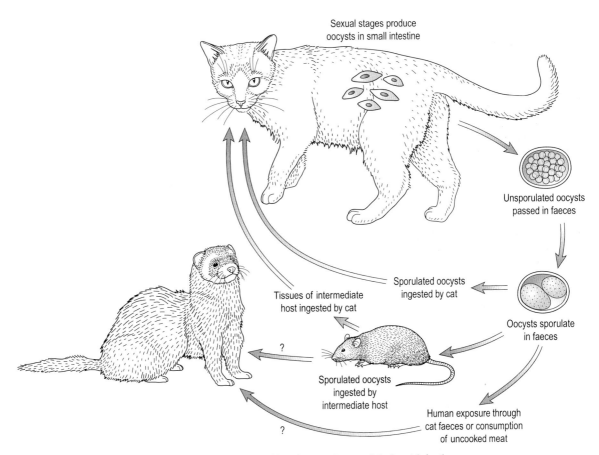

Figure 10.1 *Toxoplasma gondii* life cycle in the cat with reference to possible ferret infection.

CHAPTER TEN

Parasitic diseases of ferrets

infection. *Note* that an additional 13 adults died of chronic toxoplasmosis, which was a disaster for the project. They developed chronic progressive weakness of the posterior limbs and ataxia 6–69 months after the disease began. At post mortem, meningoencephalitis or meningoencephalomyelitis was established.

Cats, however, are the only definitive host of *T. gondii* and the only species in which the life cycle (Fig. 10.1) is completed with the enteroepithelial sexual stage.[1]

The cat excretes oocysts for 1–3 weeks after infection and these become infective 1–5 days later (depending on environmental conditions). This could pose a problem for other species like ferrets in a mixed house pet situation.[1] In zoos, it is suggested that wild Felidae be kept well away from other animals including Mustelidae.

Clinical signs: These, as indicated above, can vary considerably between species: possibly anaemia, ocular lesions (retinitis or iritis), hepatitis with clinical icterus, blindness, CNS signs, respiratory disease and diarrhoea. Additionally there may be concurrent lethargy, anorexia and fever, so there is a wide spectrum of signs. Combinations of these symptoms may occur.

I have seen a ferret with severe icterus; it had eaten a mouse and was brought in moribund but died. Unfortunately, no post mortem was possible.[5]

In cats, clinical disease is potentially more severe with co-infection of feline immunodeficiency virus (FIV).[1]

Diagnosis: (a) By possible exposure, i.e. the ferret has eaten an infected mouse. (b) In cats, diagnosis is by immunological methods used for humans.[1] It is found that enzyme-linked immunosorbent assays (ELISA) can detect *T. gondii*-specific immunoglobulin G (IgG), *T. gondii*-specific immunoglobulin M (IgM), and *T. gondii*- specific antigens in the serum. This test can also be applied to ferrets.

Treatment: Basically, treatment is with sulphonamides. *Note* that sulphaquinoxaline is toxic to ferrets! As with the cat, medication should be for at least 2 weeks, given q.i.d., and continued for some short period after clinical signs cease as a precaution.[6] *Medication*: pyrimethamine (0.5–1 mg/kg per day) plus sulfadiazine (60 mg/100 mL drinking water or 60 mg/100 g in food) with both drugs used synergistically. The drugs act against the tachyzoites but do not destroy the cyst stage. They act by blocking the metabolic pathways involving p-amino benzoic acid and the folic–folinic acid cycle.[2] If treatment is prolonged, the ferret should receive folinic acid and bakers' yeast as a supplement, as folic acid is essential for haematopoiesis. *Note*: clindamycin hydrochloride has been used on cats at dose rate of 25–50 mg/kg per day. It may not eliminate the organism but it stops replication.[7] I have used it on a ferret with a mammary abscess without reaction (see Appendix).

Prevention: Possible routes of ferret infection with *Toxoplasma* would be: (a) Ferrets catching infected rabbits, rats or mice. (b) Ferret food or housing area contamination with cat faeces. (c) Ferrets being fed uncooked infected meat. Ferrets living in a ferretarium or free-ranging in the garden could be at risk of exposure to cat faeces (see Ch. 3). Cats, however, are fastidious about burying their excreta, unlike dogs or ferrets. Dog excreta can be manually removed from the area, while ferrets will be likely to use scats trays in the ferretarium or elsewhere. Oocysts from cats' faeces can live in the environment for months or years, so there is a long-term risk.[1]

With exposure to *T. gondii*, cats and other hosts can develop an extra-intestinal phase whereby the organism is contained in a cyst. In individuals, the cysts can be activated over time to cause clinical disease and possible oocyst shedding.[1] This is not as yet recorded in ferrets but would probably be a fatal infection. To avoid contamination of their food, ferrets could be fed indoors as a routine or in outdoor cages. If ferrets free-range in garden or ferretarium, food can be placed in PVC pipes of a size suitable only for ferrets, or placed in the boltholes overnight. This also stops food contamination from bird droppings. Ferrets living in a house with cats could use the cat dirt tray. This could bring the problem closer to the ferret and ideally would require the cats' dirt tray to be placed on some raised area that the ferrets could not reach. Plenty of scats trays could be put around to deter the ferrets from going elsewhere. Ferrets housed in indoor cages would have no problem until they are let out to play in the house.

In veterinary clinics and hospitals, the ideal situation would be for separate dog, cat and ferret wards.

General dog and cat boarding establishments wanting to board ferrets should have separate facilities for each species. In Moscow, Russia, where pet ferrets are more recently established than other countries, there is a specific ferret 'hotel' where ferret owners can leave their pets while they are away.

Table 10.1 Blood values for ferret with toxoplasmosis

	Day 1	Day 14	Units
WBC	21.6	9.5	$10^3/\mu L$
Neutrophils	16632 (77%)	2565 (27%)	$/\mu L$
Lymphocytes	2808 (13%)	6460 (68%)	$/\mu L$
Monocytes	1728 (8%)	190 (2%)	$/\mu L$
Eosinophils	216 (1%)	285 (3%)	$/\mu L$
Basophils	216 (1%)	0 (0%)	$/\mu L$
RBC	8.6	11.8	$10^6/\mu L$
HGB	12.4	18.4	g/dL
HCT	39	56	%
Albumin	1.8	3.4	g/dL

WBC, white cell blood count; RBC, red cell blood count; HGB, haemoglobin; HCT, haematocrit or PCV, packed cell volume.

Important protozoan diseases

Authors' clinical example

Dr R. Gandolfi (pers. comm. 2005) has described an interesting case of toxoplasmosis in a ferret. An 8-month-old spayed female domestic ferret was examined at a local emergency clinic with a complaint of anorexia, diarrhoea and weight loss. The owners thought the animal was also vomiting but clinical signs were inconsistent. At presentation, she was febrile (T: 105.3°F), depressed, dehydrated, dyspnoeic, orthopneic and tachycardiac (HR: 230 bpm). On physical examination, she evidenced discomfort on abdominal palpation.

Initial laboratory data revealed a neutrophilic leukocytosis, microcytic, non-regenerative anaemia and decreased serum albumin. Electrolyte levels, hepatic serum enzymes, bilirubin, blood glucose and renal values were all within normal limits (Table 10.1). Survey radiographs revealed a soft tissue mass located at the anterior heart base with dorsal deviation of the trachea. An initial differential diagnosis consisted of neoplasia (lymphoma, primary lung tumour, heart-based tumour), granuloma, abscess or reactive lymphadenopathy.

Initial therapy from the emergency clinic consisted of amoxicillin at 30 mg/kg s.q., enrofloxacin at 5 mg/kg s.q., hetastarch at 10 mL i.v. and i.v. fluids 8 mL/kg per h.

The ferret was examined the next day. Radiographs revealed that the mass was enlarging and there was now a visible pleural effusion in the left hemi-thorax (Fig. 10.2).

The patient was anaesthetized by mask induction with isofluothane (2%). Thoracic ultrasound revealed a non-cavitary hilar mass, pleural effusion and normal cardiac function. Ultrasound-guided trans-thoracic fine needle aspirates were acquired. Samples were sent to a commercial laboratory for aerobic and anaerobic bacterial and fungal culture. Cytological preparations were examined immediately.

Blood samples were sent for serologic evaluation of *Cryptococcus* and *Toxoplasma*. Aerobic culture demonstrated small numbers of *Chryseomonas luteola*, a Gram-negative organism characterized as *Pseudomona*-like. No anaerobic or fungal growth was noted. The bacteria were sensitive to enrofloxacin. Serologic results were negative for both *Cryptococcus* and *Toxoplasma*.

Cytological examination revealed: severe pyogranulomatous inflammation, intracellular and extracellular organisms, elongated to slightly curved, so suspected *Toxoplasma* tachyzoites (Fig. 10.3).

Additional therapy of clindamycin at 25 mg/kg p.o. divided b.i.d. was begun based on cytology findings and enrofloxacin was continued based on culture results.

At re-check examinations:

- Day 5: *Clinical*: appetite improved and respiratory effort less pronounced. *Radiography*: mass smaller and pleural effusion resolved
- Day 14: *Clinical*: CBC and chemistries were approaching normal, neutrophilia resolved, anaemia resolved, hypoalbuminaemia resolved, lymphocytosis (moderate) and eosinophilia (moderate). *Radiography*: mass almost completely resolved
- Day 28: *Clinical*: general condition much improved.

Definitive diagnosis: with PCR positive for *T. gondii* performed on aspirated samples from Day 2 ultrasound examination.

Discussion: Toxoplasma infections in ferrets were reported as early as 1932. There are few reports of clinical cases. Infection in ferrets is thought to be by the classic oral route, either by ingestion of infective oocytes that have been excreted by the definitive host, the cat, or by ingestion of *Toxoplasma* organisms encysted in raw meat. Transplacental infection is also thought to occur. The source of infection in this case was not determined. The pet was not a 'farm-bred' individual, was housed indoors and was fed a commercial pelleted food. Information on management of clinical cases is similarly sparse, with most recommendations following guidelines for treatment in cats.

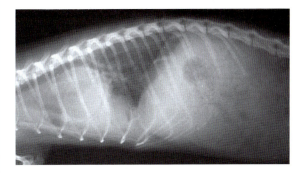

Figure 10.2 Radiological lateral view of ferret infected with toxoplasmosis. (Courtesy of R. Gandolfi.)

Sarcocystosis

Sarcocystis muris is a protozoan related to *Toxoplasma* and it has been shown experimentally that *Sarcocystis* can infect ferrets after they ingest infected mice.[8] The sporocysts voided in faeces by the ferrets could infect the mice. This parasite produces cysts in muscle tissue

CHAPTER TEN

Parasitic diseases of ferrets

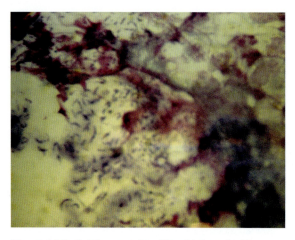

Figure 10.3 Cytology results of ferret infected with toxoplasmosis. (Courtesy of R. Gandolfi.)

and can infect man, horses, cattle, pigs, sheep, birds and reptiles. The dog is the definitive host.

Neosporosis

This is an interesting disease newly recognized in 1993 in many animals and caused by *Neospora caninum*, the cause of abortion in cattle, which had been mistaken for *T. gondii* until 1988. The disease has similar clinical signs to toxoplasmosis and the mode of infection was thought to be congenital.[9]

The dog is the definitive host. The presence of the disease in dogs, cats, rats and mice did indicate a possible future challenge to ferrets that are associated with these animals, either as pet or working ferrets. However, in an experiment, mustelids such as ermine (*M. erminea*), long-tailed weasels (*M. frentata*) and ferrets (*M. putorius*) were fed *Neospora caninum*-infected mice.[10] No *Neosporum caninum* oocysts were observed in the ferret faeces, which was fed to mice. Infection of the mice did not occur as shown by lack of *N. caninum* being detected in murine brains. It was concluded that *Mustela* species are not definitive hosts of *N. caninum*.

The disease in dogs (definitive host) has been recorded in many countries, with the major effect in puppies and older dogs being ascending paralysis from the hind legs. However, if the disease did occur in ferrets it would be another differential diagnosis for hind limb paralysis and could be confused initially with botulism. The protozoan parasite can be identified by an indirect fluorescent antibody test (IFA) on a cell culture of tachyzoites. *Neosporum caninum*, being an intracellular parasite, would kill the host rapidly by the multiplication of tachyzoites in the host cell. It is evidently the rupture of the host cell that initiates the immune-mediated disease. A possible toxin production has not been ruled out.

Treatment: Various drugs have been trialed for the treatment of neosporosis. Clindamycin has evidently been used to effectively treat polymyositis in a dog.[9]

Coccidiosis

All carnivores are susceptible and *Isospora* affects the cat and dog. It has a life cycle that involves rodents as an intermediate host. Faeces contamination could also be a risk to ferrets, especially in pet shops where young ferrets might be associated with areas that had housed cats and dogs. (However, dog infections do not appear to affect cats and vice versa so this unlikely.) *Isospora* oocysts are commonly shed from 6–16 weeks.[6]

Coccidiosis is a disease problem of mink farms, especially in young mink. The *Eimeria* associated with ferrets are *E. furonis* and *E. ictidea* and the *Isospora* is *I. laidlawii* (Fig. 10.4).[2]

In a medical laboratory, a 4-month-old ferret was found to have lethargy and diarrhoea for some time.[11] The ferret was not part of an experiment and had been weaned at 8 weeks and fully vaccinated. It had pasty dark scats around the anus and was thin, dehydrated and depressed. It was housed with a normal jill littermate in the standard laboratory stainless steel cage, with a solid floor and aspen bedding. The laboratory cages were thoroughly cleaned regularly by a heat process and bedding changed three times weekly.

The ferrets were hopper fed with ad lib dry cat food and given canned cat food once weekly. Water source was water bottles. Due to the ferret's extreme condition, it was euthanized and on post mortem the main finding was parasitic cysts of *Eimeria* in villi cells of the small intestine.

Interestingly, the companion ferret was clinically normal while the sick ferret had signs of a severe coccidiosis infection. The authors maintained that ferrets did not usually show signs of coccidiosis. They theorized that the ferret's mother shed viable oocysts into the cage and the oocysts were present for enough time to sporulate and become active. Since both young ferrets would have been exposed, the sick ferret had been somehow immunocompromised to fall to a massive bowel infection.

No other ferrets in the laboratory colony were found with symptoms, so the case was considered an isolated one and no overall treatment of stock was carried out or husbandry changed.

The presence of *E. furonis* was suspected in a 9-week-old male research ferret, which showed signs of emaciation and anorexia.[12] There was abdominal distention and slight icterus present. The ferret did not

Important protozoan diseases

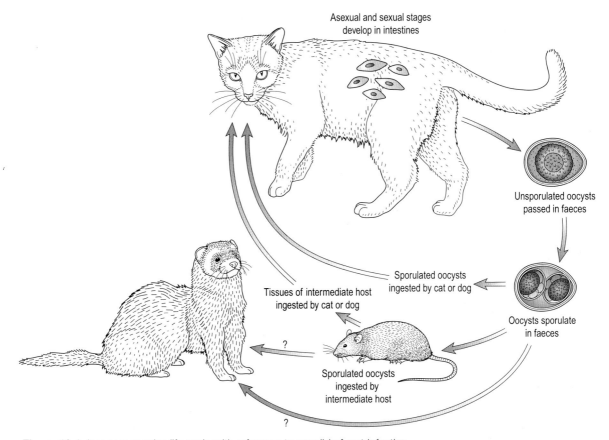

Figure 10.4 *Isospora* species life cycle with reference to possible ferret infection.

improve even on a good diet and was euthanized. The blood showed raised alkaline phosphatase (3533 IU/L), total bilirubin (4.8 mg/dL) and alanine aminotransferase moderately raised (852 IU/dL) along with hypoalbuminaemia and hyperphosphataemia (9.3 mg/dL). Blood urea nitrogen was elevated (62 mg/dL) along with a neutrophilic leukocytosis to some degree (45 000/mL), along with a regenerative left shift. A macrocytic, monochromic anaemia had occurred. The liver was enlarged with the bile duct and gallbladder epithelia having present multiple life cycle stages of *E. furonis* as meronts, gametocytes and oocysts.

Clinical signs: Coccidiosis is usually asymptomatic but in some cases, diarrhoea and tenesmus can occur. Young ferrets from pet shops can show bloody diarrhoea after purchase, with large numbers of oocysts found on faecal examination; however oocysts are often found in well-formed scats of healthy looking ferrets.

Treatment: Usually sulfonamides provide effective control, which results in ferret weight gains and healthy active kittens. Safe drugs for ferrets include sulfadimethoxine, trimethoprim-sulfadiazine, amprolium and decoquinate. *Note*: none of these drugs is actually labelled for ferret use. Infected ferrets should be treated for at least 2 weeks and faecal flotation checks carried out to confirm the parasite is cleared.[6] For large numbers of ferrets, sulfadimethoxine can be added to the drinking water but it is not really palatable and may reduce the total water intake, as it has to be given as the sole drink. The effective dose is 300 mg/kg daily, which is about 0.5 mL/kg of a 12.5% solution. Trimethoprim-sulfadiazine (cherry-flavoured) is a better choice and requires only once-daily treatment at a dose rate of 30 mg/kg of the oral suspension (48 mg/mL); thus a 400 g 7-week-old kitten would require 0.4 mL daily. *Note*: as kittens can double their weight between 7 and 10 weeks of age, this dose must be adjusted for the 2nd week to prevent under-dosing, which could lead to drug resistance.[6] Amprolium, a thiamine inhibitor, can be used on well-nourished young ferrets for about 6 weeks without toxicity problems. A daily dose of 19 mg/kg (0.2 mL/kg) of a 9.6% oral solution can be given by syringe or in the drinking water. Amprolium is not as bitter as sulfadimethoxine but does cause reduced

> **Author's clinical example**
>
> An isolated case in NSW illustrates coccidiosis in ferrets (Dr M. Thornton, Newcastle, NSW, pers. comm. 1998). Two 6-week-old kittens were bought from a breeder by a veterinary nurse, who kept them in a ferretarium and also took them frequently to work. On initial examination, they were bright and active but coccidia were found in the scats. One month after purchase, one kitten was found in the sleeping box nearly comatose and after emergency treatment, died the same day. The scats were dark and pasty, with high numbers of coccidia. Initial treatment had not been done for the original coccidia seen. The post mortem findings were unrewarding and a possible spider bite was suggested but not confirmed. American pathologist, Dr B. Williams, who has seen the result of the disease in ferrets, indicated that the parasite could have been the cause of death. He stated that coccidiosis in ferret kittens can be lethal and there are few or no histological signs (B. Williams, Department of Telemedicine, Washington, DC, USA, pers. comm. 1998). Unfortunately, the breeder did not allow the rest of the breeding stock to be checked.

water intake. However, the drug is only available in large commercial volumes and has a fairly short shelf life. *Note*: use honey or sugar-water when dealing with all unpalatable ferret medicines.

Prevention: Ferrets are becoming ever more popular worldwide and coccidiosis may become a problem of pet shops. All cages must be cleaned regularly, as coccidia oocysts become infective in a couple of days in moist warm environments. Puppies, cat and ferret kittens should have separate cages. However, ferrets would be much more at risk from same species contact for coccidiosis.

Active playful ferret kittens could spread the disease on their feet around the cage. Particular care should be taken that water and food bowls are not contaminated and are washed thoroughly in the home, veterinary hospitals and pet shops. To avoid contamination, the water/food bowls should be secured, perhaps on a slightly raised area. Hygiene, as for any disease prevention, should be observed with breeding stock and faecal flotation tests for valuable breeding stock should be encouraged.

Cryptosporidiosis

The parasite *Cryptosporidium parvum* is a widespread protozoan in the small intestine causing a self-limiting infection. The classification is under review. Recent DNA studies indicate that *C. parvum* is composed of eight genotypes at least, including zoonotic genotypes.[13] The ferret is a reservoir for the parasite but the infectivity of zoonotic types is unclear, however there is a possibility that ferrets harbour some of the zoonotic genotypes.

This disease has increased in importance as an enteric disease of animals and humans.[14] The disease is most pertinent as a danger to immune-compromised subjects, such as ferrets on long-term corticosteroid therapy for cancer treatment. *Cryptosporidium* has been isolated from asymptomatic young ferrets. Immunologically-normal animals can eliminate the parasite in 2–3 weeks. Young ferrets fed uncooked offal may show the disease. Heavy infections in ferret kittens will reduce the feed efficiency for growth and, more importantly, they are possible reservoirs for human infection and a risk as a pet shop product.[6] If the jills are fed uncooked offal they could give the disease to their offspring.

Life cycle and pathogenesis: The *Cryptosporidium* life cycle differs from other coccidia. The organism is small (4–5 mm) and difficult to detect in the live subject. The organism can infect animals from calves and humans to pigs, lambs and puppies.[14] The cryptosporidial life cycle is direct, with a direct or indirect oral infection of the host. Oocysts are shed in the faeces and are immediately infective, not requiring a maturation period. Direct contact with the shedding host is not necessary, as in many cases the oocysts can survive in the environment and are resistant to common disinfectants.

The intracellular stages in the bowel attach themselves to the mucosal brush borders and reproduce, causing a vast invasion of the brush borders and the formation of both thick- and thin-shelled oocysts. The thick-shelled oocysts occur in the faeces, while the thin-shelled oocysts cause internal hyperinfection of the mucosa, which is destroyed, leading to the breakdown of effective mucosal function and serious diarrhoea.

Cryptosporidiosis was found in two ferrets, part of a colony of animals used for various research projects at MIT.[15] Marshal Farms supplied eight 9-week-old sterilized hobs and nine 11-week-old sterilized jills. They weighed 500–600 g, three-quarters were female, and they were placed in either solid bottom polycarbonate cages individually or in larger stainless steel cages in groups of two or four ferrets. They were fed ad lib on commercial food plus water.

It happened that two female ferrets, one 4- and one 8-months-old, died the same day. They were from different shipments and housed separately with companion control ferrets. The two dead ferrets had been having dexamethasone daily. Post mortems showed bleeding in the small intestine and spinal cord.

Cryptosporidium, in several life stages, was seen by electron microscopy. A survey for the disease was then carried out on the rest of the laboratory and incoming ferrets. It was discovered that a subclinical infection of cryptosporidiosis occurred in a high percentage of young ferrets, up to 40% in the whole laboratory stock and 38–100% of the incoming stock.

The disease persisted in both the immunosuppressed ferrets in the research programme and the normal ferret colony for several weeks. *Note* the two ferrets in contact with the diseased immunosuppressed ferrets did not succumb to the *Cryptosporidia* infection, possibly due to their being immune or not receiving enough infective oocysts. The in-contacts did develop *Pneumocystis carinii* pneumonia, thus being immunosuppressed to some extent, but they may have developed antibodies to the cryptosporidia around.

The actual origin of the *Cryptospiridium* infection was a mystery but it is known that bovine *Cryptospiridium* (*C. parvum*) can cross species and the ferrets had raw beef as part of their diet. This case may highlight the danger of feeding slaughterhouse meat to ferrets (Ch. 4).

Clinical signs: The most likely clinical sign, as in dogs, is diarrhoea, also fever, abdominal pain, and constipation and/or weight loss. In animals, a 1-week-old puppy, with a history of diarrhoea of no other cause, and four out of ten cats found to have cryptosporidiosis showed chronic diarrhoea. The disease usually occurs in young animals and with ferrets can be in kittens of less than 10 weeks of age but without signs of diarrhoea.[6]

Note that zoonosis is a concern in ferrets where they are fed uncooked beef by-products such as tripe or any intestinal tissue containing C. *parvum*, as cattle are excellent reservoirs for the organism.[6] Tripe and rejected liver products were formerly fed to mink and fitch ferret farms and caused diarrhoea problems. Thus raw by-products, though probably cheap food, should not be fed to ferrets as they may be contaminated with many harmful organisms. Personally, I have always fed my ferrets meats fit for human consumption.

Diagnosis: The actual organism must be demonstrated using modified Ziehl–Neelsen stain (Giemsa's stain) on faecal smears.[14] Another technique is by the concentration of oocysts using a concentrated sugar solution and faeces sample. By this method oocysts rise to the surface and can be examined under the microscope.[6]

Treatment: Unfortunately, at the time of writing, there are still no effective drugs for treatment of cryptosporidiosis in man or animals, as the organism is highly resistant. Only the drug spiramycin has been of some benefit in human patients. Usually high fluid intake and rest is the answer.

Zoonosis aspects: This is important especially with young dogs, cats or ferrets in a household with immunocompromised individuals. We forget in Australia, that American ferrets are kept mostly indoors and some AIDS patients have been advised not to have pets of any kind. The pets could be periodically checked for infective agents and handlers should apply strict hygiene control.

Prevention: *Cryptosporidium* can be killed by formalinized saline solution or 5–10% ammonia. Evidently, according to a WHO study, only 30% of cryptosporidiosis outbreaks have been studied worldwide. (*Note*: *Cryptosporidium* is now thought to be related to *Gregarina*.)

Of the other intestinal coccidia, *Isospora belli* and *I. hominis* (now *Sarcocystis hominis*) can cause similar symptoms to C. *parvum* in immunodeficient humans but have not been recorded in any pet.[14]

Hepatozoon

Hepatozoon canis is endemic in southern Europe.[16] It is considered a travel risk with dogs under the Pet Travel Scheme (PETS) scheme in the UK.[17] However, it has been noted that parasites of the genus *Hepatozoon* have caused myocarditis and myosis in Scottish pine martens (*Martes martes*) as discovered in road kills.[18] *Hepatozoon* is an Apicomplexan protozoan, phylogenetically related to *Plasmodium* (malaria protozoan) and classified now in subclass Coccidiasina.

Hepatozoon infection has been described in amphibians, reptiles, birds and free-living mammals on several continents. In Canada, the disease has affected American mink (*Mustela vison*) and in Japan wild martens (*Martes melampus*).

So there is a possibility of polecat infection or working ferrets picking up the disease during ferreting expeditions. A tick or flea might be the parasite vector as it is with *Leishmania* and *Babesia*.

Life cycle: As an Apicomplexan, *Hepatozoon* is unusual in that its life cycle involves an invertebrate as a definitive host. The ticks *Ixodes ricinus* and *I. hexagonus* are suspect or possibly fleas or mites. In any case, the sexual phase of the life cycle occurs in the insect's gut. Interestingly, the vertebrate host becomes infected not by being bitten but by ingesting the insect with the oocysts it contains.

Schizogony occurs in many tissues of the vertebrate host with gamonts released to infect cells of the haemolymphatic system. The life cycle is complete when an arthropod feeds on the infected host.

Pathogenesis: Infections by *Hepatozoon* are usually subclinical. The four Scottish polecats with myocardiac lesions were in good body condition (other than the road trauma). One polecat had an engorged tick on its left ear while another had nasal sinus nematodes of the *Skrjabingylus* genus (see below).

Giardiasis

Ferrets are susceptible to *Giardia* spp., which are known to be endemic in all parts of the world.[1]

CHAPTER TEN

Parasitic diseases of ferrets

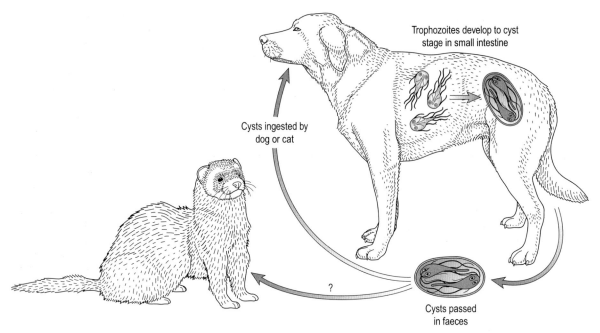

Figure 10.5 *Giardia* life cycle with reference to possible ferret infection. (*Note* that this direct life cycle diagram also illustrates the *Cryptosporidium* life cycle.) *Giardia* trophozoites are indicated in the dog (or cat) host in this case.

Giardia species were named on host specificity, see classification update below, but many parasitologists now consider that many of the names are synonymous.

Life cycle and pathogenesis: *Giardia* live in the intestine but do not invade the mucosal epithelium like *Cryptosporidium*. The motile trophozoite, only 12–17 × 1–10 μm, looks pear-shaped with a concave appearance and attaches to the mucosal wall by means of a ventral disc.[19] *Giardia* reproduce by binary fission and produce infective cysts. They are about 9–13 μm long and are infective as soon as they are passed.[14] Once ingested by a new host, each cyst wall is destroyed by the gastric juices of the upper small intestine and each cyst produces two trophozoites (Fig. 10.5).

It is unclear if all *Giardia* species are host-specific but some will infect many different hosts.[20] The hardy cysts produced from this direct life cycle can survive for months and withstand disinfectants that normally kill bacteria. The cysts spread by contaminating food or water and it is considered that just 10 cysts can cause disease in humans. It is estimated that 50% of dogs in Perth, Western Australia, carry a strain that has the potential to be transmitted to humans.[21] It is possible that a vaccine will be developed against the parasite.

Pathogenesis: This is not completely elucidated. 'Supposedly, trophozoites in the intestinal lumen adhere to or invade the intestinal mucosa where they produce 'toxins', mechanically block absorption, deconjugate bile acids, abrade microvillous surfaces, disrupt the intestinal ecosystem, destroy brush border enzymes, and/or compete for nutrients.'[14] A catarrhal enteritis has been seen histologically in dogs. In humans, there is an intestinal response to some degree with wide-ranging pathology of disease or even no detectable signs.

Clinical signs: These have not been described for ferrets.[6] In dogs, for comparison, the condition may be asymptomatic or an illness may develop 1–3 weeks after exposure with variable clinical signs, e.g. soft stools and possibly signs resembling chronic ulcerative colitis.[14] There can also be weight loss, listlessness and anorexia. In ferrets, the condition may be confused with the four prominent American ferret-wasting diseases (Ch. 9).

Diagnosis: *Giardia* can be found in the suspect scats (faeces) but the numbers of trophozoites or cysts do not necessarily correlate to the disease severity in other animals. With fresh scats, the presence of motile trophozoites is diagnostic if three smears are done at 48-h intervals (sensitivity of 43% in other animals). It is more sensitive, but time-consuming, to check for cysts using a zinc sulphate centrifugation technique, which gives 94% accuracy if done three times at 48-h intervals to allow for the intermittent cyst excretion. The zinc sulphate technique has been described in detail.[19] There are ELISA kits (enzyme-linked immunosorbent assay) as used for humans, which can be used for small animals; however they are not considered superior to the zinc sulphate technique.

Treatment: For any ferret cases, the drug used for dogs, metronidazole, can be used. It is 68% efficient. The dose would be 35 mg/kg daily. As the tablets are 200 mg, it has been found that one-quarter of a tablet daily for at least 5 days is safe for a 400–500 g ferret.[6]

Prevention: The main concern with ferrets is from pet shops, as with coccidiosis, and attention to hygiene and separation of ferrets from other pets is vital. In households with a dog or human case of giardiasis, the pet ferrets must be screened for the disease. The public health significance of the disease in dogs and cats, and therefore in ferrets, is poorly defined. Strict attention to cleaning environmental contamination is required; fortunately the cysts are not completely resistant to freezing, boiling or desiccation. Thus a 1% solution of sodium hypochlorite or 2–5% pine tar are useful disinfectants.[14] *Cautious note*: the cysts can probably survive on unsealed concrete surfaces despite disinfectants, which speaks for the remarkable resilience of these protozoan organisms.

Giardia classification update: there are multiple genotypes of *Giardia* in vertebrate hosts including man. They are called 'assemblages' and listed A to G. *Note* A and B are found in humans and animals; C only in dogs; E in hoofed animals such as cattle and pigs; F in cats; G in rats.

Recently, it has been proposed that each assemblage have new species names based on the data of molecular and biological studies of isolates in each assemblage.[22] The isolates in assemblages A, B, C and E, F and G are named *G. duodenalis*, *G. enterica*, *G. canis*, *G. bovis*, *G. cati* and *G. simondi*, respectively (N. Abe, pers. comm. 2005).

Clinical findings: *Giardia intestinalis* has been studied in the weasel but the genotype of its isolate remains unclear. A *G. intestinalis* tissue isolate from a Japanese pet shop ferret was examined genetically to validate the possibility of zoonotic transmission.[20] The *Giardia* diagnostic fragments of the subunit ribosomal RNA, beta-giardin and glutamate dehydrogenase genes were amplified from the ferret isolate and sequenced to reveal the phylogenic relationships between it and other *Giardia* species or genotypes of *G. intestinalis*; the conclusion is that the ferret isolate of genetic group A–I in assemblage A, could be a causative agent of human giardiasis and thus a zoonosis.

Leishmaniasis

The disease of leishmaniasis occurs worldwide and especially in the Mediterranean area and has been introduced into the UK in dogs.[7] With the advent of the PETS scheme in the UK for pets travelling back and forth to the continent, the risk of leishmaniasis has increased in dogs.[17] The pet ferret travelling to the continent may be equally at risk? The author notes that the PETS scheme has been extended to animals travelling between the UK and North America.

Leishmania parasites, spread by sand flies, have caused disease experimentally in ferrets but the parasitic reaction was not as profound as when the disease was introduced to the opossum. The ferret is thus not a good 'model' for that disease.[8] The *Leishmania* parasite has now been recorded in a dog in Perth, WA.[23] It has also been confirmed in the cutaneous form in four red kangaroos (*Macropus rufus*) in a zoo in the Northern Territory.

In conclusion, veterinarians might well take note of possible infection by protozoa, such as *Giardia*, *Coccidia* or *Toxoplasma*, in relation to the proliferation of the pet ferret industry round the world. Sources of infection may arise from pet shops and breeders who might not be aware of the possible risks of these organisms.

Helminthes parasites

Phylum Nematoda

The presence of infective nematodes in ferrets is not a serious problem, especially with regard to pet ferrets in the USA, which are mostly kept indoors and in cages. *None* have been found in ferrets. However, theoretically ferrets may be susceptible to some internal (and external) parasites of the dog and cat from picking up eggs and larvae and eating intermediate hosts. In working ferrets and those kept outside as pets in a ferretarium or free-ranging in an enclosed garden, infection is more likely. The heartworm (*Dirofilaria*) is an established pathogen in ferrets. In addition, there are a number of parasitic worms in rabbits, rats and mice that may affect working ferrets in the future if cross-species adaptation occurs.

Order Ascaridida: family Ascarididae (common roundworms)

Toxascaris leonina, *Toxocara canis* and *Toxocara cati* are common in dogs and cats, which can be companion animals to ferrets in indoor/outdoor situations. *Toxocara canis* occurs in dingoes and foxes in Australia.

Life cycle and pathogenesis: This involves cast fertile eggs and a paratenic host in the rat or mouse, which could put the ferret at risk.[24] *Note* that *T. canis* eggs become infective within 2 weeks after being voided in

CHAPTER TEN
Parasitic diseases of ferrets

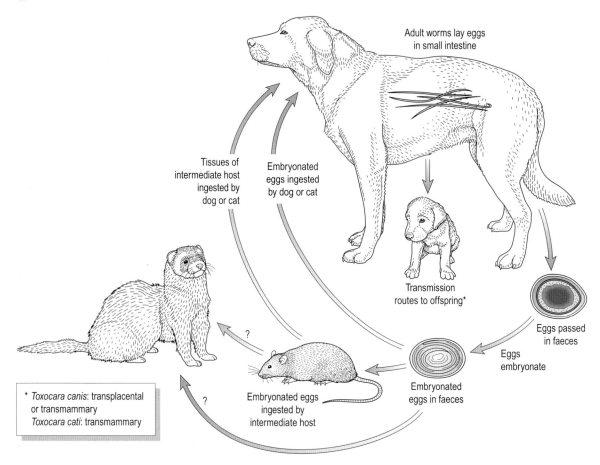

Figure 10.6 Life cycle of common roundworms with reference to possible ferret infection.

faeces. Thus an area can be contaminated, e.g. a garden where ferrets also may be kept. The eggs can remain viable in the soil for up to 2 years (Fig. 10.6).

Clinical signs: The larval forms cause damage in the lungs (*T. canis* and *T. cati*) in those animals, while *T. leonina* affects the intestine.[24] Visceral larva migrans (larvae migrating to special organs in the host body) is a concern in children and whether this condition could arise in ferrets contaminated from mice or rats is as yet unknown. In puppies and kittens, heavy infestations of roundworms cause potbelly syndrome with mucoid diarrhoea and stunted growth. Weight for weight the adult ferret might be the size of a small pup or kitten. However, at the present time the embryonated egg is thought to develop only in the target species, i.e. dog or cat. However, these factors should be borne in mind where ferrets in pet shops are in contact with puppies and kittens. *Toxascaris canis* can have transplacental expulsion of larvae so theoretically this could happen in an infected jill. *Note*: *T. leonina* does not transmit through prenatal paths or lactation.[25]

Prevention: In countries where ferrets may be kept outside in a ferretarium, there is a small risk from dog and cat faeces. Ferrets having free range in the garden of a multi-species pet household usually avoid dog faeces and cats usually bury theirs. Severe hot summers tend to desiccate dog faeces quickly, but rain could spread eggs in the garden. Dog faeces should be removed daily from the garden. Fitch ferrets have been associated with ranch mink in the USA and the possibility of worm infestation arises from food such as raw meat that can carry larvae of helminthes parasites. Normally pet ferrets would not be fed fish, as are mink and otters. However, it appears that fitch farm ferrets and mink are resistant to intestinal worms.[6]

Treatment: Some ferret owners are super-sensitive to the need for worming their dogs, cats and children and require their veterinarian to ensure that their pet ferrets

Helminthes parasites

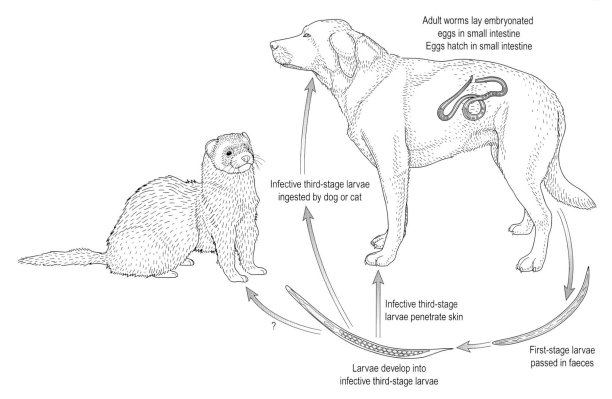

Figure 10.7 Life cycle of *Strongyloides stercoralis* with reference to possible ferret infection.

do not carry worms. After the best assurance of the low risk of worms being present, a small dose of Felex Paste (Pfizer) to ferrets to allay fears can be given. I have had no adverse reactions to this drug. A routine scat check for roundworm could be carried out at vaccination time. Now the use of drugs like selamectin (Revolution) for heartworm prevention even in ferrets reduces any danger of roundworm or even hookworm larvae establishing in the species.

Order Rhabditida: family Rhabditidae (part free-living parasitic worms or intestinal threadworms)

Strongyloides stercoralis is a parasite mostly in man around the world and also dogs, cats and foxes.[14] The ferret can be infected experimentally as shown by Eberhard.[8]

Life cycle and pathogenesis: Involves the production of an infective third stage larva that has the ability to migrate into the skin of the next host as seen in Figure 10.7.

This parasite has both a free-living and parasitic life cycle. In the latter, the female worms are found in the superficial tissues of the small intestine but without males. By parthenogenesis (without fertilization), larvae are produced and some pass out in the faeces as the free-living stage. Other larvae develop into the parasitic stage still in the gut. The free-living larvae develop in the soil and mature into free-living males and females. Mating of the free-living adults produce more larvae; some develop into free-living larvae while others go to the parasitic stage and enter a host by the skin. This is where ferrets might be infected.

The larval forms in the intestine continue the host infection by causing hyperinfection.[14] It is considered that such hyperinfection phases produce large numbers of parasites, increasing the initial exposure. It is easy to see that this situation, if it ever occurred naturally, would be fatal to ferrets. There is a possibility, especially in hot and humid climates, of zoonoses in households with infected dogs.[14]

The easy movement of the free-living third stage in moist ground is a major factor that could affect ferrets in such situations, although it is likely that ferrets would be confined indoors from these climatic conditions.

Clinical signs: Humans and dogs may show no symptoms; bronchopneumonia and diarrhoea are, however, features of the disease that might be seen in affected

CHAPTER TEN

Parasitic diseases of ferrets

ferrets. The diarrhoea appears watery, mucoid or even haemorrhagic. Anaemia with weakness, depression and haematochezia has been seen in young puppies.

Diagnosis: This would involve testing the ferret scats for larvae, using direct examination or the Baerman technique. With infected dogs, worm checks are done for up to a year after treatment to check for reinfection. The public health concern about this disease is not high at the moment though it should be remembered that infective larvae on any animal species could invade human skin on direct contact.

Treatment: The use of thiabendazole, fenbendazole and mebendazole are suggested for dogs and cats only but could probably be used in ferrets at careful low dosing.

Class Enoplea: order Trichuridae. Family Trichuridae: *Trichuris* species (whipworms)

These worms have not been recorded in ferrets but *Trichuris vulpis* could infects dogs and foxes and possibly working ferrets?

Family Trichuridae. *Capillaria* species

These are related to *Trichuris*. *Note*: *Capillaria entomelas* has been found in the small intestine of mink, beech marten and polecat and could cause haemorrhagic enteritis.[24] Keeping mink in unhygienic boxes spreads the parasite and it could be a problem of working ferrets in similar conditions of mismanagement. *Capillaria plica* of dogs and foxes affects the bladder but is relatively harmless. Foxes get the parasite from the intermediate host, the earthworm, and outdoor-living ferrets or working ferrets can eat earthworms if they are found while the ferret is digging (Fig. 10.8).

Capillaria aerophila is a parasite that can occur in the upper respiratory system of dogs and foxes and has been recorded in the cat, pine marten, beech marten, wolf and badger. Working ferrets could be at risk (Fig. 10.9).

Family Trichinellidae

It has been found experimentally that ferrets can be inoculated with *Trichinella spiralis* larvae. This was a major parasite of man through uncooked pig meat. The

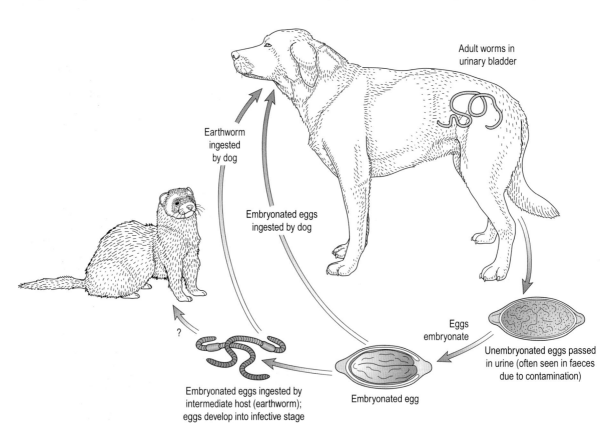

Figure 10.8 Life cycle of *Capillaria plica* with reference to possible ferret infection.

Helminthes parasites

adults develop in the mammal intestine in 3 days and produce cysts in the musculature.[8] The *Trichinella* adult would cause mild irritation and marked enteritis but the most important pathogenic effect is the presence of the larvae in the intercostal muscles. This can cause respiratory failure.

Symptoms: Variable, with diarrhoea, fever, stiffness and pain in affected muscles plus dyspnoea and oedema, which can be confused with other ferret diseases. A blood check would show a marked eosinophilia. Because of the larvae encysted in the musculature, treatment would be practically impossible.

Pathogenesis: In the animals mentioned above, infection can be mild, producing a carrier state, or severe with chronic tracheitis and bronchitis leading to bronchopneumonia. The disease is prevalent in young foxes and if working ferrets were ferreting around fox burrows they might be at risk, if faeces had been recently deposited on moist ground and the ferrets picked up eggs. Ferrets working near a badger sett could also be at risk.

There are 10 different genotypes of *Trichinella* of which seven are distinct species and affect a number of animals and birds.[26] They are not seen on mainland Australia but recorded in Tasmania in 1987 in Tasmanian devils and spotted-tail quolls. Interestingly, Webster and Kapel (2005) have demonstrated vertical transmission of *Trichinella* species across the placental barrier.[27] Vertical transmission, measured as recovery of muscle larvae in the offspring, was positive from infected ferrets, guinea pigs and mice (on high dose), but not in any fox or pig group.

Clinical signs in ferrets: They may show cough and nasal discharge, also dyspnoea with the mouth held open. Probably a single worm infestation in the ferret's upper respiratory system would be as serious as the presence of an adult heartworm. Treatment of the adult stage would be difficult.

Order Strongylida: superfamily Strongyloidea: (hookworms) family Ancylostomidae: *Ancylostoma* species: *A. canum*

This is one of four common hookworms affecting dogs, dingoes, foxes and cats. It is easily transmitted between animals and possibly rarely in man. The adult worms attach to the intestinal mucosa and suck blood.[24] The life cycle involves the production of a third stage larva that has the ability to migrate into the skin of the next host. It could be a problem for working ferrets in warm moist areas, which allow for the migration of infective larvae.

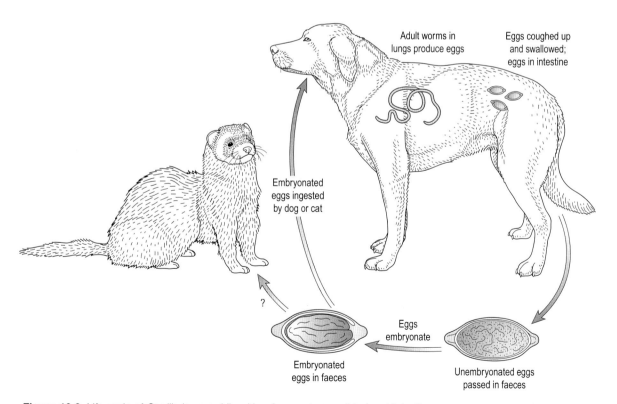

Figure 10.9 Life cycle of *Capillaria aerophila* with reference to possible ferret infection.

237

CHAPTER TEN

Parasitic diseases of ferrets

Ancylostoma tubaeforme affects cats and has a similar life cycle (Fig. 10.10).

Clinical signs: These would be a basic anaemia via the adult worm feeding on blood. Ferrets, like dogs, could possibly get an itchy skin due to larval penetration. Young animals are subject to infection by transplacental or transmammary routes as shown in Figure 10.10. Ferrets did act as experimental models for skin penetration by larvae of *Ancylostoma caninum* as found with *Strongyloides stercoralis*.[8]

Treatment: In severely affected dogs, blood transfusion is required for the anaemia, but the use of multi-worm preventives makes necessity for treatment rare. Blood transfusion for ferrets is described in Chapter 16. Routine ferret worming is possible with scaled-down dosage of pyrantel embonate (Canex puppy suspension) or piperazine citrate (Troy puppy and kitten worm syrup). Revolution for cats has been adaptable to ferrets for flea control and would affect roundworms (K. Smith, NSWFWS, pers. comm. 2005).

Order Strongylida: superfamily Metastrongyloidea: (lungworms)

Angiostrongylus cantonensis: Adult worms occur in the pulmonary arteries of rats and require molluscs as intermediate hosts to ingest the L1 stage and in which development to the L3 stage takes place. Possibly a ferret eats a rat or molluscs? Interestingly, a ferret would not be infected by eating an infected rat as the right infective stage is needed for infection. Many mammals, including humans, can be infected by eating molluscs causing neurological disorders and death. A man nearly did die eating a mollusc for a dare! So it is quite likely to happen if a ferret eats an infected mollusc (Russell Hobbs, pers. comm. 2005).

Aelurostrongylus abstrusus of the cat has a similar life cycle, with larvae infecting snails, which can be eaten by birds. I know from my ferrets that they do eat snails and I find empty shells in the sleeping box beds of ferrets living in the garden and in ferretariums. Infection is theoretically possible. Ferrets can kill rats, mice and snails in a garden. Lungworms of the *Crenosoma* genus were considered common in American mustelids[28] but have not yet been recorded in other countries. It may be that ferrets have a resistance to infection.

Life cycle and pathogenesis: Data can only be given for the cat infection but may relate to the ferret. The disease in cats is usually subclinical and self-limiting, which may be the case in ferrets. Heavy infections in cats can lead to death (Fig. 10.11). This condition has not been diagnosed in pet or working ferrets.

Clinical signs: In cats there is chronic cough, gradually increasing dyspnoea, lethargy, anorexia, loss of con-

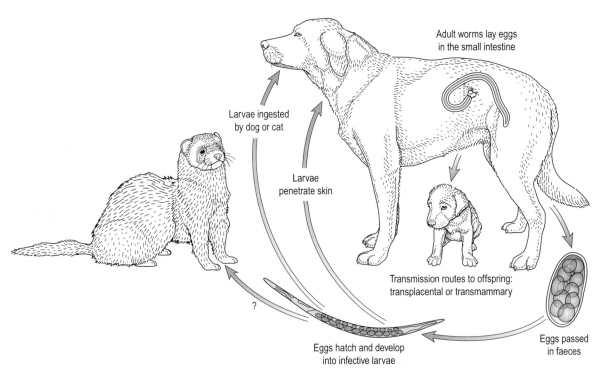

Figure 10.10 Common life cycle of the hookworm parasites with reference to possible ferret infection.

dition, pyrexia and upper respiratory irritation with sneezing and ocular/nasal discharges.[29] These symptoms are common to ferrets with respiratory diseases.

Diagnosis: Generally by blood eosinophilia, with the rest of the blood picture being normal, but parasitic eggs and larvae may be present in faecal flotation. I have yet to find eggs in ferret scats but as the snail is the intermediate host and ferrets and cats cohabit, there may be a risk in the future.

Treatment: Fenbendazole is used in cats with symptomatic infection at a dose rate of 50 mg/kg for 3 days.

Order Spirurida: superfamily Filarioidea (heartworm)

Dirofilaria immitis has been recorded in dogs, cats and ferrets. In the USA, especially Florida, it has been endemic. In one 1984 report, two 2- and 5-year-old outdoor ferrets died of the disease and only the second ferret got any treatment, with oxygen, furosemide and prednisolone for the respiratory distress.[30] Since that time, treatment and prevention of ferret heartworm has been attempted by use of ivermectin (Heartgard 30), thiacetarsamide sodium (Caparsolate), melarsomine dihydrochloride (Immiticide) and most recently moxidectin (ProHeart 6; *note* ProHeart 12 in Australia). It has been found that it takes only 6–10 adult worms to cause symptoms and death in ferrets.[31]

Life cycle and pathogenesis: With the mosquito as vector, *Dirofilaria immitis* will cause a blood-borne infection and the life cycle is illustrated by Figure 10.12.

Clinical signs: These may be vague, with anorexia and coughing and could be confused with chronic cough due to various causes. The signs would include dyspnoea, lethargy, pulmonary congestion, ascites and grade 2–3 heart murmurs with resulting right-side heart failure.[32]

Diagnosis: This was considered difficult at one time, as only 1% of ferrets show circulating microfilaria. However, according to Dr D. Kemmerer-Cottrell (DK-C) of Florida USA, where heartworm is rife, the CITE test has proved accurate. The CITE test, although still available, has been superseded by the SNAP test (IDEXX), which is effective when two adult female worms are present (S. Beatson, Vet Path Lab, Perth, pers. comm.).

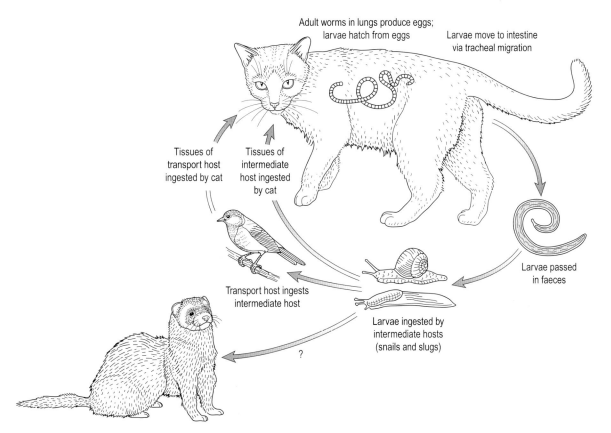

Figure 10.11 Life cycle of *Aelurostrongylus abstrusus* with reference to possible ferret infection.

CHAPTER TEN

Parasitic diseases of ferrets

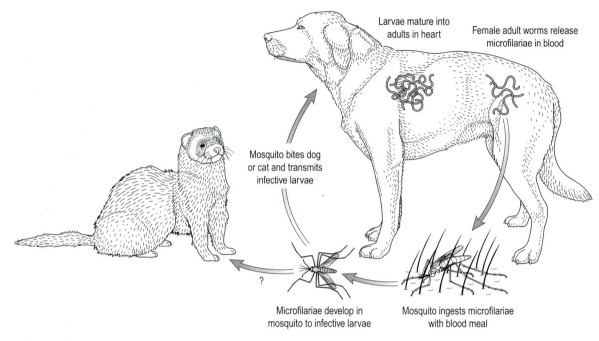

Figure 10.12 Life cycle of *Dirofilaria immitis* with definite reference to ferret infection.

Blood picture: Usually a full blood check, CBC, rarely shows eosinophilia. However, kidney function (BUN, creatinine) and liver function (ALT, bilirubin) will indicate an indirect presence of heartworm disease, if the tests are abnormal.[33] It is best to check blood profile in positive heartworm cases as a means of assessing their suitability for treatment.

Radiography: This can distinguish pulmonary congestion from other heart conditions; a pruning of vessels and right ventricular enlargement may be seen. The condition of the heart, lungs and vessels can be a basis for assessing complications during therapy.

Electrocardiogram: Carrying out an ECG or EKG would pick up abnormal heart rhythms which can add to the heartworm disease complex.

Echocardiography: Using echocardiography techniques illustrates the heart chambers and may pick out actual heartworms. Ultrasound is not particularly accurate for ferret use as it produces both false positive and false negative results. Some positive ultrasounds on suspect ferrets, by experienced operators, showed positives when the disease was not confirmed by antigen test or post mortem. Conversely, cases found positive by antigen test and post mortem were missed by ultrasound (Ch. 17).

Post mortem findings: The pathology of heartworm disease shows arteritis of pulmonary blood vessels and eosinophilic or granulomatous pneumonitis of the lungs.[33] The liver and kidneys may be involved with evi-

Author's clinical example

A heartworm case seen in Sydney, NSW

A 7-year-old sterilized albino jill was surrendered to the NSWFA Ferret Rescue to be treated for coccidiosis and mange. It developed lethargy and dyspnoea. The heart was checked revealing cardiac arrhythmia; radiographs indicated an enlarged heart and pleural fluids. The ferret died and at post mortem showed a large amount of blood in the thoracic cavity. The heart was enlarged and a mature heartworm was visible, which was extracted from the cranial vena cava. An infarct was present with haemorrhage resulting. The liver was congested with a possible tumour on one lobe. A serum sample sent for an ELISA test proved positive. The ferret was a clinical mess! (Dr B. Alderton, pers. comm. 1998).

I have recorded a 2-year-old hob ferret with heartworm, seen at post mortem, in Western Australia. The ferret had been lethargic, with loss of weight and respiratory discomfort for 2 weeks. It had been obtained from a pet shop and was suspected at first to have a non-parasitic myocardiopathy and had been on antibiotic cover for possible pneumonia. No test was done, as the ferret deteriorated and was euthanized. The heart showed the presence of six adult worms in the right auricle. Treatment would have been hopeless. It has been suggested that the larger hearts in hobs, compared with jills, allow the adult worms to reach sexual maturity (M. Finkler, pers. comm. 1999).

dence of cirrhosis in the former and glomerulonephritis in the latter.

Treatment: Sometimes not possible, as heartworms in ferrets can cause major vessel damage, rupture and sudden death, as seen in examples above. Heartworm disease, on early diagnosis, can be treated as in the dog with the Carparsolate/corticosteroid technique carried out by one specialist (DK-C, pers. comm. 1998). She states that ferrets do not have a problem metabolizing Carparsolate (*Note*: Carparsolate has been withdrawn from the drug list in USA). However, before she used a heparin or steroid adjunct, most of the sick ferrets would die due to embolism. The survival rate can be increased to about 40% with heparinization (3 days prior to Carparsolate treatment) and by using corticosteroids, the survival rate can reach 70%.

Technique: Carparsolate is given exactly as for dogs, by administration of four i.v. injections of 2.2 mg/kg 12 h apart for 2 days, via an in-dwelling 24-gauge Teflon catheter in the cephalic vein. On the first day of Caparsolate treatment, oral prednisone is given at 0.25 mg/kg s.i.d. This should continue until the patient has a negative occult test and then the ferret can be weaned off. The occult heartworm test is done at 3 months after Carparsolate treatment and, if positive, another is done at 4 months. *Note*: virtually all ferrets are negative 4 months post-treatment if the Caparsolate has worked.

It is considered that Immiticide should not be used in ferrets, although they tolerate the drug itself fairly well. However, Immiticide can cause extremely fast heartworm death (6–12 hours post-injection) with fatal embolism. A trial has indicated that there is a much higher ferret death rate with Immiticide than with Caparsolate.

A suggested alternative to adulticide treatment would be to use heartworm preventive and oral corticosteroids (prednisolone) at 1 mg once daily in the asymptomatic or slightly symptomatic patient. It may be that the survival rate for non-adulticide treatments would equal that of adulticide treatments. Additional supportive drugs such as furosemide, digitalis, enalapril, etc. can be used (see Ch. 11). Heartworm prevention can begin 1 month after the adult *Difilaria* destruction treatment.

Prevention of heartworm disease: Ferrets are mostly kept indoors in the USA, but are kept inside and outside in Australia and many other countries. DK-C is of the opinion that ferrets in endemic heartworm areas should be on preventative even if they are kept totally indoors. Australia has tropical areas where mosquitoes are prevalent and the heartworm risk is high for dogs, cats and ferrets. Many ferrets in tropical regions of Australia are kept permanently in air-conditioned houses or belong to people touring with caravans. Outside cages would require mosquito proofing, as occurs in some parts of America where heartworm is endemic (J. Marks, Lakeland, Florida, pers. comm. 1997).

Ivermectin for heartworm prevention: Heartgard 30, Merial Australia Pty Ltd, a Merck Sharp & Dohme and Rhone-Poulenc company. This chewable 68 µg form is ideal and safe for monthly heartworm prevention in ferrets, but there is no label claim regarding the product (M. Webster, Manager, Veterinary Technical Services, Merial Ltd, pers. comm. 1998). The USA chewable tablet, dog or cat, used to be used in quarters per month but are now used whole monthly for prevention. Merck studies proposed a dose rate of 6 µg/kg as protective, i.e. one-quarter of a 65 µg tablet. Merial maintain that the ivermectin is not evenly distributed in the chewable tablet, so ferrets may be getting a different dose each time. Thus, whole tablet use is recommended (M. Finkler, pers. comm. 2005). The safety margin is tremendous, evidently 200–400 µg/kg would be safe as witnessed in other species. Some honey or Ferretone paste can be used to assist acceptance. Of course, using whole tablets does make the drug more expensive for the client.

The ferret, because of its susceptibility to infection with canine heartworm, has been used initially to assess the effect of ivermectin on the early larvae stages of heartworm.[34] Thus ferrets, artificially infected with *D. immitis* 20–42 days prior to treatment, were given ivermectin at dose rates between 0.0125 and 2.0 mg/kg.[35] These studies suggest that the minimum effective dose for suppression of maturation of *D. immitis* larvae in ferrets lies between 0.0125 and 0.05 mg/kg, which is higher than the dose required for this purpose in dogs. The drug company's lack of acknowledgment of the use of ivermectin in pet and working ferrets is surprising when one regards the possible market for this drug in ferrets worldwide. This is not the only drug where acknowledgment of use in ferrets is not given by drug companies. It is stated that ivermectin can absorb water by hydrolysis, so it is considered that part of a chewable tablet could not be used and the rest saved for the following month. It is a pity that some form of drug protection could not be devised to overcome this problem for the wider economic use of ivermectin in ferrets. (The ivermectin/oil mixture below is probably more cost-effective.)

The biology, diagnosis and prevention of heartworm infection in ferrets have been considered by the American Heartworm Society, which recommends ivermectin for use in ferrets.[36] The need to have a model for canine heartworm research and to improve knowledge of heartworm in the increasingly popular pet ferret led, in 1992, to three studies.

Study 1 showed, after s.c. inoculation of third stage larvae into 24 Marshall Farms female ferrets, that adult worms were first found in the hearts 70 days post-inoculation (PI) with 93% invading the heart by 119 days. Worm recovery was seen as 1.6% at 7 days up to 79.3 % at 119 days PI.

In study 2, 10 4-month-old ferrets, five male and five female, were inoculated with third stage larvae (L3), while 10 other ferrets were noninfected controls. The biological parameters of haematology, biochemistry and urine analysis were determined with no significant changes except that the eosinophil counts were high in infected compared to non-infected ferrets. Interestingly the ferrets that lived longer than 13 weeks had 1–12 adult worms in the hearts but heart enlargements were not seen radiographically until week 32 PI. Infection was mostly in the right atrium. Angiography was the only way to see the enlargement of the cranial vena cava and the heartworms therein and thus worms in the vessels can be found by this method. The radiographs and angiograms were done under xylazine (Rompun) anaesthesia at 2.5 mg/kg i.m.

In study 3, a trial with 41 4-month-old ferrets was divided into two experiments using infected treated animals and infected untreated controls. In experiment one, 24 ferrets, 12 male and 12 female, in groups of 4–6, got ivermectin at 0, 6, 12.5, 25, or 50 μg/kg 1 month after larval infection. In the second experiment, using 17 male ferrets, the dosage was 0, 0.5, 3 or 6 μg/kg.

The results in the first experiment: none of the five control (untreated) ferrets were positive for adult heartworm antigens at 4 months PI, 2 were positive at 5 months PI and all 5 at 6 months PI. The overall effect of ivermectin was that no worms were collected from treated animals but there was a 45–65% recovery from the untreated ferrets. Ivermectin was 100% effective in preventing heartworm at the dosages given.

In the second experiment: again all the controls were negative for adult heartworm antigens at 4 months PI but four of the five controls and one of the treated animals, which had 0.5 μg/kg, were positive at 5 months PI. The outcome stated that treatment of ferrets with 3 and 6 μg/kg ivermectin was 100% effective but at 0.5 μg/kg was only 25% effective with all ferrets treated at this level found to have adult worm counts, i.e. 36.3 % recovery. None of the remaining treated ferrets were found to have worms but the control ferrets had 40–70% recovery of worms. It was concluded from this experiment that ivermectin be approved for use in ferrets for control of *Dirofilaria immitis*.[36]

Toxicity of ivermectin in ferrets: As indicated, ivermectin actually has a wide safety margin in species other than ferrets, at recommended doses of 2–500 μg/kg.[34] It is therefore unlikely to be a problem in ferrets at dose rates for heartworm protection but the drug continues not to have any mention of ferrets on the labelling. Merial Australia cannot even endorse the use of diluted ivermectin (Maurice Webster, Technical Manager, Merial Australia, pers. comm. 1998). Ivermectin is not water-soluble. I have used Ivomec (sheep 0.8 g/L) orally undiluted for six ferrets at 0.05 mL monthly dosing for heartworm prevention. I had the ivermectin in a tuberculin syringe, with sugar water before and after to take away the bitter chemical taste. I had no problems at the time. It is considered that ivermectin crosses the oral membranes so quickly that most or all is absorbed before it reaches the stomach.

DK-C has for some time used a suspension of 0.3 mL ivermectin 1% injectable in 28 mL of propylene glycol as a preventative medicine in ferrets. (The mixture is stored in a dark bottle to protect it from light.) The mixture has 100 μg/mL and of this, 0.2 mL/kg (0.02 mg/kg) is given as a monthly dose per ferret. A made-up suspension would have a 2-year expiry date. American ferret owners have good compliance giving the drug and there are no side-effects. Ferrets on this regime in Florida are protected in an area of high risk.

It is suggested that to avoid the use of propylene glycol, dilute ivermectin 1% injectable, one part to nine parts corn oil and dose the ferret with 0.1 mL per month. The dilution factor 1:9 comes to 1000 μg/mL, which equals 100 μg/0.1 mL which equals 100 μg/ferret. There is a good safety factor and the ivermectin protects against heartworms at 6 μg/kg, and incidentally ear mites at 400 μg/kg (M. Finkler, pers. comm. 1999). In his Virginia region, ferrets are kept strictly indoors. Finkler (2005) considers corn oil works with ivermectin and gives it a shelf life of 6 months if kept in a sealed dark bottle to prevent oxidation of the oil. It requires generous shaking before use.

In Sydney, where heartworm occurs, cattle ivermectin (10 g/L) was dispensed to ferret owners as 5 mL ivermectin with 45 mL propylene glycol, to be given at a dose rate of 0.1 mL per ferret monthly (B. Alderton, pers. comm. 1999). It has been queried now if studies have been carried out on the long-term efficacy of ivermectin made up this way after 1 year on the shelf (B. Alderton, pers comm. 2005). In practice, I dispensed ivermectin/oil mixture when heartworm was found in Western Australia.

One problem with ivermectin is that it is not available in small quantities for use in making up prevention mixtures so the query could be what is the shelf life when using ivermectin from a sheep/cattle pharmacy source when you are getting what is possibly the end of the can?

Other preventive drugs for heartworm:

- Milbemycin oxime, an ivermectin derivative (Interceptor, small dog) flavoured 2.3 mg tablet given daily as per small dog dose
- Moxidectin (ProHeart 6) is a macrolide similar in activity to ivermectin, acts on any adults and is given as 0.1 mL s.c. regardless of weight (American Ferret Report 2004)
- Selamectin (Revolution) is a novel semisynthetic compound of the macrocyclic lactone class and

rets showed typical symptoms of lethargy, inappetence, exercise intolerance, pleural infusion, cyanosis and dyspnoea. Laboratory evaluation showed mild anaemia and monocytosis. Hyperchloraemia was present and urinary bilirubinuria in some cases. Two ferrets had pleural effusion with between 40 and 120 mL fluids obtained by thoracocentesis. Mature heartworms were found in only one ferret.

Radiographs and ultrasound were diagnostic tools: Treatment revolved around the use of ivermectin with or without melarsomine (Immiticide). (*Note*: melarsomine was used at the canine dose rate of 2.5 mg/kg i.m. for two doses). The drug is not registered for ferrets by the FDA in America. It is a trivalent arsenical drug found to be highly effective in the treatment of adult and 4-month-old immature *Dirofilaria immitis* in naturally and experimentally-infected dogs.

Drugs:

- Ivermectin (50 mg/kg p.o. q. 30 days): all ferrets
- Prednisolone (1 mg/kg p.o. q. 24 h): all ferrets
- Melarsomine (2.5 mg/kg i.m. deep, under isoflurane sedation): some ferrets

Note at 30 days after the first melarsomine injection, the dose was repeated twice, a day apart. In addition, all ferrets had furosemide (2–4 mg/kg q. 8–12 h), diltiazem (7.5 mg/kg q. 24 h) and other heart medication as required.

The outcome of four ferrets treated just with ivermectin: Ferret 1 died in 10 days; ferret 2 died in 6 weeks. Ferret 3 gained resolution of heartworm, cleared at 6 months and was still alive 13 months after treatment. Ferret 4 had heartworms present at 16 months after treatment. Thus survival rate after treatment was considered at 50% to a 230-day period at least.

The outcome of six ferrets treated with melarsomine along with ivermectin: Two ferrets died of a type 1 anaphylactic reaction; ferret 1 immediately, ferret 2 after third injection. Ferret 3 died 1.5 days after whole treatment completed. Ferret 4 lived for over 5 months but was found by ultrasound to have worms which caused death by worm thrombosis. Ferret 5 was well 6 weeks after the second injection and ferret 6 went on to survive for over 3 years after treatment. Thus, survival rate after treatment was considered at 33.3% with an average survival time of 435 days.

Note: As bilirubinuria is a common abnormality in ferrets with *Difilaria immitis* infections, it is possible it could be used to indicate the presence of disease.

One point from this small survey is that, although with melarsomine treatment the mortality is high, those ferrets surviving appear to do so longer than those which had been treated with ivermectin alone, i.e. 453 days against 230 days.

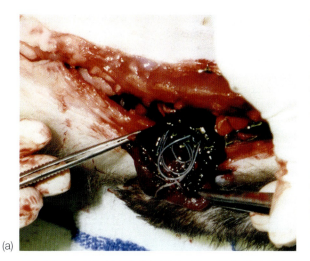

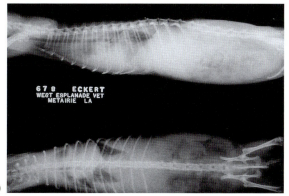

Figure 10.13 (a) Heartworm in ferret heart. (Courtesy of D. Kemmerer-Cottrell); (b) Chest fluid from heartworm. (Courtesy of Greg Rich.)

can be used at 18 mg/kg monthly for heartworm prevention. It is not having as good a success rate as ivermectin (G. Rich, pers. comm. 2005). It is now off the market in the USA as there have been some reactions in dogs.

Clinical observations on the heartworm problem in the USA

Heartworms are found on post mortem (Fig. 10.13a). Figure 10.13a shows a 3-year-old male ferret found in an abandoned house. Re-homed, it was halfway through a treatment with Carparsolate when it ate breakfast and fell over dead (DK-C, pers. comm. 2005). The disease results in pleural infusion within the chest cavity (Fig. 10.13b).

Evaluations of possible treatments: A study was carried out on a ferret population with naturally occurring *Difilaria immitis* disease.[37] Some 13 infected fer-

Antinoff Treatment Protocol based on evaluation. With a ferret found to be infected with *Difilaria immitis* and showing a positive blood test proceed thus:

1. Give ivermectin, 50 mg/kg p.o. q. 30 days, until the animal improves and the microfilaria test is negative.
2. Alongside ivermectin treatment, an initial dose of melarsomine, 2.5 mg/kg i.m. is given by deep muscle injection under isoflurane anaesthesia.
3. With the above, swelling of the i.m. site may occur and the ferret should be getting prednisolone 1 mg/kg p.o. q. 24 h, with attention to any other cardiac medication as required plus removal of pleural effusion. During the treatment time, the ferret should have quality hospitalization and cage rest.
4. One month after the first melarsomine injection, the dose is repeated under G/A.
5. After 24 hours, a final melarsomine injection of 2.5 mg/kg is given under G/A.
6. An ELISA test is done 3 months post-treatment start (TS) and then monthly. With good results, the ferret is negative to heartworm at 4–6 months after this drug course. Ultrasound can be used to check for adult worms.

Note: One vet uses the combination when there is a compromised pulmonary condition but in mild cases, with limited signs, uses only the melarsomine (Immiticide) alone (G. Rich, pers. comm. 2005).

Another survey using 28 19-week-old ferrets from Marshall Farms, New York, set out to evaluate melarsomine as an adulticide for ferret heartworm disease.[38] The ferrets were infected by subcutaneous injection of *Dirofilaria immitis* worms which all took to give the clinical disease.

Treatment was done in four groups. *Note* all injections were i.m. into the lumbar muscles using a 1 mL tuberculin syringe and 25 gauge needle. Ferret bleeding via jugular and/or cranial vena cava (Ch. 7) was under ketamine (20 mg/kg) and xylazine (2.5 mg/kg) anaesthesia.

- Group 1: Control number having only saline injections
- Group 2: Single injections of melarsomine, 3.25 mg/kg i.m. at day 0
- Group 3: Given two injections, 1 day apart, of melarsomine, 3.25 mg/kg i.m. (standard treatment schedule for dogs)
- Group 4: Single injection of melarsomine 3.25 mg/kg i.m. plus a repeat 1 month later of two injections melarsomine as for group 3 (alternate treatment schedule).

The overall results, as detected by antigen test and/or echocardiography, showed worms in the heart and near blood vessels of all ferrets in the survey. However, microfilarial counts tended to be negative or low with only apparently one ferret in each group having microfilaria. In contrast, the DiroCHEK (heartworm antigen test), in conjunction with echocardiography, was most effective in finding adult heartworms in the heart and associated blood vessels.

The treatment of heartworm ferrets with melarsomine dihydrochloride enhanced cardiomegaly and alveolar infiltrates and increased the severity of interstitial disease. (*Note* the treatment can tend to cause a more acute release of worm fragments which may cause an increase in clinical signs or changes initially.) That is, it is not the worms in the heart, but the fragments and pathology to the lungs that may well cause the majority of clinical signs (N. Antinoff, pers. comm. 2005). With the treatment, the dose rate of 3.25 mg/kg melarsomine was effective (80.6–83.3%) given either twice, a day apart, or just one injection followed by a later two injections, again a day apart, 4 weeks later. It was noted that a single injection of 3.25 mg/kg melarsomine would kill 33.3 % of adult heartworms. Interestingly, it seemed the male worms were more sensitive to the melarsomine than the female worms.

The most advanced treatment of ferret adult *Dirofilaria* infection has been explored by DK-C.[39] She trialed moxidectin (ProHeart 6) with four infected ferrets with success. Moxidectin is similar to ivermectin in activity as a macrolide and commonly used as a heartworm adulticide in dogs. Heartworm in dogs can have a life span of 5–7 years and in cats, 2 years and ivermectin can halve the parasite life span in both animals. It is presumed that moxidectin has a similar effect and may be effective in ferrets. She theorizes that the moxidectin acts on ferret heartworm adults because the worms in this species tend to be stunted in comparison with those from dogs.

Case reports on using ProHeart 6 as an adulticide

Cases 1 and 2 involved two unsterilized 2-year-old ferrets with no clinical signs of disease but a positive SNAP heartworm antigen test and positive KNOTT'S occult heartworm test. Each ferret was given 0.17 mg (0.05 mL) of moxidectin as a single dose s.c. There were no ongoing signs of heartworm disease when the ferrets were checked 2 months post-injection. At the 3rd month check, one ferret tested negative and one had a weak positive reaction. The ferret continued progress with monthly checks. A 6-month repeat injection was given and then the ferrets had twice yearly ProHeart 6 and were still well, 2 years after initial treatment.

Case 3 involved a 3-year-old castrate hob with cough and inappetence. It was a 'rescue' ferret. Clinically, the ferret had a grade I/VI heart murmur and mild pulmonary rales. CBC showed WBCs 12 500/μL (moderate elevation), eosinophilia (2.8%, 350 μL) and monocytosis (28%, 3500 μL). Everything else was normal but SNAP was very positive. A right ventricular enlargement was shown on X-ray.

In this case, treatment was prednisolone 0.5 mg q. 24 h and amoxicillin 22 mg/kg q. 12 h, plus an injection of moxidectin 0.17 mg s.c. The outcome in 1 week was reduced coughing and return of appetite. Also WBC was down to 8700/μL, while absolute eosinophils were at 2.5% (218/μL). Amoxicillin was discontinued 2 weeks post-moxidectin, while the prednisolone was still carried on. The ferret improved at monthly check-ups. At 6 month's post-initial treatment the SNAP test was weakly positive and the heart murmurs were hardly discernible, so the prednisolone was tapered off. The ProHeart 6 was continued prophylactically at 0.17 mg with the ferret still healthy after 1 year.

The final ferret case was a 4-year-old de-sexed hob with anorexia, tachypnea for 14 days and weight loss. It was emaciated with injected mucous membranes and pronounced pulmonary rales. The heart sounds were reduced in all heart chambers and pleural effusion was suspected. The SNAP test was again very positive but no microfilaria were detectable. The blood picture showed a moderate anaemia (Hct 31%) with the total WBC at 18 100/μL with an absolute granulocytosis (82%, 14 842/μL.). The BUN was moderately elevated at 59 mg/dL, and the ALT was 650 U/L. The heart was enlarged on the right side shown by X-ray.

As the ferret was so sick, thoracocentesis was used to take 30 mL of straw-coloured fluid away and the animal was put in a oxygen chamber overnight. Subcutaneous injections were given of furosemide 2.5 mg, dexamethasone 1 mg and enrofloxacin (Baytril) 4.6 mg. Nursing included giving 20 mL Hill's Prescription Diet Canine/Feline a/d by oral syringe. The next day treatment continued with moxidectin 0.17 mg s.c. then orally prednisolone 0.5 mg q. 24 h, enrofloxacin 2 mg, and furosemide 1 mg. Tube feeding continued until the ferret began eating on the 3rd day. The patient was sent home on the medical regime. The enrofloxacin was stopped at 3 weeks post-clinical admission.

The ferret was well clinically at 3 months post-clinical admission but SNAP test showed a weak positive. A second ProHeart 6 injection was given and at 9 months, the test was negative. Treatment with other drugs was stopped and the ferret would have been kept on twice yearly ProHeart 6 injections, as for dogs. Unfortunately, in the USA ProHeart 6 has been banned due to adverse reactions in dogs. This has not occurred with ProHeart SR 12 in Australia. Again as these drugs are not actually registered for use in ferrets by the American FDA, it is another failure in authorities' knowledge about their possible use in ferrets, despite problems in dogs and cats. It is hoped that the American MUMS act, Minor Use Minor Species, for the use of drugs in 'exotics' may change the situation.

It is encouraging to note that six other ferrets have been treated with ProHeart 6, with the result that only one ferret died of unrelated causes at 3 months after initial treatment but showed no parasites in the heart at post mortem. The other five ferrets were checked 4 months post-treatment and were shown to be clinically well.

Note: It is strongly advised by Merial Australia that IVOMEC Plus should not be used in ferrets, as there are no data regarding the use of the drug clorsulon in ferrets. It is considered unlikely that ferrets would become infected with *Fasciola hepatica* at which the drug is targeted. However, liver fluke can affect cattle, sheep, goats, man, horse, even kangaroo, rabbit and hare, with the snail as an intermediate host, so there may be a rare chance of working ferrets eating snails and getting infected.[26] It has been reported that *Fascioloides magna* of cattle can possibly infect ferrets.[8] *Dipetalonema reconditum* is another related parasite that inhabits the peritoneal membranes of dogs in Italy, Kenya and even Australia, with the flea as the intermediate host. *Note* that *Dirofilaria* are in the same family as *Brugia* species, which are mosquito-borne parasites in South East Asia.[8] *B. pahangi* affects domestic and wild animals and possibly man, while *B. malayi* definitely does affect man. As they have the same life cycle, ferrets could be infected from human carriers in Asian regions. Experimentally in ferrets, *Brugia* species have invoked inflammatory responses in the liver, spleen, intestine and lungs.

A digenean fluke of the family Opisthorchiidae, *Pseudamphistomum truncatum*, is a common parasite of a number of wild carnivores in Russia and Eastern Europe and has been found in UK otters (*Lutra lutra*) and mink (*Mustela vison*).[40] Snails and freshwater fish are the two intermediate hosts. The parasite invades the bile duct and gall bladder to cause cholecystitis. In Russian Belarus, the parasite infects European otters, American mink, European mink (*Mustela lutreola*) and polecats (*Mustela putorius*). It has been recorded in otters in Germany and France, while also present in European mink in Spain. It is known that the parasite affects man, dogs and cats. Man evidently has infected cats in Russia. With the latter species, there might be a possible link in the future to pet ferrets if kept in the same household.

Order Spirurida: superfamily Dracunculoidea

This superfamily includes an interesting skin parasite *Dracunculus medinensis*, affecting humans, where the female worm emerges from skin cysts. This has been

CHAPTER TEN
Parasitic diseases of ferrets

reproduced experimentally in ferrets using *D. insignis*, which is a natural parasite of weasels and other carnivores in America.

Superfamily Gnathostomatoidea: family Gnathostomatidae

Includes a parasite requiring at least three hosts in the life cycle and which can infect dogs, cats, mink, polecats and raccoons. Intermediary stages are in water *Cyclops* and various fish, frogs and crabs. *Gnathostoma nipponicum* is a natural parasite of mink that can cause larva migrans in humans as can roundworm, and it has been established experimentally in the ferret.[8]

Phylum Platyhelminthes: class Cestoda: subclass Eucestoda: Order Cyclophyllidea: *Dipylidium caninum* and *Taenia* spp.

These common tapeworms have been reported in all carnivores, which are affected by various species.[24] They now rarely cause problems in dogs and cats. The *D. caninum* life cycle requires the common flea (Fig. 10.14).

The flea is a common problem of ferrets as well as dogs and cats (see later). My concern has been picked up and stated whereby 'infection by other species can only be prevented by also controlling predatory and scavenging involving the metacestodes (larval stage) in carrion and prey animals'.[41] Polecats and feral ferrets can eat carrion in some circumstances.

However, species of *Taenia* in cats *(T. taeniformis)* and dogs (*D. caninum*) are extremely unlikely to infect ferrets (Fig. 10.15). There are several species of *Taenia* which do infect mustelids. The four *Taenia* species which infect dogs in Australia cycle through the rabbits and sheep but not rodents (Russell Hobbs, pers. comm. 2005). Working rabbiting ferrets at risk?

Clinical signs: The dog with *Dipylidium caninum* shows only anal pruritus. In the cat with *Taenia* there is loss of condition and poor coat character. Poor coat and weight might be a sign in infected ferrets if *D. caninum* managed to establish itself. No doubt intestinal blockage could occur with a growing tapeworm specimen in a ferret but we might be drawing a long bow with this scenario.

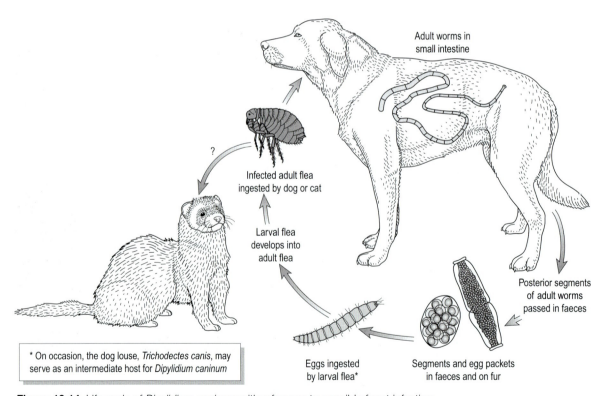

Figure 10.14 Life cycle of *Dipylidium caninum* with reference to possible ferret infection.

Treatment: For possible ferret cases, use of levamisole hydrochloride 10 mg and niclosamide 200 mg tablets (Ambex Two, Pharm Tech Pty Ltd) as a crushed tablet is recommended. Dose is 1 tablet per 2 kg, as per cat kittens; ferrets would weigh 500–1500 g.

Some other interesting possibilities of ferret infection by helminth parasites are worth mentioning here:

Class Cestoda: subclass Eucestoda: Order Pseudophyllidea: *Diphyllobothrium latum*

Diphyllobothrium affect humans through eating raw fish with the larval stages; this has been achieved experimentally in ferrets in Germany, but only as the paratenic host and not the final host, unlike dogs and cats where adult worms can develop.[8]

There is a related tapeworm of dogs and cats in Australia, *Spirometra erinaceieuropaei* (family Diphylobothriidea, same as *D. latum*). It is likely that ferrets could be paratenic hosts by eating other paratenic hosts such as lizards, frogs or rodents (Russell Hobbs, pers. comm. 2005).

Nasal worm of weasels: *Skrjabingylus nasicola* (Phylum Nematoda: Order Strongylida: superfamily Metastrongloidae)

Skrjabingylosis is the name given to a disease caused by the adult red worm, *Skrjabingylus nasicola*, in weasels and stoats in the UK, Eurasia, New Zealand and North America.[42] In America, cases are seen in the spotted skunk.

Pathogenesis: The adult worm in the nasal cavity causes irritation and swelling and severely affects the sensitive bone tissues of the skull, causing lesions which can be progressive. Where stoat (ermine) and weasel pelts are important to trappers and breeders, this disease is a great worry. On the other hand, some people concerned about wild mustelids affecting bird life welcome the disease for their control (Fig. 10.16).

The first stage larvae in weasel scats must be taken in by a mollusc. There the problem could stop, as weasels and stoats rarely eat these creatures. However, infected slugs or snails are eaten by shrews and mice that are the

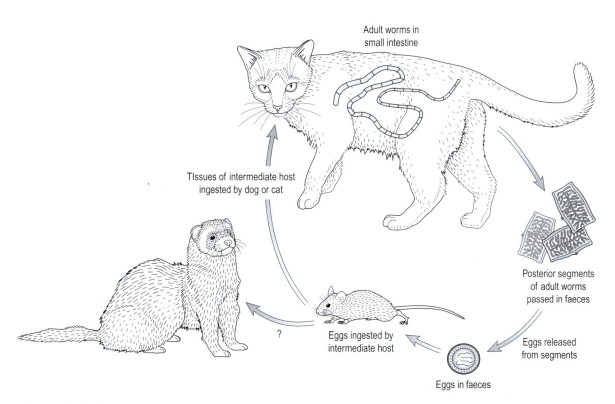

Figure 10.15 Life cycle of *Taenia* with reference to possible ferret infection.

CHAPTER TEN

Parasitic diseases of ferrets

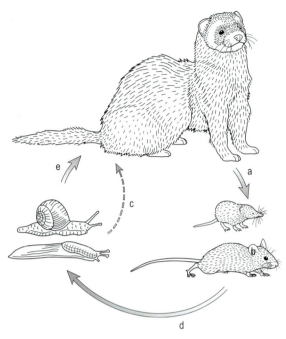

Figure 10.16 Life cycle of *Skrjabingylus nasicola* with reference to possible infection in ferrets. (After King, 1989, with permission.)[42]

prey of wild mustelids. Working or feral ferrets could thus eat snails, shrews or mice and become infected. In some cases, pet ferrets eat these things!

In another family of trematodes (Troglotrematidae), *Troglotrema acutum* occurs in the frontal and ethmoidal sinuses of fox, mink and polecat in continental Europe.[24] They have frogs as the secondary host, which working ferrets might possibly eat!

Ferret external parasites

With ferrets living in close association with dogs and cats, there is bound to be some transfer between the species, if only of the humble but ubiquitous flea. The flea can be an unwitting intermediary host or also a menace in its own right. The list of other blood sucking arthropods include mites, ticks, lice, flies, mosquitoes, sandflies and triatomine bugs which can serve as part of the life cycle of many protozoa and helminthes indicated above, which may attach themselves to ferrets under certain situations.

Fleas

There are many species of fleas, most of which have host preferences such as dogs, cats, foxes, dingoes,

Table 10.2 Host range of flea species

Flea genus and species	Hosts other than ferrets	Possible ferret significance
Ctenocephalides canis	Dog, dingo, fox, cat, man	Tapeworm contact?
Ctenocephalides felix	Cat, dog, possum	Tapeworm contact?
Echidnophaga gallinacea	Poultry, rabbit, cat	Working ferret: 'stick-tight' flea seen on ears when leaving warrens
Xenopsylla cheopis	Rat, mouse	Contact from ferret prey?
Pulex irritans	Man	Contact from ferret owner?

rabbits, poultry and ferrets plus all wild mustelids. Thus, both pet and working ferrets can get fleas, which can be the main reason for clients to present a ferret. Fleas are also vectors of disease, from the plague bacillus to tapeworms (see Internal ferret parasite section). One author considers ferrets suffer fleas and ear mites while other ectoparasites are rare.[43] It is found in drought conditions in the UK when hedgehog fleas are transferring to dogs and cats where possible and entering households. The adult flea is the parasitic stage on ferrets and it should be remembered that they are less permanently resident on any one host than lice, etc. and their host range is shown in Table 10.2.

A German survey on the presence and species of flea (*Siphonaptera*) affecting pets and hedgehogs was done with the help of 625 veterinary practices.[44] The fleas came from 294 dogs (795 fleas), 334 cats (1152 fleas), 76 hedgehogs (481 fleas), five domestic rabbits (10 fleas), one golden hamster (four fleas) and one ferret (three fleas). Interestingly, the ferret had seemingly the least fleas to find, and only *Ctenocephalides felix* at that!

Clinical signs: Ferrets get a general inflammation from fleabites and the resulting scratching plus the possibility, with heavy infestations, of anaemia in ferret kittens and sick adults.[45] Hunting ferrets will often come out of warrens with their ears covered by 'stick-tight' fleas. Jills used for hunting and then going back to breeding will sometimes lose all their kittens 4–6 weeks after birth. This phenomenon is not seen in non-working ferrets and some ferreters have wondered whether there could be any connection to the myxomatosis virus. A heavy flea infestation causes intense scratching and hair loss around the dorsal thorax and neck; scratching around the head can also be caused by a concurrent ear mite infestation in poorly maintained ferrets. Ferrets in working or breeding colonies may transmit fleas around, just as a household of cats keep an infestation going unless treated. Flea dirts on ferrets' skins are signs of infection.

Treatment: There are no chemical washes of any form registered for ferrets. Care must be taken with a small animal like a ferret regarding toxicity risks with any chemicals. Ferret owners might use any convenient dog or cat flea wash, just because they have used the same on their dog or cat, without consulting a veterinarian about toxic possibilities for ferrets. A rule of thumb is to reduce the dose used for a feline of the same weight.

It has been suggested that the most recent flea products on the market for dogs and cats could be used for ferrets but there are no manufacturers' recommendations. Dr M. Burrows in 2002 reviewed drugs against fleas and ticks such as fibronil (Frontline) lufenuron (Progam), imidacloprid (Advantage), selamectin (Revolution) and nitenpryram (Capstar) on dogs and cats.[46]

In Japan, an experimental trial was done on using imidacloprid on ferrets and rabbits.[47] Regarding the ferrets, a 3-year-old male 1000 g ferret with moderate flea infestation was given 40 mg/kg imidacloprid with the result of no fleas in the coat after 6 days but some flea faeces noted. At 20 days, the ferret was completely clear.

Similarly, a 5-year-old 1500 g ferret, indoors with dogs and a severe flea problem, was cleared in 6 days using 38.1 mg/kg imidacloprid. A 19-month-old 1005 g female ferret, with other household ferrets, with a mild flea infestation, was treated but the owner failed to return the animal for a check-up. However, safety checks with Advantage plus (feline 40) (Bayer) (10% imidacloprid + 0.5% pyriproxfen) showed no adverse side-effects on ferrets regarding body weight loss, body condition, appetite, CBC, general chemistry, urinalysis or signs on autopsy.

In the USA, it is considered that any drug approved for cats can be used on ferrets at reduced strength. Frontline spray can be used at 2 pumps per pound weight, also Feline Advantage half tube, 0.4 mL on skin (M. Finkler, pers. comm. 2005). Sprays and spot-ons are considered better than tablets to make sure of treatment.

Feline Program can be used at half strength for ferrets, in the USA dose, 45 mg given orally once a month. Lufenuron is adsorbed into the body, enters the adipose tissue and then the circulation. When taken up by a flea it inhibits chitin polymerization or deposition thus preventing egg hatching.[46] Thus there is a latent phase of 6–8 weeks before the drug kicks in to remove fleas. The lower oral Program dose for cats in Australia is 133 mg.

Advantage comes as a green pack to treat ferrets and rabbits up to 4 kg. *Note* that ferrets are usually below 2 kg in weight. The tube content is administered to the skin between the shoulder blades. *Note*: Advantage is the only spot-on registered for ferrets and rabbits. However, there have been several ferrets which have shown reaction with vomiting and skin irritation (K. Smith, NSWFWS, pers. comm. 2005). A case of Advantage toxicity has been recorded in a cat when the owner administered it *orally* by mistake. The cat had symptoms of ptyalism, gagging, increased respiratory noise, vomiting and anorexia.[48] It took time to recover. A ferret chewing on an Advantage tube might get such symptoms.

Revolution for kittens has a dose of 0.25 mL for weights below 2.5 kg. Selamectin is a semisynthetic ivermectin and targets the GABA-modulated chloride channels producing rapid insect death. It is said to have a high safety margin in cat kittens.

Capstar has only a lower dose level of 11.4 mg for cats less than 11 kg. Capstar is a systemic absorbed oral neunicotinoid insecticide that binds to nicotinic acetylcholine and causes death within 10 min by interfering with the normal nerve transmission of the insect. It said to be safe for cat kittens 4 weeks old or over but weighing at least 1 kg. It is in tablet form.

Both Revolution and Capstar should remain outsiders in the flea game until more is ferreted out about their safety for mustelids.

Frontline Top Spot (fibronil) had been used with success in Australia. Dose was half to 1 vial per ferret monthly. This is now Frontline Plus with fibronil 100 g/L and S-methoprene 120 g/L. There has been some concern that Frontline Plus is not working as effectively as the original Frontline before the insect growth regulator was added (B. Alderton, pers. comm. 2005). The Frontline spray has been used for stray ferrets at refuge homes and is most cost-effective. However, it is thought that there appears to be an increased flea resistance (K. Smith, NSWFWS, pers. comm. 2005). *Note*: Frontline can be used sprayed on a cotton bud to administer to ferret ears in suspected cases of otitis (see below).

The cost of drugs is a major concern with ferret owners though the Frontline spray is cost-effective for ferret colony or shelter situations.

Revolution used by K. Smith of NSWFWS in shelter, was one cat vial (2.5 kg) over four ferrets per month plus giving oral ivermectin monthly for heartworm. This works out cost-effective for ferret shelters and has been used often. Revolution for heartworm alone should involve the whole kitten vial but works out expensive. *Note*: Pfizer does suggest a 6 mg/kg dosage but points out that there is no actual approval for Revolution for ferrets.

Flea collars for ferrets are impractical and they could even be dangerous, with working ferrets going down warrens and getting caught up with roots. In any case, flea collars containing dichlorvos are very toxic to ferrets.[2] A vaccine against fleas is hoped for in the future.[49]

CHAPTER TEN

Parasitic diseases of ferrets

A general knowledge of the range of flea products with regard to possible toxicity in ferrets is important.

Pyrethrins: These are natural biological insecticides derived from chrysanthemum oils and of low toxicity. They have an effect on the parasite neuromuscular system giving a quick flea kill.[50] However, the effect is only transient, lasting about 4 hours, though the flea never develops a resistance to this natural drug. I have used the pyrethrin products Petgloss Shampoo (Troy) and Di-Flee Insecticidal Shampoo for Puppies and Kittens (Jurox) for ferrets. Pyrethrins are usually in synergic combination with organophosphates or carbamates. They are also combined with synergic agents such as piperonyl butoxide or N-octyl bicycloheptene, which is capable of inhibiting the insect enzymes and which would degrade the pyrethrin action by oxidative and hydrolytic means. Toxicity has been seen in cats when the sprays used contained piperonyl butoxide at 1.5% or more, where some cats showed tremors, lethargy and incoordination, which were reversed when the flea treatment was stopped.

Pyrethroids (synthetic pyrethrins): Were developed with third-generation products such as permethrin, being about 40 times more stable than natural pyrethrins and lasting for 3 weeks.[50]

Carbamates: These are anticholinesterase agents, which act by occupying the active site on the acetylcholinesterase enzyme molecule instead of acetylcholine. The effect is to cause continuous neurostimulation and paralysis of the flea.[50] The drug is not as effective as organophosphate, as the flea may recover. It is however considered a safe drug for dogs and cats. I have used it on ferrets as a flea powder for coats and putting in sleeping boxes (7-Dust, Troy). I have not used it on pregnant jills or with kittens, which may lick the powder.

Organophosphates (OPs): These drugs also act as cholinesterase inhibitors and must not be used concurrently with carbamate, as there would be a cumulative effect and possibly serious toxicity in ferrets. One OP is malathion, which is considered of relatively low toxicity to the host but deadly to fleas, by being converted into a highly toxic metabolite.[50] However, there are now safer drugs than contact OPs for use on ferrets. I have never used OPs though toxicity has been suggested to occur when the products are used grossly over-concentrated. With ferrets, I prefer to avoid any possibility of toxicity.

Methoprene: is used with pyrethrins, as it affects the flea eggs laid on the animal and disrupts the development of the flea larvae within the egg. The larvae pupate but are unable to develop further and die. It has no effect on adult fleas.

Rotenone: Occurs with sulpha as flea powder for poultry, dogs, cats, horses, calves and goats.

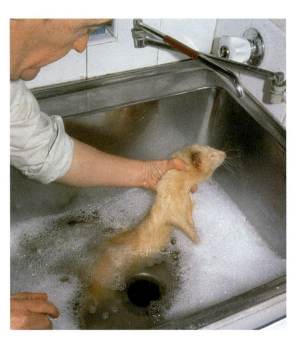

Figure 10.17 Washing ferrets for fleas.

Limonene: D-Limonene is a natural botanical insecticide from citrus peel, which has been used in sprays in the USA. It is toxic to all stages of the flea life cycle.

Herbal flea collars contain pennyroyal and eucalyptus oils; they can be hung up in closed areas such as sleeping boxes and hospital ferret cages out of ferret reach. They vaporize slowly to act as a natural flea insecticide. From personal experience in the past with my own ferrets, I have tried various methods of flea control including washing (Fig. 10.17).

Ferrets can be washed. A warm water bath is prepared and the ferret is gently immersed except for the head and then brought out and a shampoo applied. The ferret is again immersed in the water. This can be repeated and the shampoo is gradually rinsed from the coat. It is advisable to quickly dunk the whole ferret once, as it will be seen that fleas gather on the ferret's head. I have used Petgloss Shampoo (Troy) whose active ingredients are 1 g/L pyrethrins plus 10 g/L piperonyl butoxide. Di-Flee Insecticidal Shampoo for Puppies and Kittens (Jurox) has a similar formulation, but the dog/cat product contains 1g/L cypermethrin instead of the pyrethrins.

I have used Fibronil 2.5 g/L (Frontline, Rhone Merieux, Australia) in the past on my ferret colony and recorded the results.[51] The Frontline functionally inhibits gamma-amino butyric acid (GABA), the flea's main neurotransmitter. The company declares a safety factor on pups from 2 days of age and cat kittens from 7 weeks of age. I have not used it on kittens. Using the 100 mL pack Frontline, the recommended administration for a 1 kg dog or cat is six sprays. I use up to three sprays for both jills and hobs without any toxic reaction. Frontline is considered safe for pregnant and lactating bitches but I have not used it on jills in this condition. I have used it routinely otherwise and find I get ferrets clear of fleas for 6 weeks plus which compares favourably to up to 12 weeks for dogs and 8 weeks for cats. It is probably best to treat the jill and hob separately before putting to mate and isolating the jill in a clean nursery cage (Ch. 3).

Procedure: I hold the ferret, using surgical gloves, while my nurse, also wearing surgical gloves, sprays the ferret along the back and either side and rubs in the spray as the ferret naturally wriggles. There is no ferret biting or release of musk glands. I prefer to treat the ferrets in the afternoon when they have been sleeping and are relaxed. The ferrets may scratch after being sprayed and I presume there is some initial irritation from the spray, which does not persist.

Drug toxicity considerations: It is stated that any insecticide used on the animal or its environment has the capability to cause toxicity and alarming signs.[50] It is prudent for the veterinarian to be aware of toxicity of drugs to ferrets, and the general clinical signs of toxicity from possible flea products are given in Table 10.3. Drugs like chlorinated hydrocarbon products, DDT, etc. are no longer allowed as pesticides, as they enter the food chain and affect man.

In one recent trial in Denmark, the efficiency of (a) imidacloprid (Advantage), (b) imidacloprid/permethrin

Table 10.3 Insecticide toxicity signs and treatment

Insecticide group	Toxicity clinical signs	Treatment
Pyrethrins and synthetic pyrethroids	With very high doses, possible vomiting, diarrhoea, ataxia, CNS excitation, seizures, paralysis	Emesis (may induce seizures) gastric lavage; no specific antidote; seizures may be controlled by diazepam (Valium) at 2.5–20 mg i.v. as needed; barbiturates to effect. Do *not* use phenothiazines as they lower seizure threshold; calcium gluconate 10% at 2–10 mL given slowly i.v. and vitamin B complex i.m. to protect liver function; critical period 24–36 h
Carbamates	Abdominal cramping, vomiting, diarrhoea, miosis, dyspnoea, cyanosis, muscle twitching seizures, rarely tetany followed by weakness and paralysis	Atropine sulphate: 0.2–0.5 mg/kg to effect (mydriasis and reduced salivation) usually $1/4$ dose i.v. and $3/4$ s.c.; may repeat at 3–6 h for 1–2 days. Pralidoxime (2-PAM) is CONTRAINDICATED
Organophosphates (OPs)	Muscarinic: salivation, lacrimation, diarrhoea, abdominal cramping, miosis, pallor, cyanosis, dyspnoea, emesis. Nicotinic: twitching of facial and tongue muscles progressing to generalized twitching followed by paralysis CNS depression: tonic–clonic seizures, death due to hypoxia from respiratory muscle paralysis, bronchoconstriction pulmonary oedema, bradycardia	Atropine as for carbamates; 2-PAM at 20 mg/kg i.v. twice daily given over 5 min; if poisoning less than 24 h before, treatment is necessary for 1–2 days; if of longer duration may require therapy for several days Diphenhydramine hydrochloride (Benadryl) at 4 mg/kg (dogs) i.v. or i.m. (dogs or cats) every 8 h until asymptomatic; if animal becomes depressed, decrease dose to 1–2 mg/kg
Methoprene	No toxic effects recorded. There have been no deaths even at the highest oral dosing of dogs and cats	If ingested remove by gastric lavage. Do not induce vomiting treat symptomatically. If eye or skin exposed, wash directly in stream of water for 15 minutes
Rotenone	Vomiting, nausea, diarrhoea, respiratory stimulation, convulsions followed by respiratory depression, coma, respiratory failure and death	Emesis, gastric lavage before the convulsive state, warmth, quiet, assist respiration. Diazepam, calcium gluconate and B complex as for pyrethrins
D-Limonene	Has been seen in cats in USA. Hypersalivation, ataxia, and muscle tremors.	Supportive. No specific therapy

Table after Kwochka, 1987, with permission.[50]

and (c) phoxim were tested on farmed mink (*Mustela vison*) infected with the squirrel flea (*Ceratophyllus sciurorum*).[52] Results compared with untreated mink were 91.9% efficiency for (a), 89.3% for (b) and 92.2% and 99.3% for two groups of (c)-treated mink. The interesting chemical is phoxim, an organophosphorus insecticide used in sheep in Europe. Though it is said to be of high efficiency, low poison, low left-over and broad-spectrum, I wonder about the considered use of the drug for mustelids.

Ear mange

'Ear mange' is caused by *Otodectes cynotis*, the common ear mite. It has been noted, from DNA and morphological features, that the *Otodectes* mite of dog cat, fox and ferret of various hosts and geographic locations belongs to a single species *Otodectes cynotis* (Acari: Psoroptidae).[53] The ear mite in the ferret has a typical 3-week mite life cycle in the external ear. Ferrets produce a natural normal brown earwax, which can be examined on a slide at consultation. If an infestation is untreated, the outcome may be a spread of infection from the external to the middle ear and may also contribute, by tympanic membrane rupture, to an inner ear disease (Ch. 12). Clinical signs are shaking the head and sometimes rubbing it along the ground on the affected side.

Pathogenesis: This is not clear, as the mite does not bite into the skin to obtain body fluids but feeds on the epidermal debris.[24] I have theorized that a toxin may be produced by the otodectic mite which is absorbed by the ferret body. In severe infections, the ferret looks dull and stays dull like those ferrets with severe sarcoptic mange infections.

Diagnosis: By auroscope or ear swabbing at regular checks. The mite should be differentiated from *Sarcoptes scabiei* and *Notoedres cati*.

The ferret is handled firmly as suggested in Chapter 7. I found it less stressful on the ferret at examination to take an ear swab to check for ear mites. A cotton bud soaked in olive oil is used and a slide made. It is then possible to show the client the actual ear mite under the microscope. It is suggested that in the dog and cat at least, the otodectic mite has been found on other parts of the body besides the ears.[54]

Treatment: Care is required regarding possible toxicity of aural preparations in ferrets as, again, no drugs are registered for use on ferrets.[55] For dogs and cats pyrethrin, rotenone, thiabendazole and carbaryl preparations are used and applied over 4 weeks to effectively kill all newly-hatched adult mites, plus the use of a topical flea powder to remove any ectopic infestation.[54] These are considered safe drugs. For ferrets, I started by using eardrops with the minimum combination of drugs, as I was worried about toxicity, e.g. with a basic pyrethrin plus dichlorophen and piperonyl butoxide (synergist) (Troy Canker Drops). The small ear canal only allows for one or two drops of miticide. A repeat dose in 1 week and then fortnightly can eliminate the mites. Regular spot checks on ferret earwax should be advised, especially with a ferret colony, plus concurrent treatment of in-contact dogs and cats. In the USA, a selection of topical medications such as Mitox, Tresaderm, Nolvamite and Cerumite are suggested (M. Finkler, pers. comm. 2005).

A comparison of three treatments for ear mite control has been carried out.[56] Twenty-seven mite-infected ferrets were used under laboratory conditions and divided into three groups:

Group A: (five jills) received thiabendazole (Tresaderm®). Two drops into each ear once daily for 7 days, rested for 7 days, and then re-treated for 7 days.

Group B: (11 jills) received topical 1% ivermectin (Ivomec®) diluted 1:10 propylene glycol and at a dose rate of 400 μg/kg divided between each ear.

In both Group A and Group B, the ferret ears were gently massaged after the drugs were administered.

Group C: (five hobs/six jills) differed by having a s.c. injection of 1% ivermectin at a dose rate of 400 μg/kg at the same time as the group B treatment. (The ivermectin was diluted 1:4 with propylene glycol.)

The ferret groups were checked regularly for signs of depression and anorexia.

Note: the hobs were kept separate but some jills were caged in pairs. Also, as it was breeding stock, seven jills from groups A, B and C were mated with one hob of group C early during the study period of 8 weeks.

A graph (Fig. 10.18) shows the results of the experiment.

Conclusions were that topical treatment of the ferret ear canal was more efficient in destroying ear mites than the use of injectable ivermectin. In fact, the thiabendazole was equal to ivermectin. However, two applications of ivermectin against 14 in total of thiabendazole is the more economic option with ferret colonies. The authors were surprised that the injected ivermectin was less effective. The dosage, 400 μg/kg, was higher than that recommended for dogs, cats and ferrets by other authors.[56] It was noted that after 5 weeks, the infestation of the ferrets that had the s.c. injection, actually increased. It is considered that parentally-given ivermectin achieves a higher concentration in earwax. Cleaning ears before administration would help the miticide effect of the systemic ivermectin as ferret earwax impedes the ivermectin reaching the mites. The authors advise the use of topical 400 μg of ivermectin for routine mite control.

Note: for non-pregnant ferrets, ivermectin is advised topically every 3 months but jills should not be treated

Ferret external parasites

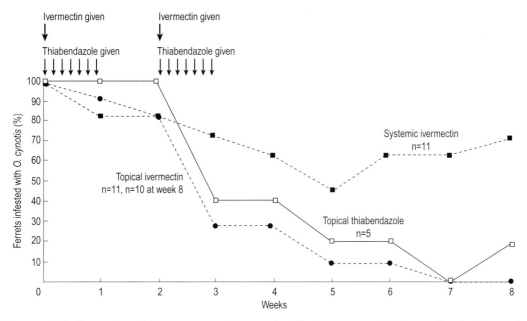

Figure 10.18 Comparison of three treatments for ear mites (*Otodectes cynotis*) in ferrets. (Graph with permission from the American Association for Laboratory Animal Science, 2005.)

during gestation. Kits over 6 weeks of age can be treated as adults.

The general use of ivermectin: This is a very good drug but again not registered for ferrets. As suggested it is found to have a broad safety margin and is advocated by some authors as the ultimate drug of choice.[6] The injectable ivermectin (MSD VET Ivomec 10 g/L) can be mixed 1:20 with propylene glycol. Then 0.1–0.3 mL (10–15 mg) can be used for each ear and repeated monthly. (Ferrets on monthly heartworm protection should have protection against ear mites.) This is possibly the best method for working ferrets exposed to both diseases. The safety factor of ivermectin is said to be such that pregnant jills can be treated in pregnancy to term and thus prevent mites in kittens.

Foot mange

Foot mange is the name I give to infections of *Sarcoptes scabiei* var. *canis* in ferrets. The disease occurs in dogs, feral dogs, dingoes, foxes and wombats, so that hunting and companion ferrets are both at risk. In outback settlements with large populations of dogs, which are unfortunately reservoirs of this disease, there is a public health aspect, as the mite is highly contagious and can affect man. Steady control of this disease in the outback is being achieved, along with the elimination of canine distemper, by better education on these diseases in animals.

This mange is one of the most important and dangerous diseases affecting ferrets and especially hunting ferrets. Sarcoptic mange in ferrets has been called 'footrot' by

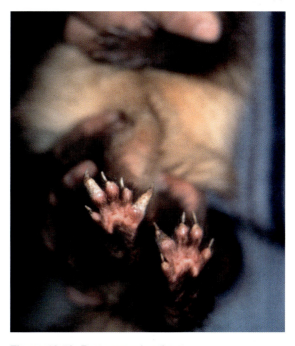

Figure 10.19 Foot mange in a ferret.

older UK ferreters, as the mange first affects the ferrets' feet. The name 'footrot' should be reserved for the disease of sheep. However, ferrets can get *Fusiformis*-type infections in dirty conditions (see Ch. 8).[45]

Clinical signs: Initially, *Sarcoptes* spp. affect the feet with yellow encrustations of material containing all stages of mite, egg, larvae and adult. The owner will suggest that the ferret looks as if it has 'trodden in something', which is a good description (Fig. 10.19). The ferret may be lame in one or more feet. The local infestation, if not checked, will spread to a general skin infection with scratching due to intense pruritus. The mite causes continuous skin damage by feeding on the skin and burrowing into the epidermis.[24]

Pathogenesis: The classic symptoms and sequelae to mange in ferrets have been described: 'The mite attacks the feet and can spread quickly to the ears, nose, eyes, tail and all over the body. It causes the feet to swell and scale off, the nails to become thick and long, scabs to appear on the body and in the ears, the hair to drop off. The animal becomes lethargic and sleeps all the time, except for brief periods to eat, drink and toilet. They finally become moribund and die'.[45] Working ferrets can be infected if fed unskinned fox meat. The mange in the fox coat quickly affects the ferrets. I have seen a working ferret with severe foot mange (Fig. 10.20) which had been untreated. The ferret had to be euthanized.

Diagnosis: By finding adults, larvae and eggs of *Sarcoptes scabiei* var. *canis* in the feet or skin scrapings.

Treatment: Must be vigorous! For ferrets in a colony or working ferrets, consideration must be given to destroying any wooden sleeping compartments. Years ago, the wood would have been treated with creosote and left for a week before replacing the ferrets. With an outbreak I had some years ago, caused by an infected ferret, I found it easier to burn the wooden sleeping boxes and start afresh. The old way to treat infected ferrets was to wash them in lime sulphur. The plant mite spray was used at 100 mL in 5 L of water in a deep sink (Fig. 10.15). The scabs on the feet were removed with olive oil if possible before washing and this sometimes required sedation of the ferret. The ferret had to be washed for at least 5 min, so the use of a kitchen timer was helpful. The sulphur wash was not rinsed off and the coat was left to dry out. It smelt but was not toxic. A weekly sulphur lime wash and keeping the ferret in a clean cage cured the problem but it could take 5 weeks.

I have always been wary of possible drug toxicity in ferrets and I have not recommended the use of malathion, carbaryl or cypermethrin compounds. However, a South Australian ferret with foot mange was treated by weekly rinses in malathion (Malawash, ICI, Australia) for 3 weeks, with the foot lesions dressed with benzene hydrochloride (Temadex, Wellcome Labs) without any toxicity signs.[57] The authors also recorded the use of amitraz (Ectodex EC, Shering Pty Ltd) as being able to cure foot mange in ferrets after one or two treatments. In the past few years ivermectin, though not registered for ferrets, has been found to be a safe drug for foot mange. Ivermectin 1% solution can be given, 0.05–0.1 mL p.o. s.c. at 14-day intervals until skin scrapings are negative and prednisone can be used to reduce pruritus at 2 mg/kg.[58] Lindane (benzene hexachloride) (Lorexane BP, a human preparation) has been used by ferreters to dress ferrets' infected feet (A. Geddes, Perth, WA, pers. comm.).

Frontline Spray (Frontline) can be used at 1 pump per kg repeated monthly for 3 months.

It has been recorded that milbemycin can be used to treat sarcoptic mange in dogs instead of ivermectin but there is no reference yet to its use in ferrets.

An odd reference to treating sarcoptic mange in dogs was made by Knight.[59] The injectable large animal registered Dectomax (doramectin 10 mg/mL, Pfizer Animal Health) was used with success with several farm and semi-rural dogs. Whether this drug (like ivermectin) could be used on severe ferret mange has not yet been tested.

Other types of mange that could affect ferrets

Notoedric mange

Notoedres cati is found on cats and rabbits so it may transfer to hunting ferrets.

Clinical signs: Similar to cats, with lesions around the head and neck and hair loss from the base of the ears and forehead and with intense pruritus.[24]

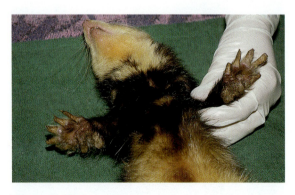

Figure 10.20 Severe foot mange in ferret leading to euthanasia.

Psoroptic mange

Psoroptes cuniculi occurs in rabbit ears, as does chorioptic mange (*Chorioptes cuniculi*) and both could possibly affect working ferrets. If a rabbit is fed to ferrets, it must be skinned to avoid mange infections.

Treatment: Use ivermectin s.c. as for foot mange.

Demodectic mange

Demodex sp. was isolated from two pet ferrets in the Netherlands.[60] The ferrets had been showing yellow discolouration of the skin and mild pruritus for 1 month. The owner, with no success, had treated them for ear mites. Apart from the skin appearance, the ferrets were in good condition. Skin scrapings and ear exudates revealed *Demodex* on both ferrets. The mites were similar to *D. criceti*, the golden hamster *Demodex* species. They were treated with amitraz (0.0125% suspension) by dipping three times at weekly intervals. The ears were treated every other day with 2 drops of solution. The result was relief of the pruritus and loss of yellow skin discolouration, but the hair did not regrow until a month after the treatment finished (after several repeat washes). Skin scrapings finally proved negative. There were apparently no side-effects of the treatment.

Other external parasites possibly affecting ferrets

Tick (ixodoidea)

Soft and hard ticks. These could affect working ferrets in the bush, from contact with vegetation, foxes, kangaroos, or rabbits in Australia. Poison ticks, *Ixodes holocyclus*, occur in eastern Australia and would be lethal to ferrets. In the dog, a rapid paralysis starts with the hind legs and moves forward.[24] In ferrets, it would mimic botulism. There is a danger of spread to Western Australia, as one poison tick came from eastern Australia on a nursery plant and affected a dog (R. Duffy, Joondalup Vet Hosp, pers. comm. 1998). In countries where ferreting is carried out regularly, the possibility of tick infestation of ferret and ferreter must be considered.

Treatment: engorged ticks must be removed completely (without leaving the head in) using a cotton swab soaked in petrol or paraffin oil. As ticks can be carriers of diseases transmitted to man, care must be taken in handling them.[2]

Lice (pediculosis)

These would be rare as in dogs and cats, as flea treatments deals with both diseases. It could occur in neglected, malnourished or poorly-kept ferret colonies. Similarly, cuterebriasis (fly myiasis) is a North American condition due to dipteran flies affecting dogs and cats. The fly life cycle includes rabbits and rodents as natural hosts. The eggs are laid in the soil and on plants by burrows and direct larval contact with the host results in cysts within the skin within 3–4 weeks. This condition might involve working ferrets which is evidently not common in America. The ferret contact would get nodular lesions usually around the head and neck like the natural hosts.[41] Treatment would be to remove the larvae but it is noted that rupture of the cyst might result in anaphylactic shock.

Conclusions

The relationship of the mosquito to the dog, cat and ferret is clearly seen.

Reference has been made in discussing the internal parasites of ferrets to their eating snails, worms, mice and rats, the possible intermediary hosts of disease. If there *is* any possibility of cross-over infection, with protozoa or helminth agents, from infected dogs and cats, then infection is only a meal away!

Special acknowledgements

The American Heartworm Society for support with the Ferret Heartworm Symposiums 1998/2003.[36,38] The parasitic life cycle diagrams are adapted from *Internal Parasites of Dogs and Cats* with permission from Technical Service Manager, Virginia Read, Novartis Animal Health, Australia.

References

1. Lappin MR. Feline zoonotic diseases. Vet Clin N Am 1993; 23:57–79.
2. Fox J. Parasitic diseases. In: Fox J, ed. Biology and diseases of the ferret, 2nd edn. Baltimore: Williams and Wilkins; 1998:375–391.
3. Thornton RN, Cook TG. A congenital toxoplasma-like disease in ferrets (*Mustela putorius furo*) N Z Vet J 1985; 34:31–33.
4. Burns R, Williams ES, O'Toole D, Dubey JP. *Toxoplasma gondii* infections in captive black-footed ferrets (*Mustela nigripes*) 1992–1998: clinical signs, serology, pathology and prevention. J Wildlife Dis 2003; 39:787–797.
5. Lewington JH. Ferrets and toxoplasma. Control and therapy. University of Sydney: Postgraduate Foundation 1992; 169:493.
6. Bell JA. Parasites of domesticated pet ferrets. Compend Contin Edu Pract Vet 1994; 16:617–620.

CHAPTER TEN
Parasitic diseases of ferrets

7. Fisher M. Endoparasites in the dog and cat: Protozoa. In Practice 2002; March:146–151.
8. Eberhard ML. Use of the ferret in parasitological research. In: Fox J, ed. Biology and diseases of the ferret, 2nd edn. Baltimore: William and Wilkins; 1998:537–549.
9. Dubey JP. *Neospora caninum*: A look at a new toxoplasma-like parasite of dogs and other animals. Compend Contin Edu Pract Vet 1990; 12:653–663.
10. McAllister M, Wills, RA, McGuire AM et al. Ingestion of *Neospora Caninum* tissue by *Mustela* species. Int J Parasitol 1999; 29:1531–1536.
11. Blankenship-Paris TL, Chang J, Bagnell RC. Enteric coccidiosis in the ferret. Lab Anim Sci 1993; 43:361–363.
12. Williams BH, Chimes MJ, Gardiner CH. Biliary coccidiosis in a ferret (*Mustela putorius furo*). Vet Pathol 1996; 33:437–439.
13. Abe N, Iseki M. Identification of genotypes of *Cryptosporidium parvum* isolates from ferrets in Japan. Parasitol Res 2003; 89:422–424.
14. Willard MD, Sugarman B, Walker RD. Gastrointestinal zoonoses. Vet Clin North Am Small Anim Pract 1987; 17:145–195.
15. Rehg JE, Gigliotti F, Stokes DC. Cryptosporidiosis in ferrets. Lab Anim Sci 1988; 38:155–158.
16. Baneth G. Diseases risks for the traveling pet: Hepatozoonosis. In Practice 2003; May:272–277.
17. Trotz-Williams L, Gradoni L. Disease risks for the traveling pet: Leishmaniasis. In Practice 2003; April:190–204.
18. Simpson VR, Panciera RJ, Hargreaves J et al. Myocarditis and myositis due to infection with *Hepatozoon* species in pine martens (*Martes martes*) in Scotland. Vet Rec 2005; 165:442–446.
19. Zajac AM. Giardiasis. Compend Contin Edu Pract Vet 1992; 14:604–608.
20. Abe N, Read C, Thompson RC, Iseki M. Zoonotic genotype of *Giardia intestinalis* detected in a ferret. J Parasitol 2005; 91(1):179–182.
21. O'Leary C. Parasite under the microscope. Health medicine. The West Australian 1999: 28 July.
22. Thompson RCA, Monis PT. Variation in *Giardia*: implications for taxonomy and epidemiology. Adv Parasitol 2004; 58:69–137.
23. Hood J. Exotic disease emerges in Perth. The Veterinarian 2003; August:15–16.
24. Lapage G. Mönnig's veterinary helminthology and entomology. London: Ballièrre Tindall; 1962.
25. Fisher M. Endoparasites in the dog and cat: Helminths. In Practice 2001; Sept:463–470.
26. Exotic Animal Diseases Bulletin No 94. *Trichinella*. Austral Vet J 2005; 83:662–663.
27. Webster P, Kapel CM. Studies on vertical transmission of *Trichinella* species in experimentally infected ferrets (*Mustela putorius furo*), foxes (*Vulpes vulpes*), guinea pigs and mice. Vet Parasitol 2005; 130:255–262.
28. Dinnes MR. Medical care of non-domestic carnivores. In: Kirk, RW, ed. Current veterinary therapy. Philadelphia: WB Saunders; 1980.
29. Wolf AM. Disorders of the respiratory system. In: Wills J, Wolf AM, ed. Handbook of feline medicine. New York: Pergamon Press; 1993:124.
30. Parrott TY, Greiner EC, Parrott JD. *Dirofilaria immitis* infection in three ferrets. J Am Vet Med Assoc 1984; 184:582–583.
31. Ryland LM, Bernard SL, Gorman JR. A clinical guide to the pet ferret. Compend Contin Edu Pract Vet 1983; 5:25–32.
32. Jenkins J, Brown S. A practitioner's guide to rabbits and ferrets. Lakewood, CO: American Animal Hospital Association; 1993:43–93.
33. Hoffman FA. Medical news. Heartworm disease. Am Ferret Rep 2004; 14(2):14–16.
34. Blair LS, Campbell, WC. Suppression of *Dirofilaria immitis* in *Mustela putorius* by a single dose of ivermectin. J Parasitol 1980; 66:691–692.
35. Blair LS, Williams E, Evanciw DV. Efficiency of ivermectin against third stage *Dirofilaria immitis* larvae in ferrets and dogs. Res Vet Sci 1982; 33:386–387.
36. Supakorndej P, McCall JW, Lewis RE et al. Biology, diagnosis and prevention of heartworm infection in ferrets. Proc Heartworm Symp. Austin: Am Heartworm Soc; 1992.
37. Antinoff A. Clinical observations in ferrets with naturally occurring heartworm disease, and preliminary evaluation of treatment with ivermectin with or without melarsomine. Proc Heartworm Symp. Austin: Am Heartworm Soc 2002; 45:47.
38. Supakorndej P, McCall JW, Supakorndej N et al. Evaluation of melarsomine dihydrochloride as a heartworm adulticide for ferrets. Proc Heartworm Symp. Am Heartworm Soc 2002; 49:53.
39. Kemmerer-Cottrell D. Use of moxidectin (ProHeart 6) as a heartworm adulticide in 4 ferrets. Exotics DVM 2005; 6:9–12.
40. Simpson VR, Gibbon LM, Khalil LF, Williams JL. Cholecystitis in otters (*Lutra lutra*) and mink (*Mustela vison*) caused by the fluke *Pseudamphistomum truncatum*. Vet Rec 2005; 157:49–52.
41. Carter GR, Payne PA. Major infectious diseases of dogs and cats. Int Vet Info Serv. Ithaca USA; 2005.
42. King, C. The natural history of weasels and stoats. London: Christopher Helm; 1989:189–193.
43. Orcutt C. Dermatological diseases. In: Quesenberry KE, Carpenter W, eds. Ferrets, rabbits and rodents: Clinical medicine and surgery; St Louis: Saunders; 2003:107–114.
44. Visser M, Rehbein S, Wiedemann C. Species of flea (Siphonaptera) infesting pets and hedgehogs in Germany. J Vet Med 2001; 48:197–202.
45. Lewington JH. Ferrets: A compendium. Vade Mecum, series C, No. 10. University of Sydney: Postgraduate Committee in Vet Ed; 1988.
46. Burrows A. Developments in flea and tick control. Treatment. The Veterinarian 2002:26–28.
47. Turuno S, Kagawa N, Saeki H. Experimental trials on the use of imacloprid against ectoparasitic insects on various exotic pets. J Vet Med 2001; 54:537–540.
48. Rich S. Advantage toxicity in a cat. Perspective 2005; 46:6–7.
49. Gower J. Vaccine puts the bite on fleas. The Veterinarian 2003; April:16–17.
50. Kwochka KW. Fleas and related disease. Vet Clin North Am Small Anim Pract 1987; 17: 1235–1262.
51. Lewington JH. Frontline for ferrets. Control and therapy. University of Sydney: Postgraduate Foundation 1996; 189:856.
52. Larsen KS, Siggurdson H, Mencke N. Efficacy of imidacloprid, imidacloprid/permethrin and phoxin for flea control in the Mustelidae (ferrets, mink). Parasitol Res 2005; 97(Suppl 1):107–112.
53. Lohse J, Rinder H, Gothe R, Zahler M. Validity of species status of the parasitic *Otodectes cynotis*. Med Vet Entomol 2002; 16:133–138.
54. Kwochka KW. Mites and related disease. Vet Clin North Am Small Anim Pract 1987; 18:1263–1284.
55. Merchant SR. Ototoxicity. Vet Clin North Am Small Anim Pract 1994; 24:971–980.
56. Paterson MM, Kirchain SM. Comparison of three treatments for control of ear mites in ferrets. Lab Anim Sci 1999; 49:655–657.

57. Philips PH, O'Callaghan MG, Moore E et al. Pedal *Sarcoptes scabiei* infestation in ferrets (*Mustela putorius furo*). Austral Vet J 1987; 64:289.
58. Tim KJ. Pruritus in pet rabbits, rodents and ferrets. Vet Clin North Am Small Anim Pract 1988; 18:1077–1092.
59. Knight G. Cheap and easy treatment of sarcoptic mange in dogs. Control and therapy. Sydney University: Postgraduate Foundation 2004; 237:1547.
60. Noli C, van der Horst HHA, Willemse T. Demodicosis in ferrets (*Mustela putorius furo*). Vet Quart 1998; 18:28–31.

CHAPTER 11

Diseases of special concern

'Many, but not all, jill ferrets will come into season early in the year and remain in this condition for many months unless mated. This has a damaging effect on the constitution of the ferret and many will simply fade away and die if denied motherhood.'

D. Brian Plummer, Modern Ferreting, 1977

This section will cover important common diseases in the reproductive, urinary and cardiovascular systems plus the disease neuronal ceroid lipofuscinosis (NCL) and the new muscular disease of disseminated idiopathic myositis (DIM).

Reproductive system diseases

Diseases of the jill reproductive system

Ferrets are subject to similar diseases and conditions affecting the reproductive system to the dog and cat. The unique condition, not experienced by female dogs and cats, affecting unsterilized ferret jills is post-oestrous anaemia (POA). It has been seen in Australia, especially where some new ferret owners are not aware of the problems and have in fact done little pre-purchase study of ferret peculiarities. The breeding season in the southern hemisphere is September–December/January (March–August in the northern hemisphere). The jill ferret, being polyoestrous and a seasonally-induced ovulator, will continue in heat maintaining a swollen vulva and high blood oestrogen levels which precipitates a bone marrow depression, anaemia (POA) and death (see Ch. 5).

Post-oestrous anaemia (POA)

In the USA, this condition has not been a problem, as ferrets are usually supplied to the pet market by Marshall Farms, New York, as young animals already sterilized at 6 weeks of age. Some private breeders however do not agree with such early sterilization, so supply to the pet market young ferrets that need to be sterilized. This procedure is usually done, as in Australia and elsewhere, at 5–6 months of age if the ferret is not going on to breeding. Opinion is now increasing against the too early sterilization of ferrets, which may bring its own problems. The sterilization of ferrets at 5–6 months was advocated for some time by American veterinarians (S. Brown, pers. comm. 1994). The condition of POA can be life-threatening.[1] Jills in heat over 1 month without being served by a hob would be at risk. The condition is an aplastic anaemia with bone marrow depression. Ferrets living outside will sometimes carry a flea burden. In the event of POA or other illness, the ferrets lose the ability to groom and the flea burden increases, adding to the sickness. Ferrets are highly susceptible to oestrogen-induced toxicity of the haematopoietic tissue like dogs. Aplastic anaemia is uncommon in domesticated species (with the exception of the cat with FeLV, which develops an erythroid hypoplasia) but has been described in six pet ferrets by Kociba and Caputo.[2]

In Hungary, the pet ferrets are normally not sterilized until 6 months of age and usually after the first litter. Consequently, ferret owners have to be aware of POA (A. Prohaczik, pers. comm. 2005).

In an experiment by Sherrill and Gorman[3] involving 20 unmated jills left in oestrus, eight died or were euthanized because of the bone marrow depression. It is interesting that the first death occurred 1 month after the start of oestrus, the last deaths 6 months after, while the 12 remaining ferrets went into anoestrous. This phenomenon can be seen in practice where some ferrets, which miss the first early September mating but then come into heat again in December display more acute cases of POA unless mated. Usually the prognosis is poor for untreated ferrets at any time in the breeding season. Breeding jills in later life, which mate but fail to conceive, may develop ovarian tumours, possibly oestrogen-induced.[4] Sherrill and Gorham found that the disease is initiated by prolonged high blood levels of oestrogens leading to a depressed bone marrow with hypocellularity and resulting temporary thrombocytosis, then thrombocytopenia, neutropenia, eosinopenia and anaemia of the normocytic, normochromic, or macrocytic, hypochromic kind.

In an earlier experiment, by Bernard et al., 20 jill ferrets were used to show the effect of oestrogen on the bone marrow.[5] Four hob ferrets were added for gender comparison. The trial involved splitting the ferrets into four groups (Table 11.1) and studying over a 4-month period. Ferrets were in natural light and on mink diet; vulval swelling was the indicator of oestrous effects.

Table 11.1 Oestrogen trial, USA

Ferret groups	Status	Treatment
1. Five jills	OVH	2 weeks on given oestrogen
2. Five jills	OVH	Non-oestrogen controls
3. Five jills plus two hobs	Unsterilized	Non-oestrogen controls
4. Five jills plus two hobs	Unsterilized	2 weeks on given oestrogen

OVH, ovariohysterectomy.

The outcome was that ferrets from groups 1 and 4 developed anaemia and post-oestrous disease, indicated by blood samples and the presence of a swollen vulva. Further, 8 out of 10 jills treated with oestrogen developed bilateral alopecia, which was permanent. *Note*: none of the hobs developed alopecia. The actual deaths are given in Table 11.2.

None of the jills of group 3 died of POA. Interestingly, the ferrets for the study had been selected in late season (mid-August) from a larger colony where approximately 30% of the jills in heat had died earlier the same season (June–July) from POA. The PCV of two dead jills had been below 10%. Thus, the surviving jills selected for the August study may have been less sensitive to endogenous oestrogen or perhaps had lower concentrations of endogenous oestrogen.

Clinical signs of post-oestrous anaemia

The haematological effects of high blood oestrogen levels are shown by clinical signs, which must be pointed out to ferret breeders. The jill's owner becomes aware of the continuing swollen vulva, which is easily traumatized. I have seen cases including one of my own jills with pale mucous membranes, depression and anorexia. Bilateral alopecia is also seen with skin ecchymosis and petechial haemorrhages (Fig. 11.1a,b). Hind leg posterior paralysis can develop, which may occur from a subdural haematoma of the spinal cord or brain. Systolic heart murmurs are usually detectable due the acute anaemia. The scats can show melaena due to gastrointestinal bleeding. A vulval discharge due to a concurrent metritis/vaginitis can occur followed by pyometra, collapse and death. *Note*: the usual cause of death is the haemorrhage associated with the thrombocytopenia. *Differential diagnosis*: spayed jills can show alopecia and a swollen vulva but here the problem is usually adrenal gland neoplasia (AGN) with involvement of vestigial ovarian tissue and seen in America as ferret adrenal disease complex (Ch. 14).[1]

Table 11.2 Oestrogen trial, USA

Group number, as Table 11.1	No. which became sick and died	No. PTS when moribund	No. PTS at end of study	No. alive at end of study
1. 5 jills	3	1	1	0
2. 5 jills	0	0	2	3
3. 5 jills + 2 hobs	1 jill	0	3 (2 jills + 1 hob)	3 (2 jills + 1 hob)
4. 5 jills + 2 hobs	4 jills	1 hob	2 (1 jill + 1 hob)	0

PTS, Put to sleep (euthanized).
Adapted from Bernard et al., 1983, with permission.[5]

CHAPTER ELEVEN
Diseases of special concern

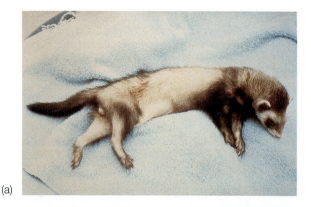

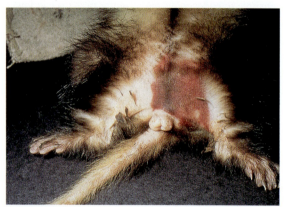

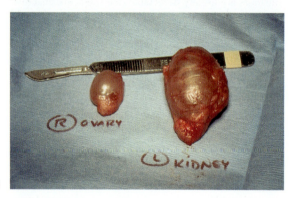

Figure 11.1 (a) Jill with post-oestrous anaemia showing alopecia and swollen vulva. (Courtesy of D. Manning, University of Wisconsin.) (b) Jill with POA showing severe ecchymosis of inner thigh and abdomen plus swollen vulva. (Courtesy of J.R. Gorham, Animal Disease Research Unit, USA Department of Agriculture.) (c) Ovarian remnant plus cystic kidney from POA affected jill. (Courtesy of G. Rich.)

In some cases, remnant ovarian tissue can lead to POA signs. The condition has been found by Greg Rich in one ferret where an ovary remnant plus a cystic kidney could be displayed postoperatively (Fig. 11.1c).

Clinical pathology
The blood picture shows severe non-regenerative anaemia, normocytic RBCs and a depressed PCV below 25% (if below 15% the condition is considered irreversible) plus neutropenia and thrombocytopenia (S. Brown, pers. comm. 1993). When the PCV goes below 20% and/or the platelets are at 50 000/mL or lower, clinical signs appear with the low PCV/platelets resulting in a decreased total serum protein level even in cases of significant dehydration.[6] In a prolonged oestrus, the hypocellular bone marrow only contains 10–20% of haematopoietic cells; the remaining cells are made up of adipocytes, RBCs and haemosiderin-containing macrophages.[3]

Post mortem
The characteristic features are pale tissues and generated haemorrhages in a ferret which has lost weight. There is extensive blood seepage in the stomach, small and large intestines while the skin has subcutaneous ecchymoses and petechiae.[3] The latter also occur in the heart. Further haemorrhage is observed in the omentum, urinary bladder, uterus and periovarian fat. Subdural haematoma or haematomyelia occur in the thoracic, lumbar and sacral skeletal regions and become the cause of ataxia and paraplegia. The vulval discharges and pyometra experienced by the ferret are caused by an *E. coli* pyometritis and/or a *Corynebacteria* vaginitis. The possibility of bronchopneumonia can be due to *Klebsiella* species.[2]

Diagnosis
This is indicated by the obvious vulval swelling and associated alopecia in the unsterilized jill. A blood PCV of less than 20% is conclusive. It is possible to do vaginal cytology but not usually necessary.[7] The jill when seen may be well into POA and signs of pyometra and pneumonia plus CNS conditions may confuse the picture. The prognosis is poor.

A partial alopecia and melaena can occur in pregnant jills and one author states that at some time in oestrus all jill ferrets will have at least a mild anaemia.[6] I have recorded a pregnant jill with partial alopecia around the eyes, all four feet and ventral abdomen but not the tail.[4] As in POA, the jill had apparent petechial haemorrhages in these regions giving her a 'blue 'effect but the phenomenon disappeared after a week. After weaning the kittens without trouble, the jill was put to a vassy (vasectomized hob) and at 20 days post-mating went into the 'blue' period again. She was not sick as in POA. She regained her normal skin tone and hair after about a week indicating some hormonal upset which was reversed naturally.

Prevention of post-oestrous anaemia

Some breeders like to delay the use of jill ferrets for a breeding season. If the jill is not spayed and comes into heat at 6 months of age, oestrus can be terminated by the use of proligestone (Covinan, Intervet), a second generation progestogen. This is given in September as oestrus commences (March in the northern hemisphere) when the jill has been on heat for 10 days. This drug technique was trialed by M. Oxenham with the Wessex Ferret Club, UK in 1984 with success.[8] Proligestone is given at 0.5 mL s.c., which causes reduction of vulval swelling in 3–4 days. If there is a slow vulval size reduction, a repeat of 0.25 mL s.c. is suggested.

Some interesting points were seen in the Oxenham trial. The mating season starts in March (northern hemisphere) and the first 10 jills were given the dosage in March 1984 and their progress was followed over the next six mating seasons during which a further 182 similar doses were given to a total of 131 jills. Table 11.3 shows the numbers injected yearly. A number of jills received more than one annual injection and these figures are shown in Table 11.4. It was seen that some jills returned to oestrus between May and August following the injection from the 1986 study. The phenomenon occurred in the following years in some jills. This response is recorded in Table 11.5.

With the seven in the first column in Table 11.5, six jills received injections the following year and did not return to oestrus. This was probably a biological variation. Some of these jills had second injections the same year, which suppressed oestrus for the rest of the summer with no ill effects. None of the jills that returned to oestrus for the rest of the season had any signs of illness. Three of the 11 jills (Table 11.5) were accidentally mated, with the May and June matings fertile but with a litter size of four and three respectively. The third mating in July resulted in sterile pseudopregnancy. Fertility the year following the injection appears unaffected and eight litters were recorded, producing 65 kittens, an average of 8 per litter (range 3–13). *Note*: some hair loss can occur around the area of the injection site; this was seen in some of the trial jills and may be due to drug irritation. No cases of pyometra have been recorded in jills in the UK using proligestone and I have not seen any in Australia while using it for some years. The Oxenham trial shows admirably how a ferret society can cooperate with the veterinary profession to improve knowledge about preventing a serious ferret disease like post-oestrous anaemia.

Chorionic gonadotropins can induce ovulation followed by a pseudopregnancy of 40–50 days, so this may be useful if the ferret breeder wants to breed the jill mid-season.[9] Drugs available are human chorionic gonadotrophin (hCG) (Chorulon, Intervet) dose at 20 IU i.m. or buserelin (Receptal, Hoechst) at 0.25 mL i.m. Both are given when the jill has been on heat for 10 days. The hCG can be repeated at 7 days if regression of the vulval swelling is slow.[7] A vasectomized hob (vassy) is the non-drug method of taking a jill out of heat to save from

Table 11.3 The Oxenham and Wessex ferret club hormonal trial (with permission)

Year	1984	1985	1986	1987	1988	1989	Total
No. of jills injected	10	12	26	33	64	47	192
No. of jills injected first time	10	4	18	24	45	30	131

Table 11.4 The Oxenham and Wessex ferret club hormonal trial (with permission)

						Total
No. years each jill injected	1	2	3	4	5	
No. jills	89	32	4	3	3	131

Table 11.5 The Oxenham and Wessex ferret club hormonal trial (with permission)

No. times jills have returned to oestrous	1	2	3	4
No. jills	7	2	1	1

CHAPTER ELEVEN
Diseases of special concern

mating later and protect against POA. The vasectomy operation is described in Chapter 19.

A unique feature of pet ferrets in Russia is the lack of veterinarians in some regions to do the spay operation. To eliminate a prolonged oestrus, ferret owners arrange for matings in the late oestrous phase to minimize any chance of pregnancy but preventing POA. An outcome of this is more than half the Russian pet ferrets originate from home breeding instead of from breeders. This type of breeding has increased since 2002 while the supply of pet ferrets from fur farms has declined.

Treatment of post-oestrous anaemia

This is possible in early cases but when the PCV is below 15% the case is critical. The method of choice is ovariohysterectomy to remove the source of endogenous oestrogens and can be done with the jill on heat. The spaying operation should not be attempted if the PCV is 15% or lower because of the possibility of irreversible bone marrow damage.[1] One author[10] has recorded the treatment of a sick 500 g entire jill ferret having a PCV of 7%. The jill had been on heat for more than 4 months and was treated with an ovariohysterectomy plus 13 blood transfusions over a 5-month period, in addition to intensive care, anabolic steroids, corticosteroids, antibiotics plus vitamins and a high calorific diet. It even had to be treated for a concurrent sarcoptic mange. The ferret was able to have transfusions easily from other unrelated ferrets, as there is no problem with blood types (Manning, pers. comm. 1998). The blood was given via a 23 gauge jugular catheter (mixed with sodium citrate). Even a bone marrow graft was given. On final blood transfusion, the PCV on a successful treatment went up to 30%. It is interesting that the ovariohysterectomy was carried out using xylazine (4 mg/kg s.c.) plus 5 minutes later ketamine (30 mg/kg s.c.) was given (Ch. 13).

Chemical means to treat POA can be by megestrol acetate which has been used to delay oestrus but there may be a risk of pyometra.[11] This reference was in 1979 and I used a 5 mg Ovarid tablet on a sick jill ferret in 1977 with success.

Vaginitis

In one American ferret-breeding establishment, vaginitis was common in jills left in heat for more than 2 weeks and may be an indication of an impending POA. It also occurs in pregnant jills or occasionally post-parturient jills.[12] Clinically, there is an obvious vaginal discharge and the jill's hindquarters are wet with discharge in severe cases. If the condition were to go untreated, the vaginal/vulval outer margins become necrotic. A vaginal swab will usually pick up a *Staphylococcus/Proteus* infection. An ascending vaginitis in pregnant or oestrous jills may cause a secondary cystitis and rapid formation of uroliths within 2 days, with the urolithiasis having palpable stones. Urethral obstruction by uroliths causes urinary straining. *Note*: these breeding ferrets would be on a prepared dry food which may be an additional factor in urolithiasis, while breeders in other countries may be using fresh meat, where the condition is uncommon. Urease-producing bacteria like *Staphylococcus* and *Proteus* are highly likely to lead to urolithiasis.[12] Treatment must be by broad-spectrum antibiotic and may require surgery for bladder stones (see later).

In Australia, I have seen vaginitis in jill ferrets kept in cages where grass seeds or awns are in the bedding. They are usually easily removed and the infection treated with clavulanic acid/amoxicillin drops. In New Zealand fitch farms a similar situation arose in caged ferrets and was considered uncommon but on one farm rose to 77%.[13] Again the vaginitis was due to hayseeds and barley straw in the bedding. The infective agent was found to be a *Streptococcus*. In breeding colonies, the bedding adhered to the vulva during the jill's oestrus because of mucous secretion. The clinical signs were again a yellow mucopurulent vulval discharge, which could lead to secondary metritis and signs of septicaemia. Pathological signs included a non-destructive purulent vaginitis and cervicitis with secondary ulcerative purulent metritis in some cases. The treatment followed the usual lines of removing the foreign material from the vagina and using long-term penicillin. The effect of the disease on the fertility of fitch ferrets appeared to be minimal, with most of the affected jills conceiving and having healthy litters. The problem was then avoided by not using hay for bedding.

Author's clinical example

My 1-year-old sable jill, Wendy, was in her second heat. She was not mated and went into severe depression and anorexia with a vulval swelling, which remained and became traumatized. There was a sterile vaginal discharge. I had had no experience with POA to date. To treat Wendy I used 0.05 mg megestrol acetate solution made by dissolving a 5 mg Ovarid tablet in sterile water.[4] I gave 0.5 mL of solution p.o. once daily using an insulin syringe. Results were dramatic with the vulval swelling decreasing from the second day of treatment and she was normal by the 7th day when the treatment was stopped. The drug was not repeated and she went on to breed normally. Having to treat POA should be avoided by *prevention* in all cases!

Reproductive system diseases

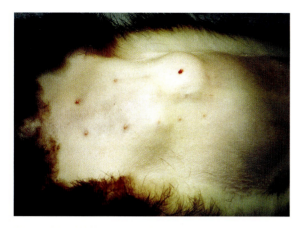

Figure 11.2 Abdominal swelling pyometra in 5-year-old female ferret. (Courtesy of G. Rich.)

Pyometra

This can be a major disease with some unsterilized jills, stemming from a possible POA. Pyometra in the ferret is like the dog and cat and can occur in breeding colonies and laboratory ferrets worldwide. Ferret breeders in Australia, New Zealand, UK and Europe see pyometra in older jills in pseudopregnancy (Fig. 11.2). I have seen it associated with an ovarian tumour in an older jill of mine.[4] Pyometra can be a major finding in POA.

Clinical signs

The ferret may show a purulent vaginal 'open' discharge or have a 'closed' pyometra which is worse. The jill will be lethargic, depressed, and possibly toxic and may or may not be febrile. With an associated POA, the signs of bone marrow depression will be evident. The enlarged uterus is palpable and if rupture of an open or closed pyometra occurs, peritonitis is fatal. A culture of the vaginal discharge will show organisms such as *E. coli*, *Staphylococcus* and *Streptococcus* or possibly *Corynebacterium*, the usual organism associated with pus.

Treatment

If POA is involved an attempt can be made to cycle the jill out of oestrus, using Covanan or HCG injections. It is suggested that she be mated[6] but I would be wary of infecting the hob. Once the jill is stabilized however, an ovariohysterectomy can be performed with fluid replacement against shock and antibiotic cover. Blood transfusion may be required for very acute cases as described by Ryland[10] and is discussed in Chapter 20.

The parallel event of pyometra in the dog and cat compared to ferrets has been seen by stump pyometra

> ### USA clinical example
>
> From a breeding colony, a 2-year-old 700 g jill was presented with severe diarrhoea, vaginal discharge and anorexia. She had been mated 2 weeks before presentation and during the previous mating had developed mastitis and required the kittens removed to a foster mother. She was thin and lethargic with a temperature of 104°F, total WCC of 2700 × 10/L and BUN 40 mg/dL. As the vaginal discharge was apparent, the jill was hospitalized, given antibiotic and spayed the next day. The anaesthetic procedure consisted of 0.1 mg acepromazine, then 20 mg ketamine followed by halothane by mask as shown in Chapter 16. The uterus was grossly enlarged despite the fact that there had been continuous drainage and it contained about 20 mL of pus. The jill recovered from the operation, temperature down to 101°F the next day and she was sent home on clavulanic acid/amoxicillin drops to fully recover. It was interesting that the diarrhoea showed no signs of intestinal parasites or diet upsets and stopped immediately the jill was spayed.

D. Kemmerer-Cottrell, Florida, USA, pers. comm. 1999.

in ferrets after the sterilization operation[7] but I have not seen this in any ferrets to date. A cystic ovarian remnant has been recorded in a severely ill spayed jill showing anaemia, swollen vulva and bilateral abdominal masses.[14]

Aggressive treatment for pyometra in a breeding jill

The use of Lutalyse (prostaglandin, Pharmacia & Upjohn, Animal Health) has been recommended by Bell[15] as used on a ferret in 1999. In 2000, the jill was breed with success delivering healthy kittens. Lutalyse acts by destroying the corpus luteum after a false pregnancy. Consequently, the uterine tissue is expelled. When this drug is used in a case of pyometra, it causes myometrial contraction and expulsion of the pus.

The treatment regime involved the rehydration and administration of antibiotics to counter the pathogenic bacteria, usually *E. coli*. The use of trimethoprim, amoxicillin, enrofloxacin or chloramphenicol was suggested perhaps after sensitivity tests. Usually there is no time for this due to the acute effect of the pyometra. Any of the drugs are usually effective. Lutalyse was given at 0.1–0.2 mL per jill by i.m. injection. This was followed by oxytocin in 1 hour or so, when a large amount of infective material was expelled and the jill brightened. Finally an anti-prostaglandin (Banamine, flunixin meglumine) was given. This drug has analgesic and anti-inflammatory possibilities. After a couple of days, the uterus was checked by palpation to judge size. A second course of Lutalyse was not needed. It must be judged if the Banamine, antibiotics and fluid cover are required for a few more days.

Note that Banamine is a drug which can cause bowel ulcers in ferrets and other animals. It is not clear if the ferret jill is particularly susceptible. It may be another stress factor in the very sick jill. The list of drugs actually labelled for ferret use is small, see Appendix.

Diseases of the hob reproductive system

Grass awn injury

With hay bedding, grass awns can get caught in the prepuce and cause irritation and infection in the same way as was seen in the jill's vulva. They require removal sometimes under a general anaesthetic and then given antibiotic cover. The prepuce can be lubricated with an antibiotic/cortisone ear cream, e.g. Panalog (Novartis). Hobs get a similar condition in the dry mating season when they mark their territory, if living outside, by moving along the ground and pressing their groin area down and urinating as they move along. This is the equivalent of dogs marking trees. They get grass seeds lodged in the groin tissue and even the prepuce and will require medical and surgical attention. Damage or infection to the penis may result in extrusions (Fig. 11.3).

Testicular tumours

Sertoli cell tumours have been recorded in six ferrets ranging in age from 4–6 years and showing unilateral or bilateral enlargement of the testes.[6] One affected ferret had additionally an interstitial tumour and seminoma.

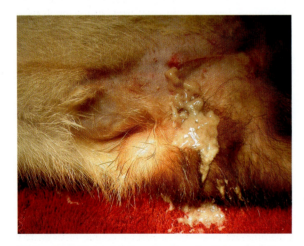

Figure 11.3 Extrusion from ferret penis, fed on biscuit diet. (Courtesy of G. Rich.)

These conditions have not been recorded in Australia to date. I have only seen testicular sac cysts, which were non-pathogenic, in two older vasectomized hobs. One author has recorded a ferret Sertoli cell tumour, which caused total alopecia and intense pruritus; it was possibly secondary to hyperoestrogenism and could be cured by castration.[7] Compare my two hobs' alopecia event (Ch. 14). *Note* that feminization or androgenization can occur with testicular tumours in other animals but are not yet recorded in ferrets.

Prostate problems

Enlargement of the prostate, showing possible infection, or sterile cysts, has been a feature of American neutered ferrets with adrenal disease,[7] now suggested to be ferret adrenal disease complex (FADC) (C. Johnson-Delaney, pers. comm. 2005). Excessive production of the male hormone precursor androstenedione via the adrenal tumour is the cause and is dealt with by adrenalectomy.[1] Infection or cystic enlargement of the prostate has not been recognized in either neutered or entire hobs in Australia to date, with no urinary blockage clinical cases seen as yet.

Prostatic enlargement by hormone, infection or cystic development is a common cause of urethral obstruction in the sterilized male ferret, more so than urolithiasis. This has been the finding in the USA. The prostate acquires single or multiple variable-sized fluctuant cysts. A prostatic cyst histologically has large amounts of keratin resulting from squamous cell metaplasia of the prostate gland.[7] The prostate enlargement can be associated with transitional cell tumours of the bladder.[1]

Clinical signs

Any disruption of urination causes the male ferret acute discomfort. It cries in pain when attempting urination. A check for FADC is required in prostate cancer (Ch. 14). With radiology, a prostate abscess may look like the bladder as it can be very large, but seen on lateral view the bladder is found depressed by the prostate mass. If available, ultrasound is a useful positive diagnostic tool in this condition to show prostate enlargement.[7] Urine analysis shows a high leukocyte count consistent with infection.[1]

Treatment

The enlarged prostate associated with FADC will regress after the removal of the affected adrenal gland. With infected tissue however, treatment involves surgical removal of the prostate mass, which is not an easy operation. The infective greenish material of a prostate abscess is cultured and the ferret must be placed on a broad-spectrum antibiotic of choice for many weeks.[1] For treating the hormone-affected prostate without surgery, the best medical treatment is flutamide, which was tested by Rosenthal and is used now extensively by Brown and others in the USA (S. Brown, pers. comm. 1999). This human drug acts as an anti-androgen at the level of the prostate, by blocking the effect of excessive androgen hormones being produced by the adrenals via receptors in the prostate tissue, thus preventing stimulation of the prostate tissue. The dose rate for ferrets is 10 mg/kg q. 12 h p.o. The drug is expensive and would require special compounding for use in ferrets; it could however be used to avoid costly prostate surgery (Ch. 18). Thus in cases of prostatic disease where there is no obstruction of the urinary tract and no evidence of infection, flutamide can be very effective in slowing or reducing the prostatic condition. If surgery has been carried out, the drug will prevent recurrence but would have to be given for life. The prognosis of this condition is variable as it may not be possible to remove all the cancer to stop recurrence. It may even be necessary to perform a cystotomy on the sick ferret as well.[1]

Diseases of the urinary system

Disease problems of the urinary tract have been rarely, if at all, recorded in the past in Australian pet and working ferrets, though renal failure does occur in aged ferrets. The condition of urolithiasis is rare in Australia, possibly due to differences in ferret diet from other countries, notably the USA.

The kidneys

Enlargement of one or both kidneys can occur in ferrets over 3 years of age. This can occur in pet or laboratory ferrets.[1,6] The enlargement can be associated with cysts (Fig. 11.4), which can be single or multiple with usually no clinical signs or perhaps associated with renal failure.[16]

Seizures can warn of kidney failure involving cystic kidneys and this was seen in one 3-year-old neutered hob emergency case.[17] The ferret had a history of repeated seizures and when presented was weak, ataxic and disorientated. Being thin, the ferret could be palpated easily and showed a 4–5 cm long mass in the mid-abdominal area, which on radiology and subsequent post mortem of the ferret was found to be one of two cystic kidneys. The enlarged kidneys had typical irregular surfaces with multiple translucent fluid-filled cysts of the cortex and medulla. The ureters were patent which ruled out bilateral hydronephrosis. If one kidney only had been affected it could have been removed and the ferret could have survived. The cystic spaces were lined by cuboidal epithelium but there were some normal glomeruli and tubules in the affected kidneys, though fibrous thickening of the renal tissue was progressing. The aetiology of cystic kidneys is considered as hereditary, developmental or acquired.[17]

Kidney failure occurs secondary to the renal cyst disease so with suspect cases a check of renal functions is required. This should include a complete blood count, urine check and serum chemistry plus ultrasound and even intravenous pyelographs if possible.[7] It is noted by one author[17] that bilateral multiple cortical renal cysts must be distinguished from those of kidney polycystic disease. The latter is seen in man and is hereditary. Both diseases have early irregular renal cyst distribution but polycystic disease is known to have cysts in other organs such as the liver. Besides other animals and fish where polycystic disease is recorded, it has been noted in the mustelids in striped skunks.[18]

Diagnosis

The phenomenon of 'flattening' in ferrets is one indication of abdominal pain and could be due to many problems including cystic kidney disease. One such case has been described as, 'Flattening occurs in ferrets when they lie down flat on the stomach with outstretched neck'.[19] The pose registers discomfort and is seen to be done on cool surfaces for pain relief.

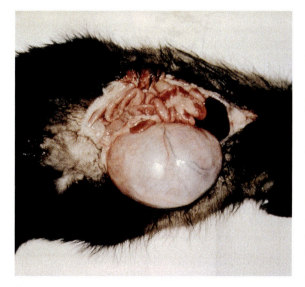

Figure 11.4 Renal cyst in a 3-month-old ferret. (Courtesy of G. Rich.)

One 2-year-old spayed jill with a poor appetite, weight loss and a history of 'flattening' was examined, seen to be alert and active but had one enlarged kidney.[20] The blood picture and urinalysis were normal. After radiograph confirmation that the ferret had one enlarged kidney, three times the normal size, it was removed and the animal made an uneventful recovery and could be maintained on one kidney. Histology of the removed kidney found several renal cysts plus damaged renal tubules.

The author[20] suggests a 2–5 % incidence in his USA practice, more in jills than hobs and in ferrets over 3 years of age. Ferrets can live with renal cysts but sooner or later, there are clinical signs leading to renal failure. The renal pain can be manifested in the ferret 'flattening' as described. Some ferrets only show signs at the renal failure stage with poor appetite, polydipsia and lethargy. With a possible unilateral cystic kidney, treatment by nephrectomy is only feasible if the other kidney is clear of disease. Surgery is possible on cystic kidneys as demonstrated by Rich (Fig. 11.5). The hole was stitched up with 5-0 PDS.

The renal disease syndrome

Renal disease in ferrets mirrors that encountered in dogs and cats and is just as demanding in treatment. It has been suggested that renal disease in ferrets is considered similar to the cat disease but there are differences. Due to the smaller-sized animal involved in medicating for the disease, plus toxicity factors of drugs, the prognosis in treating ferrets is guarded.[21]

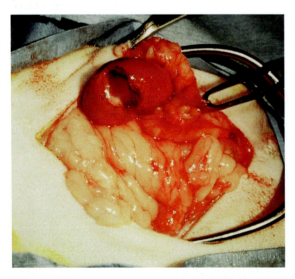

Figure 11.5 Renal cyst surgery of a 2-year-old ferret. Hole stitched with 5-0 PDS. (Courtesy of G. Rich.)

There are two general renal disease syndromes:

1. Acute renal failure: A rapidly-progressing form that may be reversible.
2. Chronic renal failure: A slow progressive form that is usually not reversible.[22,23]

Also, progressive renal failure and chronic interstitial nephritis are terms associated with the outcome of renal disease. Pyelonephritis is an acute infection of the kidney. In general, acute renal failure may be overcome but there may be kidney damage which gives rise to a stressed kidney, then progressive renal failure leading to chronic renal failure or chronic interstitial nephritis.

It is useful to consider renal disease in cats as with young adult cats it can involve lower urinary tract inflammation and urethral obstruction.[23] In young ferrets, urethral obstruction in some sterilized hobs has been seen in the USA but not to date in Australia. It is considered to be a diet problem by some authorities (J. Bell pers. comm. 1998). In older cats, the problem is usually a progressive loss of renal function and older ferrets show similar problems. This has been seen in Australia and other countries. With ferrets from 6–10 years, the renal problems of ageing occur which might be exacerbated by climate where ferrets are kept outdoors all the time. Outdoor ferrets in the UK and New Zealand, for instance, are not stressed by heat through living in a colder climate. Ferrets being outside in a hot climate should have facilities to go below ground away from the heat or be kept in cool sheds. They usually sleep by day and are active in the evening and night (Ch. 3).

Acute renal failure (ARF)

The ferret shows clinical signs of polydipsia and polyuria and moves into depression, inappetence, weight loss and rear leg weakness.[7] Vomiting is not a feature of the disease, though ferrets can vomit like dogs and cats. Oral ulcers and 'uraemic' halitosis may be noted later and I have had cases in ferrets over 6 years old. The ferret may show dehydration and pallor. On examining the kidneys, using ferret 'scruffing' technique, a guarding of the abdomen is experienced if the ferret is in pain. One or both kidneys may be enlarged and this will show radiographically. A blood profile and urine check is required for complete diagnosis. Examination of the urine for urine sediments is useful. Ultrasound and pyelographs can be considered if available. There are some veterinary hospitals in Australia where ferrets can be referred for the latter procedures besides universities, which cuts costs to the ferret owner over this dangerous disease diagnosis.

Blood investigation of ARF

The damage done in kidney disease is reflected in the degree of azotaemia in most animal species. Azotaemia is the accumulation of protein metabolites in plasma when the kidney function is compromised. Both serum creatinine and blood urea nitrogen (BUN) are used to show the degree of azotaemia and kidney function in cats and dogs.

Serum chemistry in ferrets differs from dogs and cats in that the serum creatinine findings do not parallel elevations of the BUN in renal failure.[7] This was commented upon by Kawasaki.[24] Later estimations of glomerular function rate decided that the serum BUN and creatinine reading to determine renal insufficiently are questionable as the BUN can be influenced by non-renal factors. It is stated that the increase in serum concentrations of both substances do not actually appear until the kidney is 75% damaged.[25] It has been considered that creatinine elevation for ferrets is much lower that that of dogs and cats, as the normal mean value is lower (0.4–0.6 mg/dL) and the range is narrower (0.2–0.9 mg/dL). It may be that renal tubular secretion or enteric factors may be more prominent in affecting creatinine metabolism in ferrets than in other animals.[16] It is now thought that the normal values have actually been set too high and that they are accurate but the published 'normals' up to this point have been based on some cat data and are therefore not accurate (K. Rosenthal, pers. comm. 1999). A list of up-to-date normals, including creatinine has been included in the appendices.

The BUN factor is not considered an accurate measure of kidney failure though it is recorded as being raised in clinical cases. Moreover, the renal assessment of factors such as hyperphosphataemia, hypocalcaemia and hyperkalaemia at respective readings of (>10), (<8) and (>6) are better suited for guidelines of disease.[1] Diagnosis of renal disease is, therefore, better based on clinical signs, urinalysis, clinical pathology and possibly renal biopsy.

A study by Esteves et al.[25] derived clearance tests in ferrets for glomerular filtration rates (GFR) using endogenous creatinine, inulin and exogenous creatinine. The 24- and 48-hour collection times were done for endogenous creatinine and exogenous (i.v. admin.) creatinine plus (i.v. admin.) radio-labelled inulin. The 24/48 hour results did not differ significantly. A ferret colony of 27 ferrets ranging in age from 9 months to 7 years was used for the trial.

The mean results (over a 24-hour period):

a. Endogenous creatinine   2.50 mL/min per kg body weight
b. Inulin   3.02 mL/min per kg body weight
c. Exogenous creatinine   3.32 mL/min per kg body weight

It was noted that the GFR appeared to decrease with advancing age, as measured by the inulin and exogenous creatinine, while for the endogenous creatinine there was no apparent age factor. The cause was undetermined.

Azotaemia, for convenience, could possibly be pigeon-holed into prerenal, primary renal and post-renal as for cats.[23] The causes of renal damage relating to the cat kidney can indicate what possible renal damaging factors can occur in the ferret, shown in Table 11.6.

Note that dehydration could occur in hot climates where outside living or working ferrets in cages could possibly get compromised kidneys in heat stress. Ferrets quickly die when left in cars on hot days. Ferrets seen urinating and then lapping their urine might be habitual or they might be going into stress in a hot climate situation. As has been noted urethral obstruction occurs in sterilized hobs, and even pregnant jills, in the USA and may be nutrition-related.

Table 11.6 Azotaemia factors with possible reference to ferret kidney disease

	Pre-renal		Post-renal
A	Reduced renal perfusion Dehydration Shock 　Septic, hypovolaemic, haemorrhagic, hypoadrenocorticoidism	A	Urethral obstruction Muco-crystalline plugs Urolithiasis Granulomatous urethritis Neoplasia
B	Excessive urea production Gastrointestinal haemorrhage	B	Bilateral urethral obstruction Neoplasia
		C	Urethral trauma Gunshot wounds Automobile accident

Table adapted after Senior, 1993.[23]

CHAPTER ELEVEN
Diseases of special concern

Treatment

This is based on treating cats and the feline renal products are supposed to be suitable for ferrets.[1] The aim of the treatment is to remove the offending cause, instigate fluid therapy and discontinue any nephrotoxic drugs.[10] This latter point is important with ferrets, where nephrotoxic antibiotics must be avoided and taking into consideration that new drugs are not labelled for use in ferrets, the field is wide open. Toxicity effects with ferrets can be a constant worry.[21] Sick ferret rehydration requires lactated Ringer's solution or, if hyperkalaemia (high potassium) is present or suspected, the use of 0.9% normal saline is necessary.[23] Even when water is available for sick ferrets, oliguria occurs and may persist after rehydration. In cats the correction of metabolic acidosis is only necessary with pH <7.2 or serum <14 mm/L. The hyperkalaemia can be managed temporarily with sodium bicarbonate, glucose/insulin and calcium gluconate administration.

A diuretic course should be given with sick ferrets with oliguria. Furosemide (frusemide) is recommended at 1–2 mg/kg p.o., i.m. or i.v. b.i.d. A diuretic given hours or days after the initial onset of ARF will not decrease the severity of renal damage but polyuric animals are easier to manage.[23] Beware of over-hydration with fluid therapy and diuretic use, which can lead to pulmonary oedema where there is a persistent oliguria. To prevent excess sodium, the i.v. fluids should be changed to 2.5% dextrose in 0.5% saline or 5% dextrose in water.[23] Maintenance fluids should thus have low sodium (<70 mmol/L) and high potassium (>20 mmol/L). The rate of administration should be slowed to replace the insensible losses + urine production + gastrointestinal losses (diarrhoea and vomiting); in the ferret this could be around 100 mL/kg per day. Thus a maintenance rate of 4 mL/kg per hour, at least, plus any additional losses is required (Ch. 16). Peritoneal dialysis can be attempted in cases where persistent oliguria leads to dangerous hyperkalaemia, extreme azotaemia and severe metabolic acidosis, but even treating cats the results are relatively poor.[23] This can be due to the severity of renal damage in ARF, which prevents a return to normal renal function and possibly due to complications associated with any dialysis, e.g. peritonitis. *Note* that polyuria could occur in ferrets, as in cats. In an ARF situation where drugs like gentamycin or amphotericin B are used over a long period, they can be nephrotoxic.[21] Care should be taken to avoid such drugs if possible.

Development of polyuria after initial oliguria can indicate a recovery phase in disease. With the polyuric phase, fluid therapy should prevent dehydration and diuresis associated with hypokalaemia. *Note:* the long term use of furosemide (frusemide) can lead to hypokalaemia. A frequent body weight check is required in renal disease cases and appropriate changes in fluid administration carried out to prevent dehydration, which would lead to further renal damage. Sick ferrets, especially working ferrets or ones normally living outside, would be best kept in during hot weather to prevent stress on the kidneys due to dehydration. Ferret owners are best advised to weigh their pet ferrets weekly as a general check anyway.

An adequate potassium supplement will prevent hypokalaemia, e.g. Animalac Supplement (Troy). A suitable low protein cat diet can be used for sick ferret renal cases and Whiskas Low Protein canned food is a possible choice but giving it depends on ferret acceptance. It also has plant fibre content which ferrets find hard to digest. The Hill's Prescription Diet Feline k/d may be a better choice but some ferrets might consider it too bland. It might need to be pepped up with a savoury chicken stock. The product characteristics of the k/d diet are reduced phosphorus, calcium, protein, sodium, magnesium, increased non-protein calories, a B vitamin addition and an overall dietary acid load reduction. The resultant pH is more alkaline at 6.6–6.9. The fibre content is low at 0.8% which is within the Willard recommendations (Ch. 4). It is important to note that the k/d diet is contraindicated in struvite urolithiasis management. The feeding of k/d diet for cats is given at five-eighths of a tin for a 2.5 kg cat. The nephritic ferret possibly will be below normal weight, which is jill 500–900 g, adult hob up to 2000 g.

One author states that low protein diets are a controversial subject with renal disease.[26] Another opinion is that protein should not be lowered below 30% because there can be other health problems. This has been seen in cats with skin and hair conditions and muscle disease. It has been discovered in cats that too low a protein diet causes additional problems at the time in their life when they need to a have a certain level of protein to maintain healthy tissues (S. Brown, pers. comm. 1998). The important thing is for the ferret, or cat, to have high quality meat protein and the diet fat level should be kept up to 25–30% or body-wasting can occur. The vegetable content of the diet should be low or non-existent and thus low protein foods with any plant protein are not really suitable. Though it is not important in recent understanding of renal disease to restrict the protein, the salt and phosphorus should be restricted (M. Finkler, pers. comm. 1998). He suggests using aluminium hydroxide as a phosphorus binder in those cases of hyperphosphataemia.

Chronic interstitial nephritis (CIN) or chronic renal failure (CRF)

The ageing ferret, like the ageing dog and cat, can suffer from CIN (CRF). No doubt the recurring effects of

ARF can result in CRF in the future for the ferret. CIN is a slow progressive loss of kidney function, the cause of which might not be clear. Ferrets can present signs compatible with glomerulonephropathy and this may indicate Aleutian disease (AD) as seen in the USA, UK and New Zealand. Glomerular nephritis is very common in aged ferrets in the USA and may have gone unrecognized in many countries to date.

Clinical signs

The uraemia produces a mild polydipsia and polyuria in advanced cases. Depression and lethargy with weight loss, oral ulcers and halitosis, pale mucous membranes occur plus diarrhoea and even vomiting. On palpation, the kidneys feel reduced due to nephrosis over time. The blood check would indicate anaemia and serum examination shows an increase in kidney enzymes, increased phosphate (hyperkalaemia) and decreased calcium (hypocalcaemia). Urine analysis shows increased protein, blood cells and more dilute urine. The cat shows a differential in symptoms between ARF and CRF; this can be placed in a table form and related to the symptoms seen in ferrets with renal disease (Table 11.7).

Treatment

In the CRF cat cases, the emphasis is again on rehydration, removal of toxic irritants and supply of a low protein, low phosphorus diet as for ARF.[23] A similar plan can be carried out for ferrets, but as suggested above, the protein should not be below 30% in the diet.

Table 11.7 General ideas on the differentiation of acute and chronic renal failure

	ARF	CRF
Onset of signs	Recent	Prolonged
General body condition	Good	Poor
Urine volume	Low[a]	High
Red cell mass	Normal	Anaemic
Serum K	High (can be normal)	Low (can be normal)
Urine sediment	Active	Benign
Response to supportive Rx	Recovery[b]	No recovery
Renal size	Normal or enlarged	Small[c]
Renal biopsy	Necrosis	Fibrosis/atrophy

[a]Some forms of ARF develop polyuria not oliguria, e.g. gentamicin nephrosis.
[b]When the insult causing ARF is massive recovery is not possible. [c]The kidneys are enlarged in many forms of CRF, e.g. polycystic kidney disease. Table after Senior, 1993.[23]

Again, with aged ferrets, antibiotics are used with caution with regard to nephrotoxicity. A good point from cat management is that dietary changes should be done gradually over a few days. Adjustment to new metabolic excretion rates require more time in CRF so that the extracellular fluid (ECF) volume and composition may not be properly maintained when dietary changes are too abrupt.[23] In addition, there should be no sudden environmental changes that alter the quality or pattern of food and water intake. This idea could relate to ferrets. Ferrets can vomit like cats and this could be controlled by use of cimetride 10 mg/kg q. 8–12 h, p.o., s.c., i.m. or i.v.

With cats it is found that a reduced protein intake in ARF or CRF causes decreased polydipsia and polyuria, improves the feeling of well-being and lessens azotaemia and proteinuria, but the author does state that the protein given should be of high metabolic value to the body.[23] This links up with ideas of Brown et al. regarding ferret treatment and not reducing protein below 30%. The source of protein is considered important as it has been found that dogs fed low protein diets where the sole source of protein was egg albumin had a more severe metabolic acidosis. Whether the phenomenon would occur in cats, or ferrets, is questionable.

The management of anorexia in sick ferrets can be just as frustrating as dealing with cats or dogs. Gradual change over to a new lower protein/low phosphorus diet has been indicated and warming the food or adding highly flavoured (low sodium) gravy or chicken fat helps. Sometimes hand feeding is the only answer. An example is given of a home-cooked low-protein/low-phosphorus diet for nephritic cats, which could be suitable for ferrets.

A possible home-cooked low-protein/low-phosphorus diet as a suggestion for nephritic ferrets (after D. Senior using half the weights that he uses for cats) is given here:[23]

- 57.5 g liver
- One large egg (50 g) hard-cooked
- 175 g cooked rice with no added salt (1 cup)
- 7.5 g vegetable oil (half tablespoon)
- 2.5 g calcium carbonate (half teaspoon)
- plus vitamin/mineral supplement (e.g. Animalac, Troy)

Procedure: Dice and braise the liver, retaining fat. Combine all ingredients and mix well. Add water to improve texture and palatability. Result is 292.5 g at 1397 kcal/kg as fed.

Secondary hyperparathyroidism (SH) is a feature of cat and dog CRF with the finding of hyperphosphataemia. It occurs when the glomerular filtration rate (GFR) falls to approximately 20% of normal, resulting in impaired renal phosphate excretion. Phosphate retention causes renal mineralization, SH and a potential increase in kidney damage.[27] *Note* that mineralization is common in dog/cat renal cases with CRF and may be an important factor in progression and perhaps also in ferrets. Hyperphosphataemia caused an inhibition of activity of the hydroxylase kidney enzyme, which contributes to the decreased production of calcitrol, the most active form of the vitamin D_3. The decrease of calcitrol brings on the SH.

Secondary hyperphosphataemia, which has been attributed to hyperparathyroidism, has been noted by Finkler, though he is of the opinion that not all ferrets develop it. It is a function of the timing in the course of the disease when a blood test is run (M. Finkler, pers. comm. 1998). He also states that 15% of dogs with chronic renal failure have hypercalcemia without hyperphosphataemia.

The parathyroid hormone (PTH) may be an important uraemic toxin and possibly involved in anaemia, neurotoxicity, dyslipoproteinaemias, insulin resistance, promotion of soft tissue calcification, renal osteodystrophy and increased renal damage.[27] PTH causes severe toxic injury to the kidneys because of the high number of PTH receptors in renal cells. There can be an uptake of calcium into the cells and eventually a precipitation of calcium phosphate into tubule lumen and a vicious circle may be set up with renal destruction. Clinical studies have not completely demonstrated this possibility, but there was one study providing good evidence for the effect of phosphorus restriction in CRF in dogs.[27] Some clinical studies in cats have shown that Whiskas low protein/low phosphorus diet (Waltham) does bring about a significant decrease in PTH in naturally-occurring CRF. This could be of value in ferret cases but, as noted earlier, the Whiskas diets do contain vegetable matter, which is not good for digestion in compromised sick ferrets. *Note*: if a special diet does not correct the hyperphosphataemia or secondary hyperparathyroidism, oral phosphorus binding agents have been used in dogs and cats (Table 11.8).

Alternatively calcitrol on a once-daily basis at extremely low doses (1.5–3.5 ng/kg body weight) will inhibit PTH production directly and does reduce serum PTH levels without a significant hypercalcaemia.[23] *Note*: in various studies, not with ferrets however, it has been shown that a reduction of dietary protein intake does bring about clinical benefits in uraemic animals. Besides reducing the level of protein catabolism, the dietary protein restriction helps by:

a. Reducing the intake of dietary phosphorus
b. Decreasing the protein-related solute load, thus lessening the severity of polydipsia and polyuria
c. Decreasing the acid load, thus helping to alleviate metabolic acidosis.[27]

However, there are problems associated with excessive protein restriction, as pointed out earlier by Brown, such as those listed here:

a. Uraemia, as a catabolic state, may adversely affect several aspects of protein metabolism
b. Increased urinary losses of protein or of specific amino acids can occur in renal failure
c. In CRF, the protein requirements for dogs and cats, and probably ferrets, have not been established. It is likely that they may be different or higher than those of healthy animals. Thus, consideration should be made to providing high quality protein sources for use in restricted protein diets to prevent essential amino acid deficiencies. Very low protein diets may not be accepted easily by dogs, cats[27] or ferrets. With CRF dogs, the protein intake is recommended at not less than 1.9 g/kg body weight daily unless further restrictions are required to control uraemia (~11 g protein/400 kcal metabolizable energy (ME) from a 10 kg dog diet).[27] CRF cats have a greater risk of protein malnutrition due to the inability to downregulate hepatic enzyme activity associated with protein catabolism, even when the dietary protein intake is low.[27]

In CRF ferrets the effect of reducing protein intake has not been fully studied.[16] It is surmised that restriction of dietary protein before clinical signs of CRF would delay the progression of renal damage.[27] Could this concept be applicable to ferrets? Could it be postulated that feeding ferrets at a lower food weight, instead of continuous ad lib feeding, may take stress off the kidneys? However, evidence is not clear about this concept for dogs and cats. It could be speculated that the idea might be one of the answers explaining why working ferrets in temperate climates, which get fed once daily or even

Table 11.8 Binding agents used with chronic renal disease

Compound	Starting dose	Comments
Aluminium hydroxide, carbonate oxide	30–90 mg/kg per day, dogs/cats	Liquid most effective (recommended by Finkler)
Calcium acetate	60–90 mg/kg per day, dogs/cats	Most effective calcium-containing agent. Risk of hypercalcaemia with all calcium salts, however

Diseases of the urinary system

Author's clinical example
Chronic renal failure in a ferret

Dave Such's sable 5-year-old hob, Caesar, was presented in January 1998 being listless and having bad breath, bleeding gums and very dirty teeth. He was slightly dehydrated. In the first instance he was treated with clavulanic acid/amoxicillin (Clavulox drops, Pfizer) and s.c. fluids while dental treatment was discussed and blood tests advised. Caesar did not improve on initial treatment but relapsed further with obvious polydipsia and polyuria and began convulsions. He was dehydrated, had lost weight and had pale mucous membranes. He had mouth ulcers, bleeding gums and halitosis. His kidneys felt small on palpation. It proved difficult to get enough blood for a full blood test but urine sample indicated the severe CRF that had been suspected.

Caesar was scheduled for oral attention and pre-treated for 24 hours with fluids and more antibiotics. Under gaseous anaesthesia, his teeth were cleaned and ulcers treated. He was discharged the next day after recovering with a package treatment for renal disease, which would be carried out by his concerned owner.

Dr Edleston advised continuing Clavulox drops plus Hills k/d diet and fluids to be given s.c. to prevent dehydration. As happens with CRF cases, Caesar would not eat the Hills diet so a home diet was devised.

Dave Such's homemade diet for nephritic ferret, Caesar

Morning meal: Half egg yolk mixed with Di-Vetelact supplement, with 2 drops of Pentavite vitamin/mineral supplement. Not all eaten but also given chicken breasts thinly sliced (about 20 g meat).

Evening meal: Heinz baby mixed cereal, about 3 teaspoonsful plus one teaspoonful of Di-Vetelact. All would be eaten. (A mixed cereal diet might be questionable.)

Caesar was maintained on this diet and the convulsions stopped but he did have slight twitching bouts at times. Caesar progressed well after 3 weeks and gained weight being well-hydrated. He became bright and alert though he did have his 'off days' and was sleeping a lot as most older ferrets do anyway.

Caesar finally died on the 14 April 1998 at 8.45 p.m. A much-loved pet.

Dr R. Edleston & Dave Such (New South Wales Ferret Society), pers. comm. 1998.

every few days, seem to live longer than house-bound ferrets. Ferrets kept as outdoor/indoor pets could be considered as being somewhere in between.

The minerals potassium, calcium and sodium are generally affected by CRF[27]:

a. Thus hyperkalaemia caused by an obligatory potassium loss, as seen in the cat, is possible in ferrets and would require dietary replacement of the mineral
b. The blood calcium concentration in CRF can be low, normal or high, so calcium supplementation would be helpful in hypocalcaemia but contraindicated in the presence of hypercalcaemia
c. The kidneys play a primary role in sodium homeostasis, so in CRF, as the glomerular filtration rate falls, the surviving nephrons have to increase their secretion of sodium to cope with the increased delivery rate. This must decrease in efficiency as the disease progresses.

With CRF, there would be a deficiency in water-soluble vitamins, so the dietary levels must be kept up in sick animals of all species.

The clinical example, left, shows how devotion to the pet is a critical factor in getting any sort of results with renal disease cases. Four months of concentrated effort! A client's 5-year-old ferret, Rambo, had a similar condition, but as he was very averse to hand feeding he had to be euthanized. Rambo had been bright before his owner boarded him for 2 weeks at a ferret-boarding establishment. The ferret showed severe mouth ulceration, weight loss and lethargy. It was possible that the mouth ulceration was in part due to the ferret chewing at the wire of the cage.

Pyelonephritis (PYN)

This condition has been recorded in laboratory ferrets in the USA by Fox[6] and in the UK.[28] It is usually the result of an ascending urinary infection with septicaemia or possible calculi involvement. The acute case can show anorexia, fever and depression. *E. coli* is the common causative agent. PYN is possible but rare in pet ferrets and must be treated aggressively.[26] It has not been recorded in working ferrets.

Diagnosis

This is by finding blood, leukocytes, renal tubular or white blood cell casts plus the causative bacteria in the urine.[6] Lower urinary infections may be confused with this condition.

Treatment

Involves fluid therapy and the use of broad-spectrum antibiotics, keeping again in mind the nephrotoxicity of some drugs. Trimethoprim-sulfa drugs (5 mg/kg once daily) and ampicillin or amoxicillin (10 mg/kg b.i.d) are useful. Chloramphenicol has been a drug of choice with ferrets. The injectable form chloramphenicol succinate (30–50 mg/kg b.i.d., i.m., s.c.) can be given orally as there is no palmitate available. (Given in a sugar solution as it is very bitter.) A full 7-day treatment or more with any drug is essential to remove infection.[6]

Hydronephrosis

This occurs when the excretory passage from the kidneys is blocked by physical ligature of the ureter, also cystitis, prostatic enlargement due to neoplasia, calculi, other neoplasia and herniation of the bladder. An unfortunate case of one ureter being tied off by mistake during an ovariohysterectomy operation on a 1-year-old jill was recorded in detail.[20] However, the ferret could maintain itself with one kidney after the affected one had been removed.

Urolithiasis

This has apparently been a common occurrence in USA pet ferrets.[1] It has also been recorded in farm mink[29] and laboratory ferrets.[30] In Australia and New Zealand to my knowledge the condition is very rare, possibly due to the difference in our ferret diets, as shown in Chapter 4. The disease is characterized by solitary or multiple renal cystic calculi or possibly sandy material in the bladder or urethra. A urethral blockage is the outcome and can be very acute in sterilized hobs and less acute in sterilized jills. In the latter, large stones can develop in the bladder before symptoms arise.

Struvite (magnesium ammonium phosphate) uroliths occur with or without a urinary tract infection. The aetiology of struvite disease is not clear but it is considered that diet is a likely factor as seen by work at Marshall Farms.[12] The normal pH of hob and jill ferret urine is 6–7.5.[7] A diet that contains mostly plant source protein will produce a urine pH above 6.0, the point at which struvite crystals will form; with an animal protein diet, the metabolic processes form acid urine. Ferrets fed on cat food can be at risk of struvite formation[12] because most generic cat foods and cat chow contain a corn base. Ferrets on pelleted dog food are at risk as the food contains a high fibre and vegetable content (Ch. 4). In Australia, New Zealand and Europe where working and pet ferrets are on a fresh meat diet, any urolithiasis is rare. Working ferrets are less likely to get urolithiasis anyway compared with sterilized pet ferrets. Note that by keeping ferrets off dry ferret or cat food this problem can be avoided. It is suggested that high quality cat food such as Iams, ANF Tami Premium and Science diets, as in the USA, will not induce struvite formation as they are meat-based diets.[12]

USA clinical examples

Triple phosphate crystals have been recovered from a 3-year-old ferret with cystitis and cultured to yield *Staphylococcus* (Fig. 11.6). The ferret was fed on cat food (G. Rich, pers. comm. 2005). Another ferret had bladder stones removed (Fig. 11.7) and was put on antibiotics with a diet change from a grocery store brand of ferret diet to Totally Ferret (Ch. 4) and showed great improvement.

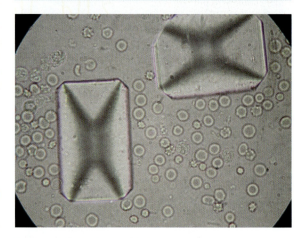

Figure 11.6 Triple phosphate crystals from ferret with cystitis. (Courtesy of G. Rich.)

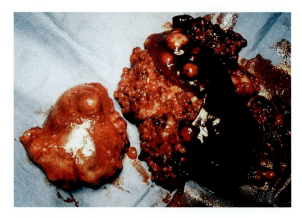

Figure 11.7 Bladder stones from ferret on poor commercial ferret meal diet. (Courtesy of G. Rich.)

Aetiology

Pregnant or lactating jills can succumb to uroliths because of diet or by urease-producing *Staphylococcus* or *Proteus* species, as the jills are constantly mobilizing minerals. With sterilized hobs, urolithiasis is mostly from a dietary cause.

Diseases of the urinary system

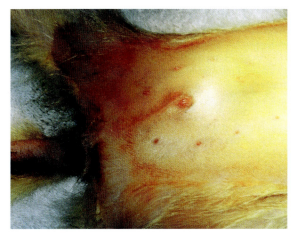

Figure 11.8 Urethral swelling/blockage due to adrenal gland disease. (Courtesy of G. Rich.)

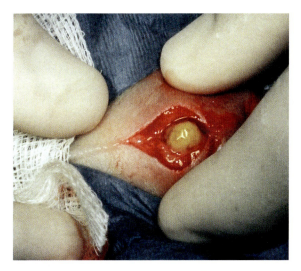

Figure 11.9 Urethral swelling at pelvic flexure with stone being extracted. (Courtesy G. Rich.)

Clinical signs

These can be very alarming in the sterilized hob, with severe distress at the urethral blockage, violent straining and screaming in pain (see also Prostate disease).[12] The swollen bladder will be palpable. American vets claim that sterilized pet ferrets with the condition do not get aggressive to humans like cats,[12] but I should be wary of handling a sterilized working ferret in this condition.

Jill ferrets, on the other hand, will often not show signs for some time until the bladder stone reaches a large size. They may show intermittent straining for some days or weeks before they get in real distress.

Ferrets are said to have a higher pain threshold than other animals and tolerate discomfort better but care must be taken with examining working ferrets that are naturally quick to react to any situation. With a jill, the fur round the hindquarters shows tell-tale signs of wetness from urine dribbling and the vulva may be scalded. The jill's bladder stones are usually easily palpable and seen on radiographs.[1] In addition jills in heat may get a wet peritoneal area and urolithiasis after a prolonged heat because the open vulva and wetness invites an ascending infection.

Another case of a 5-year-old male ferret on cat food has been recorded (Fig. 11.8). It was not a prostatic-induced adrenal disease ramification (G. Rich, pers. comm. 2005). Swelling at the pelvic flexure showed presence of a stone on surgery (Fig. 11.9).

Treatment

In the male ferret with urinary blockage the situation is life threatening. Catheterization is difficult, though not impossible, in the male ferret due to the J-shaped os penis (baculum) but is described in Chapter 20. However, trauma from the operation may induce an ascending infection. Also, the penis may be quickly filled with fine struvite material after the initial pressure is relieved. For that reason, a cystotomy is preferable.[12] The bladder can be first decompressed using a 22–25 gauge needle, removing most of the struvite content and flushing out with saline and repeated or a full cystotomy done (S. Brown, pers. comm. 1997). This is obviously less stressful to the ferret. It may be possible to retrograde flush via a catheter in the prepuce. *Note*: the prepuce is pinched as the back flushing is done and possibly clears struvite grains. If a cystotomy is carried out, the bladder is then flushed with saline, an antibiotic drug is left in the bladder and the ferret is put onto a fresh meat diet. In the USA, some cases of urolithiasis are so severe that a perineal urethrostomy is required.

With the jill, surgery would be required to remove the bladder stones. With the jill there is more time to prepare in contrast to the sterilized hob. Brown did not find calculolytic diets useful.[1] Ferret emergency procedures were needed (Ch. 20). When the jill undergoes surgery, the urethra is checked as stones too large for the jill to expel via the vulva will get lodged and must be repositioned into the bladder by gentle manipulation. Thus they can be removed with the cystotomy. It is advisable to operate on pregnant jills quickly as they may sometimes develop a prolapsed rectum and vagina with resulting fatal haemorrhage due to tissue damage (D. Manning, pers. comm. 1998). The situation of stone formation can be avoided by a good diet!

It is considered that sterilized hobs and jills, pregnant or not, will tolerate the anaesthesia and the kittens

CHAPTER ELEVEN
Diseases of special concern

> **Author's clinical example**
>
> **Urolithiasis in the ferret using a calculolytic diet**
>
> A young unsterilized jill was fed on cat biscuits and meat for some time and presented showing straining on urination. The jill was radiographed and a distinct bladder stone was seen. The owner could not afford surgery and long-term treatment using Hills Canine Prescription s/d diet was commenced. The stone was dissolved after several months and then the jill switched to Science diet Feline maintenance dry diet that was fed permanently.
>
> B.L. McDonald, St. Andrews Veterinary Clinic, Sydney, NSW, pers. comm. 1998.

carried by a pregnant jill will not be compromised. The ferret's postoperative care would involve use of broad-spectrum antibiotics such as clavulanic acid/amoxicillin (Clavulox palatable drops) 0.25 mL b.i.d., or a trimethoprim-sulfa combination at 15–30 mg/kg q. 12 h, p.o. or s.c. after urine and stones culture. The latter drug is useful as it will concentrate in the urine and most pathogenic urinary organisms are sensitive to it. The drug tablet has to be made up in solution. Paediatric drops can be used for ferrets if available. Dietary changes away from the offending vegetable protein type food should be gradual, with the ferret given a wide selection of high quality cat food as ferrets might reject a sudden change.[12] It is suggested that warming pelleted foods may be acceptable. In a suspect urinary case, I have used diced lamb hearts covered in a chicken stock, which was licked up before the meat was eaten. As a diet, eggnog with 20% fat level, is made with whipped cream, milk and egg yolk with a tablespoon of raw pureed liver added to each 6 oz; this is highly palatable to the ferret. The diet provides a concentrated source of calories, especially for those affected pregnant or lactating jills and remarkably will lower the urine pH, even when the original diet is still fed.[12] Fresh water should of course be available to ferrets at all times but in my experience ferrets do not drink to excess, unless sick, and do get a fair amount of fluid from fresh meat. There are specialized diets such as the Hill's Prescription Diet range with Canine s/d used as an aid to the dissolution of struvite urolithiasis and initial control of struvite crystalluria.

I would consider a whole fresh meat diet would have avoided this crisis. It might be difficult to get clients to move away from dry foods for ferrets, which of course are considered 'convenient' as they are for feeding dogs and cats. As has been stated regarding ferret nutrition, many USA veterinarians dealing with ferrets are reconsidering the feeding of dry food over the long term with regard to other possible conditions besides urolithiasis (S. Brown, pers. comm. 1998).

The Australian Cosi Pets milk, which I have used, states on the label 'Vets advise that excessive dry foods without adequate fluid intake can result in kidney disorders'. The main goal is to get ferrets, or cats, to drink enough water with dry foods! Any lack of water for ferrets, e.g. bowls getting knocked over while owners are away all day, could contribute to dry food induced kidney disorders, especially with ferrets on ad lib feeding. Ferrets get water from moist fresh meat. It is interesting to note that only two cases of cystic calculi have been recorded in New Zealand fitch (ferret) farms which were maintained on a commercial wet meat diet.[13]

Cystitis

This can be a primary condition without the formation of bladder stones (see above) and is possibly a result of descending or ascending infection.[1] One author considers that in ferrets cystitis is more likely to be associated with urolithiasis.[7]

Symptoms

These would be the characteristic frequent urination, sometimes painful, and urine staining around the vulva in jills and hindquarters and around the penis with hobs. Haematuria can occur but with unsterilized jills there may be some blood associated with the ferret heat. If the bladder is palpated it appears thickened by the disease.[7]

Diagnosis

Requires urinalysis to detect red and white cells present and culture will be required for pathogens. One author advises full blood analysis on all ferrets over 3 years of age as routine health check (S. Brown, pers. comm. 1998). In Australia, I have only seen renal problems in ferrets 5–6 years old with associated kidney disease.

Treatment

As with general cystitis in dogs and cats, the best results will depend on the urine culture findings, bacteriology sensitivity and a suitable antibiotic course for 2 weeks. If possible, radiographs and perhaps use of ultrasound may be required in some cystitis cases to check for specific causes such as bladder cancer, abdominal masses, or even prostate enlargement in sterilized hobs.[7]

Trauma to the ureter

Urinary tract trauma is relatively common in veterinary medicine involving the kidneys, urethra and/or bladder.

Damage to the ureters is less likely and clinical signs of ureter rupture are mostly non-specific so that the animal can be come seriously ill while awaiting a diagnosis. A US study was carried out on unilateral ureteral rupture involving eight dogs, one cat and one ferret.[31] The 4-year-old male castrate ferret was not seen clinically till 60 days after the trauma (no reason given) while the other animals were taken to be examined hours/days after the event but no longer than 7 days. The ferret showed no specific urinary tract signs and there appeared to be no abdominal distension or discomfort. A concurrent injury turned out to be a diaphragmatic hernia which was apparently not mended probably because of the anaesthetic risk. A right ureteronephrectomy was successful where the right ureter had been found torn. Abdominal radiology or ultrasound was not done on this case nor excretory urography attempted. The ferret went on to recover and was not seen as a follow-up and presumed to be okay.

Trauma causing rupture of the ureter is documented in humans as:

a. Crushing of the ureter into the transverse processes of the lumbar vertebrae
b. Excessive tension on the ureter when there is severe stretching between the two 'fixed' ends
c. Movement of the kidney against the relative immobile uteropelvic junction
d. A combination of spinal hypertension and sudden acceleration/deceleration.

The question of how trauma affected this particular ferret with the resulting diaphragmatic hernia, but no broken bones, is interesting and may be of a kind where a house ferret gets caught in some sort of in-house fall. In dogs and cats, surgical repair of a diaphragmatic in the first 24 hours has a high mortality risk. The ferret after 60 days may have adapted to the condition.

Cardiovascular disease

This is considered a common complaint in ferrets over 3 years of age in the USA.[32] It was also said that some 3-year-old ferrets were considered almost geriatric and prone to certain conditions (S. Brown, pers. comm. 1998) both of which can occur in either sex and to date the exact causes are unknown. Genetics may play a part (Ch. 5). Dilated cardiomyopathy progresses slowly over time, while hypertrophic cardiomyopathy initiates sudden death by left ventricular hypertrophy.

The ferret heart

In the normal ferret, the heart rate can be between 160 and 250 bpm and will vary with rate of excitement, with sinus arrhythmia commonly seen. In many ferrets, murmurs are always abnormal with the exception of a high pitched Grad 1-11 innocent murmur found in juveniles which disappears with age (M. Finkler, pers. comm. 2005).

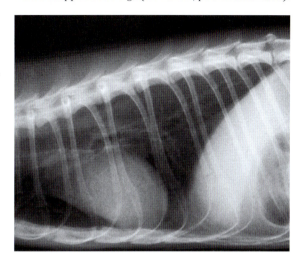

Figure 11.10 Normal ferret chest. (Courtesy of Tom Kawasaki.)

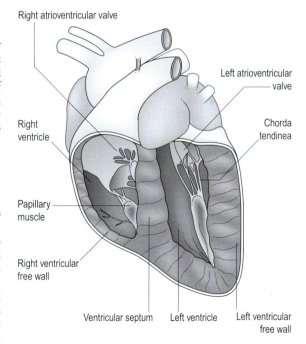

Figure 11.11 Normal heart section drawing. (Courtesy of Tom Kawasaki.)

CHAPTER ELEVEN

Diseases of special concern

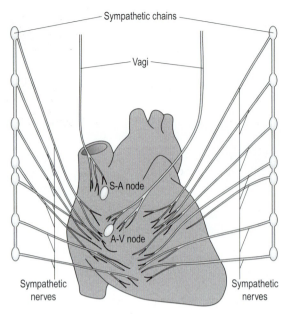

Figure 11.12 Cardiac vagi and sympathetic nerve complex. (Courtesy of Tom Kawasaki.)

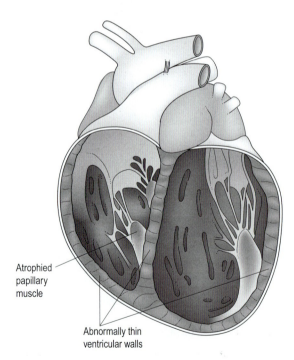

Figure 11.13 Heart dilated cardiomyopathy (DCM) section. (Courtesy of Tom Kawasaki.)

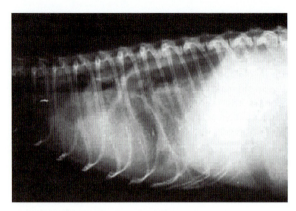

Figure 11.14 Radiograph of DCM; lateral. (Courtesy of Tom Kawasaki.)

Normal heart radiology is seen in Figure 11.10. A cross-section of the heart is shown in Figure 11.11. The ferret heart and lungs are also seen in Figure 2.21a,b (Ch. 2). The cardiac nerve supply is shown in Figure 11.12.

Dilated (congestive) cardiomyopathy (DCM)

This is seen in 80% of ferret cardiac cases (Fig. 11.13). It has been found by one author that the addition of taurine to high quality feline and musteline diets over the last few years reduced the incidence of cardiomyopathy in the USA.[1] However there is no firm evidence that taurine deficiency is implicated in ferret heart problems according to Finkler.[26]

I have seen only one case of ferret cardiomyopathy. An older ferret, Pandy, showed initial signs of weight loss, dyspnoea, enlarged heart on radiology (e.g. Fig. 11.14) and systolic heart murmurs. Despite treatment, it died.

Clinical signs

The classic signs can include general lethargy, weight loss, dyspnoea, with splenomegaly and ascites or even sudden death that can be seen in American pet ferrets over 3 years of age.[1] Additionally there can be weakness, difficult breathing, poor capillary refill, thrombus, hypothermia, pleural effusion but not usually coughing unless there is concurrent heartworm disease (Ch. 10). Systolic heart murmurs occur (gallop rhythm) and these are due to the rapid filling of the dilated left ventricle, which causes the 3rd heart sound and a pronounced atrial contraction producing the 4th heart sound. *Note*: at the left 5th intercostal space, one can palpate a stronger or weaker than normal precordial heart beat,

Cardiovascular disease

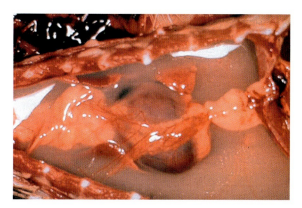

Figure 11.15 DCM pleural effusion at post mortem. (Courtesy of Tom Kawasaki.)

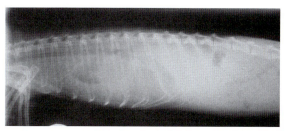

Figure 11.17 Congestive heart failure case; lateral radiograph. *Note* the pleural effusion obscuring the cardiac silhouette and producing leafing in lung lobes. The trachea is elevated dorsally. (Courtesy of M. Burgess.)

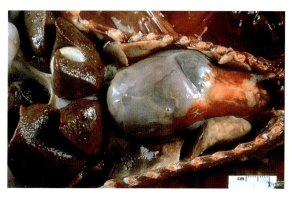

Figure 11.16 DCM at post mortem. (Courtesy of Tom Kawasaki.)

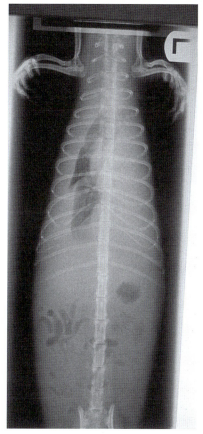

Figure 11.18 Congestive heart failure radiograph; dorsoventral view. *Note* this patient has ascites, which obscures most of the abdominal detail except for gas in bowel. (Courtesy of M. Burgess.)

which has a longer duration than in the non-affected animal.[32] In addition one can pick up jugular pulsations with any ventricular arrhythmias or tricuspid valvular insufficiencies or even failure of the right heart muscle. The ferret lethargy is associated in time with hypothermia, cyanotic membranes and a weak femoral pulse.

A severe combination of pleural effusion and ascites (Figs 11.15, 11.16) may be confused with that caused by heartworm (Ch. 10) or neoplasia (Ch. 13). Cytology of pleural fluid as a differential diagnostic tool is therefore considered essential by Miller.[32] The outcome of a congestive heart failure case is illustrated in radiographs in Figures 11.17, 11.18.

The cause is now thought to be either genetic, immune or inflammatory response and is noted more in male ferrets over 3 years of age. The heart muscle as illustrated is thin and weak. *Note*: the cardiac output (heart rate multiplied by the stroke volume) is affected by the weak muscle tone.

Diagnostic techniques

On auscultation, one finds tachycardia with murmurs, diagnosis being assisted by radiography, electrocardiography (ECG) and ultrasonography.

277

CHAPTER ELEVEN
Diseases of special concern

Radiology

The normal ferret heart lies at an angle between the 6th and 8th ribs with the apex situated to the left of the median, shown on lateral view (see Fig. 2.22b), and about 1 cm anterior to the diaphragm. Radiograph findings would indicate cardiac enlargement in the diseased animal plus other conditions, e.g. the presence of thoracic lymphoma, pleural effusion and lung and blood vessel involvement in cardiomyopathy effects. Spleen and liver enlargements are sometimes seen in cardiac cases. *Note*: if the heart touches the diaphragm curve it usually indicates cardiac enlargement. A characteristic of dilated cardiomyopathy is said to be a loss of translucent area between the heart and the sternum giving a 'floating heart' appearance (Fig. 11.14).[1]

Electrocardiography (ECG)

As with dogs and cats, ECG is an essential tool in detecting ferret arrhythmias and conduction disorders using the P-QRS-T morphology. The ferret ECG differs in that the P waves are normally small like the cat, but the tall, wide QRS complexes amplitudes and sinus arrhythmia are similar to the dog ECG (Fig. 11.19). In ferrets suffering dilatative cardiomyopathy, sinus rhythm, atrial and ventricular arrhythmias, atrial premature contraction (APC), ventricular premature contraction (VPC) and different degrees of A-V block have been detected.[32] The S wave is seen in leads II, III, or aVF indicating right ventricular enlargement (RVE), ventricular premature contractions (VPC); bradycardia or tachycardia (Fig. 11.20).

If possible, the ferret ECG is recorded without resort to sedation but this is sometimes not possible, so light isoflurane anaesthesia is advised. The ECG clips will have to be adapted for ferrets with the teeth on the alligator clips flattened and/or covered with gauze (Fig. 11.21).[33]

Experimental values for ferrets were obtained under anaesthesia, which can be compared with anaesthetic ideas (Ch. 16). The ECG values of 52 clinically normal ferrets obtained by Bone et al.[34] are shown in Table 11.9, with the ferrets under ketamine and ketamine–xylazine combination. The latter procedure proved best in obtaining a stable ECG base line, due to fewer muscle tremors

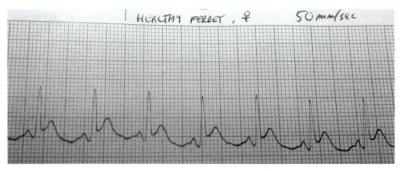

Figure 11.19 Healthy ferret ECG from aVF line. (Courtesy of Tom Kawasaki.)

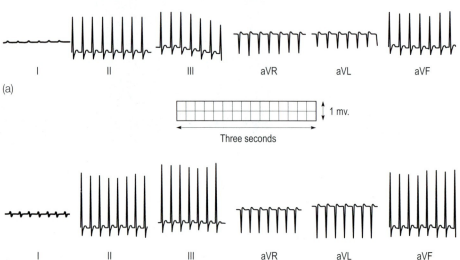

Figure 11.20 Electrocardiograms in (a) a normal ferret and (b) a ferret with right ventricular hypertrophy. A grid in the centre of the figure is calibrated from measurement of one millivolt and a 3-second strip in these photographically enhanced images of the original recording.

Cardiovascular disease

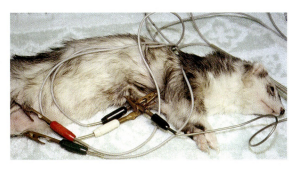

Figure 11.21 Ferret set up for ECG. (Courtesy of Tom Kawaski.)

and more relaxed ferrets under the combination. In another study by Smith and Bishop[35] recording ECGs on weanlings, normal adults and ferrets with right ventricular hypertrophy, the young ferrets were anaesthetized using ketamine (15 mg/kg i.m.) but with halothane (1%) after intubation. The adults were anaesthetized by sodium pentobarbital (25 mg/kg i.p.) and readings were taken with the subject in right lateral recumbency. The recording were taken using leads I, II, aVR, aVL and aVF. The ECGs obtained of normal and affected ferrets are shown in Figure 11.20. All ferrets showed (a) *normal sinus rhythm* while diseased ferrets showed (b) disruption of heart cycle. Ferrets with cardiac disease commonly show a sinus tachycardia and less commonly a sinus bradycardia and conductive disturbances.[33]

Abnormal rhythms are ventricular premature contractions (VPC), atrial premature contractions (APC) (Fig. 11.22), second and third degree AV block (Fig. 11.23). Sternal positioning produces larger QRSs than right lateral positioning (Finkler, pers. comm. 2005). An interesting series of articles on general interpretation of ECG in small animals was produced by Martin in 2002.[36]

Echocardiography (ultrasonography)

Ultrasonography in the ferret is described in detail in Chapter 17. This is the most modern and specific tool for diagnosing cardiomyopathy and other cardiac disease. Normal values for ferrets are shown in Table 11.10. It is the best method for hypertrophic cardiomyopathy.

M mode echocardiography allows quantitation of chamber size and wall thickness besides an assessment of the indices of systolic function. Both dilated cardiomyopathy and hypertrophic cardiomyopathy can be checked by echocardiography; they both show a dilated left atrium. In the case of DCM there is a thin-walled hypocontractile left ventricular free wall and interventricular septum. The HCM case has a thickened left

Table 11.9 Electrocardiographic data for 52 clinically normal ferrets[a]

Parameter	Mean ± SD (range)[b] (n = 25)	Value[c] (n = 27)
Age (months)	10–20	Average, 5.2
Male:Female ratio	All male	1.25
Body weight (kg)	1.4 ± 0.2	NA
Heart rate (beats/minute)	196 ± 26.5 (140–240)	233 ± 22
Rhythm		
Normal sinus	NA	67%
Sinus arrhythmia	NA	33%
Frontal plane MEA (degrees)	+86.13 ± 2.5 (79.6–90)	+77.22 ± 12
Lead II		
P amplitude (mV)	NA	0.122 ± 0.007
P duration(s)	NA	0.024 ± 0.004
PR interval (s)	0.056 ± 0.0086 (0.04–0.08)	0.047 ± 0.003
QRS duration (s)	0.044 ± 0.0079 (0.035–0.06)	0.043 ± 0.003
R amplitude (m V)	2.21 ± 0.42 (1.4–3)	1.46 ± 0.84
QT interval (s)	0.109 ± 0.018 (0.08–0.14)	0.12 ± 0.04

[a]All ferrets were sedated with ketamine–xylazine. [b]Data from Bone et al., 1988.[34] [c]Data adapted from Fox, JG. Biology and diseases of the ferret. Philadelphia: Lea & Febiger; 1988:170, and J. Edwards unpublished data, 1987. NA, not available; MEA, mean electrical axis.
Table from Stamoulis et al., 1997, with permission.[33]

CHAPTER ELEVEN

Diseases of special concern

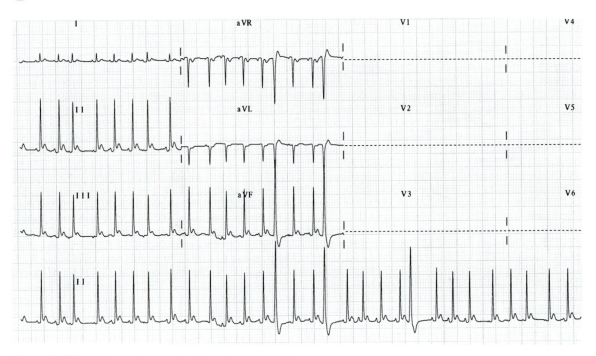

Figure 11.22 Atrial premature contractions. (Courtesy of Tom Kawasaki.)

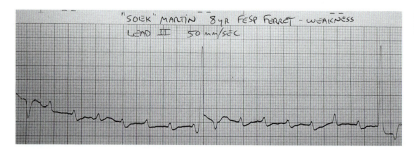

Figure 11.23 A complete AV block. (Courtesy of Tom Kawasaki.)

Table 11.10 Mean echocardiographic values for 34 normal adult ferrets

Parameters	Mean value
Left ventricle, end-diastolic	11.0 mm
Left ventricle, end-systolic	6.4 mm
Left ventricular posterior or free wall	3.3 mm
Fractional shortening	42%
End-point septal separation	None

Data from N. Sitinas, N. Beeber and M. Skeels, unpublished data, 1992. Table from Stamoulis et al., 1997, with permission. (See also Ch. 17.)

ventricular free wall and/or interventricular septum and normal to increased ventricular contractility, while a thickened basilar interventricular septum appears to obstruct the left ventricular to aortic tract during ventricular systole.[32] Additionally, studies of aortic valvular insufficiency have been made on ferrets using colour flow imaging.[33]

Treatment prospects

The aim of any treatment is to regulate heart rate and rhythm, after load and contractility. A specific diagnosis is required to relate to an appropriate treatment routine. Ferrets with DCM should have rest and low sodium diet.[16]

Furosemide (frusemide) at 0.25 to 1.0 mg/kg p.o. s.i.d./b.i.d., perhaps up to 2 mg/kg. Furosemide therapy can be enhanced by thiazide diuretics at cat doses.

Enalapril: This drug is used at 0.25–0.50 mg/kg q. 24–48 h if kidneys are healthy. Start at 0.5 mg/kg q.

48 h and attempt to obtain maintenance dosage of 0.05 mg/kg q. 24 h. If the dose is tolerated, increase on daily basis but if ferret is lethargic adjust to once every 3 days.

Why use enalapril? In the normal ferret when there is low blood pressure, the kidney is stimulated to release the enzyme rennin which acts on catalyzing the conversion of angiotensinogen to angiotensin I, which is converted by an angiotensin-converting enzyme (ACE) in the lungs to angiotensin II. This latter powerful vasoconstrictor helps readjust blood pressure to vital organs. It increases aldosterone production and sodium resorption while stimulating myocardial fibrosis and remodels the heart. There are many receptors on the heart for this hormone. Thus, in the normal animal it is compensatory but in the heart-diseased animal it is deleterious. Enalapril maleate (Merial) is an ACE inhibitor, blocking the angiotensin II and thus aldosterone production, vasoconstriction and myocardial reconstruction (T. Kawasaki, pers. comm. 2005). (*Note*: enalfor (Merial) is the Australian equivalent of enalapril and not registered for ferrets.)

Digoxin: used as elixir at 0.005–0.01 mg/kg s.i.d up to b.i.d. There have been no clinical trials on digoxin in ferrets but Rosenthal suggests 0.01 mg/kg daily with adjustments with further dosage by serum evaluation.[16] The digoxin routine is started at once daily and then adjusted to possibly every other day or double daily dose if required. Serum levels can be monitored.[33] As with dogs, the dosage is based on lean body weight assuming normal 15% body fat but ferrets tend to lose weight quickly with many conditions when ill. The sick ferret must be monitored, if possible by regular blood checks on digoxin serum levels and by use of ECG, radiographs and echocardiography techniques. Ferrets should not be stressed by these procedures on a too regular basis if the prognosis of useful life is only months.

With excessive pleural effusion a thoracentesis is done and fluid submitted to the laboratory.[33] In acute heart failure an oxygen tent can be used (Ch. 20) and furosemide (frusemide) at 2–4 mg/kg s.c. or i.m q. 8–12 h. Should continue with digoxin at reduced dose, 1–4 mg/kg, also p.o.

Note: Chitty in the UK had some success with using pimobendan (Vetmedin), a dog drug, in two ferret cases of DCM where ACE inhibitors were not working well. Dose rate was 0.5 mg/kg b.i.d. The ferrets picked up under drug medication but died a few months later, most likely from the condition and not drug-caused (C. Chitty, pers. comm. 2005).

Hypertrophic cardiomyopathy (HCM)

This condition requires further study and is basically sudden death of the ferret by heart muscle failure. This

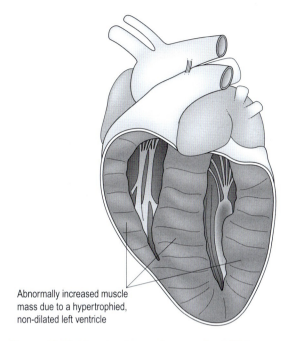

Figure 11.24 Hypertrophic cardiomyopathy (HCM). (Courtesy of Tom Kawasaki.)

could happen following a routine surgery (M. Finkler, pers. comm. 2004). The HCM condition could be genetic with the heart muscle effects being thickening, stiffness and non-compliant tissue. It has been noted that 9% of normal cats have HCM (T. Kawasaki, pers. comm. 2005). HCM is shown in a cross-section of the heart Figure 11.24.

Clinical signs

These are vague and may be a left-sided or sternal systolic murmur, detected in acute cases with echocardiography showing left ventricle hypertrophy. Depending on the acuteness of the cardiac defect, systolic sounds may be normal or greatly increased tachycardia.[33]

Diagnosis

Auscultation reveals arrhythmia and murmurs while less than 10% of cases are demonstrated by radiography as cardiomegaly. Echocardiography is the best method, revealing the left ventricular free wall and interventricular septum thickened (T. Kawasaki, pers. comm. 2005).

Treatment prospects

If possible, treatment is usually initiated to improve diastolic function and reduce congestion. Rest again is

CHAPTER ELEVEN
Diseases of special concern

essential. The technique is to start with a low drug dose. A check is made for any adverse reactions, which in ferrets could result in arrhythmias (including heart block) with general lethargy and inappetence.[33] With ferrets propranolol (Inderal) is a beta-blocker to slow the heart rate down and is used at 2.5 mg/ferret p.o. b.i.d. atenolol (Tenormin) is used at 6.25 mg/day and furosemide dosage is at 0.25–1.0 mg/kg p.o. s.i.d/b.i.d. Enalapril dose is 0.005–0.01 mg/kg p.o. q. 24–48 h.

The calcium channel antagonist drug diltiazem (Cardizem, Dilacor, Tiazac) is used at one-eighth of a 30 mg tablet s.i.d/b.i.d. Nitroglycerine ointment is used at one-eighth of an inch twice daily for the first 24 hours (M. Finkler, pers. comm. 2004).

Nitroglycerin (as 2% ointment) is a venous dilator and useful in emergency treatment to reduce pre-load and aids in reducing pulmonary oedema. (*Note*: be careful hypertension does not occur.) However, the prognosis for hypertrophic cardiomyopathy is considered poor with 6 months maximum survival. Post mortem will show hypertrophy of heart muscle as shown in the four cut sections Figure 11.25.

Valvular heart disease (VHD)

This is apparently a more common disease in older ferrets in the USA and is similar, but not as frequent, as endocardiosis in dogs in which there is chronic fibrosis and nodular thickening of the free ends of the atrio-ventricular valves. This leads to distortion of the valve cusps so that valve leakage occurs, resulting in a massive incompetence and congestive heart failure.

Clinical signs

These are variable but usually a definite murmur covering the whole systole and registered at the left apical region (may progress to a complete congestive heart failure as in dogs). In addition, moist rales can be detected on lung auscultation. The radiology and ECG checks are variable while the echocardiograph shows left or right atrial enlargement and mild dilation of the affected ventricle. Like hypertrophic cardiomyopathy, the systolic sounds in valvular heart disease may be normal or greatly increased. Using Doppler echocardiography techniques found that the mitral or tricuspid valves show regurgitation; in some cases both are affected. *Note* that the degeneration of the valves is seen at post mortem as being abnormally thick, like those of the dog with endocarditis. In addition, the heart atria are visibly dilated.[33] The blood flow and relevant valves association is shown in Figure 11.26.

The regurgitation from mitral valve insufficiency is recorded over the left apical region while the tricuspid regurgitation is noted in the right parasternal area. Varying degrees of aortic valvular insufficiency can be found in ferrets. The abnormality can be in 50–60% of ferrets but the reason is a puzzle. The auscultatory murmur is found along the left sternal border though is not usually heard. The cause is considered to be possibly acquired

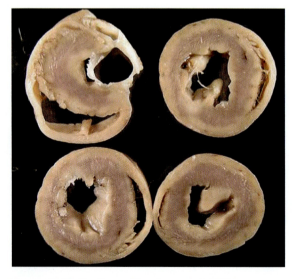

Figure 11.25 Sections of heart muscle in HCM. (Courtesy of Tom Kawasaki.)

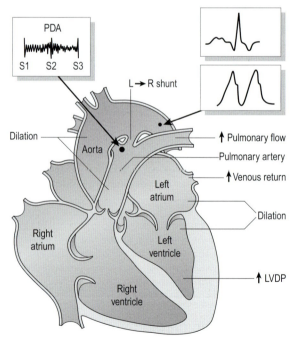

Figure 11.26 Patent ductus arteriosus; drawing showing heart blood flow. (Courtesy of Tom Kawasaki.)

endocardiosis and mucopolysaccharide deposits. It does not require treatment unless the left ventricle is volume-overloaded (T. Kawasaki, pers. comm. 2005).

Treatment prospects

Initially use furosemide and enalapril, which act to reduce regurgitation and congestion. When the systolic function is impaired or if supraventricular arrhythmias occur, the ferret can go onto digoxin therapy.

Myocarditis

This has actually been seen in association with *Toxoplasma*-like organisms in ferrets, producing multifocus necrosis of the myocardium (Ch. 10). It is also noted that Aleutian disease syndrome can cause a fibrinoid necrosis and mononuclear cell infiltration into the ferret heart arterioles[33] (Ch. 8). In the presence of sepsis, inflammatory lesions can be seen in ferret hearts and could occur in hob ferrets if fighting in the mating season with resulting severe trauma.

An atrial tumour has been recorded in a ferret as in Figure 11.27.

Lymphoma can occur in many organs and infection of the mediastinal lymph nodes will in time compromise the heart and lungs. Associated cardiac problems include thrombus, retinal atrophy (Ch. 12) and cardiomyopathies. *Note* that infection of the heart by *Dirofilaria immitis* is a serious condition in ferrets (Ch. 10).

Of the DCM and HCM conditions, the disease of dilated cardiomyopathy, as described earlier, is the more common in the USA and can be illustrated by the following three cases:

1. DCM in an 8-year-old sterilized hob ferret was recorded[37] and compared with a normal ferret of the same age, sex and approximate weight. The diseased heart was larger in size, both ventricles were dilated and the interventricular septum and both ventricular free walls had thinned. Other pathological lesions were areas of myocardium destruction and replacement with fibrous tissue, a yellow-brown liver, due to haemosiderosis, and cysts of yellow fluids in both kidneys (not related to the DCM). Haemosiderosis was also found in the bronchial lymph nodes, lungs and spleen which parallels signs of dilated cardiomyopathy in other species.

2. In a combination of diseases, a 3-year-old silverpoint male ferret was treated for possible intervertebral disc disease. It recovered somewhat with treatment, but in 5 weeks developed sneezing

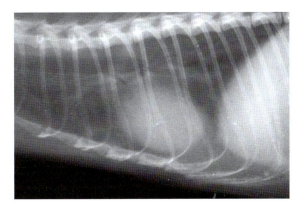

Figure 11.28 Cardiomyopathy radiology, lateral view. (Courtesy of Tom Kawasaki.)

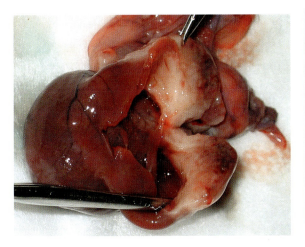

Figure 11.27 Atrial tumour. (Courtesy of Tom Kawasaki.)

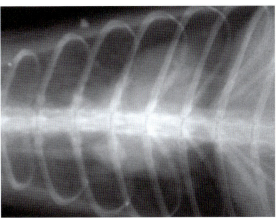

Figure 11.29 Cardiomyopathy radiology; dorsoventral. (Courtesy of Tom Kawasaki.)

and dyspnoea and showed signs of DCM.[38] It died despite treatment and on post mortem, the heart chambers were found to be markedly enlarged and the brain showed meningitis with *Cryptococcus* invasion (Ch. 12).
3. A 5-year-old ferret showed lethargy and weight loss. With radiology (Figs 11.28, 11.29) plus a confirming ultrasound, DCM was diagnosed. The ferret was treated with enalapril and furosemide resulting in the animal returning to stable health to be maintained on the drugs (G. Rich, pers. comm. 2005).

Diseases of the central nervous system

Neurological conditions affecting the ferret include rabies and canine distemper (Ch. 7) and *Cryptococcus* (Ch. 10). Posterior paralysis is associated with Aleutian disease, botulism and metabolic insulinoma. Trauma to the spine can result in paralysis and one case of disc decompression has been recorded in Australia (B. McDonald, pers. comm. 1998). Disc compression affecting the spinal cord and treatment has been recorded by Lamb et al. in the UK (Ch. 19). Conditions such as chordoma and plasma cell myeloma have been noted.[39] A list of neurological problems is given in the appendices.

Neuronal ceroid lipofuscinosis (NCL)

A 'new' condition affecting the ferret CNS was recorded by Geraghty and France, University of Sydney Veterinary School, Sydney NSW in late 1990s. NCL has been seen in several Sydney ferrets. Clinical signs first appear in adults of both sexes and include gradual onset hind-limb paresis progressing to incontinence, behavioural changes and often blindness. There is no treatment although affected animals can be kept for some time before requiring euthanasia.

Confirmation of the diagnosis requires histopathological examination of nervous tissue in which the intracytoplasmic granules typical of this disease in other species are seen in neurons at virtually all sites (brain, spinal cord and peripheral ganglia).

NCL is an inherited disease involving accumulation of macromolecules within neurons due to an enzyme deficiency; it has been extensively studied in a number of species including dogs, sheep and humans, although these appear to be the first recorded cases in ferrets. The manifestation in ferrets differs somewhat from that most often seen in other species since it is of late onset and the early clinical signs are more typical of a thoracolumbar spinal lesion than diffuse neurological disease.

Differential diagnoses might include botulism, tick paralysis, distemper, Aleutian disease and spinal injury. The onset and course of NCL in ferrets, however, is far more gradual than would typically be seen in any of these conditions. The heritability of NCL in ferrets is at present unknown since pedigree information has been unavailable in all cases so far studied (F. Geraghty, M. France, pers. comm. 1998). There have been no other sightings of this disease condition to date.

Disseminated idiopathic myositis (DIM)

A strange muscular disease phenomenon in ferrets has arisen in the USA.

Introduction

In mid- to late 2003, Drs Burgess and Ramsell saw, in fairly quick succession, four cases of what appeared to be a new disease syndrome in the pet ferret. The hallmarks of this illness were high fever and an unusually high neutrophil count, far above what ferrets normally would generate even with severe sepsis. That, and the total lack of response to any conventional therapy they initiated, led them to believe that they were indeed dealing with a disease process they had not previously encountered. Dr Mike Garner at Northwest ZooPath in the Seattle, Washington area, agreed after viewing histopathology specimens. He noted a suppurative myositis involving nearly all muscle groups in the body, including the heart. Two years later the exact cause of this devastating disease syndrome is not understood, but over 40 confirmed cases have been compiled in the USA and extensive tests have been performed. The following is a summary of what is known to date.

Presenting signs and history

Affected ferrets are young, typically 3–21 months old at time of onset of clinical signs. Cases have occurred in ferrets from various breeders, and in both male and female ferrets of various colour types. Many (single) cases occurred in multiple ferret households; at this time, other ferrets in those households remain nonsymptomatic even months after exposure to the ill ferret. Affected animals appeared healthy and normal until acute onset of illness. Owners typically report sudden onset of lethargy, variable anorexia, reluctance to move and variable signs of pain when handling their pet (vocalizing, wincing, tensing of muscles). Some owners note that the ferret 'feels warm' to the touch. Paresis and ataxia may be noted. Vaccine history is variable; some ferrets had received multiple distemper immunizations and/or rabies immunization. Distemper vaccines used were Fervac-D (United Vaccines, Madison, Wisconsin, USA), Purevax (Merial, Athens, Georgia, USA) or Galaxy D (Schering-Plough, Omaha, Nebraska, USA). Rabies prophylaxis utilized Imrab 3 (Merial, Athens, Georgia, USA). All ferrets had received at least one distemper vaccine at their breeder facility of origin. Dietary history was also variable; affected animals had been fed a variety of different diets from different manufacturers; in reviewing all cases known to date, no dietary link could be made based on types of food fed.

Clinical signs and physical examination findings

Onset of clinical signs is typically acute, and usually includes fever (103–108°F) and lethargy. Patients may become weak and demonstrate paresis or ataxia in some cases. Pain response may be elicited on palpation in many cases, especially over the rear portion of the body (lumbar region). Anorexia may be present initially or in later stages of the illness; weight loss and dehydration may occur due to decreased food and water intake. Stool characteristics are inconsistent but may include diarrhoea of variable color. Some patients begin to show a preference for soft food instead of kibble, perhaps due to waning appetite or to masseter muscle pain. Tachycardia and/or heart murmurs may be present. Mild serous nasal/ocular discharge may be seen. Pinpoint orange discolourations may be present on the skin of the trunk. Mentation typically remains normal even in weak patients, but occasional seizures have been documented. Some individuals have one or more enlarged peripheral lymph nodes, but not a generalized lymphadenopathy. Some weak and debilitated patients showed evidence of secondary sepsis shortly before death, evidenced by a sudden decline in condition, red-flushed mucous membranes, hyperpnoea, sudden increase in body temperature and weakness. Predictably, histopathology in these patients revealed occasional rod bacteria in some tissue samples, consistent with sepsis, but these were not found in most individuals who died of DIM.

Clinical pathology findings

Severe leukocytosis consisting primarily of neutrophilia is the most significant finding in DIM cases. Although the white cell count may be normal very early in the disease process, the neutrophil count typically shows progressive and dramatic elevations within the first 10–14 days of the illness. The normal total WBC range in ferrets is 2500–7500 (8000)/μL. Even in cases with severe sepsis, the total white cell count rarely exceeds 14–16 000/μL. Ferrets with DIM generate neutrophil counts of extraordinary magnitude, often as high as 40–60 000/μL; one case exceeded 100 000/μL. This finding alone suggests an unusual disease process at work, as ferrets usually seem incapable of producing these neutrophil counts in response to any septic condition we have encountered.

Ferrets with DIM may also demonstrate mild to moderate anaemia, often non-regenerative in the early stages of the disease, later becoming regenerative. Serum chemistries are in general unremarkable and inconsistent from case to case; one finding worth noting is that even with severe myositis (histopathologically confirmed) this disease does *not* typically produce CK elevations.

Histopathology findings

Histopathology performed by Dr Mike Garner (see p. 212) revealed significant findings. Most prominent was a widely disseminated suppurative to pyogranulomatous polymyositis, involving most muscle groups of the body, even periocular and cardiac muscles. The oesophagus appears to be the most heavily affected tissue; lumbar and rear limb muscles are also severely inflamed. Cardiac myositis is prominent as well. Granulomatous to pyogranulomatous lymphadenitis has been noted in ferrets who demonstrated peripheral lymphadenopathy. No infectious agents were visualized in lymph node or muscle specimens. As mentioned previously, a few cases wherein secondary sepsis was suspected did demonstrate a low number of rod bacteria in various tissue specimens post mortem. These bacteria were not present in muscle or lymph node specimens and were considered consistent with secondary sepsis due to debility; culture revealed common bacterial species with little resistance to common antibiotics. Other findings include pneumonia, splenic extramedullary haematopoiesis and myeloid hyperplasia of the spleen and/or bone marrow. In addition to standard cytologic staining, tissues were also examined using Warthin–Starry (silver) stain, B&B stain, Gimenez stain, acid-fast stain, fungal cytochemical stains and protozoal histochemical stains. None have revealed infectious agents in the lesions. Electron microscopy was performed on two cases with negative findings.

Miscellaneous tests

Radiography and ultrasonography have yielded no significant findings. Laparotomy typically reveals no gross abnormalities. Urinalysis is unremarkable. Virus isolation was performed on one case with negative findings. One case was rabies tested and was negative. Viral serology for Aleutian disease virus and canine distemper virus was also performed on a few cases and results were negative.

Attempted treatments

Numerous antibiotic regimens utilizing most classes of antibiotics have consistently failed to produce clinical improvement or resolution of leukocytosis. These include penicillins, cephalosporins, fluoroquinolones, doxycycline, clarithromycin, azithromycin, trimethoprim-sulfa, aminoglycosides, metronidazole and chloramphenicol. Similarly, antifungal agents, steroidal and nonsteroidal anti-inflammatory drugs, vitamins, antihistamines and supportive care have all failed to produce prolonged clinical improvement. Immunosuppressive therapy utilizing high dose prednisone, cyclophosphamide or cyclosporine has failed to produce consistent response. One of our cases seemed to respond to alpha interferon and was in total clinical remission for 1 month, but later relapsed and died. One suspected case (not definitively confirmed with histopathology) seems to be currently stable on a combination of cyclosporine and ketoconazole. However, nearly all cases progress in severity and die or are euthanized; progression varies from days to several months. All histologically confirmed cases to date have died.

Discussion

The aetiology of DIM is not currently known. The general disease process is a strong inflammatory response aimed primarily at muscle groups, affecting young ferrets. Therefore, there is an immune-mediated component; whether there is an infectious agent inciting the inflammatory response is less clear. Contagion between exposed ferrets has not been demonstrated. There may be genetic factors predisposing some ferrets to this condition, even if an infectious agent is partially responsible. In other species, dysregulation of neutrophils and dysfunction of adhesion molecules have sometimes been shown to cause dramatic elevations in white cell counts.

Vaccine-induced immune response must be considered as well; some vaccines in humans have been shown to induce myositis, polyarthritis, uveitis and autoimmune reactions.[40–42] Granulomas or abscesses can be induced locally by vaccine adjuvants.[40] Ferrets tend to have a fairly high incidence of vaccine reactions including anaphylaxis. All confirmed DIM cases to date have received at least one dose of canine distemper vaccine.

The suppurative to pyogranulomatous nature of the inflammation suggests a bacterial or rickettsial aetiology, but no such organisms have been detected in muscle or lymph node lesions. The complete lack of response to numerous antibiotics also makes these aetiologies less likely. Rickettsia may elude detection more easily than bacteria, so cannot be completely ruled out. Negative electron microscopy and virus isolation studies are inconclusive. Low viral numbers and difficulty with detection of some viruses can produce negative results even in the face of viral infection. Only a few cases have had EM and virus isolations studies, so no conclusions can yet be drawn regarding a viral aetiology at this time. Prions and protozoa tend not to incite a neutrophilic inflammation; fungal infection is unlikely due to lack of visualization of fungal elements with special staining.

Suggested diagnostics and treatments

Young ferrets (ages 3–21 months) which present with acute onset of fever, lethargy, weakness or lumbar pain must be considered as possible DIM cases. The main rule-outs would be acute bacterial sepsis (such as that induced by an intestinal foreign body with bowel perforation or suppurative hepatitis, etc.) and possibly acute coronavirus infection. Canine distemper virus could also mimic these initial signs, but is far less common and should only be considered in unvaccinated ferrets. One or two enlarged firm peripheral lymph nodes would also be suspicious for DIM; lymphoma would be a differential diagnosis.

Initial therapy should include appropriate supportive care, and broad spectrum antibiotics such as enrofloxacin (5–10 mg/kg i.m or p.o. b.i.d) and amoxicillin (10–20 mg/kg s.q., i.m. or p.o. b.i.d); these can help prevent secondary sepsis in severe DIM cases as well. Failure to respond rapidly to antibiotic therapy, combined with failure to localize an infectious event such as a bowel blockage or hepatitis, should increase the index of suspicion for DIM.

Initial diagnostics should include a CBC and complete serum chemistries, including serum lipase, globulin, glucose, ALT, GGT, BUN, creatinine, CK, albumin, calcium and phosphorous. Serum lipase elevation may suggest gastroenteritis (see Inflammatory bowel disease, Ch. 9); severe ALT and GGT elevations may suggest suppurative hepatitis (see Hepatitis, Ch. 9). Moderate to severe leukocytosis with neutrophilia is consistent with DIM, especially if other findings are mostly normal. If neutrophilia is not present or is not extreme, i.e. <12 000/µL, then a follow-up CBC should be performed 5–7 days after the initial blood profile; in many cases the neutrophilia will have markedly increased during that time. Neutrophil counts exceeding 14 000/µL are highly suspicious for DIM.

In cases with non-responding idiopathic pyrexia and/or pronounced neutrophilia, a muscle biopsy should ideally be performed when the patient is stable enough for a brief anaesthetic procedure. The best muscles to biopsy ante-mortem, based on severity of pathology in past cases, would be rear leg or lumbar muscles. Oesophageal muscle has the most consistently severe lesions but is not practical to biopsy except on post mortem exam. If peripheral lymphadenopathy is present, a lymph node biopsy should be performed. Biopsy samples should be preserved in formalin, with additional samples sent for bacterial culture and sensitivity if possible. The author recommends samples be sent to Dr Mike Garner at Northwest ZooPath (near Seattle, Washington, USA) as he has been evaluating tissues samples from multiple cases from the time they first recognized the syndrome. Ideally, the practitioner submitting tissues should contact Dr Garner regarding any need for additional tissue samples (besides formalin-fixed tissues) that he may use for other testing modalities.

Based on evidence to date, the most promising treatment protocols may involve immune-suppressing or immune modulating therapies; however, case numbers are limited using treatments such as cyclosporine + ketoconazole and no solid conclusions regarding the efficacy of such therapy can be drawn. That said, the nearly 100% mortality rate in confirmed DIM cases leads us to the conclusion that little stands to be lost in trying new treatments. Research is ongoing to unravel the aetiology (and possible prevention or treatment) of this severe and emerging disease syndrome.

References

1. Jenkins J, Brown SA. A practitioner's guide to rabbits and ferrets. Lakewood, CO: The American Animal Hospital Association; 1993.
2. Kociba G, Caputo CA. Aplastic anaemia associated with estrus in pet ferrets. J Am Vet Med Assoc 1981; 178:1293–1294.
3. Sherrill A, Gorham J. Bone marrow hypoplasia associated with estrus in ferrets. Lab Anim Sci 1985; 35:280–286.
4. Lewington JH. Ferrets. Vade Mecum, Series C No. 10, University of Sydney: Postgraduate Foundation; 1988.
5. Bernard SL, Leathers CW, Brobst DF, et al. Estrogen-induced bone marrow depression in ferrets. Am J Vet Res 1983; 44:657–661.
6. Fox JG, Pearson RC, Bell JA. Diseases of the genitourinary system. In: Fox JG, ed. Biology and diseases of the ferret, 2nd edn. Baltimore: Williams & Wilkins; 1998:247–272.
7. Hillyer EV. Urinogenital diseases. In: Hillyer EV, Quesenberry KE, eds. Ferrets, rabbits and rodents: Clinical medicine and surgery. Philadelphia: Saunders; 1997:44–52.
8. Oxenham M. Oestrous control in the ferret. Vet Rec 1990; 10:148.
9. Oxenham M. Ferrets. In: Beynon PA, Cooper JE, eds. Manual of exotic pets. London: British Small Animal Veterinary Association Publications; 1996:97–108.
10. Ryland LM. Remission of estrus-associated anaemia following ovariohysterectomy and multiple blood transfusions in the ferret. J Am Vet Med Assoc 1982; 181:820–822.
11. Howard JW. Control of oestrus in ferrets. Vet Rec 1979; 104.
12. Bell J. Infectious diseases of ferrets. Orlando: Proc North Am Vet Conf; 1993.
13. Animal Health Division. Diseases of fitch. Surveillance. New Zealand: Ministry of Agriculture and Fisheries; 1984: 11:2.
14. Gentz EJ, Veatch JK. Cystic ovarian remnant in a ferret. J Small Exot Anim Med 1995; 3:45–47.
15. Bell J. New medical treatment for pyometra in the breeding jill. Medical news. Am Ferret Rep 2000; 11(3):8–9.
16. Rosenthal K. Ferrets. Vet Clin North Am Small Anim Pract 1994; 24:1–23.
17. Dillberger JE. Polycystic kidneys in a ferret. J Am Vet Med Assoc 1985; 1:74–75.
18. Ryan CP. Polycystic disease of the kidney in a striped skunk and Mongolian gerbil. Vet Med Small Anim Clin 1981; 76:1351–1354.
19. Weiss C. The 'flat ferret' syndrome. American Ferret Association. Am Ferret Rep 1996; 7:11.
20. Nelson WB. Hydronephrosis in a ferret. Vet Med 1984; April.
21. Lewington JH. Antibiotics in use for ferrets: A review. University of Sydney: Postgraduate Foundation. Control Ther Ser 1996; 193:901–902.
22. Cowgill L, Adams LG. Renal failure: acute & renal failure: chronic. In: Tilly LP, Smith FWK Jr, eds. The 5-minute veterinary consult, canine and feline. Baltimore: Williams & Wilkins; 1997: 1016–1018.
23. Senior D. Disorders of the urinary system. In: Wills J, Wolf A, eds. Handbook of feline medicine. Oxford: Pergamon Press; 1993:193–211.
24. Kawasaki T. Creatinine unreliable indicator of renal failure in ferrets. J Small Exot Anim Med 1993; 1.
25. Esteves M, Marini RP, Ryden EB, et al. Estimation of glomerular filtration rate and evaluation of renal function in ferrets. Am J Vet Res 1994; 55:166–172.
26. Finkler M. Practical Ferret Medicine and Surgery for the Private Practitioner. Roanoak, Virginia: Roanoak Animal Hospital; 1999.
27. Markwell PJ. Dietary management of renal failure in dog and cat. Waltham Focus 1998; 8:16–21.
28. Hammond JJ, Chesterman FC, eds. The ferret. In: UFAW Handbook on the Care and Management of Laboratory Animals. Edinburgh: Churchill Livingstone; 1972.
29. Fraser CM, ed. Urinary infections and urolithiasis in bacterial diseases of mink. In: The Merck veterinary manual, 7th edn. Rahway: Merck; 1991:1052.
30. Nguyen HT, Moreland AF, Shields RP. Urolithiasis in ferrets (*Mustela putorius*). Lab Anim Sci 1979; 29:243–245.
31. Weisse C, Aronson LR, Drobatz K. Traumatic rupture of the ureter:10 cases. J Am Anim Hosp Assoc 2002; 38:188–192.
32. Miller MS. Ferret cardiology. Proc North Am Vet Assoc 1993; 735.
33. Stamoulis ME, Miller MS, Hillyer EV. Cardiovascular disease. In: Hillyer EV, Quesenberry KE, eds. Ferrets, rabbits and rodents: Clinical medicine and surgery. Philadelphia: Saunders; 1997:63–76.
34. Bone L, Battles AH, Goldfarb RD, et al. Electrocardiographic values from clinically-normal anaesthetized ferrets (*Mustela putorius furo*). Am J Vet Res 1988; 49:1884–1887.
35. Smith SH, Bishop SP. The electrocardiogram of normal ferrets and ferrets with right ventricular hypertrophy. Lab Anim Sci 1985; 35:268–271.
36. Martin M. ECG Interpretation in small animals. (1),(2),(3) In Practice 2002; March, April, May.
37. Lipman NS, Murphy JC, Fox JG. Clinical, functional and pathologic changes associated with a case of dilative cardiomyopathy in a ferret. Lab Anim Sci 1987; 37:210–212.
38. Greenie PG, Stephens E. Meningeal cryptococcosis and congestive cardiomyopathy in a ferret. J Am Vet Med Assoc 1984; 184:840–841.

CHAPTER ELEVEN
Diseases of special concern

39. Antinoff N. Musculoskeletal and neurologic disease. In: Hillyer EV, Quesenberry KE, eds. Ferrets, rabbits and rodents. Clinical medicine and surgery. Philadelphia: WB Saunders; 1997: 126–130.
40. Green CE. Immunoprophylaxis and immunotherapy. In: Green CE, ed. Infectious diseases of the dog and cat. Philadelphia: WB Saunders; 1998.
41. Jani FM, Gray JP. Influenza vaccine and dermatomyositis. Vaccine 1994; 15.
42. Hanissian AS, Martinez AJ, Jabbour JT, Duenas DA. Vasculitis and myositis secondary to rubella vaccination. Arch Neurol 1973; 3:202–204.

CHAPTER 12

Diseases of the ferret ear, eye and nose

'Those who go poaching with ferrets choose a moonlight night; if it is dark it is difficult to find the holes.'

Richard Jefferies, The Amateur Poacher, 1879

The domestic ferret (Fig. 12.1) is highly adapted to nocturnal hunting but the organs of special sense; the ears, eyes and nose of the ferret have conditions that challenge the practitioner. The term 'rare occurrence' for a number of problems might make the practitioner dismiss the subject to the back of a list to be studied – until the 'rare occurrence' occurs in one's own pet ferrets. I had the occurrence of idiopathic otitis interna, galactose-induced cataracts and nasal/meningeal *Cryptococcus neoformans* in my ferret colony. For that reason, I have a sharp interest in these diseases and will illustrate here the practical results of the three 'rare occurrences'.

The special anatomy of the ferret ears, eyes and nose is not dealt with specifically as a whole in any ferret book to date. Basic comparative anatomy can be found in *Guide to Dissection of the Dog* by H.E. Evans and A. de la Hunta, 6th edn. 2004. Details of the neuroanatomy of the optic tract and of the nasal conchae are in the excellent 2nd edn. of James Fox's *Biology and Diseases of the Ferret* (1998), which details the physiology of the visual and auditory systems in respect to their use in biomedical research, as a model of those senses in humans.

The ferret auditory sense

Ferrets are unfortunately still used in biomedical research and have been involved in experiments on hearing, including the effects of viruses on the inner ear,[1] e.g. Reye's syndrome in humans. The question of deafness in ferrets worries ferret owners, but usually ferrets have acute hearing and a keen sense of smell for hunting, while their sight is more adapted to their nocturnal habit.

Deafness

In the domestic ferret, deafness is fairly common especially in animals having some degree of whiteness in their coats (Ch. 5). It is described as the Waardenburg syndrome and is a dominant genetic defect resulting from the underdevelopment of the inner ear. In North America, it is estimated that approximately 75% of all the ferrets with blaze and panda colourations are affected. 'Blue-eyed' ferrets are also affected. Deafness can be confirmed with the brain stem auditory evoked response (BAER). This syndrome is supposed to be different to that in albino ferrets, which although able to hear, have an abnormally small hearing mechanism in their middle and inner ear (Dr C. Whiteside, Calgary Zoo Animal Health Centre, pers. comm. 2005).

A ferret jill has been recorded as deaf when repeatedly ignoring a crying kitten (Amy Flemming, pers. comm. 1999). She has recorded the condition in a Western Australian black-eyed white hob taken to the USA and considered it the Waardenburg syndrome. Normally, the ferret kitten gains its hearing ability at about 32 days old, in contrast to cats, which hear at 6 days; this is determined by response to a loud clap. It is found that both the auditory and visual senses appear to become functional at about 30 days and this relates to the interaction of the two systems.[2] The BAER test is used on cats, dogs and many other species and would be

CHAPTER TWELVE

Diseases of the ferret ear, eye and nose

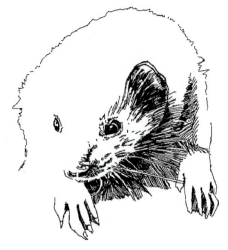

Figure 12.1 Ferret face (by Debbie Squance, 1999).

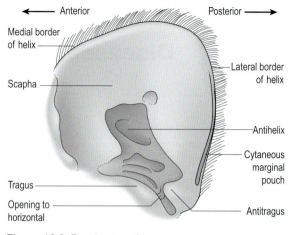

Figure 12.2 Ferret external ear.

the same for ferrets in terms of physiology and pathology (Dr Strain, Louisiana State University, pers. comm. 1999).

Features of ear anatomy

The external ear (Fig. 12.2) of the ferret consists of an auricle (pinna) and an external ear canal, which differ markedly in shape from that of the dog and cat. The ferret pinna is set close to the head and half-moon-shaped, some 2 cm wide in adult hobs and pointing forward, as the animal requires excellent hearing for hunting rabbits (ferreting). Some ferrets have a flatter, wider pinna, large compared with the head size and this is possibly a congenital breeding fault.

There is no distinct tubular ear canal as in the dog and cat. A screen of fine hairs around the anterior margin protects the whole ear canal. One interesting feature, the lateral margin of the ear canal has a more pronounced recession, intertragic incisure-like, which is more tube-shaped than seen in the cat and some 5 mm

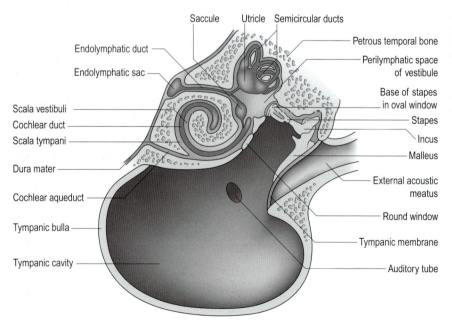

Figure 12.3 Diagram of the structure of the middle and inner ear of the dog. (From Getty R, Foust HL, Presley ET, Miller ME. Macroscopic anatomy of the ear of the dog. Am J Vet Res 1956; 17:364–375, with permission.)

Diseases of the ferret ear

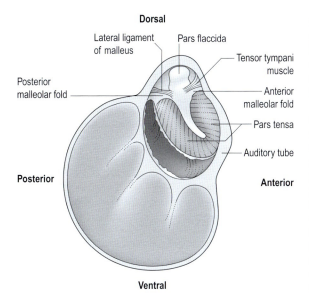

Figure 12.4 Diagram of the medial face of the lateral wall of the left tympanic cavity of the dog. (From Spreull JSA. Otitis media in the dog. In: Kirk RW, ed. Current veterinary therapy V. Philadelphia: WB Saunders; 1976, with permission.)

long. It gives the impression of a miniature aural resection.[3] Almost opposite, medial, to the base of the intertragic incisure, is the opening of the horizontal canal, which passes anteromedially to the tympanic membrane. There is hardly any depth to it. One feels that some foreign material might easily get into the 'resected' ear canal when the ferret is digging. However, whether the shape of the ferret external ear makes it prone to otitis has not been shown.

The middle and inner ear can be compared with that of the dog in general structure and this is shown in Figures 12.3 and 12.4.

Diseases of the ferret ear

Otitis externa

This can occur in the case of fight wounds involving the pinna caused by hobs fighting in the mating season, or in advanced cases of foot mange in all ferrets. Treatment of the former involves antibiotics and possibly surgery with the ferret sedated or anaesthetized. A primary otitis externa of the ear canal caused by ear mites (*Otodectes cynotis*) is common in ferrets as in dogs and cats (Ch. 8). Treatment is with an acaricide drug. Yeasts such as *Malassezia* can be associated with ear mites as opportunistic pathogens and need to be treated by a wide-spectrum aural preparation. Care must be taken with handling the small ferret ear and possibly ototoxic drugs should be used for a minimum time only. Olive oil is safe to soften earwax and normal saline can be used by pipette to flush the ear canal.

Severe *Malassezia* infections can cause crusting and necrosis of the pinnae in association with ear mites and they may spread to the ferret face. In eight ferrets seen in the UK, despite treatment with betamethasone, neomycin and monosulfiram, the infected areas of the pinnae had to be cut away (G. MacGregor-Skinner, pers. comm. 1998). The infected areas showed inflammatory cells and yeasts beneath the corneum but no acanthosis. The suggested treatment is by oral ketoconazole, 5–10 mg/kg b.i.d. and topical dressing with miconazole, polymyxin B and prednisolone. All ferrets, dogs and cats in contact should be treated. The length of treatment should be monitored for any possible toxic effects of drugs used.[4]

Otitis media

This can be caused by ear mite infection (*Otodectes cynotis*); inflammation of the tympanic membrane can cause inner ear infections. In New Zealand fitch farms, otitis media was found to be common in adults in a 1984 survey with four farms showing an incidence ranging from 0.3% to 30%.[5] In these cases the fungus *Absidia corymbifera (syn. ramosa)* appeared to be the causative agent along with ear mites. *Absidia corymbifera* is normally not found in ears but is in the environment, so the pathogenesis of the disease is unclear.

Presumably, there is an external ear canal contamination by fungi from the bedding if it is hay or straw. I personally do not like ferrets bedded in straw or hay for many reasons but with large numbers of animals, the husbandry can be difficult to standardize without resorting to these materials. Mouldy bedding must be removed frequently. *Absidia corymbifera*, probably in combination with the external ear canal ear mite, can cause a dermatomycosis and tympanic membrane inflammation and even rupture, with invasion of the middle ear and possibly the cranium, meninges and brain. The clinical signs may not be specific and with high numbers of ferrets in fitch farms, might have gone undiagnosed. Signs of head shaking with ear mites and ear scratching give an indication, plus possibly a discharge from the ear. The ferret may be lethargic and depressed. The lymph nodes in the region commonly show a lymphadenitis. With inner ear involvement, the head tilts to the side of lesion and there may be loss of balance with circling, leading finally to prostration and death from toxaemia.

CHAPTER TWELVE

Diseases of the ferret ear, eye and nose

The ear pathology shows debris in the external auditory canal with mites and fungi present. Pus is possibly in the middle ear and tympanic bulla, with the tympanic membrane sometimes ruptured, and if not, badly inflamed. Necrosis and granulomatous inflammation of the petrous temporal bone can be evident, and the disease can lead to a granulomatous meningoencephalitis with vasculitis and thrombosis. The fungal lesions can be found in the temporal and pyriform lobes of the cerebrum and in the adjoining areas of the cerebellum and brain stem. The disease can be confirmed by checking the ear mites and fungal hyphae under the microscope or by a lymph gland aspirate or at postmortem. It should be noted that there appears to be a complex relationship between mite and fungus and of course fungi are encouraged to grow where antibiotics have been used. This is a difficult problem, as antimycotics used to kill the fungus are either required long term or are ototoxic or nephrotoxic. It is a question of which is doing the most damage, the mite or the fungus. In the case of ear mites, I wonder if there is a toxicity factor, which makes the ferret moribund. Fungal diseases in many cases have a preference for brain tissue, where the blood supply is of course high and the fungus reaches the brain by the quickest route, via either the ear or nasal cavity (see *Cryptococcus* infections). Routine treatment for ear mites should be carried out on all ferrets living inside or outside (Ch. 10). In laboratory and breeding establishments, strict hygiene should be maintained to prevent this dangerous disease combination of ear mite and fungus.

Otitis interna

This is suggested as an uncommon disease of ferrets. The causative agent might be difficult to pin down, but is possibly spread from otitis media. In reference to a laboratory ferret colony infested with ear mites, one ferret showed signs of circling and ataxia and possibly had secondary otitis interna from the middle ear *Otodectes* infection.[6] The ferret was cleared of mites and given chloramphenicol for bacterial infection and the condition resolved, but no recovery time was given. Otitis interna is possible in ferrets and is alarming, as it can be dramatic in appearance. It is also termed idiopathic otitis interna (IOI) where the cause is not certain. The vestibular system is disturbed and the common signs in dogs and cats are head tilt, circling and nystagmus.[7] It is stated that because of the dramatic and characteristic clinical signs associated with otitis interna, it is more commonly and easily diagnosed in dogs and cats than otitis media. This is also the case with ferrets, though the incidence is low but very alarming to the ferret owner when it does occur.

Author's clinical example

These signs were seen in my 5-year-old vasectomized albino hob, Hoppy, with IOI (Fig. 12.5). No mites were seen in aural swabs. In comparison, dogs with acute cases are severely disorientated, may circle around, fall on the affected side and be practically unable to walk normally. In Hoppy's case, he showed a sudden onset of incoordination, circling to the right, head tilt to the right, inability to right himself and a horizontal nystagmus. On examination, the right tympanic membrane appeared reddened compared with the left. After several days, the signs become less pronounced and the nystagmus may disappear. This occurred with Hoppy, who vomited once, was depressed and felt hot on first examination. There was no effect on the hearing centre.[9] A full blood check showed a lymphopaenia.

The actual vomitus on culture revealed *Salmonella*, which was suspected to be from a kangaroo meat source and could initiate a systemic infection of the inner ear. Hoppy did not have a full *Salmonella* illness with continuous vomiting and diarrhoea (Ch. 8). In dogs, in addition, to otitis media, there may be signs of facial nerve paralysis, otitis externa or keratitis, but this did not happen with Hoppy.

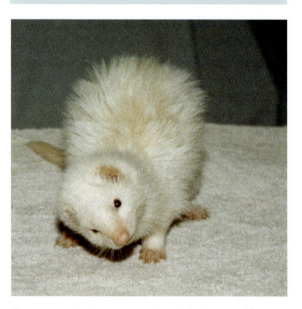

Figure 12.5 Albino vasectomized hob, Hoppy, with idiopathic otitis interna (IOI).

Aetiology

It is sometimes not known which organisms are commonly involved in otitis interna but they possibly arise from a concurrent otitis media. The most common

Table 12.1 Distinguishing signs of peripheral and vestibular inner ear disease

Signs	Peripheral	Central
Head tilt, circling, rolling, falling, positional strabismus	+	+
Spontaneous nystagmus	Horizontal or rotary	Horizontal, rotary or vertical
Positional nystagmus	Type does not vary with position	Type varies with position
Gait	Leans to side of lesion	Mild to severe ataxia weakness
Conscious proprioception	Normal	Delayed or absent
Other cranial nerves affected.	VII	V, VI, VII
Cerebellar signs	–	Hypermetria, head bobbing, Intention tremors

+, may be present; –, absent
Table from Shell, 1988, with permission.[8]

route of infection of the inner ear apparatus is via the tympanic membrane. Working ferrets could get ear mites from infected rabbits taken down the warrens. It is possible that otitis media may be clinically silent or the signs overlooked in the dog and cat.[8] This could be the same with ferrets. Clinical signs of idiopathic otitis interna are a head tilt to the affected side, spontaneous horizontal or rotatory nystagmus and asymmetric limb ataxia with preservation of strength.
Table 12.1 shows signs, which distinguish peripheral from vestibular disease of the inner ear in the dog and cat. They might equally relate to symptoms seen in ferrets. Table 12.1 should be kept in mind when considering ferret inner ear disease, as it is liable to nervous disorders similar to the dog (e.g. canine distemper) or the cat (*Cryptococcus neoformans*). Other disorders that affect the otic nerves or the brain stem[8] are given in Table 12.2.

Radiology of the tympanic bulla in cases of IOI is essential considering the anatomical relationship of the inner and middle ear. Thus a middle ear infection can be 'silent' but spread to the inner ear causing vestibular signs.[8] With my IOI case, the skull of the affected ferret was compared to an unaffected hob of the same size. It showed an increased density of the tympanic bulla on the affected side in the sick ferret, which indicated otitis media.[9]

Treatment

The treatment of idiopathic otitis interna parallels that of otitis media. The middle ear is checked to be clean of fluids before treatment commences using an auroscope and radiology.[8] Consideration must be given about ototoxicity of drugs in animals and man. One author advised treating dogs and cats using possibly cephalosporins, chloramphenicol or trimethoprim-sulfa drugs.[8] The course is of 3–4 weeks duration. There is now a range of potentially ototoxic agents tabled[10] mainly considered toxic to humans and stimulating animal tests. The list is evidently growing. I have used chloramphenicol (0.25 mL b.i.d.) over 3 weeks as a drug of choice. Unfortunately, the syrup form is not available but the injectable drug can be given by mouth with a strong sugar solution against the bitter taste. Chloramphenicol has caused ototoxic symptoms with a guinea pig but only when applied directly to the tympanic membrane.[10]

Theoretically, antibiotic cover should be based on a culture from the external or middle ear and blood checks may be required for suspected blood-borne pathogens. With Hoppy, vomitus and meat were cultured, giving *Salmonella* growth, indicating a possible blood-borne infection to the ear.[9] In severe cases of otitis interna

Table 12.2 Disorders which affect the otic nerves or brain stem

Peripheral vestibular disease possibilities (conditions affecting the vestibule cochlear nerve or inner ear structures)	Central vestibular disease possibilities (conditions affecting the brain stem nuclei)
a. Otitis media	a. Canine distemper: remember ferrets can get canine distemper from dogs, foxes, dingoes
b. Idiopathic vestibular syndrome (in old dogs so perhaps old ferrets?)	b. Reticulosis
c. Ototoxic drugs	c. Vascular accidents
d. Trauma	d. Trauma
e. Neoplasia	e. Neoplasia
f. Metabolic polyneuropathies	

CHAPTER TWELVE

Diseases of the ferret ear, eye and nose

associated with otitis media in dogs, the protocol is to correct the otitis media, even to the extent of an incision of the inflamed tympanic membrane (myringotomy). The process allows for exudate samples to be obtained and the middle ear cavity irrigated. There is no record of this being attempted with a ferret. It is stated that the tympanic membrane remarkably seals over once the otitis media is resolved.[8] In general treatment of IOI, the systemic corticosteroids can be used but are best avoided. The drug would help in the short term to reduce inflammation of the vestibular, cochlear and facial nerves. Topical corticosteroids may be dangerous if the tympanic membrane is ruptured, so toxicity of topical ear drugs should be borne in mind at all times with prolonged use. The structure of the middle and inner ear has been revised with relevance to the treatment of idiopathic otitis interna and is shown in Figures 12.3 and 12.4.

Initiation of an inner ear crisis

The three considered routes of infection or toxic damage to the inner ear are:

1. Across the tympanic membrane by an inflammatory response due to a foreign body or mite infestation. No doubt the otodectic mite inflames the tympanic membrane and possibly extrudes toxins, which I consider dulls the ferret. Inflammation, necrosis and rupture of the tympanic membrane can be a sequel.[8] The eardrum must be examined and with the ferret this would possibly require a general anaesthetic.
2. The auditory tube, which connects the nasopharynx to the middle ear, can be a passage for pharyngeal infections to the ear. Human influenza and para-influenza viruses give rise to inner ear disease in humans.[1] Thus ferrets, which are susceptible to human influenza and other respiratory diseases, could get infected ears by that route. Bacterial organisms such as haemolytic *Streptococcus* and other organisms involved in ferret 'snuffles' could be culprits.
3. Blood-borne infections cannot be ruled out. I have experienced that with my ferret Hoppy.[9] Hobs with IOI conditions may have been with jills having vaginal infections of a haemolytic *Streptococcus* or *Staphylococcus*, so these organisms could be the basis of infection through intercourse and the hob then grooming itself.

Prognosis: This is good if the IOI case is caught early enough. There might be resulting minor vestibular deficits with a slight head tilt, like Hoppy, or mild ataxia remaining after the antibiotic treatment.[9] In chronic cases there might be chance of osteomyelitis of the osseous bulla and petrous temporal bone with a graver prognosis. If the infections ascend the vestibular, cochlear and facial nerves to the brain stem, a brain stem abscess or meningitis may arise, causing similar effects to fungal invasion with *Cryptococcus neoformans* (see nasal section). The central vestibular signs of depression and loss of strength occur and can progress to the rapid death of the ferret (Table 12.2). In other animals, a bilateral otitis interna has been shown to destroy the auditory receptors and produce irreversible deafness.[10] This could also occur in ferrets.

Note: there are two possible aetiological effects here. The *Otodectes cynotis* mite caused inflammation of the tympanic membrane plus a toxin excretion or there was a toxicity effect of the Apex drops which contain polymyxin B sulphate 10 000 units, nitrofurazone 2.6 mg, neomycin sulphate 5.0 mg, lidocaine hydrochloride 2.5 mg and pyrethrins 0.5 mg. Neomycin is one of the aminoglycoside antibiotics, which are potentially ototoxic and nephrotoxic if used over long periods.[12] Others are streptomycin, kanamycin and gentamicin, which should be avoided in ferrets. The ototoxic effect results in the degeneration of the hair cells with hearing loss and/or vestibular dysfunction. Ototoxicity is a serious and complex problem with all animals and man. There are many suspect ototoxic agents in the literature and they have been highlighted in studies with guinea pigs, dogs, cats and chinchilla rabbits, basically concerned with the risks of ototoxicity in humans. One author is of

Author's clinical example

An 8-month-old de-sexed sable jill, Pipa, was treated for ear mites with Apex ear drops (Apex Laboratories, NSW) twice daily for a few days.[11] She had shown distinct signs of ear rubbing on the floor and the pinnae and periauricular regions were erythematous. She was seen 14 days later with ear mites still present and given a repeat dose of Apex drops. In another 14 days, Pipa was seen with vestibular signs of circling, falling to the left and general incoordination. The left head tilt was pronounced and she had a 40.8°C temperature. On examination of the ear, only a few mites were seen but there was a bulging tympanic membrane of the left ear so a diagnosis of otitis media and otitis interna was made. The ferret was switched to treatment for mites with Ivomec (ivermectin 10 mg/mL MSD) at 400 µg/kg s.c. and amoxicillin/clavulanic acid combination (Clavulox palatable drops, Pfizer) for the possible infection at 12.5 mg/kg p.o. b.i.d. As a result, the temperature returned to normal in 48 hours and the neurological signs improved over 2 weeks to a complete recovery of the ferret.

the opinion that toxicity in small animals is rare but warns that we should be cautious when using ototoxic agents.[10]

The ferret ophthalmic sense

The ferret's eyesight is poor compared with its senses of smell and hearing. It is really a nocturnal animal like its polecat ancestor.[13] Studies of the ferret visual system have been orientated to such problems as the influence of photo-periods on reproduction, albinism and its effects on ocular development and various studies on ferret neuro-ophthalmic development and basic investigation relevant to human eye problem research.[14] The visual systems are studied using the very immature state of newborn ferret visual systems.[15]

The examination of the ferret eye is carried out similarly to the dog and cat and tests can be performed except the Schirmer tear test. The eye is examined with the help of a magnifying headband lupe and for internal eye examination, an ophthalmoscope in a dark room.

One author advocates the use of indirect ophthalmoscopy plus a 30- or 40-dioptre (D) condensing lens.[14] I have had ferrets examined by an eye specialist who used a slit lamp biomicroscope.

Ferret eye anatomy

The development of the ferret eye has been studied in detail in the past. Two authors examined the development of orientation selectivity in the visual cortex.[16] They concluded the maturation of orientation selective response requires neuronal activity and that normal development requires light stimulation.

Features of ferret eye anatomy (Fig. 12.6) include a well-developed third eyelid, which can be used for a third eyelid flap for ulcer treatment as in the dog and cat.[17] The cornea is relatively large in relation to the eye structure and the lens is nearly spherical and placed back in the posterior eye chamber.[14] The pupil is a horizontal elliptical slit, not like the vertical slit in the cat, and more efficiently protects the eye from strong sunlight. The retina is similar in form and vascular

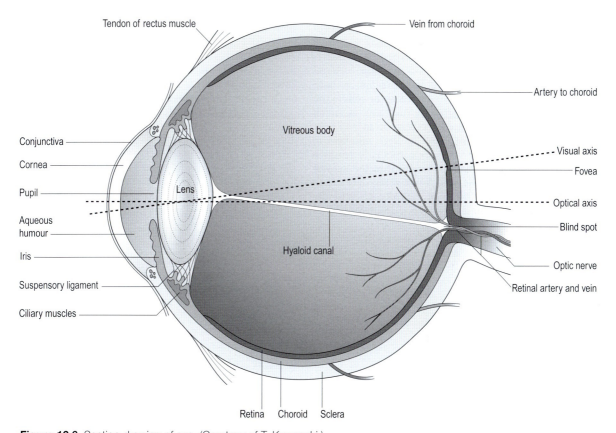

Figure 12.6 Section drawing of eye. (Courtesy of T. Kawasaki.)

CHAPTER TWELVE

Diseases of the ferret ear, eye and nose

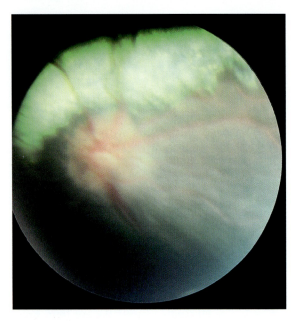

Figure 12.7 Normal sable retina. (Courtesy of T. Kawasaki.)

The ferret, along with other mustelids, using the combination of a large cornea, spherical lens and a tapetum lucidum highly receptive to dim light, is well-adapted to nocturnal living. The tapetum gives the 'eye shine' glow to nocturnal animals caught in a torch beam.

Range of vision

The ferret has binocular vision, directed downwards and slightly more lateral than the polecat (*M. putorius*). The more sideways position is due to the consequences of juvenilization of the face during domestication (Ch. 6). All polecats have larger eyes than ferrets. The steppe polecat (*M. eversmanni*) has eyes slightly higher on the head to be able to scan the sky for raptors.[22] The binocular vision of the ferret is compared to other mustelids in Figure 12.8.

The visual field is only a narrow range directly in front of the ferret's face and gives a blind spot directly in front of its nose as shown by the drawing by Fara Shimbo (Fig. 12.9). The ferret can orientate its head so that the maximum visual field is maintained.[23]

Dr Carolyn King in New Zealand also outlined the adaptation of the main senses of the mustelids. The short pointed face of weasels, for instance, allows both binocular vision forward and a wide arc of monocular vision on each side.[21] One author suggests ferrets are supposed to have mostly monocular but very little binocular vision.[24] King is of the opinion that, from their facial conformation, there is no difference in the range of vision between weasels, stoats and ferrets. The eye that sees well in dim light achieves this ability at the expense of sharp acuity in bright light.[21] Thus, most carnivores see movements rather than pictures but they can be sharp-eyed on focusing in on prey. So waving a finger in front of a ferret in daytime can be dangerous. The ferret sees and responds to moving objects at speeds of 25–45 cm/s, being that of a mouse in a hurry![14] When

pattern to the dog (Fig. 12.7).[18] The tapetum is well-defined with the 7–10-cell layer containing high zinc and cysteine content and the myelinated optic disc is relatively small.[19] A study of the tapetum lucidum established that the structure is the same in both pigmented and albino ferrets.[20] The receptor cells in the retina, cones and rods differ in function, as in all animals. The cones are used for perception of bright light and colours and are found in large numbers in diurnal species, while the rods are particularly sensitive to low intensity light and are numerous in the eyes of nocturnal animals.[21] Thus the ferret retina has a high proportion of rods; in the photoreceptor layer of the ferret the rods predominate in the ratio of 50–60:1.[15]

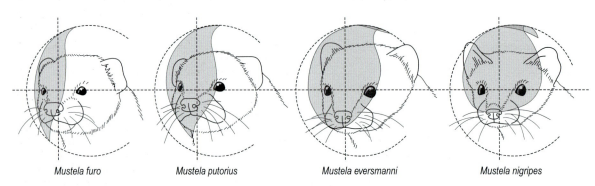

Mustela furo   Mustela putorius   Mustela eversmanni   Mustela nigripes

Figure 12.8 Approximate binocular visual fields in ferrets and polecats. (Courtesy of F. Shimbo.)

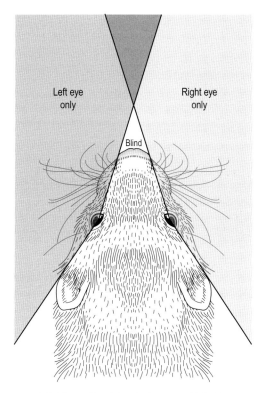

Figure 12.9 Binocular vision in ferret and blind spot. (Courtesy of F. Shimbo.)

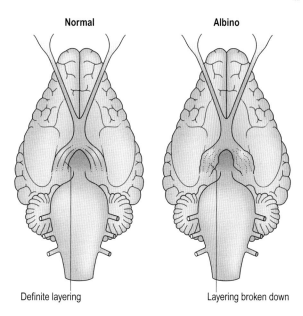

Figure 12.10 Ventral view of ferret brain showing optic chiasma and indicating suspect embryonic damage area in albino ferret. (Courtesy of F. Shimbo.)

the object is moving faster or slower the ferret is not stimulated to act but once the object is seen, the ferret goes for the anterior portion as a hunting animal would to its prey. The feral ferrets of New Zealand and the European polecat will hunt mostly by their sense of smell. The hearing and olfactory senses are more 'dominant' than sight. I have seen two free-running hob ferrets in the mating season engrossed in following the scent trails of two jills in daytime. They would pass within 20 cm of each other and not get visual contact stimulation, but when the scent of one reached the other, it would stop abruptly and attack at speed and they would have to be separated. It is said that the ferret's visual range is limited to ground level and it hunts by rapidly moving the head up and down and from side to side.[14] The ferret does this when in open ground and it goes back more to its mustelid fear of being caught in open country, where a hawk will easily take a stoat or weasel. Ferrets are heavier to be picked up by raptors, though we do have large ravens in our area, which caw loudly and make my ferrets bolt down a pipe!

The ferret's ability to see objects clearly depends of course on the optical properties of the eye, which involves the retinal sensitivity, as with other animals, and the state of the central nervous system optical processing of visual images. The retinal activity is usually the controlling factor. Optical abnormalities can occur with the ferret eye and the optical quality of this special sense organ is considered moderate. In detail, ferrets appear to be 6.8 D (range 5–8 D) hyperoptic or farsighted. Of 12 ferrets studied, four revealed astigmatism of 0.5 D or greater. Additional faults can be found in the refraction between the two eyes because of the large spherical lenses. This may show up in dim light when the pupil is dilated.[14] The ferret higher visual pathways have been extensively studied over the years.[15] On the question of perception of form, work has been done on the weasel, which can appreciate different letters in form discrimination tests (Herter 1939) to get a food reward or not from differently-labelled boxes.[21] It is said that in ferrets the image brightness might be the factor, as objects brighter than the background stimulate a more effective prey-catching behaviour than darker images.[14]

There is a difference in the layering in the visual centres of the brain between the normal ferret and albino as seen in Figure 12.10. The genetics of this has been studied with regard to crossed eyes in albinos of various species. The weak eyesight of the albino ferret is due to extreme disruption of the lateral geniculate nucleus (LGN), that part of the brain responsible for integrating input from each side of each eye to allow

CHAPTER TWELVE

Diseases of the ferret ear, eye and nose

binocular vision. In the normal pigmented ferret, the LGN is made up of orderly layers, where input from either the right or left side of each eye is received in an orderly sequenced manner. In the albino ferret this layering breaks down, the layers may be mixed, broken into leaflets, or parts missing entirely.

The brain does try to compensate whereby the erroneous input from the LGN is simply censored by the visual cortex or there is actual 'rewiring'. This was discovered by Guillery et al. (1977) in Siamese cats and also confirmed in ferrets. Thus the brain compensates by 'censoring' jumbled information;[23] Figure 12.10 indicates this.

Colour vision

The possibility of colour vision in mustelids has been raised by some authors.[22,21] The stoat and weasel for instance have retinas of mixed rods and cones typical of diurnal animals. German investigators (Herter 1939, Gewalt 1959) attempted to test for colour appreciation with common weasels but the tests were inconclusive. The stoat, however, which has a similar retina to the weasel, has been tested and can see at least red and possibly also yellow, green and blue. The ferret has not been studied as have the stoats and weasels but its retina has been compared with that of the cat and has a similar density of rods and cones and there is a suggestion that the ferret may be able to detect colour.[14] Bob Church advises that both polecats and ferrets see shades of grey while ferrets may see reds but polecats see blues and reds (Ch. 6). In any case, the detection of colour is of no real advantage in nocturnal hunting animals like mustelids. The ferret eye, in association with the visual nervous system linked to the pineal gland, is involved with reproduction and also endocrine problems. The ferret oestrous cycle is related to photo-period length. It will begin with extended photo-periods in spring and the cycles can be adapted to increasing or decreasing litters per year.[2] A blind ferret would not start oestrous. It is theorized that an artificial regime of extended photo-periods may be the cause of adrenal gland neoplasia in ferrets (see Ch. 14).

Ferrets are extremely variable when tested for depth perception. I agree with Fara Shimbo that most ferrets hate heights. They may climb up but are afraid to drop down. Fara has had experience with polecats (see Fig. 1.2) and she has found that they become hysterical when held with their head downwards. Likewise, when holding a ferret, it is best with its head upwards, against one's chest, so that it does not look towards the ground.[23]

Diseases of the ferret eye

Congenital problems can include microphthalmia, cataracts and dermoids. Infections of the eyes can occur in kittens (Ch. 5). Upper molar abscesses can show up as swellings into the eye orbit (Fig. 12.11). In the young ferret, the condition of Mittendorf's spot has been seen on examination of the vitreous body. It manifests as a small grey or white area just inferior and nasal to the posterior pole of the lens. It is a perinuclear ring which represents the remains of the lenticular attachment of the hyaloid artery. It has no effect on vision (Fig. 12.12) (T. Kawasaki, pers. comm. 2005). There can be signs of the hyaloid artery remnant. The position of the hyaloid canal is shown in Figure 12.6.

Conjunctivitis

Conjunctivitis is a common visible sign of eye impairment and can be of bacterial or viral origin. Ferret kittens

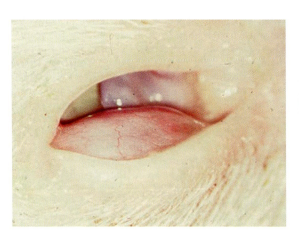

Figure 12.11 Tooth abscess effect. *Note* swollen conjunctiva. (Courtesy of T. Kawasaki.)

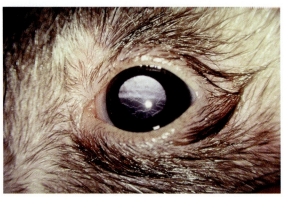

Figure 12.12 Mittendorf's dot. (Courtesy of T. Kawasaki.)

can get infected eyes with panophthalmitis from *E. coli* infections, which have been described in Chapter 5. Conjunctivitis is a major sign of infections of both canine distemper and human influenza (Ch. 8).

Chronic conjunctivitis treatment

An interesting case of an 8-month-old de-sexed male ferret with acute right eye conjunctivitis led to treatment using nasolacrimal flushing to remove an obstruction.[25] The discharge had been occurring for 3 days. An asymptomatic ferret had been added to the household; a suspect carrier? However the ferret showed no other disease symptoms; fluorescein staining was negative for ulcers and there was no foreign body found under topical anaesthesia. Thus the ferret was initially sent home on gentamicin with betamethasone topical ophthalmic drops to be administered t.i.d. The ferret eye did improve on the medications but symptoms recurred once they were stopped. It was re-checked and it was decided to do a nasolacrimal flush with culture and sensitivity of the infected tissues and radiology. Figure 12.13 shows the initial problem. The duct flushing was carried out under G/A and magnification technique.

A blunted 27 gauge needle was attached to an extension set with a 35 cc syringe containing sterile saline. *Note*: a Dremel tool with an appropriate grinding stone or nail file can be used to blunt the needle, which is sterilized in an autoclave. This set-up was used to can-

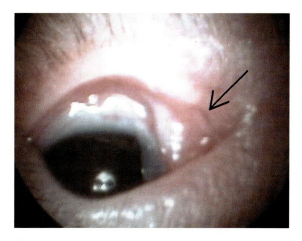

Figure 12.14 Dorsal punctum leads to nasolacrimal duct (arrow). (Courtesy of M. Conn.)

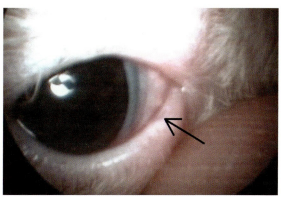

Figure 12.15 Ventral punctum leads to nasolacrimal duct (arrow). (Courtesy of M. Conn.)

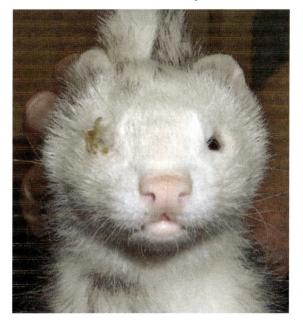

Figure 12.13 Young male ferret with unilateral mucopurulent ocular discharge. (Courtesy of M. Conn.)

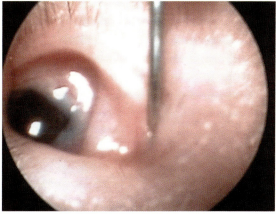

Figure 12.16 The dorsal punctum is cannulated. (Courtesy of M. Conn.)

nulate the upper dorsal punctum (Fig. 12.14) and the lower ventral punctum (Fig. 12.15).

Note: the added flexibility of movement that the extension set provides allows for the precise placement of the needle into the tiny structures and is obviously superior to attaching a syringe directly to the needle.

The dorsal and ventral punctum communicated with each other but no saline was seen dripping from the nose (nasal meatus) indicating that the nasolacrimal duct was obstructed.

The surgeon devised a technique to flush open the duct by applying intermittent pulses of saline into the dorsal punctum (Fig. 12.16) while the ventral punctum (Fig. 12.17) was held shut by a cotton tip applicator. It took several attempts but a clot was released through the right nare and saline rushed through the nasal meatus (Fig. 12.18). Skull radiographs showed normality. There was no indication of damaged turbinates as in 'snuffles' (Ch. 8). The ferret went back on its original medication for 2 weeks and made a complete recovery.

Physical irritation of the cornea

Laboratory ferrets suffer from dust irritation from bedding, which is usually sawdust or pulped paper waste. Pet and working ferrets are normally bedded down with old towels, etc. Cat litter in scats trays can be a problem, especially if the ferret 'noses' into it. I prefer using newspaper in scats trays which stops the problem.

It is suggested that blindness in otters in the UK can be caused by herbicides. It is surmised that otters moving through contaminated vegetation could get contact with chemicals, which may affect their eyes.[26] However, blind otters can survive presumably by using the senses of smell and hearing. This could possibly happen to wild mink in the UK and working ferrets.

Nutritional problems occur in vitamin/mineral deficiencies, but are rare (see Table 12.3).

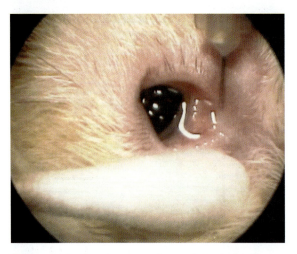

Figure 12.17 The dorsal punctum is flushed while the ventral one is held shut by a cotton bud. (Courtesy of M. Conn.)

Table 12.3 Some eye conditions caused by vitamin/mineral deficiencies in the diet

Deficiency	Resulting eye condition
Riboflavin vitamin B	Corneal vascularization and opacification
Biotin	Conjunctivitis
Vitamin A	Conjunctival discharge, lens opacification (cataract) and night blindness

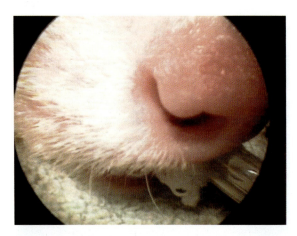

Figure 12.18 The nares are inspected to demonstrate patency of the duct through the nasal meatus. (Courtesy of M. Conn.)

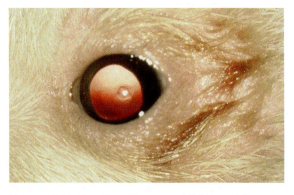

Figure 12.19 Eye ulcer. (Courtesy of T. Kawasaki.)

Author's clinical example

My 18-month-old 2kg hob ferret, Jason, was initially treated under ketamine anaesthesia for a right eye injury resulting from a ferret fight.[27] He was hospitalized and the deep ulcer was treated on an hourly basis using a drop of Mucomyst Formula 30 from an eye-dropper. This formula is more effective over the first 42–72 hours. Jason was held in a towel and did not resist treatment, which continued for 7 days when the ulcer was considered cured. As it was the mating season, he was placed then with a jill but had a recurrence of pus in the eye. A repeat eye check under ketamine showed the ulcer had cleared but an infection site was found on the inner side of the lower eyelid. A small drainage hole was made at the base of the eyelid and the eye was flushed with saline. The eye was consequently dressed daily with neomycin eye cream (Neosporin, Glaxo-Wellcome Ltd) and he was given 0.25 mL terramycin i.m. daily. He was better in 3 days and returned to the ferretarium. This was a complicated eye injury but illustrates a method of treatment.

Corneal ulcers

Corneal ulcers (Fig. 12.19) can occur in ferrets, especially with hobs fighting in the mating season or squabbling ferrets in a colony. Pet ferret toenails should be clipped against causing this sort of damage. Treatment in ferrets may require initial sedation or even anaesthetic for primary examination. Check the eye for ulcer with fluorescein stain. Use non-steroidal eye antibiotic creams or drops. *Note* that old mink are susceptible to the development of a cloudy, oedematous cornea, which is secondary to a corneal endothelial degeneration.[24] The ulcers can be superficial or deep and I have had success with a deep corneal ulcer in a ferret using Mucomyst Formula.

The Mucomyst Formula 30 can be an expensive way of treating eye ulcers but is recommended in deep ulcers (Dr Z. Chester, Vet Ophthalmologist, Perth, WA, pers. comm. 1998). Its disadvantage is that it has to be made-up and used immediately. There are a number of ophthalmic drugs that can be used on superficial eye ulcers now in the ferret, as for the dog and cat. Chloramphenicol is a drug of choice and is in the Mucomyst Formula, Table 12.4. *Note*: Mucomyst eye drops are now available.

Chlorsig drops (chloramphenicol 5 mg/mL plus hypromellose 3 mg/mL; Sigma) are excellent topically for superficial eye ulcers in the ferret and Clavulox palatable drops (Pfizer) is a useful oral medication. Topical eye medication for ferrets can also be given one-handed by 'scruffing' the ferret (Ch. 7).

It is possible to use the nictitating membrane for a '3rd eyelid flap' in the ferret.[17]

Uveitis

It is considered that anterior uveitis is commonly caused by trauma or may be a secondary problem to ulcerative keratitis.[14] It can be associated with cataract formation but is uncommon and mild in comparison with that of dogs. I had a 7-year-old black-eyed white jill, Heidi, with a left side cataract and uveitis. She had eye irritation and squinting and was prone to rub the affected eye side of her face along the ground. Hair loss occurred around the eye and treatment was by twice-daily application of an eye cream containing 10 mg/g chloramphenicol plus 5 mg/g hydrocortisone acetate (Chloroint, Ilium) over the eye globe. The situation stabilized, hair regrowth occurred and the irritation stopped. Uveitis or chorioretinitis can be a feature of many diseases of other animals that can affect ferrets. It is further suggested, but not proved, that the ferret has a possible retrovirus

Table 12.4 Mucomyst Formula 30 for use on eye ulcers

Drug	Amount mixed in 30 mL water	Final (%) drugs in mixture	Action	Remarks
Chloramphenicol 20% (Solymycin, Intervet)	1.5 mL	1%	Antibacterial	
Acetylcysteine 20% (Mucomyst, Mead Johnson)	10.0 mL	7%	Anticollagenase	Concentrations above 10% are irritating
Atropine 1%	7.5 mL	0.25%	Cycloplegic	For pain
Methopt (Sigma)			Prolongs corneal contact time	

The total amount dispensed is 30 mL, which must be stored in the refrigerator and should keep for 6 weeks. (Formula as adapted from G. Severin (1973), in Bloggs JR. The eye in veterinary practice. Melbourne: V.S. Supplies Ltd; 1975.)

CHAPTER TWELVE

Diseases of the ferret ear, eye and nose

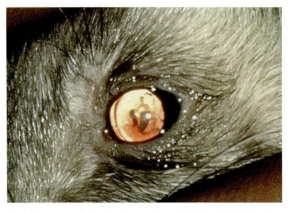

Figure 12.20 Cataract. (Courtesy of T. Kawasaki.)

that can cause uveitis, as it has been found that some ferret viral agent does cross-react with feline leukaemia virus on an immunoassay test. In comparison to the ferret, mink can be experimentally infected with Aleutian disease (AD) and develop iridocyclitis.[14] It would thus be prudent to do a full work-up on suspect ferrets with uveitis that does not relate to the usual causes of trauma, ulcerative keratitis and lens-induced uveitis.

Cataract

The condition of cataract (Fig. 12.20) is considered second to retinal atrophy. However, in my opinion, the list of possible cataractogenic agents is being constantly added to and can include modern foodstuffs and pharmaceuticals (Ch. 4).[28]

This is an opacity of the lens sufficient to cause a reduction of visual function and to date involves known and unknown factors. The lens experiences an insult in the form of white multifocal punctate opacities, which can be widely scattered in the posterior and subsequently anterior cortical/subcortical matrix. Cataracts do occur in the ferret and they can be hereditary, secondary to a dietary problem or idiopathic.[29] An interesting suggestion is made regarding ferret diet and cataracts. In the high fat diet that ferrets are supposed to have, the reactive oxyradicals generated from rancid fats could induce cataracts (Ch. 4). This occurs by aggregating crystalline lens proteins and inactivating the lenticular enzymes that usually repair oxidative damage. Oxyradicals may also effect damage by exceeding the buffering capacity of the lens antioxidants, vitamins C, E and the carotenoids. Some vitamin deficiency/excess effects are seen as cataracts experimentally in animals,[29] as shown in Table 12.5. It is said that because the ferret eats to a calorific requirement and not to a nutrient need, if the diet fat is increased without a corresponding protein increase, it can fall into a protein deficiency.[29] In this way, could cataract formation occur in ferrets as indicated in other animals?

Cat kittens have been fed arginine-deficient milk replacements with resulting lens opacities.[30]

It has been possible to produce cataracts in orphaned puppies experimentally when they were fed a commercial bitch's milk replacement (Esbilac).[31] The author states that cataract development in hand-reared puppies at least is not limited to commercial milk replacements. He found pedigree Shar Pei pups fed on a home formula developed cataracts to a significant degree. Formulation of the milk food was 2.5 cans of evaporated milk, one

Table 12.5 Nutritional deficiencies/excesses experimentally induced in relation to animal cataracts

	Animals with cataracts
Nutrient deficiency	
Riboflavin	Rats, mice, pigs, chicks, salmon, cats
Calcium	Dogs, rats, rabbits
Tryptophan	Pigs, rats, guinea pigs
Vitamin E	Rats
Methionine	Fish, rats
Protein	Pigs (query ferrets?)
Arginine (not experimentally induced)	Dogs and wolves
Nutritional excess	
High galactose	Rats and man (query ferrets?)
High xylose	Rats
Excess of polyunsaturated fats acids in diet if protein not increased leads to steatitis	Ferret in protein deficiency leads to cataracts?

cup water, two egg yolks, two tablespoons of corn syrup and one-third inch of rice cereal. He examined the breeding stock yearly but was unable to find a cataract, so surmising that inheritance was not involved. Esbilac was also used in another group of pups when the bitch died after a caesarean operation. Some pups were fed by a surrogate mother and some used the milk substitute.

Ferret nutrition has often been compared with that of mink, on which it has been somewhat traditionally based (Ch. 4). The presence of cataracts in mink on their diet is negligible but this may further reflect that ferret nutritional requirements, and therefore possibly cataractogenic factors, are different for the two mustelids.[29] Trauma, infection or metabolic factors can also be involved with ferret cataracts.[2] I have experienced cataracts in black-eyed white ferrets from a possible enzyme deficiency.[32] Eye opacities have been recorded in ferret kittens along with a number of other possible congenital or hereditary conditions.[33] A ferret colony used for laboratory research in the UK showed a low incidence of five ferrets with unilateral cataract, which made eating from a bowl difficult, and one case of bilateral cataracts.[2] In a major ferret-breeding establishment, they saw some congenital cataracts that were evident when the kittens were weaned. The jills were removed from the breeding colony (around 27 000 animals) when possible (J. Bell, Marshall Farms, New York, pers. comm. 1993). In another laboratory colony of ferrets, cataracts were found in two genetically-unrelated ferret populations using slit lamp biomicroscopy. Ferrets at around 1 year of age had a variety of lens defects (34 of 73 ferrets) ranging from fine multifocal punctate opacification to mature cataracts. When checked at around 18 months of age, many of the remaining ferrets had also developed fine multifocal punctate opacities on the posterior lens cortex. In a second group of 15 adults and 47 6-month-old ferrets, it was found that 31 of the youngsters were considered normal but 16 had some form of opacification.[2] This indicates a slow progressive cataract formation in some ferrets; this could have a variety of causes, including genetic and nutritional.

It has been stated that there are three disorders of sugar metabolism now recognized as causing cataracts.[28]

1. *Hyperglycaemic cataract*: Low concentrations of blood glucose affect the metabolic glucose utilization pathways, e.g. hexokinase enzyme activity, and it has been found in rats that this leads to cataracts.
2. *Diabetic cataract*: This is due to excessive blood glucose and over-stimulation of the metabolic glucose utilization pathways.
3. *Galactose-induced cataract*: I once supplemented the feeding of my ferret colony with the milk supplement Divetelact (Sharpe Laboratories, NSW, Australia) given as a morning drink. The meat meal was at night. The supplement contained, among other things, biotin, which in deficiency, can lead to baldness in ferrets if they are fed excessive eggs. Divetelact has, however, at least 95% of its lactose converted into its two components, glucose and galactose. Thus, the supplement is contraindicated in animal species which show intolerance to lactose in that they get diarrhoea due to the supplement.[33] None of my ferrets had shown this reaction. Possibly, there was no lactose intolerance in my ferrets but rather an inability to metabolize galactose once it was free of the lactose (D. Manning, Wisconsin Medical School, Wisconsin, USA, pers. comm. 1993). However, some of them did get signs of impending or actual cataract (1993). If one or both of two vital galactose-metabolizing enzymes are absent when the lactose is split, the galactose remains in the blood stream and can be a possible cataractogenic agent.

Author's clinical example

Of nine ferrets in a ferretarium colony, one, Sammy, a sable hob, only 2 years old, showed a distinct right eye cataract and slight left eye opacity. He was one kitten of a litter from a black-eyed white hob (BEW) and a sable jill. The whole colony was examined using a normal ophthalmoscope and slit ophthalmoscope, by Dr Z. Chester (Tables 12.6, 12.7). The ferrets were sedated with ketamine i.m.

The common factor with these ferrets was that they were fed Divetelact supplementation daily, with the pregnant and nursing jills also getting the supplement. It has been found, in relation to the dietary or physiological excess of some monosaccharides in animals and humans, that the long-term blood rise of either D-glucose or D-galactose may lead to cataract development.[28] That was of concern to me. Trials on carbohydrate malabsorption have been carried out on dogs.[34] A trial of feeding Divetelact to my ferrets and doing blood tests was carried out in conjunction with the University of Western Australia Biochemistry Department, Perth (November 1992). The ferrets were bled from the tail at 20 min and 120 min after a morning drink of Di-Vetelact and no meat (Table 12.8).

Figures 12.21 and 12.22 show the difference in graphs between Sammy, with prominent cataract of right eye and Josie, who was clear of cataracts and also cleared the blood galactose efficiently.

Table 12.6 Ferret colony ophthalmology examination results

Ferret colony member	Lens examination result	Comment
Sammy: sable hob	Right lens prominent cataract Left lens slight opacity	Sammy: brother to Tippy
Snowy: BEW hob	Left lens slight opacity	Snowy: father of Sammy and Tippy
Sophie: sable jill	Focal retinal haemorrhage Lens clear	Sophie: mother of Sammy and Tippy
Tippy: BEW jill	Right lens slight opacity	Tippy: sister to Sammy
Smudge: BEW jill	Lenses clear	Smudge: daughter of Tippy and Tuppy
Tuppy: albino hob	Lenses clear	Tuppy: mated with Tippy
Josie: sable jill	Lenses clear	Not related
Midge: sable jill	Lenses clear	Not related
Penny: silver mitt jill	Lenses clear	Not related
Whitey: albino hob	Prominent bilateral cataracts	Recent stray ferret kept for contrast as not claimed

Table 12.7 Family relationships of black-eyed white ferrets in relation to possible galactose-induced cataracts

Date	Jill	Hob	Offspring kept
1984	Jenny (silver mitt)	Goldie (BEW from Canberra)	Susie (BEW jill)
1988	Susie (BEW)	Simon (silver mitt)	Snowy (BEW hob)
1990	Sophie (sable)	Snowy (BEW)	Tippy (BEW jill) Sammy (sable hob)
1990	Tippy (BEW)	Tuppy (albino)	Smudge (BEW jill)

Table 12.8 Results of blood tests on galactose levels in ferrets

Ferrets with high blood galactose levels at 120 min	Ferrets with low blood galactose levels 120 min	Comments
Sammy (sable) Snowy (BEW)	Josie (sable) Midge (sable)	Of all ferrets, only Josie and Midge showed to be clear of blood galactose and also cataract
Tippy (BEW)		Difficulty in getting blood sample. Lower reading
Smudge (BEW)		Classic galactose blood graph suggesting lack of enzyme action
Penny (silver mitt)		Stray ferret. Had been on long-term Di-Vetelact
Tuppy (albino)		Stray ferret. Had been on long-term Di-Vetelact
Whitey (albino)		Whitey was classic bilateral cataract with no history as stray ferret recently acquired

Note: Sophie died in accident before trial.

Aetiology

Galactose-induced cataract is said to be due to the lack of either galactokinase or hexose-1-phosphate uridyl transferase, enzymes essential for pathways in sugar metabolism. Where the galactose is continuously supplied, the absence of one or both enzymes would cause a dramatic rise in blood galactose levels and this was seen in some of my ferrets.[32]

Of course, this small sample cannot be in any way be considered a proper research trial but to me as a practitioner, it rang alarm bells, so I stopped using Di-Vetelact and advised others not to use it on a long-term basis for ferrets. I hoped for some comment or even that offers to further research the phenomenon might arise from a publication of the results.[32] However, it appears in the research world that trials are done on ferrets for the benefit of people but not ferrets! It is suggested that

The ferret ophthalmic sense

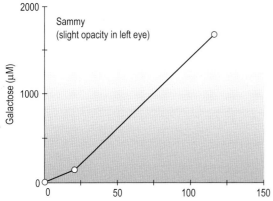

Figure 12.21 Sammy had right eye cataract and slight left eye opacity.

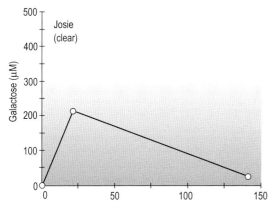

Figure 12.22 Josie had no cataract.

possibly an overload to the biochemical system could occur, with high levels of galactose swamping a deficient system when a large volume of Di-Vetelact drink is taken on an empty stomach (Professor P. Hartmann, Department of Biochemistry, UWA, Perth, Australia, pers. comm. 1992). This theory points to giving meat and milk products together, though milk in adults need not be given regularly and some ferreters only give milk to breeding stock. In a review of cataractogenic substances it was considered that the concept currently under investigation (1980) suggested 'that the deleterious effects of a variety of antagonistic agents (including poor nutrition) occurring at low exposure over a period of time, would summate to cause many of the cataracts clinically seen'.[28]

Galactose-induced cataract update

A 1994 check showed that Sammy and Snowy had no further degeneration of their eye condition after being taken off Di-Vetelact. Tippy showed no degeneration and likewise her daughter, Smudge, was clear of cataracts. Penny and Whitey had died, but four new members were added to the ferret colony: Tyke (sable hob), Lucky (sable jill), Nipper (sable jill) and Heidi (BEW jill), all young unwanted ferrets and found to be clear of cataracts. In 1999, Lucky and Heidi were still with the colony. Lucky was still clear of cataracts but Heidi was showing a definite left eye cataract – a black-eyed white genetic problem? One author advised that although he has seen cataracts in ferrets, it has been bilateral cataracts in a young ferret and there have been unilateral cataracts in rather old ferrets (like Heidi). He suggested that if the link between galactose intolerance and cataract formation was a metabolic one then the bilateral disease would be more common. He suggested the presence of a predisposing microbial problem (? virus) that might be exacerbated by the presence of galactose in circulation (D. Manning, pers. comm. 1993). Possibly a small trauma could be indicated followed by a sub-clinical infection. My original 1992 ferrets were on the same diet and none showed external signs of infections at the time.

The relationship of the black-eyed white ferrets involved was interesting from the genetic prospect but, as indicated earlier, research trials would be required using many ferrets to draw any conclusions (Ch. 5).

The questions in research could be along two possible lines:

1. Is there an increased likelihood that ferrets consuming milk regularly for long periods develop cataracts at a higher incidence than seen in those that do not?
2. Is there any known end-product or side-product of galactose metabolism that is likely to play a role in the development of this disease?

If trials on these questions prove positive, then there would be something to consider for the future, especially as at the present moment, the genetic picture of Australian ferrets cannot be changed by importing new blood lines. Overall, it is sad and alarming to find blindness in ferrets as it is in any animals. Investigations into any causes would be worthwhile in the future. *Note*: my silver mitt jill, Squeak, from the breeding of silver mitt hob, Boysie, with BEW jill, Patch, now has a right eye cataract (2005).

Mature cataracts can cause uveitis, which results in miosis, mild corneal oedema and squinting, as illustrated earlier. The uveitis can be severe with keratic changes and one author has seen cataract-induced uveitis to cause glaucoma or anterior lens luxation, or both, in ferrets.[15] Thus, the ferret eye with mature cataracts should be checked for signs of uveitis and treated with topical corticosteroids or topical non-steroidal anti-inflammatory drugs. The cataract-induced uveitis may be chronic and require extended treatment over months or even years (see uveitis segment above). Otherwise, there may be complications leading to glaucoma and surgery may be required to remove the lens.[14] This surgery is possible to carry out but there is too much postoperative inflammation with the small eye (M. Finkler, pers. comm. 1998).

Retinal atrophy

This disease occurs in ferrets with the same clinical and ophthalmoscopic signs as in the dog and is considered by one author as possibly 3–4 times more common than cataracts.[35] He states that the retinal atrophy is usually associated with a cataractogenic luxated lens and is easily detected despite the small size of the ferret eye (Fig. 12.23); usually in ferrets over 3 years of age.

The distinguishing ophthalmologic features are characteristic hyper-reflectivity and an avascular fundus (Fig. 12.24). The possible aetiology of retinopathy of this nature includes heredity and possible nutritional deficiency. In the cat, the condition is associated with aminosulphonic acid/taurine deficiency and this may well be the case with ferrets.[36] Taurine is naturally synthesized in most animals by the liver and the highest concentrations occur in excitable tissues including the heart,

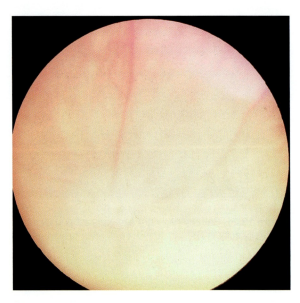

Figure 12.24 Vascular attenuation stage. (Courtesy of T. Kawasak.)

retina, CNS and skeletal muscle.[37] One can supplement with taurine in affected cases if some blood vessels are present. Taurine deficiency in the retina of the cat results in bilateral degeneration in the area centralis with tapetal discolouration and hyper-reflectivity causing eventual blindness. For diagnosis, the hyper-reflectivity and vascular attenuation can be seen without the aid of a mydriatic. In the early stages there is mild to moderate tapetal hyper-reflectivity, which increases as the tapetum degenerates with the blood vessels fading from view. The retinal glow increases and blindness ensues. Suspect ferrets can be clinically examined and a mydriatic drug is used for confirmation of the retinal atrophy. It is suggested that pupil dilation is essential with albino ferrets and the ophthalmic examination is best carried out at + (black) 5–8 dioptres.[38] It is difficult to be aware that a ferret may be blind and one exercise to check this is to place the ferret in a strange room or surround and watch its action. With ferrets running in the garden in the evening, I have often observed them passing and apparently not seeing each other. It is usually the hob ferrets that are busy following a jill scent trail and are so engrossed that they do not perceive other passing ferrets; the sense of smell is more dominant than the sense of sight. A blind ferret could maintain itself in its own environment but with ferrets living in a garden or ferretarium, blind ferrets would be in danger of falling into ponds or water bowls (Ch. 3). Treatment is not possible, but Finkler does suggest taurine supplementation with Felovite II or FurRovite produced by Marshall Farms, New York.

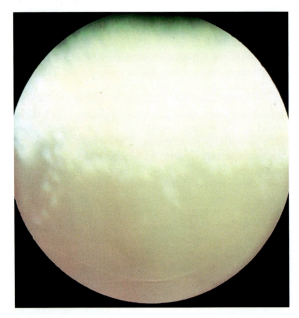

Figure 12.23 Progressive retinal atrophy. There are stages in-between normal and this condition. (Courtesy of T. Kawasaki.)

Other possible eye conditions

Glaucoma (Fig. 12.25), lens luxation (Fig. 12.26), entropion (Fig. 12.27), keratitis and keratitis sicca are rare conditions in ferrets though one case of Horner syndrome has been recorded.[38] A persistent hyaloid artery, of the hyaloid canal may be seen but is not harmful. A case of ferret distichiasis has been recorded (T. Kawasaki, pers. comm. 2005).

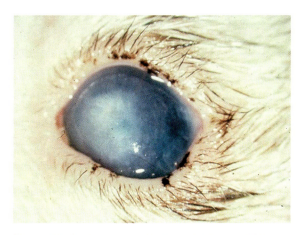

Figure 12.25 Glaucoma. (Courtesy of T. Kawasaki.)

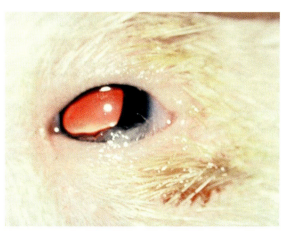

Figure 12.27 Entropion. (Courtesy of T. Kawasaki.)

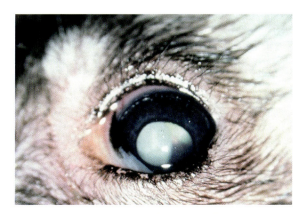

Figure 12.26 Luxated lens. (Courtesy of T. Kawasaki.)

The ferret olfactory sense

The ferret's sense of smell ranks in importance with its sense of hearing.[13] Marking territory and scenting another animal's presence and path is common to many mammals and more so to the mustelids, who follow prey persistently by its scent trail.

Features of ferret nasal anatomy

The nasal organ of the ferret is shown in cross-section in Figure 2.13. The nasal cavity is formed by the maxilla and nasal bones dorsally and laterally, with the maxillary and palatine bones supplying the cavity floor, similar in shape to a long-nosed dog. The bony nasal aperture is composed of two entrances to the nasal cavity, which is composed of two symmetrical halves as in the dog.[39] The ethmoid bone complex is located between the brain case and the facial part of the skull. It consists of the ethmoid labyrinth, the cribriform plate, and the median bony plate of the nasal septum. The ethmoid labyrinth is composed of many delicate scrolls, as in the dog, that attach to the cribriform plate and occupy the fundus of the nasal cavity. Bony scrolls, the conchae, project into each nasal fossa and with their mucosa act as baffles to warm and clean inspired air. The nasal cavity is one of the first lines of defence therefore, as in other animals, against pathogenic invasions. On the other hand, it can supply a vascular environment for pathogens to grow and spread if they do overcome the body's defenses. The conchae are divided into a small dorsal and large ventral portion in the ferret, as in the dog. The olfactory mucosa lining the conchae that house the olfactory nerve cells allow infection to invade the brain via the cribriform plate of the ethmoid complex. The ethmoid plate in the ferret does not completely pass ventrally to the cartilage of the nasal septum to divide the nasal fossa, as it does in the dog.

A longitudinal section of the brain and olfactory organ is shown in Figure 2.16.

CHAPTER TWELVE

Diseases of the ferret ear, eye and nose

Diseases of the olfactory system

Any disease problem affecting the olfactory system can put the hunting ferret in crisis. The nasal cavity involvement is prominent in infections such as canine distemper and human influenza in ferrets and is the gateway to infections of the lungs leading to pneumonia. The ferret is susceptible to 'snuffles', which is an upper respiratory condition similar to the snuffles seen in cats and involves nasal discharges and culture of various contributing possible pathogenic organisms of the nasal cavity (Ch. 8). A particularly nasty nasal worm of weasels, stoats, and skunks, *Skrjabingylus nasicola*, which affects the skull and causes pressure on the brain, might affect ferrets (Ch. 10).

Cryptococcosis

I would like to highlight a particularly dangerous nasal disease, which I have come across in ferrets, cryptococcosis, caused by the fungus *Cryptococcus*. The fungus *C. neoformans* previously had two varieties; var. *neoformans* and var. *gatti*. The development of the PCR technique (DNA sequencing) has now changed classification in many fields, as here. *C. neoformans* var. *neoformans* consisted of serotype A, now *C. neoformans* var. *grubii*, and serotype D, now *C. neoformans* var. *neoformans*. *C. neoformans* var. *gatti* (sometimes referred to as *C. bacillisporus*) consisted of serotypes B and C but now has been raised to a new species, *C. gatti*.[40,41]

The organism occurs worldwide and can infect a variety of hosts.[42] It can cause exterior nasal lesions, internal nasal infection and spread to the brain and lungs. I have recorded three cases of *C. neoformans* var. *neoformans* in ferrets, involving the CNS and also the lungs.[42,43] A case of an exterior nasal cryptococcosis infection was recorded by Richard Malik, involving *C. bacillisporus* (R. Malik, pers. comm. 1998). Many cases have historically been seen, mainly in the cat, by Wilkinson.[44,45] Other cases in Australia alone include the dog[46] and the parrot.[47] Besides infecting large farm animals, it infects native Australian animals such as kangaroos, wallabies and koalas. It can also affect humans,[48] being endemic in Australia and a list of other countries. *C. neoformans* var. *neoformans* (synonym *Torula histolytica*) usually affects immunocompromised subjects with the organism being the most common cause of fungal meningitis. It presents in humans as fever and headache.

Cryptococcus neoformans is a dimorphic fungus, which occurs worldwide in soils and bird droppings. *C. bacillisporus* is geographically restricted and is associated with the flowers and bark of Australian gum trees. Unlike *C. neoformans* var. *neoformans*, *C. bacillisporus* affects immunocompetent hosts.[48] Infection is by inhalation from the environment. It affects the nasal cavity and can spread to the brain and lungs. *C. neoformans* is said to quickly invade the central nervous system and other regions such as eyes, lymph nodes and skin.[49] It is not clear whether encephalitis occurs via the blood stream or locally through the cribriform plate. Considering the acute CNS signs in my hob ferrets, I think the direct cribriform route is very likely.

Clinical signs

Basically, with intra-abdominal infection, the ferret is found dead. There can be posterior paralysis associated with meningitis and rhinitis. Symptoms are well-documented as being common for cats but also seen in dogs.[49] In human cases, the clinical signs are typically meningitis or encephalitis[48] while most other animals show upper respiratory distress first.[50] In my two cases, respiratory signs led quickly to CNS signs.

In the cat, the disease shows unilateral or bilateral nasal discharge with sneezing and a firm swelling over the bridge of the nose. Sometimes small growths occur inside the nares.[51] The infection can spread from the nasal cavity to the draining lymph nodes, a condition noted in a ferret.[4] There may be infected papules and nodules on the head and skin and ulceration and drainage can occur. The cat shows CNS signs demonstrated by depression, disorientation, seizures, head pressing and posterior paralysis. In severe cases there are cranial nerve deficiencies and motor neuron lesions which produce ocular abnormalities such as pupillary dilation, chorioretinitis, optic neuritis and retinal detachment[49] (compare ferret eye diseases).

The dog will show more characteristic CNS and ocular disease, which could be compared with my ferret cases. In the dog, dissemination of the fungus is more widespread to other organs than in the cat. The CNS signs in the dog include head tilt, nystagmus, circling, disorientation, head pressing, varying degrees of paresis or paralysis, incoordination and seizures (compare ferret ear diseases). Chorioretinitis and optic neuritis are the most common eye symptoms, as in the cat. Skin lesions can also occur in dogs. Thus, some or all of these clinical signs recorded in the cat and dog can be applied to possible cases of *Cryptococcus* in the ferret. Cryptococcosis can occur in the skin form and alarmingly in the CNS/lung form.[43]

Diagnosis

Malik has used impression smears from skin lesions, nasal exudate smears, aspirates, biopsy, BAL specimen, antigen test (LCAT) and CSF cytology. Culture medium is a Sabouraud/Birdseed agar at 28°C. The LCA test has been reviewed by Malik et al.[52]

In 1996, when I had two ferrets sick with cryptococcosis, the LCAT test was carried out by the WA Agriculture Department and delays caused problems. It took at least 3 days to get a result. The diagnosis for CNS/lung forms in ferrets must be done quickly to have

Author's clinical examples

Ferrets with CNS infection

In Perth, I had two hob ferrets with clinical signs consistent with *Cryptococcus neoformans*. Neither hob had shown any early signs of the 'snuffles', like the condition that can occur in some jills (Ch. 7). 'Snuffles' could be compared with the early signs of cryptococcosis in cats. Both hobs lived outside in the garden and ferretarium but also came indoors.

1. Alby, 2-year-old albino hob (sick: 28 Sept. 1996–1 Nov. 1996, i.e. southern hemisphere spring). Initially, he showed signs of 'snuffles' with paroxysmal sneezing and serous or purulent nasal discharges. No temperature rise or anorexia but in a few days he showed a distinct stiffness around the neck when being picked up. This was put down to a possible fight as ferrets usually go for the neck. He improved on antibiotics clavulanic acid/amoxicillin (Clavulox palatable drops, Pfizer) but became less active. Alby regressed with neck spasms when handled and slight incoordination. This moved to lassitude but he was still eating fresh meat. Alby became progressively lethargic and when moving began circling to the right (but without the head tilt of inner ear disease). He remained on antibiotics. Blood tests were done as he further regressed, with body weight falling from 1240 to 1000 g. The LCAT test on the blood took 3 days to get a result, which was positive for *Cryptococcus*. Alby's condition was such that I reluctantly put him to sleep.

2. Tyke 3-year-old silver mitt (sick 5–24 Feb. 1997, i.e. southern hemisphere summer). Initially, he showed lethargy and then signs of 'snuffles' with sneezing which showed blood flecks. As I had been caught once, he was immediately LCAT-tested. He was started on the antibiotic routine for 'snuffles' with clavulanic acid/amoxicillin (Clavulox palatable drops, Pfizer) plus directly on ketoconazole (KTZ) (Nizoral) at 50 mg/ferret daily dose (S. Brown, pers. comm. 1996). *Note* the 200 g Nizoral tablet cannot be dissolved in water but is made up in suspension in 2 mL of water. Of this shaken suspension, 0.5 mL was given twice daily using a tuberculin syringe and followed by a sugar solution. The LCAT test results took 6 days.

Tyke continued eating but lost weight from 1060 to 930 g. He had a 'dull' look but was not pyrexic. He continued with some occasional mild sneezing and stayed on both medications daily plus vitamin B injection daily. However, by 6 days he was brighter in the eye and became more alert in the evening and even attempted to play. We were used to ferrets sleeping during the day anyway. He was kept daily in the hospital for observation and indoors in the family room at home at night. The LCAT test result was inconclusive. The KTZ was reduced to 0.25 mL daily for a few days and then every other day after that, as I was worried also about drug toxicity. He continued on antibiotics. The LCAT test was repeated, though I was sure I had another cryptococcosis case. Tyke kept on eating and became more active in the evening, so we were encouraged, but he was not really normal and slept a lot. The LCAT test again proved inconclusive but was not taken as negative! A normal blood profile showed mild to moderate hepatopathy and pre-renal azotemia. KTZ is known to be hepatotoxic but in Tyke's case had been used for 6 days and then reduced. In cats, the treatment is supposed to go on for at least 4–8 weeks after the clinical signs have resolved.[49] Toxicity is seen in cats so I was assuming that ferrets with a small body weight would be more at risk. Some 18 days after the initial treatment, Tyke relapsed, becoming incoordinate and falling to the side, like Alby did. He was also restless, with vague staring eyes and poor eye reflex. When placed outside on grass he was incoordinate and showed back arching (Fig. 12.28). It was all so sudden and alarming after his improvement, but Tyke died. I was convinced in my mind that he had succumbed to cryptococcosis and possibly drug toxicity. Such is the frustration of inexperience!

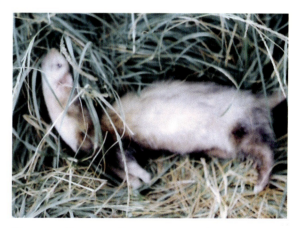

Figure 12.28 Tyke suffering from meningitis from *Cryptococcus* infection showing back arching.

any chance of success. *Note*: with the LCAT test it is possible that a negative test does not rule out cryptococcosis, especially in localized areas.[49]

Differential diagnosis: Consider cryptococcosis with chronic diseases. i.e. chronic rhinitis, 'snuffles' (Ch. 8), CNS conditions, inner ear disturbance, pneumonia, pleurisy, intra-abdominal mass or lymph node enlargement.

Pathology

In Alby's post mortem of lung tissue, there were variable changes in tissue with areas of atelectasis and multifocal areas of increased cellularity, predominantly pyogranulomatous with neutrophils and macrophages present within alveolar septa. With the increase in cells were scattered cryptococcal organisms especially around the larger airways. Fox has recorded two pathology cases showing internal lesions.[4] In one mature hob ferret found dead in the UK, the post mortem showed masses of yeast-like organisms (10 μm in diameter and surrounded by a mucoid capsule) in a jelly-like substance on the abdominal organs seen on close histological examination. In another 3-year-old hob with cardiomegaly, the histological examination revealed signs of lesions in the heart, lungs and liver related to congestive cardiomyopathy and heart failure plus meningitis with yeast-like organisms (cryptococci bodies) in the inflamed meninges. The presence of thick-walled budding yeasts in the pneumonic lungs was indicative of cryptococcosis. *Note* the three cases recorded of ferret cryptococcosis were all hobs. At the microscopic level, it is seen in the cat that there is a relative lack of tissue response on the part of the host. The yeast cells evidently multiply rapidly and push aside the neighbouring tissues without signs of an inflammatory response.[44]

Regarding the laboratory tests for my ferrets, the long wait for results contributed to the disaster; nowadays Vetpath Labs, Perth, WA have the test at hand and can do it in 20 minutes from receiving the blood. With cats and dogs, the test is said to be 95% sensitive with a specificity of 100%. Nowadays the disasters with Alby and Tyke may have been avoided but the treatment of the disease after pathogen confirmation is not easy and can be drawn out over months or years.

After the loss of the two hobs, I did an immediate spot LCAT test on one of my four jills, Lucky, who had previously shown a distinct 'snuffles'. The LCAT test then proved a distinct negative. Lucky was still part of the ferret colony in 1999. I was of the opinion that cryptococcosis in the CNS form is a hob disease. Ironically, a few weeks after Tyke died, an adult ferret hob came in with lassitude and a stiff neck observed when it was picked up that day. The hob had recently been sterilized and lived alone in the garden. The client was reluctant to go to much expense and I put the hob immediately on KTZ with instructions on how to treat. The client did not bring the ferret back but on contacting by telephone, I found they were satisfied as the ferret had recovered in 2 weeks on the medication. (An open case.)

Drugs used for treating cryptococcosis

There are five drugs available for treating fungal diseases in cats and dogs primarily and they differ in efficiency, cost and toxicity.[50]

1. Ketoconazole (KTZ): (Nizoral 200 mg tablets). This is the cheapest drug; although it does work well in cats, it often results in vomiting and inappetence. The tablets have to be made-up in suspension for ferrets and the dosage given with food like cats. It caused no vomiting with my two cases but can be hepatotoxic over the long treatment that is usually required for mycotic infections. Ferret dosage is one-quarter of a tablet per day.

2. Itraconazole (ITZ): (Sporanox). This is now the drug of choice for cats and ferrets. It is more effective than KTZ, generally has fewer side-effects and is given once daily. It is expensive compared with KTZ but much less so than fluconazole (FCZ). It can be used on ferrets with external nasal fungal growths, after cutting away the lesion as much as possible. Cat dosage is one 100 mg capsule per day. One-quarter capsule for ferret daily, i.e. 25–33 mg p.o. in Energel (R. Malik, pers. comm. 1998).

3. Fluconazole (FCZ): This would be the drug of choice in ferrets with CNS involvement, but is a high cost drug. (Cat dosage is one 50 mg capsule every 8 hours (4 kg cat), adjust for ferret weight. Note that ITZ costs $22 per week to treat a cat, pre-2000, while using FCZ it would cost $85 per week. ITZ and FTZ are in capsule form.

4. Flucytosine: (Tablet form 250 mg). Like KTZ it is a useful effective anti-cryptococcal drug but because of rapid resistance development when used alone, it is kept to improve the efficiency of the other antifungal drugs. It would have to be given in suspension for ferrets.

5. Amphotericin B: This is a powerful drug but is unfortunately nephrotoxic.[44] It is used for CNS fungal involvement but must be given i.v. or s.c., so cannot be used for home patients. Amphotericin B is made by adding 10 mL of sterile water to a 50 mg vial of Fungizon (Squibbs) to produce a 5 mg/mL colloidal solution.[50]

Note: drugs which are metabolized in the liver should not be used in conjunction with KTZ, ITZ or FCZ. In addition, flucytosine and amphotericin B are not useful for CNS infections as they are unable to cross the blood–brain barrier.

Two Canadian ferret cases were recorded in Vancouver.[53] A 19-month-old castrated house pet ferret was used to being taken for walks on a lead and known to be a digger around trees. In June 2001, it had a sudden development of a firm hairless, ulcerated mass on the second digit of the left hind leg. Phalanges 1, 2 and 3 were excised but no follow-up antifungal treatment occurred. Histology however found organisms suggestive of *C. neoformans* in the inflammatory area though the bone was unaffected. Using immunohistochemistry the organism was identified as yeast cells of *C. neoformans*. The quick surgery seemed to be a success with the ferret showing no evidence of recurrence after 4 months.

Author's clinical example

There have been five cases of cryptococcosis in ferrets in the Sydney area to date.[40] In contrast to my CNS cases, Dr Malik was treating a case of an invasive mycotic rhinitis in a 5-year-old castrate ferret, Mario, due to *C. bacillisporus,* which is associated with eucalyptus trees in Australia. The ferret, Mario, was presented in July 1998 to the NSW Ferret Society Ferret Refuge with snuffling and sneezing and with a lump on the bridge of its nose where the infective agent had penetrated through the nasal bone to the surface (Fig. 12.29). Sydney University offered to help Mario with the fungal drugs as a ferret trial.

The lesion was debulked under general anaesthesia, a blood LCAT test (titre 1024) and biopsy were taken confirming *C. bacillisporus* which was susceptible to ITZ. *Note* in dogs and cats, this fungal infection is difficult to treat. Mario was put on a quarter of a 100 mg capsule of itraconazole (ITZ) once daily. The medication was given in various kinds of meat and he was under the care of a member of the Society. The ferret stabilized without any reaction to the drug in a week and the dose was increased to one-third of a capsule per day (i.e. 25 mg daily going to 33 mg daily after 3 weeks).

The ferret's appetite was not decreased by the medication; if it had been, the medication would have been stopped. *Note*: at 171 days after starting treatment, the signs of the disease disappeared, with the antigen titre falling from 1024 to 128. ITZ was reduced to 25 mg and the LCAT stayed between 16 and 32 from 10 months after start of therapy. (ITZ is less toxic than KTZ but by how much ferret-wise?)

Mario's activity level improved. He began grooming himself and the snuffling and sneezing decreased. It took nearly 6 months to clear the nasal infection. The ferret was recorded as doing really well in May 1999 though still on ITZ capsules (Dave Such, NSWFWS, pers. comm. 1999). The treatment was stopped at 3 years when there was a fear of systemic toxicity. However, Mario went sick 3 months later when an abdominal mass was detected and then he was put to sleep. The cranial abdominal mass was found to be a cirrhosis bile duct carcinoma. Interestingly, no cryptococcal organisms were found on PM in the nasal cavity, CNS or other tissues.[40]

The cost of this treatment over many months would be possible for ferret owners but if the CNS was involved, the use of expensive fluconazole (FCZ) would be required.

The four other ferret cases cited, numbered 2, 3, 4 and 5 had mixed results.

Ferret 2: Lived with its brother case 1 (Mario). The ferret was a 6-year-old male, Luigi, and kept with the welfare society from July 1998. It had a chronic nasal haematoma and 'snuffles' and had been bitten (June 1999), presumably caused by ferret fighting which would have a stress factor. Luigi showed lethargy a month later and his physical condition also included mild splenomegaly, superficial cervical and popliteal enlargement, snuffles effects and hair loss from caudal flanks, pelvic limbs and tail on both sides. He had a scaly, dry and inflamed skin.

Primarily, Luigi was treated with a blanket ivermectin (300 µg/kg s.c.) and doxycycline course (12.5 mg orally b.i.d. for 4 weeks), though skin tests were negative for mite and ringworm. By August 1999, the ferret had weight loss (from 1.5 kg when taken in to 1.35 kg), had increased alopecia and a suspicious swelling at the angle of the right jaw. When the lump was incised (under isoflurane/nitrous oxide) and lab tested it was found to be a *C. bacillisporus* infection. Though treatment was started with ITZ, because of the worsening skin condition, Luigi was put down. The post mortem confirmed the diagnosis.

Malik asserts that Mario had a cryptococcosis primarily from a rhinitis, which spread to the nasal bridge while in Luigi it was a cryptococcosis of both retropharyngeal lymph nodes with an accompanying skin condition.[40] The skin condition was an immune-mediated dermatopathy.

Ferret 3: A 2-year-old castrated sable hob, which showed dyspnoea, lethargy and weakness in January 1999. It only weighed 0.9 kg but a heartworm test was negative. Due to its poor condition for a radiograph the ferret was sedated (ketamine 25 mg/diazepam 1.5 mg s.c.) and also put on halothane with 100% oxygen intubated. Chest X-rays were taken, frothy tracheal material was noted. The radiographs showed severe diffuse alveolar disease with pleural effusion. The ferret became cyanotic and despite extra oxygenation died in 2 hours. On post mortem, capsulated yeasts were found in the lungs and infection by *C. bacillisporus* was confirmed by immunohistochemistry.

Ferret 4: Is interesting as being the first 2–3-year-old spayed jill with cryptococcosis to my knowledge. I had been of the opinion that it was more a ferret hob disease. The jill showed lethargy and anorexia over a few days and had been gagging. On further examination, the jill showed an abnormal 'panting' respiration mode, having slightly cyanotic mucous membranes and a sausage-shaped abdominal mass. Body weight was only 650 g. Again, anaesthesia was used for radiology and an exploratory operation. Unfortunately, the jill died under anaesthesia. Post mortem showed a 5 × 1 cm soft mass enclosing a part mesenteric lymphadenomegaly with enlargement of the

CHAPTER TWELVE

Diseases of the ferret ear, eye and nose

liver and abdominal clear fluid. Encapsulated yeasts were found in the intestinal mass with foamy macrophages. *C. neoformans* var. *grubii* (formerly *C. neoformans* var. *neoformans* serotype A) was found as the disease cause with a primary site in the intestine and then in enlarged lymph nodes, lungs and liver.

The final Australian ferret, case 5, was again a castrated hob ferret aged 5 years. It weighed 1.25 kg in April 2001 and it showed a swollen distal left forelimb, poor appetite and lethargy. It had a history of chronic 'snuffles' and an antibiotic-resistive temperature episode in December 1999. The affected foot was twice the size of the opposite one and showed swollen metacarpal and phalangeal regions when the ferret was held from the ground, and was thought to be the result of a penetrating injury. The cellulitis was treated with amoxicillin-clavulate and carprofen for 2 days, with improvement. The ferret could place the leg as the swelling reduced and it regained its appetite. Curettage was carried out but the lesion was found to be ulcerated to 1 cm. A smear impression stained with DiffQuik showed a pyogranulomatous inflammation and suspect *Cryptococcus* organisms. The diagnosis was cryptococcal antigen in serum >2048. The ferret was treated with ITZ (25 mg p.o. daily) for 5 weeks until the lesion was no longer present and was continued on ITZ until 6 months when the antigen titre was negative. The LCAT was monitored till February 2002 when the titre was <2. Unfortunately, further contact with the patient was lost.

From Dr Richard Malik, University of Sydney, NSW.

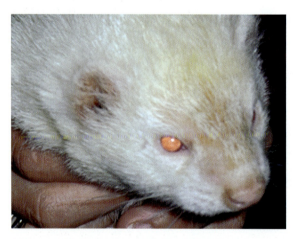

Figure 12.29 Mario with nasal *Cryptococcus*. Notice brownness of nose. (Courtesy of B. Alderton.)

Another ferret, a 3-year-old hob, was found to have hind limb weakness, swelling of the distal left hind leg and an enlarged popliteal lymph node. The ferret was inappetent and thin. A biopsy of the node found a cryptococcal lymphadenitis and *C. neoformans* var. *grubii* by immunohistology. The ferret was immediately treated with fluconazole (FLZ) at 12 mg orally b.i.d. The ferret improved in 4 months but had a lame leg. The present-day condition of the two Canadian ferrets is unknown due to lack of owner contact. The ferrets were part of an outbreak of cryptococcosis in Vancouver Island in 2000–2001 involving multispecies with cats, dogs, dolphins, two ferrets and a llama.[53]

Discussion: These Sydney and Vancouver *Cryptococcus* cases along with my own show the extent of cellular damage and protracted nature of this deadly disease.

It can affect:

1. Nasal cavity intrusions
2. Local lymph nodes
3. Meningoencephalitis direct from nasal cavity
4. Soft tissue, especially distal extremities
5. Granulomatous pneumonia with or without pleurisy
6. Intra-abdominal infections.

Unfortunately, the signs of cryptococcosis may take time to show making treatment difficult except in the case of nasal cavity infection, a direct entry to the brain. The obvious initial infection is via the upper and lower respiratory tract, skin or subcutis normal mucosa or wounds, followed by the gastrointestinal tract. It can be a disease of ferrets living outside, which can be a worry, and in chronic cases can take from weeks to months to show. Some authors consider that early dissemination of cryptococcus to the CNS is not a feature of infection in ferrets.[40] It is considered that ferrets appear similar to cats but unlike dogs and humans where a spread to the meninges or brain can occur after the development or recrudescence of a respiratory infection. I personally maintain, having had ferrets die from the condition, that once the fungus is taken into the nasal cavity it is highly likely to go straight to the brain in perhaps broken nasal capillaries from sneezing bouts.

The other problem in treating ferrets with cryptococcosis is the danger of drug toxicity in itself over the long period required to kill the fungus!

In North America, British Columbia in Canada seems to have become an endemic region for cryptococcosis in the same way that southern California is known for coccidioidomycosis and the Mississippi area for blastomycosis.[54] A survey of 15 dogs, 20 cats, one cockatoo and the two unfortunate ferrets indicates the trend.

We know the *C. neoformans* association with eucalyptus trees (Australia, South America and California) and *C. neoformans* var. *neoformans* is associated with pigeon droppings. This latter has been my worry with the ferrets I lost to cryptococcosis. *Note*: *C. neoformans* var. *gattii* (serotype B) causes disease in Australian koalas.

The problem on Vancouver Island is related to climate with rain forest where fungal organisms have been cultured from many tree barks, e.g. fir, alder, Garry oak, maple, cedar and pine.[54] The incidence of cryptococcosis in the area has increased dramatically since 2000. It should be noted that the island is a tourist drawcard for Americans who may travel with their pets and that might include ferrets. Considering the pet ferret involvement, one had respiratory tract signs including nasal discharge while the other had signs of acute abdominal discomfort and an abdominal mass could be palpated. *Note* that the ferrets were trained to walk on a leash and lived in the suburban areas of the island.

Histology was studied of six infected animals, dogs and cats and five of the animals showed meningitis from cryptococcosis. No information is given on the infected ferrets but on serological testing of 22 out of 48 animals, the titres varied from 1:2 to 1:20 000, with one of the ferrets having the latter value. Cultures were not performed on the ferrets. However, 19 of 38 animals were recorded to be alive in 2004 after treatment with antifungal drugs.[54] *Note* the affected animals in the British Columbia survey had clinical signs associated with the CNS, which differentiated them from Australian reports of *C. neoformans* var. *gattii* (serotype B) infections and the *C. neoformans* var. *neoformans* infections of other parts of North America. My affected ferrets had definite CNS signs.

General epidemiology
Cryptococcus is called the 'silent killer' and is found in the bark of natural host trees such as the common red gums, Tuart (*Eucalyptus gomphocephala*) and flooded gums (*Eucalyptus rudis*) as *C. bacillisporus*. Tuart harbours the disease in Western Australia but we do not have these trees in our garden. The fungi are in the flowers and no doubt can be taken by the wind. Horses grazing under host trees have been infected. In Sydney, NSW, the infection of cats with the fungus is more apparent in spring and summer when the gum trees lose their bark.[50] The ecology of *Cryptococcus* has been studied in the light of possible human infection.[55,56] Australia has exported eucalyptus trees to various countries around the world and infections of cryptococcosis in humans have arisen. The disease is prevalent in warm to hot climates but rare in continental Europe and the UK.[50] *Cryptococcus neoformans* var. *neoformans* is found in weathered pigeon droppings, where creatinine, a constituent of avian urine, enhances its growth.

Note there are different environmental factors between the Australian and British Columbia scenes. In Australia, the *C. neoformans* var. *gattii* (serotype B) exists in its highest concentration in dead plant material in the hollows of eucalyptus trees whereas in British Columbia the organism is found in living tree bark and in the air. In Australia, it is considered that *C. neoformans* var. *grubii* is in the inner city and possibly *C. neoformans* var. *gattii* in rural regions.[54] Research in Australia points to *C. neoformans* var. *gattii* (serotype B) growth not being influenced by differences in temperature, climate or latitude. Moreover, disease in mammals appears to be directly related to the concentration of the fungal species in the environment.

Cryptococcus has a wide spectrum of possible sources from even healthy human skin, oropharynx and gastrointestinal tract plus soil, fruit juice, milk, butter, grass and several species of insects.[44] That man and animals can contract the disease, though supposedly rarely, from this broad spectrum of sources is well known, but the actual method of establishment of the fungus as a disease entity is poorly understood. In humans, it is suggested to be likely that immune-suppressed people can succumb.

In the USA, it is the most common fungal disease in AIDS patients and is usually acquired by the pulmonary route and then disseminated to the CNS to cause meningitis (D. Manning, pers. comm. 1997). There is no clear evidence that *Cryptococcus* is transmitted from animals to man. However, AIDS patients in the USA have given up their pet ferrets for fear of a remote possibility (S. Brown, pers. comm. 1997). It is advised that care should be taken with hygiene when handling infected animals of all species.

In America, a case of meningeal cryptococcosis was picked up in a ferret suffering from cardiomyopathy, which was actually treated for a suspect intervertebral disc disease as it had posterior paralysis and listlessness. It died some 5 weeks after being first being seen when showing sneezing, serous nasal discharge and dyspnoea. The post mortem showed the heart involvement and the CNS infection by *C. neoformans*.[57]

On my enquiry, the region does have a number of pigeons around but Scooter was a house ferret. There was no history of 'snuffles'.

I regret that my ferret Pip (6-year-old sable) died within 2 days in June 2006, of severe pulmonary cryptococcosis. He had no 'snuffles' signs but had respiratory distress for 2 days previously, showing 'flattening' but had not lost weight (1600 g). I have no answer for the acute infection. Perhaps getting into the compost heap to dig? Though *Cryptococcus neoformans* is of course ubiquitous.

Curtis recorded the first case of *Cryptococcus* infection in cats in Western Australia in 1951 in his own pet cat,[58] as mine was in the ferret. Like other mycotic diseases, *Cryptococcus* is a more likely disease factor in tropical and subtropical regions of the world with warm humid climates. Cats acquire it in the summer months, the same timing as with my ferrets.

If protected from sunlight and drying, *Cryptococcus* can remain viable in contaminated bird droppings for 2 years.[49] My garden ferretarium is shaded by tall trees and thus attracts birds (Ch. 3). The high cover of shady

CHAPTER TWELVE

Diseases of the ferret ear, eye and nose

USA clinical case

Hanley et al. (2005) in Wisconsin had an interesting case involving an 18-month-old sterilized male ferret, Scooter, which showed a history of regurgitation but was otherwise normal.[41] The ferret weighed 1.07 kg and was in good condition with a good coat. The presence of a markedly enlarged right submandibular lymphadenopathy led to a fine needle aspirate under isoflurane anaesthesia. Radiology with blood and biochemical checks was carried out.

- Blood findings – monocytosis 640 cell/μL (normal range 0–432 cells/μL)
- Hypocalcaemia 8.0 mg/L (normal range 8.6–10.5 mg/L)
- Hypophosphataemia 5.0 mg/dL (normal range 5.6–8.7 mg/dL)
- Hypoproteinaemia 5.2 g/dL (normal range 5.3–7.2 g/dL)
- Hypoalbuminaemia 2.7 g/dL (normal range 3.3–4.1 g/dL).

The FNA revealed *Cryptococcus neoformans* which by further characterization was revealed as a melanin positive strain of *C. neoformans* var. *grubii* (serotype A). Fortunately, no other organs were affected. The route of entry was unknown but it was thought that some infection did occur elsewhere.

Diagnosis: On cytological evidence, a granulomatous lymphadenitis with a moderate reactive hyperplasia to the fungus was suggested.

Treatment: Itraconazole was the drug of choice and given at 15 mg/kg p.o. q. 24 h as a suspension. This follows the cat dosage of 5–10 mg/kg p.o. q. 12 h or 20 mg/kg p.o. q. 24 h. The treatment of this disease needs to be early, as I well know, and of a lengthy period. With this ferret, treatment lasted 10 months apparently with no side-effects. The owners were to monitor the ferret progress with a re-check in 3 weeks.

The submandibular gland decreased to one-third the size after 3 weeks treatment and the ferret physical and fundic examination was normal. Of interest, itraconazole capsules were given for continuing treatment. Each capsule contained around 700 beads and the owner could open the capsule and count out 105 beads and give daily in the food. It made it easier for treatment over the long period.

Progress: At 6 weeks, the lymph node was normal and at each subsequent visit, the *Cryptococcus* antigen titre decreased until it was negative at 10 months after presentation. A great result!

The ferret's ALT had been elevated to 231 U/L from 76 U/L but was still in the normal range (82–289 U/L) so treatment was continued till it dropped to a negative titre whereby it was stopped. *Note* that the patient was checked periodically using the latex *Cryptococcus* antigen agglutination test (LCAT) to check on continuing freedom from the fungus.

Conclusions to case: The infective source of cryptococcosis was not found and no human contacts suffered the disease. The ferret came from an enclosed animal shelter and had not moved from interstate. Latency periods are known in humans and koala cases for the disease and could be possible in ferrets.

Comment: A good case result. Cost-wise, the ITZ was about US$10/week, thus a total cost about US$400–500. There were no drug side-effects and the chemical profile taken 3 weeks before stopping the medication showed no elevation of liver enzymes. A check-up (August 2005) reported Scooter doing well.

trees tends to keep the ground temperature down; the trees are needed to protect the ferrets from high temperatures. Thus the conundrum. I had had ferrets since the early 1970s without trouble, but in 1996/97, I had two cases of *Cryptococcus*. The danger factor is just an unlucky chance contamination. In Western Australia, there is a high incidence of human mycotic infections but few in cats (S. Beatson, Vetpath Labs, Perth, WA, pers. comm. 1996). We also had two cats and two dogs with no cryptococcosis problems. In Queensland, seven cases of *Cryptococcus* in cats were recorded in 3 years[44] and one interesting dog case in South Australia. Dog infections can resemble ferret CNS cases. In this case, the dog showed clinical signs of depression, cough, disorientation, right pupil miosis and left eye mydriasis, indicating lung and CNS fungal involvement. The owner kept pigeons, the probable source of infection.[46]

My first recorded case also involved birds.[42] An aviary owner had the idea of keeping a ferret in his finch aviary, with the purpose of keeping local mice away, which were attracted by the seed. The ferret became sick with a 'snuffles' and died after some weeks, whereupon a post mortem showed the presence of cryptococcosis thick-walled yeast-like organisms in the lungs. Aviary watching is not a job for ferrets!

Obvious facial granuloma and nasal distortions have been seen in cats with cryptococcosis. Some ferret strains here and in the USA show a distinct 'Roman' nose, which must not be confused with a mycotic disease. In the USA, immune-suppressed dogs with ehrlichiosis are good candidates for cryptococcosis. The possibility of tick-borne infections, like ehrlichiosis, in ferrets have not been recorded except for a possible dog paralysis tick (*Ixodes holocyclus*) in NSW. The possibility of ticks affecting working ferrets here, in New Zealand or the UK and European continent, could occur. Ticks are often found on working ferrets in the UK but apparently do no harm.[59]

C. *bacillisporus* in immunocompetent humans is no real threat as it can be treated. There is insufficient data as to whether the fungus behaves as a primary pathogen or opportunist in the ferrets treated by Malik et al.[40] Cats with immunosuppression caused by FeLV or FIV, or otherwise debilitated or under corticosteroid therapy, have a high chance of falling to a *Cryptococcus* infection. Lymphomas in ferrets are equivalent to FeLV, so possibly ferrets with this condition can be susceptible to the fungus. An investigation into ferrets having retrovirus-induced cancers is referred to by Pearson and Gorham.[60] Concurrent viral infections that could affect ferrets and make them immunosuppressed have been described (Ch. 8). 'Snuffles' may arise from nasal disease and a depressed ferret may be more susceptible to mycotic invasion of the nasal cavity. In ferrets undergoing chemotherapy for cancer treatment with corticosteroids, it is theoretically possible for them to be more open to mycotic infections (S. Brown, pers. comm. 1998).

Infection methods

It is said that some animals and man can have colonization of the nasal cavity with *Cryptococcus* species without clinical disease and could become subclinical carriers or develop the disease later. The exact mechanism of CNS infection is not known but is thought to be as a result of invasion of the cribriform plate or along the optic nerves. With the experience I had of two ferret cases I would suggest, with the sudden meningitis that occurred, the cribriform plate entry is very likely. This is a practitioner's view.

Increase of CNS signs is due to the virulence of the fungal strain and the fungal capsule structure is of interest. Thus, opsonins and a cell-mediated immune response are required to attach the fungal capsule to macrophages, so that if macrophages are deficient the organism cannot be overcome. Thus, immunosuppressed animals are at risk. I felt concern over my hobs, Alby and Tyke. The common factor was the 'snuffles' and they were both put under antibiotic cover with no avail. With hindsight, they should have gone onto prompt antifungal treatment. So, changes in the immune system's recognition of capsular antigens could alter response to the organism. Perhaps genetics and species differences might play a part in the virulence of *Cryptococcus*.[61]

There is no sex difference in cats with cryptococcosis but with my ferrets, hobs were infected with the CNS disease. The reason? One author, discussing dogs and cats, states that the risk factor for *C. neoformans* is high in an animal 'excessively nosing about in contaminated soil or droppings'.[49] That exactly describes hob ferrets' behaviour! They will nose around the scats tray or where jills have passed scats out in the garden or ferretarium.

Thus, this condition may not be a problem with hob ferrets indoors or in sheds, etc. Jill ferrets, however, do not nose around in the soil excessively, if at all.

According to some authors, cryptococcal infections occur more in young dogs because they actively dig, sniff around and roll in rotten vegetation while older cats appear to be infected by aerosol infections when dirt is dry as in summer conditions in hot Mediterranean climates.[61]

Some ferrets in a garden situation do eat snails and slugs at times. As these creatures can 'slide' over bird droppings, they could be a source of infection.

Prevention

We are told that the cryptococcosis is a rare disease, being rare in dogs but more common in cats, so where does that put the ferret? On the other hand, I have had numerous hob ferrets in the garden and ferretarium for years with no problem and so have other ferret owners. So what has happened? Speaking of Western Australia, one factor might be our hot summers and perhaps the fact that over the past few years we have had summer water restrictions and my back garden is a good example and now has less groundcover. Ferrets really nose into the naked soil! There are also numerous wild birds, including pigeons and doves.

With *Cryptococcus* so well distributed, it is difficult to think of preventive measures. Perhaps:

a. Having no gum trees in the garden.
b. Breeding colonies kept under cover all the time in sheds, etc. This does happen elsewhere and the UK and NZ but I do not like to see ferrets caged all the time.
c. Ferrets kept strictly indoors. That has its own problems unless handled sensibly (Ch. 14).
d. Ferrets outside but on well-grassed areas or with groundcover plants keeping the ferrets from direct contact with the soil. When ferret breeding, I used thick newspaper sheets under scats trays in toilet area to stop hobs nosing in soil where jills toilet. Use of grass clippings, etc. as temporary ground cover. I make the effort to leave branch cuttings with leaves in the ferretarium and allow weeds to grow. This is broken down and makes a 'jungle' effect for the ferrets and keeps their noses off the dirt. Ferrets will however dig to some extent.
e. Keep water bowls, food bowls and scats trays covered against bird droppings contamination.
f. Keep ferrets in just during summer months.
g. Vaccination against the disease is unfortunately not available but would eliminate (a) to (d) makeshift ideas. An autogenous vaccine used on a sick cat appeared to work in conjunction with flucytosine.[45]
h. At the present time, I am installing a hawk bird scarer in the tree in ferretarium 1.

CHAPTER TWELVE
Diseases of the ferret ear, eye and nose

i. *Note*: I had bird faeces from the ground in ferretarium 1 tested for *Cryptococcus* growth in November 2005, with a negative result (J. Jardin, Vet Path Laboratories, Perth).

Prognosis: With cats, the treatment can take up to 6 weeks but the prognosis is good provided there is no CNS involvement. It is always poor to guarded in the case of dog infections. The picture is not clear with ferrets, although Malik et al. have recorded success over some time with Mario.[61] Hanley et al. also had success as seen above.[41] I am still not happy with the toxicity of drugs over a long period regarding ferrets but the outcome seems to have been good in recent cases. Skin granulomatous infections may well be cleared over time as seen in case examples but ferrets with CNS involvement, much like dogs with meningoencephalitis cases, would require a guarded prognosis in relation to the disease. Cryptococcosis may well become more prevalent in the future due to possible climatic changes from global warming.

Nasal neoplasia

A nasal tumour was discovered in a Japanese ferret which had ramifications with spread to the eye orbit (Yasutsugu Miwa, pers. comm. 2005). The 4-year-old castrate was presented with exophthalmos of the left eye. Other than the bulging eye, the ferret had shown sneezing but otherwise was healthy. The swelling had been developing for 4 months. The eye was ulcerated and other ophthalmologic values were intraocular pressure (IOP) right eye, 26 mmHg and left eye 28 mmHg. Iris blood vessels were congested and the optic disc was red and swelling. Ultrasound revealed a retrobular tumour.

From an FNA and cytology a lymphoma was suspected and a course of prednisone was started, giving 1 mg/kg b.i.d. for 7 days, then 1 mg/kg s.i.d. for another 7 days. This had no effect but the owner decided on surgery. An orbital enucleation was done for diagnosis and prevention

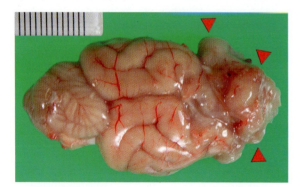

Figure 12.30 Brain tumour image at post mortem. Arrows indicate tumour. (Courtesy of Yasutsugu Miwa.)

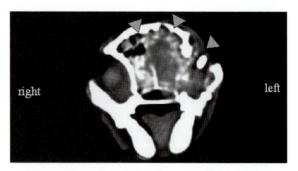

Figure 12.31 Ferret brain tumour CT scan. Arrows indicate tumour spread. (Courtesy of Yasutsugu Miwa.)

of future eye trauma like corneal rupture. With the eye removed, the ferret went home after hospitalization and lived for 5 months. A post mortem and histopathology found a mass located in the orbital cavity and outside the globe (Fig. 12.30). It consisted of oval epidermal cells, with clear nuclei, arranged in diffuse sheets, tubules, cords or glands. The glands contained eosinophilic material. Infiltration into the orbit was seen with cell mitotic figures and adipose tissue was located between the globe and the mass. A first diagnosis was made of a craniopharyngioma. However, based on the CT image (Fig. 12.31) and the location of the mass a corrected diagnosis was made of adenocarcinoma originating from the paranasal sinuses. Hence, the early sneezing fits?

References

1. Rarey KE. The ferret as a model for inner ear research. Lab Anim Sci 1985; 35:238–241.
2. Whary MT, Andrews PLR. Physiology of the ferret. In: Fox JG, ed. Biology and diseases of the ferret, 2nd edn. Baltimore: Williams & Wilkins; 1998:103–148.
3. Lewington JH. Examination of ferret ear. Control and therapy. University of Sydney: Postgraduate Foundation 1990; 152:195–196.
4. Fox JG. Mycotic diseases. In: Fox JG, ed. Biology and diseases of the ferret, 2nd edn. Baltimore: Williams & Wilkins; 1998: 393–403.
5. Animal Health Division. Diseases of fitch. Surveillance. New Zealand, Ministry of Agriculture and Fisheries 1984; 11:2–27.
6. Fox JG. Parasitic diseases. In: Fox JG, ed. Biology and diseases of the ferret. Baltimore: Williams & Wilkins; 1998: 375–391.
7. Christman CL. Disorders of the vestibular system. Compend Contin Edu Pract Vet 1979; 1:744–751.
8. Shell LG. Otitis media and otitis interna in diseases of the ear canal: etiology, diagnosis, and medical management. Vet Clin North Am Small Anim Pract 1988; 18:855–899.
9. Lewington JH. Idiopathic otitis interna of the ferret. Control and therapy. University of Sydney: Postgraduate Foundation; 1989; 151:183–184.
10. Merchant SR. Ototoxity. Vet Clin North Am Small Anim Pract 1994; 24:971–980.

11. Dipold T, Roberts L. Ear mites and otitis media/interna in a ferret. Control and therapy. University of Sydney: Postgraduate Foundation 1996; 192:809.
12. Lewington JH. A review of antibiotics in use for ferrets. Control and therapy. University of Sydney: Postgraduate Foundation 1996; 193:901–902.
13. Lavers RB, Clapperton BK. Ferret. In: King CM, ed. The handbook of New Zealand mammals. Oxford: Oxford University Press; 1990: 320–330.
14. Miller PE. Ferret ophthalmology. Semin Avian Exot Pet Med 1997; 6:146–151.
15. Jackson CJ, Hickley TL. Use of ferrets in studies of the visual system. Lab Anim Sci 1985; 35:211–215.
16. Chapman B, Stryker MP. Development of orientation selectivity in ferret visual cortex and effects of deprivation. J Neurosci 1993; 13:5251–5262.
17. Lewington JH. Third eyelid flap for treating a corneal ulcer in a ferret. Control and therapy. University of Sydney: Postgraduate Foundation 1994; 178:675.
18. Kern TJ. Ocular disorders of rabbits, rodents and ferrets. In: Kirk R, ed. Current veterinary therapy, No. 10. Philadelphia: WB Saunders; 1989: 681–685.
19. Wen GY, Sturman JA, Shek JW. A comparative study of the tapetum, retina and skull of the ferret, dog and cat. Lab Anim Sci 1985; 35:200–210.
20. Tjalve H, Frank A. Tapetum lucidum in the pigmented and albino ferret. Exp Eye Res 1984; 38:341–351.
21. King C. The natural history of weasels and stoats. London: Christopher Helm; 1989.
22. Shimbo FM. A Tao full of detours: The behavior of the domesticated ferret. Boulder: FURO; 1992.
23. Shimbo FA. The ferret book. Boulder: Tercel; 1984.
24. Kirschner SE. Ophthalmologic diseases in small mammals. In: Hillyer EV, Quesenberry KE, eds. Ferrets, rabbits and rodents, Clinical medicine and surgery. Philadelphia: Saunders; 1997:344–345.
25. Conn M. Resolution of chronic conjunctivitis in a ferret with a nasolacrimal duct obstruction. Exotic DVM 2004; 6:1.
26. Chanin P. The natural history of otters. London: Christopher Helm; 1985.
27. Lewington JH. Ferrets: A compendium. Vade Mecum Series C10. University of Sydney: Postgraduate Foundation; 1988.
28. Rathbun WB. Biochemistry of the lens and cataractogenesis: Current Concepts. Vet Clin North Am Small Anim Pract 1980; 10:377–399.
29. Miller PE, Marlar AB, Dubielzig RR. Cataracts in a laboratory colony of ferrets. Lab Anim Sci 1993; 43:562–568.
30. Remailard RL, Pickett JP, Thatcher CD. Comparison of kittens fed queen's milk with those fed milk replacer. (Report of original article). J Am Vet Med Ass 1993; 202:12.
31. Martin CL, Chambreau T. Cataract production in experimentally-orphaned puppies fed a commercial replacement for bitch's milk. Am Anim Hosp Assoc 1982; 18:115–116.
32. Lewington JH. Ferrets: possible galactose-induced cataract development. Control and therapy. University of Sydney: Postgraduate Foundation 1993; 172:545–546.
33. Ryland LM, Gorman JR. The ferret and its diseases. J Am Vet Med Assoc 1978; 173:1154–1158.
34. Bird PH, Hartmann PE, Kelly SE, et al. Carbohydrate malabsorption assessed using bioluminescence assays to measure simple sugars. Austral Vet J 1990; 67:341–342.
35. Kasasaki T. Retinal atrophy in the ferret. J Small Exot Anim Med 1992; 1.
36. Millichamp NJ. Retinal degeneration in the dog and cat. Vet Clin North Am Small Anim Pract 1990; 20:799–835.
37. Fettman M. Trace elements and miscellaneous nutrients. In: Adams HR, ed. Veterinary pharmacology and therapeutics. Ames: Iowa State University Press; 1995:731–733.
38. Finkler M. Practical ferret medicine and surgery for the private practitioner. Roanoke, Viriginia: Roanoke Animal Hospital; 1999.
39. Evans H, Delahunta A. Miller's guide to the dissection of the dog. Philadelphia: WB Saunders; 1971.
40. Malik R, Alderton B, Finlaison D et al. Cryptococcosis in ferrets; a diverse spectrum of clinical cases. Aust Vet J 2002; 80:749–755.
41. Hanley CS, MacWilliams P, Giles S, Paré J. Diagnosis and successful treatment of *Crytococcus neoformans* var. *grubii* in a domesticated ferret (*Mustela putorius furo*). Unpublished article; 2005.
42. Lewington JH. Isolation of *Cryptococcus neoformans* from a ferret. Austral Vet J 1982; 58.
43. Lewington JH. Cryptococcosis in the ferret. Control and therapy. University of Sydney: Postgraduate Foundation; 1997; 195:923–924.
44. Wilkinson GT. Feline cryptococcosis: a review and seven case reports. J Small Anim Pract 1979; 20:749–768.
45. Wilkinson GT, Bate MJ, Robins GM, et al. Successful treatment of four cases of feline cryptococcosis. J Small Anim Pract 1983; 24:507–514.
46. Nicholls J. Cryptococcosis, pneumonia and encephalitis in dogs. Control and therapy. University of Sydney: Postgraduate Committee 1989; 150:165.
47. Doneley B. Cutaneous cryptococcosis in an African grey parrot. Control and therapy. University of Sydney: Postgraduate Committee 1991; 161:335.
48. Ellis DA. Brief notes on cryptococcosis. Mycology Unit Newsletter. Adelaide: Women's and Children's Hospital; 1999.
49. Barlough JE. Cryptococcosis. In: Tilly LP, Smith FWK Jr, eds. The 5-minute veterinary consult. Baltimore: Williams & Wilkins; 1997:488–489.
50. Malik R, Martin P, Wigney DI, et al. Cryptococcosis in cats: diagnosis and treatment. Feline Medicine and Surgery. University of Sydney: Postgraduate Foundation 1998; 30:101–105.
51. Pelt DR Van, Lappin MR. Pathogenesis and treatment of feline rhinitis. Vet Clin North Am Small Anim Pract 1994; 23:807–823.
52. Malik R, McPetrie R, Wigney DI, et al. A latex cryptococcal antigen agglutination test for diagnosis and monitoring of therapy for cryptococcosis. Austral Vet J 1996; 74:358–364.
53. Duncan C. Multispecies outbreak of cryptococcosis in southern Vancouver Island (2000–2001) British Columbia. Can Vet J 2002; 43:792–794.
54. Lester SJ, Kowalewich NJ, Bartlett KH, Krockenberger MB, Fairfax TM, Malik R. Clinicopathologic features of an unusual outbreak of cryptococcosis in dogs, cats, ferrets and a bird; 38 cases. J Am Vet Med Assoc 2004; 225:1716–1722.
55. Ellis DH, Pfeiffer TJ. Natural habitat of *Cryptococcus neoformans* var. *gattii*. J Clin Microbiol 1990; 28:1642–1644.
56. Sorrell TC, Ellis DH. Ecology of *Cryptococcus neoformans*. Rev Iberoam Micol 1997; 14:42–43.
57. Greenlee PG, Stephens E. Meningeal cryptococcosis and congestive cardiomyopathy in a ferret. J Am Vet Med Ass 1984; 184:840–841.
58. Curtis AJ. A case of torulosis in a domestic cat. Austral J Med Tech 1951; 1:71–74.
59. Porter V, Brown N. The complete book of ferrets. Bedford: D&M Publications; 1997.
60. Pearson RC, Gorham JR. Viral disease models. In: Fox JG, ed. Biology and diseases of the ferret, 2nd edn. Baltimore: Williams & Wilkins; 1998: 487–497.
61. Malik R, Martin P, et al. Successful treatment of invasive nasal cryptococcosis in a ferret. Aust Vet J 2000; 78:158–159.

CHAPTER 13

General neoplasia

'Ferrets can contract many diseases and disorders other than those already mentioned. Among them are cancerous tumours, ...'

Fred J. Taylor's Guide to Ferreting, revised edn. 1988

Neoplasia is rare in Australian ferrets compared with American ferrets, as we have ferrets only in the thousands while the USA/Canadian pet ferret population is up to around 10 million. However, pet ferrets are becoming increasingly popular in Australia. Numbers have also risen in other countries around the world. This brings on an increased awareness of possible neoplasia.

One of the suggested causes of ferret neoplasia is genetic predisposition (Ch. 5). Australian ferret genetic lines have not been added to since the 1920s. Private breeders carry out ferret breeding and we have no large commercial organizations. In New Zealand, pet ferrets have been banned since the late 1990s, but there are two commercial breeding establishments. Mystic Ferrets and Southlands Ferrets supply ferrets for the research and pet markets around the world (not Australia). Private breeders in the USA import ferrets from around the world, including Australia and New Zealand, to enlarge their gene pool, which was at one time restricted to ferrets from Marshall Farms. At time of writing, it appears that the USA has more different types of neoplasia recorded and problems that do not exist elsewhere.

The recording and incidence of neoplasia in Australia has been very low; one reason has been that ferret owners have been reluctant in the past to bring their ferrets to the veterinarian. This situation is changing now, as the ferret becomes more popular as a pet, besides being a working animal. Veterinarians worldwide should make sure they report neoplasia in ferrets and perform post mortems. It would be advantageous for universities to assist practitioners with reduced fee pathology, to encourage ferret owners to seek help, allowing a database to be built up for the future.

Ferret neoplasia in the USA

The common neoplasms seem to be lymphoma, various skin neoplasms and the two major endocrine conditions of adrenal gland neoplasia and insulinoma; the latter two are discussed in Chapter 14. The overall incidence of ferret neoplasia in the USA is not considered high. However, at the time of writing, there is still concern with the major neoplasms affecting the adrenal glands, pancreas and haematolymphatic system which are still prevalent and require intense treatments. Various surveys have been undertaken in the USA of ferret neoplasia in laboratory and pet ferrets,[1-3] and the subject has also been discussed in the UK.[4] With such low numbers of ferrets, no surveys have as yet been done in Australia.

It is noted that the apparent scarcity of spontaneous cancers in ferrets may be due in part to their relatively short lifespan, which is seen particularly in laboratory ferrets, as these still make up the bulk of the northern hemisphere ferret population. However, for various reasons, including neoplasia, the pet ferret population does not seem to be very long-lived in the USA. It has been pointed out that compared with laboratory ferrets, those kept in zoos do not have a higher incidence of neoplasia. This is despite zoo ferrets living a more normal, longer life and the probability of neoplasm development being supposed to increase with age.[1] The suggestion has been made that because there is a low incidence of neoplasia in ferrets, they are in some way genetically resistant to such disease. However, without a greater database on ferret neoplasia, that assumption is unreliable. Dillberger and Altman found that over a 4-year period, 12 cases of ferret neoplasia were diagnosed in a particular laboratory; a literature review yielded 83 further cases in ferrets, polecats and even black-footed ferrets.[1] They concluded that ferrets have a similar risk of cancer to other animals.

The position of a malignant tumour in the body may dictate an acute or chronic effect. The position of a neoplasm in the neck or cranial mediastinum produces acute symptoms on enlargement of the growth as shown in the following two examples.

The thyroid can be the site of adenocarcinoma as illustrated by a 2-year-old de-sexed jill, living indoors, which was seen with a midventral cervical mass that developed over 2 weeks (Fig. 13.1a,b).[5] (The site of the normal thyroid is shown in Figure 2.19.)

Two other household ferrets were normal, all were vaccinated and fed on commercial food. The tumour was palpated as a 5.5 × 5 cm prominent immobile mass to the left of midline. It filled the cervical region from the angle of the jaw down to the thoracic inlet. The ferret developed signs of severe dysphagia. Radiology found the trachea deviated ventrally and to the right of the midline as in Figure 13.1b. Radiology and ultrasonograms of the ferret's chest found no spread of disease.

Regarding thyroid activity, the serum thyroxine concentration was normal at 35 mmol/L. *Note*: to check if the tumour mass was endocrinologically active, a sophisticated soft tissue nuclear scintigraphy was carried out using technetium 99m pertechnetate sodium which gave negative results so that treatment of the mass with radioiodine was ruled out. Instead, one of the cancer treatment protocols (see later) was initiated. The outcome was that the tumour regressed and within 2 weeks was down to one-tenth of its original size. The ferret improved and the dysphagia stopped, showing the positive side to the protocol procedures in ferrets. However, 4 months after the initial treatment the tumour recurred and the ferret was put to sleep. Histology showed that the mass was a thyroid adenocarcinoma with metastases to the cervical lymph nodes and liver.

Lymphoma

Any enlargement of organs in the ferret anterior cranial thoracic region can quickly give rise to distress due to the relative narrowness of the chest. A common occurrence is some form of lymphoma. These growths are seen in young ferrets (lymphoblastic type) and old ferrets (lymphocytic type) in the USA and may have a viral origin.[6] It is sometimes hard to tell well-differentiated lymphoma cells from normal lymph node cells. Also, since the neoplasm is not usually homogenously distributed throughout the lymph node, false negatives have been seen in both ferrets and dogs (Levine, Honolulu Zoo, pers. comm. 2005).

Lymphoma are considered the most common neoplasms and the disease spectrum involves peripheral and visceral lymph nodes, spleen, liver, mediastinum, bone marrow and kidney while the small intestine and skin

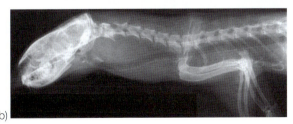

Figure 13.1 (a) Post mortem photograph of ferret showing the mass. (b) *Note* the displacement of trachea by neoplastic mass. (Courtesy of JW Carpenter, MV Finnegan and Vet Med 2003.)

CHAPTER THIRTEEN
General neoplasia

are not usually sites for this tumour type.[7] In an account of 13 spontaneous cancers in laboratory ferrets in the UK, six were found to be lymphoma.[6] In American households with numbers of ferrets and also cats, it has been suggested that lymphoma may multi-infect from Aleutian disease virus (ADV) or feline leukaemia virus (FeLV) but one study did not find these viruses associated with lymphoma.[8]

In an American laboratory ferret colony, three cases of mediastinal lymphoma with signs of acute morbidity with splenomegaly plus hepatomegaly with a large thoracic mass were found.[9] Examples of thoracic neoplasia are given with lymphoma cases in Figures 13.2, 13.3 and a fibrosarcoma in Figure 13.4.

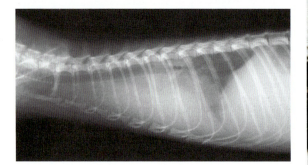

Figure 13.2 Chest lymphoma. (Courtesy of G. Rich.)

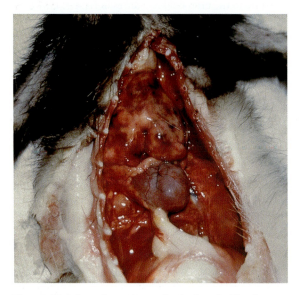

Figure 13.3 Lymphoma in mediastinal cavity. The ferret was presented with dyspnoea and died within 24 hours. Radiograph and post mortem revealed lymphoma. (Courtesy of G. Rich.)

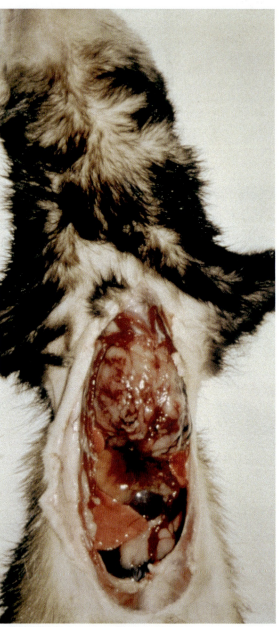

Figure 13.4 Fibrosarcoma in the thoracic cavity. The ferret was presented with dyspnoea. Using ultrasound as a guide, a needle aspirate revealed hard fibrous/cartilaginous tumour. Ferret was euthanized. (Courtesy of G. Rich.)

Figure 13.2 is of a 4-year-old ferret, which showed severe dyspnoea, weight loss, lymphocytosis on peripheral smear with a white blood cell count of 11 400 (68% lymphocytes).

In another American survey,[3] 62% of lymphomas were detected in sterilized male ferrets, which is the usual case. In Australia, with older working hob ferrets, any enlargement of the submandibular lymph glands could be mistaken for sites of an abscess build-up from fight wounds, especially with hobs in the mating season or even working ferrets, which can get bitten around the head and neck. A retrospective study of clinical and pathological findings in 60 cases of confirmed lymphoma in ferrets revealed that of the cases studied, three had been found dead and one died just before examination.[10] Of the rest, 21 had chemotherapy while seven had surgery and the remaining 28 had no treatment. Unfortunately, eight ferrets could not be completely followed-up. However, a survival time >2 months was more likely for ferrets over 3 years old. Mean survival time after diagnosis was 6 months in cases of high-grade lymphoma and 8 months for ferrets with low-grade lymphoma. Of the 21 ferrets that had chemotherapy, three died from complications of the treatment and five could not be followed-up, but a mean survival time was given as 10.6 months for the rest. Of the seven ferrets that had surgery, four had the spleen removed, two had lymph nodes removed and one had a skin tumour excised. No chemotherapy was given to these ferrets. The mean survival rate for them was 12 months. Of the 28 ferrets not treated, 16 were euthanized after diagnosis while four ferrets over 4 years old did live for several years (mean range 1.3–5.2 years).

Thus, the clinician has the option to advise treatment and/or surgery or perhaps advise no treatment. My jill ferret with splenic lymphosarcoma survived for 6 months on alternative medicine post-operation (see Australian neoplasia). The internal spread of lymphoma can occur as it does in other animals. In 5-year-old ferrets, stage 2 lymphomas arise in the abdominal organs and it is suggested that they may have occurred due to chronic inflammation of the intestine. This brings speculation that a dietary factor might be involved and composition of the diet, particularly fibre content, may in some way be a predisposing factor. Further, certain lymphomas in humans have been shown to be associated with chronic *Helicobacter pylori* infection. In ferrets, lymphoid hyperplasia in the gastric mucosa and gastric lymph nodes are also features of chronic *Helicobacter mustelae* infection (Ch. 9). With regard to possible chemotherapy for lymphoma, Brown maintains that mediastinal lesions respond well but the gastrointestinal lymphomas do not, which could suggest that gastrointestinal lymphomas may be initiated by inflammation of unknown cause and it is postulated that the condition could be aggravated by excess dietary fibre.

Lymphoma in young ferrets

Ferrets between 4 and 6 months old can develop malignant lymphomas rapidly.[7] I have seen a sudden death in a 3½-month-old ferret with a malignant thymus lymphosarcoma. Signs of any lymphoma can be as non-specific as anorexia, weight loss and lethargy, plus enlargement of glands such as lymph nodes and spleen. A young ferret may have hind leg weakness with a spay-legged appearance. If there is dyspnoea, radiographs will show the presence of a mediastinal mass if lymph glands are involved. Besides the thymus, the multicentric lymphoma typically involves the CNS, the musculature and gonads.[7] The presence of a gastric lymphoma will cause a foreign body reaction with anorexia, possibly vomiting, depression and dehydration. The lymphoma may be palpable. Usually by this stage, the lymphoma has spread rapidly throughout the body. A blood profile shows leukaemia with atypical lymphocytes in less than half of young ferret cases. Fox has illustrated the distribution of clinical signs of neoplastic conditions in the ferret at various ages and clearly shows the high percentage of mediastinal cancers in ferrets 1 year old or younger (Fig. 13.5).[2]

Thymic lymphoma in adult ferrets

Two cases of thymic lymphoma were seen in 5-year-old ferrets.[11] One case is interesting to comment on, regarding the disease and associated problems with a ferret of this age. A ferret at 4 years of age had been diagnosed with an enlarged spleen and opacity over the heart base by radiology. When presented as a 5-year-old, cardiomyopathy was diagnosed with pleural effusion. From 1 year old, the ferret had been having vomiting periods,

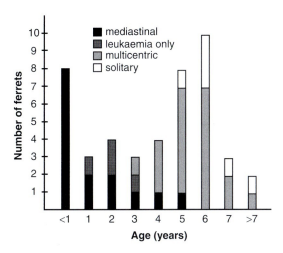

Figure 13.5 Distribution of clinical signs against the age of the ferret with lymphoma. (From Erdmann S, Xiantang Li and Fox JG. Haematopoietic diseases in biology and diseases of the ferret. Baltimore: Williams & Wilkins 1998:233, with permission.)

CHAPTER THIRTEEN
General neoplasia

possibly associated with eating, and since 3 years old, it had episodic dyspnoea, wheezing, enlarged spleen and chronic anal sac impaction. It underwent a bilateral anal sacculectomy (Ch. 18). In all my years of having ferrets I have never had ferrets with anal sac troubles. Could it have been related to the diet?

The ferret was treated with Lasix for the cardiomyopathy at 4 mg every 12 hours plus KCl elixir. Then, several days after the X-rays, echocardiography found a cystic mass in the cranial mediastinum as well as left ventricular hypertrophy but without pulmonary signs of congestive heart failure.

The splenomegaly was considered as a malignant lymphoma and the mediastinal mass as a possible thymoma. The ferret continued to be treated at regular visits for lethargy, vomiting and diarrhoea but with presumably no change of diet. Then after 8 months, the patient developed a hind limb paresis. This was considered to be either a malignant lymphoma, intervertebral disc disease (Ch. 19) or arterial thrombosis.

The blood picture showed a normal leukocyte count of 10 000 cells/μL and left shift (band = 202 cells/μL) and lymphocytosis of 5151 cells/μL. Other values were normal except for alanine transaminase increase to 327 U/L. Treating the paresis with prednisolone gained some improvement in movement but the lymphadenopathy became general accompanying a weight loss. The ferret was euthanized.

Post mortem found the cranial mediastinum mass to be a thymic lymphoma, some 3.5 × 3.0 × 2.0 cm, with characteristic multilobular structure with petechiae and prominent vasculature.

Mark Burgess has indicated how a thymic lymphoma can spread in the chest as illustrated by Figure 13.6.

It is said that the presence of upper respiratory infections can be a feature of chronic lymphoma. 'Snuffles' occurs sporadically in some Australian ferrets including my own (Ch. 8) and could be an indication of cancer. Similarly, an ongoing gastrointestinal disease may be present. Both conditions respond to antibiotics but only while treatment is being carried out. Thus a lymphoma may be an underlying cause.

Lymphoma in adult ferrets

The adult ferret can slip into a chronic lymphoma state gradually with it being put down to 'old age'. I had a case of my own with a 7-year-old hob, Sammy, showing submandibular lymph node enlargement. I did not notice it at once but then decided, as the ferret was active, to leave it. I am still not sure if I could have gained much for the ferret with surgery and/or chemotherapy at that age. The clinical signs again can be inappetence, lethargy and weight loss. It is advisable to get ferret owners to keep a check on their ferret's weight, especially when the animal is over 5 years old. Older ferrets may get vomiting and tenesmus, as occurs in young ferrets. Splenic enlargement can be common and the enlarged spleen is palpable (see Fig. 7.3). The cause may be extramedullary haematopoiesis without malignancy, so it is considered that splenic aspiration is not diagnostic, especially in older ferrets.[7] With the high splenic cancer incidence, I would be inclined to remove the spleen in older ferrets (Fig. 13.7).

I had a jill with an enlarged spleen condition which, when held with a normal ferret of the same age and size for comparison, showed a prominent left-side swelling of the abdomen. It was a splenic tumour (see Fig. 7.3).[12] In the older ferret a chest cough due to mediastinal lymph node enlargement may be confused with heart disease. Along with these signs can be general icterus, paralysis, plus possible palpable abdominal masses besides the spleen, where the kidneys, adrenals and pancreas can be involved.

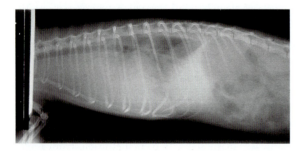

Figure 13.6 Thymic tumour. (Courtesy of M. Burgess.)

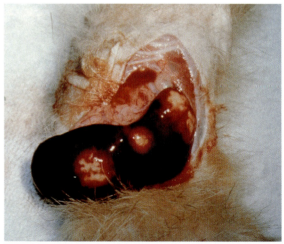

Figure 13.7 Lymphoma of spleen. (Courtesy of M. Finkler.)

Diagnosis

In a definitive appraisal, this would be by cytology and histology of the internal organ involved but generally, the palpation of enlarged lymph nodes in the absence of pyrexia can indicate neoplasia.[3] The popliteal lymph node is reasonably accessible for complete removal so as to check for the presence of systemic lymphoma. It can be dissected out, it is usually near the surface, and is found as a dark red or brown node possibly surrounded by fat.[13] It has been recorded in one American practice that 23 of 73 lymphadenectomies (32%) carried out because of persistent lymphocytosis were reported as lymphoid hyperplasia, but biopsies in 50 of 73 ferrets (68%) were positive as lymphoma.[3] A complete blood count is advised as routine for ferrets over 1 year old. The American experience with lymphoma in ferrets makes veterinarians hypersensitive to the disease being present early in life. In Australia, I have had only my own 3½-month ferret with cancer and others recorded have been in ferrets 5 years or older. I doubt at the present time that the average Australian ferret owner would agree to yearly blood testing of their ferrets.

Treatment

The use of surgery and/or chemotherapy in ferrets for cancer treatment follows that for the dog and cat. Ferrets tolerate the prolonged chemotherapy treatment well at the drug levels worked out for them.[13] Before embarking on the treatment protocol, full blood chemistry should be done, remembering to give the ferret a 4–6 hour fast to check glucose fasting levels. Radiology should be done to check for any suspicious abdominal or thoracic masses. Echocardiography check is useful if available. Needle biopsies of any enlarged organs, e.g. spleen, can be carried out but are considered of limited value, so exploratory operations are more valuable.

Back in 1998, it was estimated that in the USA, ferrets over 3 years of age were already suffering from insulinoma, adrenal gland neoplasm or even cardiomyopathy and possibly early renal disease when diagnosed as a lymphoma case. Have things improved?

Protocols for cancer treatment in ferrets

Two major protocols have been extensively used by Dr S. Brown (Midwest Bird & Exotic Animal Hospital, Westchester, IL) and Dr K. Rosenthal (Animal Medical Centre, New York). A third protocol has been devised by Dr J. Mayer of Tufts University School of Veterinary Medicine. An interesting fourth protocol from Dr P. Selleri in Rome is included for consideration.

Protocol 1 (Dr S. Brown)

This involves the use of prednisone, vincristine (Oncovin–Lilly) and cyclophosphamide (Cytoxan–Mead Johnson) (Table 13.1). Vincristine is given intravenously and requires the ferret to be anaesthetized and an indwelling catheter put in place, which is kept patent by flushing with heparinized saline. As a precaution, a blood profile is carried out within 24 hours of giving the cytotoxic drug, and if the WBC count is seen to fall below 1000, the drug is discontinued. This also applies if the PCV falls below 30% or if the ferret is obviously sick.[3]

Protocol 2 (Dr K. Rosenthal)

This involves the use of Protocol 1 drugs plus asparaginase (Elspar–Merck) and methotrexate (Lederle or Mexate–Bristol) and possibly doxorubicin (adriamycin–Atria)[13] as developed by Dr K. Rosenthal (Table 13.2).

Table 13.1 Time sequence for Protocol 1 for ferrets

Week	Day	Drug	Dose	Comments
1	1	Prednisone	1 mg/kg	Given b.i.d. and continued daily p.o.
	1	Vincristine	0.12 mg/kg	Given i.v.
	3	Cyclophosphamide	10 mg/kg	p.o. or s.c. (not given on same day as vincristine)
2	8	Vincristine	0.12 mg/kg	Given i.v.
3	15	Vincristine	0.12 mg/kg	Given i.v.
4	22	Vincristine	0.12 mg/kg	Given i.v.
	24	Cyclophosphamide	10 mg/kg	p.o. or s.c.
7	46	Cyclophosphamide	10 mg/kg	p.o. or s.c.
9		Prednisone	1 mg/kg	Now decrease dose to zero over 4 weeks

Note the ferret should have a CBC check weekly during and after therapy (then at 3-monthly intervals). b.i.d., bis in die; i.v., intravenous injection; p.o., given by mouth; s.c., given subcutaneously. (Table after Brown, 1997, with permission.[3])

CHAPTER THIRTEEN

General neoplasia

Table 13.2 Time sequence for Protocol 2

Week	Day	Drug	Dose	Comment
1	1	Asparaginase	400 IU/kg	Given i.p. but once only
1	1	Prednisone	2 mg/kg	Given b.i.d. p.o. and continued
1	5	Vincristine	0.07 mg/kg	Given i.v. 5 days after asparaginase
2		Cyclophosphamide	10 mg/kg	Given p.o.
3		Vincristine	0.07 mg/kg	Given i.v.
4		Methotrexate	0.5 mg/kg	Given s.q.
5		Vincristine	0.07 mg/kg	Given i.v.
6		Cyclophosphamide	10 mg/kg	Given s.q.
7		Vincristine	0.07 mg/kg	Given i.v.
8		Methotrexate	0.5 mg/kg	Given s.q.
Use same protocol at 2-weekly intervals for 6 months.		Asparaginase must not be used for at least 6 months after first use		
Check WBC at 1 or 2 weeks		Doxorubicin can be used as rescue agent if protocol fails		

Note: Doxorubicin (adriamycin, Adria) must be given i.v. and has been used as a rescue agent for both protocols above when there is a recurrence of disease after a remission period. It is useful for single agent therapy being given at 1 mg/kg i.v. It can be used along with prednisone at 1 mg/kg b.i.d. (Table after Brown, 1993, with permission.[13])

It should be noted that the vincristine dosage depends on which other drugs are used in combination. One veterinarian uses 0.75 mg/m² or 0.12 mg/kg i.v. when used in combination with cyclophosphamide and prednisone. She uses 0.07 mg/kg i.v. with prednisolone, asparaginase, cyclophosphamide and methotrexate (A. Lennox, pers. comm. 2005). The latter dose is the same as 0.5–0.75 mg/m² which is used by J. Meyer. He uses no vincristine on ferrets. (See Protocol 3.)

Discussion

Use of these two protocols with lymphoma is highly work-intensive and long term; the veterinarian and client must balance up the expense and possible outcome of the procedure. However, Brown is of the opinion that it is worthwhile treating lymphoma cases, especially those with cancers in the mediastinum, spleen, skin and peripheral lymph nodes. According to her experience, those ferrets with internal liver, intestinal or bone marrow sites, or multifocal lesions in any organs, plus, remarkably, the solitary mandibular lymph nodes, show a poor response to treatment. Generally, Protocol 2 is now used in major American hospitals as standard procedure for lymphoma; although it is longer than Protocol 1, it gives a better success rate. The hospital makes sure the client is aware of the length of the procedure, the drugs involved and the cost and that the owner's compliance with instructions is a major factor.

Some technical points

1. All ferrets have bone marrow biopsy done prior to chemotherapy to assess risks.
2. The CBC is drawn immediately the ferret enters hospital and the cephalic vein is not used for this procedure. Water can be given to the ferret and a treat (Nutrical, etc.) but no food.
3. The ferret is weighed as routine on admittance.
4. With the blood profile, if the WBC is over 2000 and the PCV is above 30% then the ferret is in good clinical condition for treatment. However if the WBC is between 1000–2000, Neupogen, a drug that stimulates white cell production, should be given and the clinician can decide based on other signs whether to commence treatment. If the WBC is below 1000, chemotherapy is not given but Neupogen is given with other supportive care (Brown, pers. comm. 1998). The ferret is checked in 3–4 days with another WBC count.
5. *Note* chemotherapy should not be attempted until the WBC rises above 2000. Furthermore, if the PCV is below 25%, then Neupogen is administered and

chemotherapy is discontinued until the PCV rises above 30%.
6. It is considered that around the 3rd–4th week of therapy the ferret will lose weight. The ferret can be helped with a supplementary diet either by syringe or bowl. The use of Feline A/D Total Recovery Diet or meat baby food is recommended, mixed with heavy cream or blended beef liver.[3] Feeding should be 4 times daily. It is known that ferrets depend more on fat for energy rather than carbohydrate, plus a high quality protein meat (Ch. 4).
7. Other supportive nutritional supplements recommended by Brown are as follows: vitamin C at 50–100 mg/kg p.o. q. 12 h, Pau d'Arco at 3–5 drops p.o. q. 12 h, Pycnogenol at 15 mg p.o. q. 24 h, echinacea at 3–5 drops q. 12 h.
8. It may be necessary to take other biochemistry tests on the ferret, also radiographs and to give other supportive care over the long period of chemotherapy.

Administration of chemotherapeutic agents

The use of dangerous anti-tumour drugs requires i.v. administration under a general anaesthetic (Ch. 16). In the American hospitals cited above, the anaesthetic of choice is isoflurane, masking the ferret down without the use of any premedication. A 23- or 24-gauge butterfly catheter is placed in the cephalic vein (Ch. 20) and is flushed with 3 mL saline before giving the drug. The chemotherapeutic agent is diluted with 3 mL of non-heparinized saline, with the exception of doxorubicin, which should be diluted with 5 mL of non-heparinized saline. The drug is administered slowly with a follow-through of 3 mL saline to flush.[3] The leg is bandaged and the ferret left to recover in a warm cage. The ferret can then be fed and released to the client.

One veterinarian suggests only sedation of the ferret for chemotherapy, with ketamine i.m. or s.c. before giving the agent into the cephalic vein (using a 1 mL tuberculin syringe and 26- or 28-gauge needle while holding the ferret). He never masks down with isoflurane for any routine procedures (M. Finkler, pers. comm. 1998).

With sick ferrets on continuous medication by intravenous injection, the jugular vein has been used over a long period with a so-called vascular port.[14] This technique has been used in humans, dogs and pigs. The system is made up of a 4-F silicone rubber catheter connected to a moulded plastic injection port with as self-sealing septum. This vascular access system was used on an 8½-year-old 685 g spayed jill with large superficial cervical, popliteal and axillary lymphoma and intra-abdominal lymphoma. The interesting point is that the ferret had the vascular port for 33 weeks while under protocol 2 and it collapsed 5 days after vincristine medication and was put to sleep. One wonders in the time frame of treatment about the progressive toxicity of the drugs used.

Toxicity effects of drugs used on ferrets are to be looked out for and can occur after 1–2 days of treatment, beginning with at least lethargy, anorexia, vomiting and possible hind leg weakness. Hair loss occurs, especially the whiskers. The progression is to dyspnoea and complete collapse. Important note: veterinarians should be personally aware of the toxicity of the drugs used and wear gloves when handling them and caution staff on procedures. Safe disposal of used materials, needles, etc. is essential.

Protocol 3 (Dr J. Mayer)

Unlike the first two protocols, this method of treating sick ferrets has been especially developed for ferrets, where repeated i.v. access is not an option (Table 13.3). The method involves totally oral and s.c. drugs so there is no need for invasive procedures. However, it extends over a significantly longer period of 26 weeks (J. Mayer, pers. comm. 2005). The chemotherapy drugs are used based on metabolic scaling, using the surface area of the animal in square metres. This method is more accurate than body weight. At the time of writing, Dr Mayer has 20 ferrets doing well on the protocol with remission achieved at around 10 weeks.

Staging protocols for ferret lymphoma treatment could include CBC+ platelet count, chemistry profile, urinary analysis (culture if indicated), freezing serum for later viral assay, thoracic radiographs (two views), abdominal ultrasound, bone marrow aspirate and histopathology.

It is considered that oral chemotherapy with prednisolone is extremely effective and remissions have been seen within 4 days after the initial treatment (J. Mayer, pers. comm. 2005). However, remission will only last for about 3 months and then the lymphoma comes back as multi-drug resistant (MDR) and spreads fast. If is considered that a ferret is doing really well months after treatment one should not relax prednisolone treatment and in fact the dosage should be high, 1–2 mg/kg. It has been noted that the MDR lymphoma can be treated with success by radiation therapy, which may be the future way to go for this deadly disease.

Protocol 4

An interesting protocol for treating adrenal tumours in ferrets has been proposed by Dr Selleri. The technique has been used in human medicine against thyroid, parathyroid, kidney and liver neoplastic masses and in dogs for cancerous adrenal glands.

CHAPTER THIRTEEN
General neoplasia

Table 13.3 Time sequence for Protocol 3

Protocol 3, Time sequence	Drugs used
Week 1	L-ASP, CTX, PRED
Week 2	L-ASP, CBC*
Week 3	L-ASP, CYTOSAR, Cytosar × 2 days
Week 4	CBC*
Week 5	CTX
Week 7	MTX, CBC
Week 8	CBC*
Week 9	CTX
Week 11	CYTOSAR, LEUK
Week 12	CBC*
Week 13	CTX
Week 15	PCB
Week 16	CBC*
Week 17	CBC
Week 18	CTX
Week 20	CYTOSAR, LEUK × 2 days.
Week 23	CTX
Week 26	PCB
Week 27	CBC, CHEM
If not in remission, continue weeks 20–26 for 3 cycles	
Drugs	**Dosage**
KEY to Protocol 3:	
PRED, Prednisone	2 mg/kg p.o. daily × 1 week then q.o.d.
L-ASP, L-asparaginase	10 000 IU/m² s.q.
CTX, Cytoxan elixir	250 mg/m² p.o. GIVE WITH 50 mL/kg of LRS s.q. once.
CYTOSAR, Cytosar	300 mg/m² s.q. × 2 days (dilute 100 mg with 1 mL H_2O)
MTX, Methotrexate	0.8 mg/kg i.m.
LEUK, Leukeran	1 tab ferret p.o. (or ½ tablet daily for 2 days)
PCB, Procarbazine	50 mg/m² p.o. daily for 14 days
LRS, Lactated Ringers Saline (Hartman's)	

Dose reductions: If CBC* indicates severe myelosuppression, reduce dosage by 25% for all subsequent treatments of the previously used myelosuppressive drug. (Courtesy of Dr Joerg Mayer, DMV, MSc. Tufts University School of Veterinary Medicine, N. Grafton, MA.)

The protocol requires expert ultrasonography and involves injection of the tumour with 0.1–0.2 mL of sterile alcohol (96%). Alcoholization causes thrombosis and necrosis of the mass. Once the needle is inserted, the amount of alcohol injected depends on the size of the gland. Different sites in the gland are used and care is taken not to pull the tip of the needle out of the adrenal capsule. The amount of alcohol injected every time may change due to observation of the glandular parenchyma by echogenicity. With a small glandular mass, the needle is inserted only once. However, it is found that a single treatment is not usually effective so the patient is checked with ultrasound 2–3 weeks later and the process repeated if the patient is still symptomatic.

The treatment has been used on over 30 ferrets and to date there have been no complications. The protocol is considered useful in those animals that cannot go into surgery (P. Selleri, Rome, pers. comm. 2006).

There are mixed feelings in the veterinary profession as to the use of this technique on ferrets though its use has been recorded in thyroid surgery in the cat. Dr J. Mayer considers ferrets with FADC might benefit from the technique and broached the subject at the 2006 North American Veterinary Congress, causing debate (J. Mayer, pers. comm. 2006).

The question of drug toxicity with ferrets is interesting in a case of metastatic squamous cell carcinoma (SCC) where the veterinarians chose the drug bleomycin for its low acute toxicity, ease of administration and the fact it had been used in dogs and cats, to treat a 5-year-old castrated male ferret. Bleomycin is derived from *Streptomyces verticillus* and is classed as a water-soluble anti-tumour antibiotic.[15]

The 900 g ferret had a neoplastic mass of $1.8 \times 1.0 \times 0.6$ cm on the right lower lip, which had recurred after excision 14 days earlier. A biopsy confirmed a squamous cell carcinoma.

Treatment: Bleomycin was started at a dose rate of 10 U/m^2, s.m. once weekly. However, in 3 weeks, the mass increased to $2.4 \times 1.1 \times 0.9$ cm. The bleomycin was upped to 20 U/m^2, s.c. once weekly. The tumour size then decreased to $2.0 \times 0.7 \times 0.5$ cm over 3 weeks. The dosage was kept constant but by 2 months, there were signs of the tumour regrowing. The ferret was put to sleep.

Note: Difficulty in treatment of invasive neoplasms can be frustrating to clinicians. Of course, many squamous cell carcinomas (SCC) are invasive to bone and untreatable cumulative drug toxicity must surely be a factor. A ferret with an inoperable tumour mass was treated with the drug melphalan but within 10 days of treatment it died of haemorrhagic diarrhoea.[15] With the bleomycin case, the ferret had a cumulative dose of 150 U/m^2 but unfortunately no post mortem was possible to determine toxicity. It is stated that the ferret dosage of bleomycin was less than that used for pulmonary fibrosis in the dog. However, on a body weight basis, there must be concern.

The incidence of neoplasia in ferrets outside North America appears to be small and relates to the population difference in ferret numbers as pointed out earlier. We can only take note of the cases that appear prevalent in the USA and consider whether they are occurring in ferrets in Australia and elsewhere to any degree. Considering the overall picture, the details of occurrence of ferret neoplasia in the USA are now given, with reference to the types of neoplasms that are seen by one major veterinary hospital dealing exclusively with ferrets and small pets other than dogs and cats.

American neoplasia cases 1990–1997

Details of American ferret neoplasia are seen in Tables 13.4–13.7. (Courtesy of Dr Susan Brown, Midwest Bird and Exotic Animal Hospital, Westchester, Illinois, USA, pers. comm. 1999.)

With reference to the American tables for the 1990–1997 survey: pancreatic islet cell adenoma 180, lymphoma 132, adrenocortical carcinoma 110 and adrenocortical adenoma 54, dominate the list. The situation of neoplasia numbers in America appears to show by a survey of 1525 cases over a similar period (1990–2000) that pancreatic islet cell tumours, lymphoma, adrenocortical carcinoma and adrenocortical adenoma are still in high proportion to other ferret neoplasia.[16] Another survey of neoplasia in the USA is yet to be done (Bruce Williams, pers. comm. 2005).

A review of interesting neoplasia in American ferrets

Various authors have reported on the cases of lymphoma types in American pet ferrets.[10,17]

C-cell carcinoma

I find one case of ferret C-cell carcinoma interesting.[18] A Marshal Farms 10-week-old sterilized male ferret was taken into a zoo for education purposes. It was vaccinated against CD and rabies and fed dry cat food daily and fresh meat twice weekly. By about 31 months of age the ferret was thin, showing a poor appetite and hair coat loss. A more palatable cat food (Max Cat Adult, Nutro Products) was tried and Nutraderm, a skin and hair coat conditioner was applied. This brought about an improvement in a few weeks.

When the ferret was 45 months of age, it was found semi-conscious but it rallied on its own. For up to 8 weeks afterwards, the ferret had diminished appetite, reduced activity and poor hair coat. On examination, the ferret weighed 962 g, a drop from 1350 g 12 months

Table 13.4 Ferret neoplasia cases, 1990–1997, differentiated by sex

Total cases	Males	Females	Sex unknown
480	231	217	32

Table 13.5 Ferret neoplasia cases, 1990–1997, grouped by age

<1 year	1 year	2 years	3 years	4 years	5 years	6 years	7 years	8 years	9 years	Unknown
5	15	40	80	66	86	38	17	4	2	127

CHAPTER THIRTEEN
General neoplasia

Table 13.6 Histopathologically confirmed neoplasms in 480 cases 1990–1997

Tumour type	Site	No.
Adenoma, benign cystic	Face	5
Adenoma, sebaceous gland	Skin	15
Adrenocortical adenoma		54
Adrenocortical carcinoma		110
Adrenocortical carcinoma	Metastasis to the liver	1
Adrenocortical carcinoma	Metastasis to the spleen	1
Apocrine gland cystadenoma	Skin	2
Carcinoma and adenocarcinoma	Popliteal lymph node (metastatic probably of endocrine origin)	1
Carcinoma and adenocarcinoma	Ceruminous gland	1
Carcinoma and adenocarcinoma	Epithelial	1
Carcinoma and adenocarcinoma	Ocular globe	1
Carcinoma and adenocarcinoma	Prostate	1
Carcinoma and adenocarcinoma	Pancreas	1
Carcinoma and adenocarcinoma	Pancreas with omental metastasis	1
Carcinoma and adenocarcinoma		
Carcinoma and adenocarcinoma		
Carcinoma and adenocarcinoma		
Carcinoma and adenocarcinoma	Mammary gland, cystic	1
Carcinoma and adenocarcinoma	Mammary gland, acinar	1
Carcinoma and adenocarcinoma	Multicentric (liver, intestine, omentum)	1
Carcinoma and adenocarcinoma	Salivary gland	1
Carcinoma and adenocarcinoma	Prepuce	3
Chordoma	Tail	4
Dermatofibroma, benign	Prepuce	1
Dermatofibroma, benign	Skin	3
Dermatofibroma, benign		
Dermal discrete cell	Skin	2
Epithelioma	Skin (sebaceous gland)	3
Fibrolipoma	Skin	1
Fibroma	Skin	2
Fibrosarcoma	Bone	1
Fibrosarcoma	Cervical vertebrae, SC	1
Fibrosarcoma	Mouth	1
Fibrosarcoma	Multicentric abdominal	2
Fibrosarcoma	Ovarian remnant	1
Haemangioma	Digit	1
Haemangioma	Mesentery	1
Haemangioma	Skin	5
Haemangioma	Liver	1
Haemangiosarcoma	Liver	1
Histiocytoma	Skin	1

Table 13.6 Histopathologically confirmed neoplasms in 480 cases 1990–1997 – cont'd.

Tumour type	Site	No.
Insulinoma (pancreatic islet cell adenoma)		180
Insulinoma (pancreatic islet cell adenoma)	Metastasis to the liver	11
Insulinoma (pancreatic islet cell adenoma)	Metastasis to local lymph nodes and mesentery	2
Lipoma	Skin	1
Lymphoma		132
Malignant nerve sheath tumour		1
Mast cell tumour	Skin	23
Mast cell tumour	Lung	1
Mast cell tumour	Lymph node (popliteal)	1
Mast cell tumour	Multicentric (liver, lymph node, lung, gall bladder)	1
Mesothelioma	Mesentery	1
Osteoma		1
Papilliferous adenoma	Vulva	1
Sarcoma	Skin	1
Schwannoma (neurilemoma)	Leg	1
Spindle cell tumour		1
Squamous cell carcinoma	Face	4

before. It had normal temperature but showed on palpation a soft tissue mass in the right thyroid region. The zookeeper had noted the ferret coughing or choking at times.

Blood serum evaluation showed all normal, including calcium, except: elevated lactate dehydrogenase at 1837 IU/L (range 241–752 IU/L), elevated (marginally) globulin at 3.1 g/dL (range 22.9 g/dL) and fasting glucose level at 65 mg/dL (range 107–138 mg/dL). The thyroid total T4 was at 1.0 µg/dL (range 1.01–8.29 µg/dL) but the sample was insufficient to give a complete thyroid profile.

On surgery, the red vascular tissue mass was found to be 3×2×2 cm and impossible to remove from the thyroid regions so the ferret was put to sleep. The trachea was deviated to the left by the enlarged thyroid mass while the left thyroid appeared normal. On abdominal post mortem, the adrenal glands were both enlarged (5–6 mm) but the pancreas was 'grossly normal.' On histology however, the pancreas had a discrete non-encapsulated tumour with mildly aplastic islet cells.

On histology, the right thyroid mass had features characteristic of an endocrine neoplasm and more likely of C-cell origin rather than a thyroid follicular epithelium origin. In addition, one adrenal gland showed multiple neoplastic foci which resembled adrenocortical adenoma as seen in ferrets by Fox. It was considered by the authors that the features in this case mimic those observed in human multiple endocrine neoplasia syndromes (MEN). This leads on to genetic possible involvement with the unique gene locus (MEN-I) (Ch. 5).

The authors also considered that the glucose fasting level of 65 mg/dL suggestive of hypoglycaemia, where the symptoms are of weight loss, anorexia, etc. were probably due rather to pancreatic islet tumour than C-cell carcinoma. The hair loss seen in this case could be indicating abnormal increase in adrenal gland steroid output (Ch. 14).

Teratoma (adrenal)

The adrenal gland is subject to unusual hormonal stimulation as indicated in Chapter 14 and is a site of adrenocortical adenoma and adenocarcinoma. Furthermore, the presence of adrenal teratoma of pet ferrets has been described.[19] Teratoma are not common neoplasia in animals or humans but are strange because they contain tissue of many germ cell lines. These could be:

- Ectoderm – skin, nervous tissue and oral and nasal tissue lining
- Mesoderm – being connective tissue, bone, cartilage, muscle and even urinary, cardiovascular and reproductive tissue elements
- Endoderm – including gastrointestinal, glandular tissue and respiratory tissue.

CHAPTER THIRTEEN
General neoplasia

Table 13.7 Multiple system involvement in ferrets, 1990–1997

Tumour type	No. of animals
Adrenocortical adenoma, mast cell tumour (skin)	1
Adrenocortical carcinoma, mast cell tumour (skin)	1
Adrenocortical carcinoma, lymphoma	1
Insulinoma, adrenocortical carcinoma	44
Insulinoma, adrenocortical carcinoma, lymphoma	2
Insulinoma, adrenocortical carcinoma, mast cell tumour (skin)	2
Insulinoma, adrenocortical carcinoma, mast cell tumour (lung)	1
Insulinoma, adrenocortical carcinoma, dermal discrete cell neoplasms	1
Insulinoma, adrenocortical carcinoma, prostatic carcinoma	1
Insulinoma, adrenocortical carcinoma, vulvar papilliferous adenoma	1
Insulinoma, adrenocortical adenoma	25
Insulinoma, haemangioma (mesentery)	1
Insulinoma, haemangioma (subcutaneous)	1
Insulinoma, lymphoma	7
Insulinoma, mast cell tumour (skin)	2
Total ferrets with multiple neoplasms	91

The four ferrets affected showed some interesting highlights and can be compared regarding age of incidence of presenting symptoms. These are shown in Table 13.8.

The adrenal glands were found to be composed of various germ cell lines.

The histogenesis of teratomas is debatable with thoughts of a gonadal development or an extragonadal source.[19] It is said that extragonadal teratomas could likely originate from diploid plenipotent progenitor cells that escape embryonal organizers during migration. Could the process be associated with development of ferrets sterilized too early? (see Ch. 14).

Splenic tumours

As noted previously the spleen is a common site of splenomegaly in mature and older ferrets with enlargement up to 10 cm. Neoplastic conditions seen are lymphosarcomas and myelolipomas.[20] The latter can occur in animals and humans but are rare and benign. They are neoplasia of mature adipose and haematopoietic tissue in variable proportions and they do not cause disease unless of great size or associated with the adrenal glands. Tail hair loss and an enlargement of the spleen featured in one 5-year-old ferret.[20] The ferret was suffering a mild hypochromic anaemia and became progressively worse with weakness and collapse. Interestingly the ferret was anaesthetized with ketamine (30 mg/kg i.m.) and xylazine (2 mg/kg i.m.) before being put to sleep with carbon dioxide. Post mortem revealed a spleen 9 × 3 × 2 cm which was 2–3 times the normal size.

Diagnosis is usually on histopathological findings while their origin is uncertain. *Note* there can be one or many discrete nodules in the spleen which are neoplastic. Most enlarged spleens consist of a mixture of marked congestion and extramedullary haematopoiesis with erythrocytic, leukocytic and megakaryocytic lines.[21]

Table 13.8 Adrenal teratoma in four ferrets

Ferret details	History and physical on inspection	Clinical highlights by palpation etc.	Post mortem highlights	Interesting features
3-year-old male	Anorexic and weak	Abdominal and thoracic masses. Pleural effusion	Lymphadenomegaly. Splenomegaly. Pleural/peritoneal l effusion	Neoplastic enlarged right adrenal gland
Adult ferret	Persistent fever	Leukocytosis	Adrenal glands of 2.5 cm	Both adrenals neoplastic
Adult silver mitt 1 year old	Anorexia and swollen abdomen	Dark brown fluid from abdomen. Cystic mass in abdomen	Cystic mass in abdomen hangs from dorsal aspect of abdomen	Neoplastic mass related to adrenal cortex
Spayed 4-month jill	Clinically normal	Mid-abdominal mass	Firm dorsal mass above colon	No left adrenal gland seen

Table relates to data from Williams et al., 2001.[19]

Kidney tumours

The kidney is a rare site of primary neoplasia. A 2-year-old pet ferret presenting with anorexia, weight loss and lethargy and a large intraabdominal mass was palpated and confirmed by X-ray. On laparotomy, a lobulated mass was found replacing one kidney. It was found to have a ureter attached and was designated as a transitional cell carcinoma from histology.[22] The lobulated cystic mass with a poor capsule had developed in the perirenal connective tissue and adjacent adrenal gland. Interestingly, no renal tissue could be seen in the mass though the ureter was present. It was suggested that the neoplasia came from a blind ending ureter i.e. renal agenesis. The opposite kidney was normal. As a pet ferret in 1990, the animal was considered to have had no exposure to renal carcinogens. It is hopeful that in present times the range of household 'contaminants' has not increased (Ch. 15).

Adrenal tumours

These are the subjects of Chapter 14. It is interesting to note that a survey of metastatic tumours to the adrenal gland, from various sites, in domesticated animals has been carried out regarding canine, feline, equine and bovine adrenals but not Mustelidae.[23]

Skin cancers

The skin is one region which American authorities suggest is a quite common site of cancers, squamous cell carcinomas (SCC) being the most prevalent. One report, however, found that after removal of a SCC there was no evidence of metastasis within 4 months.[24]

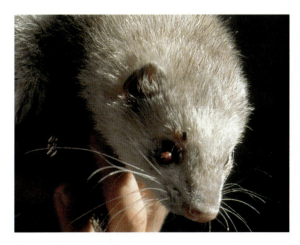

Figure 13.8 Ferret, Ferdie, with squamous cell carcinoma of eyelid.

I have recorded a SCC on the eyelid of a 5-year-old sterilized sable male, Ferdie (Fig. 13.8). The SCC was removed, using ketamine/halothane anaesthesia, leaving the eyelid intact and the cancer did not recur for 18 months.[25]

The occurrence of cutaneous epitheliotropic lymphoma (CEL) has been recorded.[26] It occurred in an 8-year-old 1000 g sterilized jill which originally was presented with a general progressive dermatitis which was pruritic and not responsive to ivermectin, antibiotics or corticosteroids. Histology revealed the disease.

The ferret was treated conservatively for 18 months with 1.1 mg/kg prednisone orally twice daily but only slightly improved, then got worse. Its clinical condition is worth considering regarding the outcome.

Re-examined 20 months after diagnosis, all medication was stopped for a month and the ferret was re-evaluated by a veterinary dermatologist. The ferret was underweight, but well hydrated though it showed a diffuse generalized alopecia and erythema. On the head, dorsal and ventral body, plus limbs, interdigital and peri-inguinal areas, footpads and tail were found patchy or circular excoriations, erosions, with serous or haemorrhagic crusts and ulcerations.

Differential diagnosis regarding the skin condition and pruritus was put as: – other cutaneous or systemically spread neoplastic conditions, adrenal adenoma/adenosarcoma, mastocytosis, infectious elements, Aleutian disease, FeLV, dermatophytosis/ectoparasitism, *Otodectes* (general), sarcoptic, demodectic mange, allergic skin disease and drug sensitivity. A full investigation procedure came to the conclusion that the CEL was possibly of T-cell phenotype origin.

An additional diagnosis of renal disease, being chronic renal failure plus bacterial cystitis with possible pyelonephritis was found. The ferret was treated with isotretinoin at 2 mg/kg p.o. every 24 hours and though it was not a cure, it was well tolerated and could be used as a palliative treatment in such cases. A cover of amoxicillin was also given for the treatment which resulted in decrease in the signs and some fine hair growth on the head, dorsum and limbs by 60 days post-initial treatment.

The owner declined further treatment of the ferret which was euthanized and histology found a severe multifocal, acute, suppurative pyelonephritis and cutaneous epitheliotropic lymphoma. This disease is most difficult to treat in other animals and man as it is in ferrets.

Mastocytomas (mast cell tumours)

In contrast to CEL, the mast cell tumour is a non-invasive skin tumour similar to tumours in cats. They

CHAPTER THIRTEEN
General neoplasia

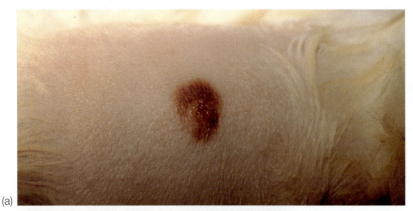

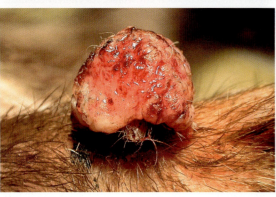

Figure 13.9 (a) Mast cell tumour on flank of an albino ferret. (Courtesy of M. Finkler.) (b) Basal cell tumour (sebaceous epithelioma). (Courtesy of Greg Rich.)

can be removed surgically and do not re-grow. As with mast cell tumours in dogs and cats, the cause is unknown (K. Wyatt, Murdoch University Cancer Care Unit, pers. comm. 2005).

Finkler has recorded a mast cell tumour as shown in Figure 13.9a. The tumour appears flat and hairless with a hyperkeratotic plaque which is pruritic. Histologically the tumour is a well-demarcated unencapsulated mass in the superficial dermis and consists of well-differentiated mast cells.

In a review of 142 ferrets (1987–1992) of which 57 were found to have skin neoplasia, 59% of these were basal cell tumour cases.[27] The others were 16% mastocytoma plus 11% fibroma but, unlike other surveys, there were no squamous cell carcinoma cases in the group. The basal cell tumours did contain some squamous features but could not be classified on the accepted classification as squamous cell carcinoma.

Basal cell tumours arise from primitive pluripotential cells of the epidermis and can differentiate into various cellular types such as sebaceous or squamous cells.[2] They are generally benign (Fig. 13.9b).

A spontaneous leiomyosarcoma of 3.0 cm in diameter was found on a 2-year-old female ferret's left shoulder and was removed under acetylpromazine/ketamine anaesthesia. Diagnosis confirmed a leiomyosarcoma by histology, lack of muscle striation with PTAH staining plus strong positive staining for desmin and muscle actin but negative staining for haemoglobin. Staining sections by the immunohistochemical technique using an avidin-biotin complex immunoperoxidase method makes it easier to diagnose poorly differentiated tumours.[28] Leiomyosarcomas are thought to originate from the blood vessel wall smooth muscle cells.

Piloleiomysarcoma

With regard to the hair coat, seven ferrets, 2–6 year olds, were described as having piloleiomysarcoma of the arrector pili muscle.[29] One jill and six males were examined, with two being entire hobs. It was noted by the authors that tumours were found only in 2.5% of 288 ferrets examined between 1993 and 2000. The masses identified had the structure of a well-demarcated but non-encapsulated proliferation of large spindle- to strap-shaped cells arranged in interwoven bundles as seen histologically. The neoplastic lumps were 0.5–2.0 cm in diameter and found either round the head or the trunk with no limb involvement. They had been noticed between 2 weeks and 4 years before coming to surgery. Follow-up of three ferrets after complete excision surgery showed survival rates of 2 years, 18 months and 5 months. The latter case is still alive after two operations at time of case report. *Note* a subcutaneous leiomyosarcoma has been recorded in a ferret with a similar histology, etc. to the hair follicle tumours.

Apocrine tumours

The fourth most common neoplasia after AGN, insulinoma, and lymphoma are those which affect the integument such the mast cell tumour (30%) above, sebaceous gland adenoma (22%), haemangioma (13%), benign cystic adenoma (9%) and adenocarcinoma of the prepuce.[30] *Note*: the tumours that account for 22% of skin tumours are dermatofibroma, fibroma, fibrosarcoma, histiocytoma, sarcoma and squamous cell carcinoma.

A perianal apocrine gland affected by an adenocarcinoma has been recorded in a 5-year-old spayed jill. This case treatment combined surgery and radiation therapy.[30] The ferret showed a perianal mass, which was investigated by fine needle aspiration (FNA) and shown to be a cancer on cytology examination. Initially the ferret had a mass 0.5 × 0.5 cm in the right perianal area. It had had skin mast cell tumours removed 12 months previously. Otherwise the ferret was healthy under normal clinical tests.

After 14 days, the mass had grown to 2.0 × 2.5 cm. It was abutting the colorectum and vulva, so radiation therapy was used on the site with the ferret under 2–2.5% isoflurane and oxygen. An isocentric (80 cm) cobalt teletherapy unit was used. This was done over 25 days giving a maximum dose of 4800 cGy.

However, around 5 weeks after radiation treatment, the original site showed another enlarged mass. This time surgery was used, with careful regard to the colon site, and what was found appeared to be an anal sac. (American ferret breeders usually do not now remove musk glands before ferret sale.) Histology showed no neoplasia. Remarkably, the ferret went on to ferret adrenal disease complex (FADC) and insulinoma and had operations for them both. Then, 1 month after the adrenal gland/insulinoma operation, two masses were discovered in the inguinal lymph nodes area, and removed and classified as aggressive apocrine gland tubular adenocarcinoma. The ferret was then checked by radiology and ultrasound for metastasis and chemotherapy was suggested to the owner who opted for an oral prednisone course of 1 mg/kg p.o. q. 12 h.

Within 3 months, the ferret was showing stranguria and dyschezia with symptoms caused by the enlarged sublumbar lymph nodes. Radiation therapy was again instigated which did in time reduce the size of the lymph nodes so that the ferret could toilet naturally. However, 1 month after the end of radiation therapy the stranguria returned and the lymph nodes were again enlarging. The owner decided on ferret euthanasia and refused a post mortem investigation.

Note: This is rather a sad case with the ferret already in the adrenal gland neoplasia/insulinoma bracket of its life getting a general neoplasia crisis. It was considered that a more conclusive diagnosis of adenosarcoma would have been possible with a biopsy rather than FNA. This ferret case was always one with a guarded prognosis.

A case of anal sac adenocarcinoma was reported in a Japanese pet ferret (Yasutsugu Miwa, pers. comm. 2005). The ferret was presented with masses associated with the anus. One 2 × 3 cm mass was above the anus and another 2.4 × 3.5 cm, below the anus (Fig. 13.10).

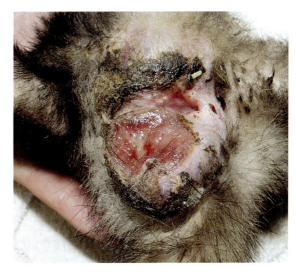

Figure 13.10 Anal adenoma before treatment. (Courtesy of Yasutsugu Miwa.)

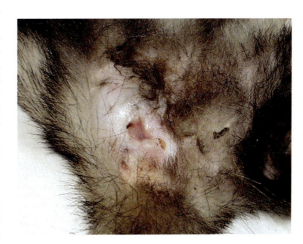

Figure 13.11 Anal adenoma after treatment. (Courtesy of Yasutsugu Miwa.)

The masses were removed by cryosurgery and the wound healed as shown (Fig. 13.11). Unfortunately, the tumours did recur later.

In an American adult pet ferret of undetermined age, it was found that a swollen, inflamed and dilated anus with faecal incontinence was caused by a squamous cell carcinoma.[31] The anus at rest was enlarged to 5 mm and showed pink rectal mucosa. Defaecation was involuntary and the scats soft. On palpation, the anal ring showed firm subcutaneous tissue and the ferret received a course of antibiotics for a possible anal sacculitis. The lesion continued to grow over the next month, the ferret lost weight and was put to sleep.

On post mortem, a firm neoplastic structure was found in the anal ring which measured 4.4 cm in diameter and 0.6 cm in depth. Histology revealed an invasive neoplasia which also incorporated the anal sac. *Note*: squamous cell carcinomas are rarely seen in the ferret perianal region. The involvement of the anal sac epithelium was considered very unusual for any animal species according to the author.[31]

Skeletal neoplasia

Chordoma are uncommon tumours, which arise from notochord remnants and can occur in ferrets, mink and other animals including humans. The tumours are slow-growing and locally aggressive with a probability of recurrence after surgery.[32] Interestingly, tumours of sacrococcygeal or vertebral origin are known to metastasize to bone, lung, lymph node and skin. In humans, chordoma appear more in males and it is considered that ferrets with the tumour could act as 'models' for human disease.

In a histological study of 20 ferrets,[32] it was found that a typical tail tip chordoma consists of a multilobulated mass of central bone and cartilage with a surround of pale lobules of vacuolated polygonal cells known as physaliferous cells. The zonal patterns of the latter cells are unique and the presence of bone and cartilage may have occurred in a number of ways during development from the notochord.[32] It is considered that the components could represent notochord-induced cartilaginous and osseous differentiation within the tumour. The mean age of these affected ferrets was 3.4 years, the females outnumbered the males and half the jills were spayed.

I have recorded only a skin tumour on the tail of a 6-year-old sable Jill, Nipper (Fig. 13.12), but no histology was done. It was not in a chordoma situation but probably a sebaceous gland type. It did not recur after excision. (She also had a splenic lymphosarcoma as indicated in Table 13.8.)

Tumour types on tails besides chordoma include sebaceous gland carcinoma, sweat gland carcinoma and papillary cystadenoma. These have been sporadically recorded over the years in the USA, as with Burgess' example of a tail lymphoma in a ferret (Fig. 13.13).

A 4-year-old healthy hob was found to have a basic chordoma, a smooth 1.5 × 1.1 cm lobular firm mass at the end of its tail.[33] The thinly-haired, pink and white tumour had increased in size over 1 year. Fine needle aspiration (FNA) showed a cytology of larger physaliferous cells and smaller chondrocyte cells. The tumour region was amputated and a cure was obtained. An earlier account had recorded chordoma in a 4-year-old unsterilized sable jill and a 3-year-old castrated fitch male.[34] In the jill, the 1 cm diameter mass surrounded the last coccygeal vertebra. Under microscope staining the tumour was well circumscribed, but not encapsulated, being partially divided into delicate bands of fibrous tissue lobes. Among the oval to polyhedral cells present there were small grey blue cells with clear vacuoles, which were considered neoplastic. *Note* that two out of these three ferrets were unsterilized and all were under 5 years of age. The authors pointed out that at the time (1988) four of seven (57%) chordoma were recorded in mink and ferrets which were only 1% of the total animal population under veterinary care. The authors suggested that mustelids may be at greater risk of chordoma than other animals.[34] The tail tumours did not recur after amputation. Chordoma can be locally invasive but

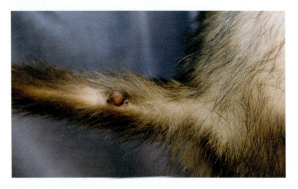

Figure 13.12 Tumour on tail of 6-year-old jill, Nipper, possible basal cell.

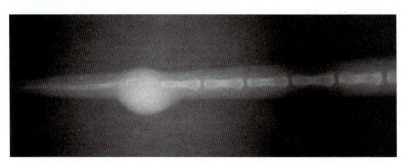

Figure 13.13 Tail lymphoma. (Courtesy of M. Burgess.)

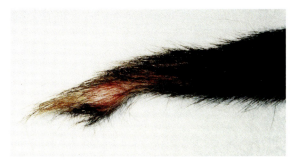

Figure 13.14 Chordoma. (Courtesy G. Rich.)

asymptomatic types can be missed at post mortem if the vertebral column is not examined.

Chondrosarcoma in four pet ferrets had been described even earlier but unfortunately, the ferrets' ages were not given.[35] After partial tail amputation these tumours did not recur. Rich has recorded a chordoma in a 5-year-old ferret as indicated in Figure 13.14.

Cervical chordoma have been found in ferrets whereas previously, they had only been seen at that site in the rat and cat and some humans.[36] One 5-year-old sterilized albino pet ferret had a 4-month history of ataxia in the hind legs leading to paresis with loss of limb action. The ferret had lost weight and was put to sleep. A post mortem showed a mild generalized muscular atrophy especially over the hind limbs. The atlanto-occipital joint was disarticulated to reveal a soft whitish-grey 1.5 × 1.0 cm amorphous mass. The material spanned the articular space and involved the articular facets to extend into both the foramen magnum and vertebral canals of C1 and C2. Further features were a moderate right ventricular dilation (Ch. 11), hepatic congestion and spondylosis of the lumbar spine. On histology, the grey mass had the features of a chordoma.

The other 4-year-old male sable ferret presented with a ventral cervical mass, which on radiology was causing a ventral deviation of the trachea. The ferret was surgically examined under general anaesthesia. A yellowish-white coarsely nodulated 2 × 5 cm mass was found loosely attached to the periosteum of the ventral aspect of C2 and C3 vertebrae. The mass was able to be removed but the ferret had to be put to sleep 4 months later when the tumour recurred. On post mortem, a spherical yellowish-white mass was found along the ventral aspect of vertebrae C2 and C3. *Note* a separate 1 cm nodular mass occurred firmly attached in the subcutaneous tissue adjacent to C2 and C3. On histology, the material was a chordoma.

Other neoplasia in Japan

With pet ferrets imported from the USA, the incidence of neoplasia has become apparent in recent years. (Anal gland neoplasia has been noted above.) A lymphoma was seen by CT scan as a small mass attached to the thoracic wall (Fig. 13.15). The patient had undergone surgery for splenomegaly but there was no indication of neoplasia of the spleen. A preoperative radiograph had shown a small mass in the lung area without clinical signs. The mass enlarged in 4 months and based on the CT images, FNA was done under the echo guide and the lesion diagnosed as a lymphoma (Yasutsugu Miwa, pers. comm. 2005).

Another ferret showed an unusual lymphoma of the front footpads which were swollen (Fig. 13.16).

The diagnosis of lymphoma was again done by cytology. In addition, the mandibular lymph glands were swollen on both sides and the axillary lymph node on the right side.

Sakai comments on neoplasia in a 5-year-old castrate ferret showing a subcutaneous mass in the right lateral thoracic wall.[37] The mass had gradually increased in size to 7.5 × 4.5 × 4.5 cm in 1 year, so that surgical resection of the mass plus the right axillary lymph node was carried out. It was found that the mass was quite clearly demarcated but the surrounding muscle tissue was affected, leading to the excision of affected tissue along with the tumour. The tumour showed a fibrous makeup with an area of necrosis in the centre of the mass. Using histology, immunohistochemistry and presence of numerous mitochondria and myofibrils (~15 nm in

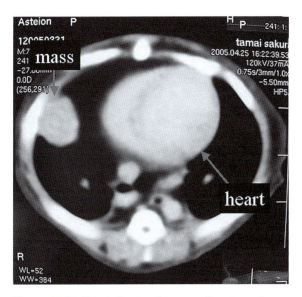

Figure 13.15 Ferret chest wall tumour. (Courtesy of Yasutsugu Miwa.)

CHAPTER THIRTEEN

General neoplasia

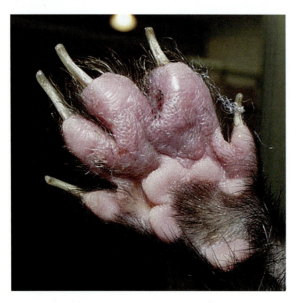

Figure 13.16 Ferret foot lymphoma. (Courtesy of Yasutsugu Miwa.)

diameter) the authors designated the tumour as a rhabdomyosarcoma as illustrated by Fox.[2]

Nakanishi et al. record a gastric adenocarcinoma with ossification in a 6-year-old female ferret which had a firm mass 2 cm in diameter in the region of the stomach.[38] The mass was composed of a neoplastic proliferation of well-differentiated epithelial cells, as seen on post mortem, with a tubular or glandular pattern. Osseous metaplastic foci were found which showed a positive immunohistochemical reaction against bone morphogenetic factor, protein 6, which is an osteogenic factor.

Neoplasia in Russia

Russian pet ferrets appear, at the present time, not to suffer neoplasms to the extent of USA or Japan. It may be because of their upbringing from European stock and the feeding of raw meat (Dmitry Kalinin, Russian Ferret Society, pers. comm. 2005).

Neoplasia in Australian ferrets

Since having ferrets from 1971, I have personally recorded very few cancers in my own ferrets and others. One reason was that there were not the numbers of ferrets seen compared to the American situation with pet ferrets and it took time for ferret owners to get accustomed to visiting their vet regarding health problems. Working ferrets were not experiencing cancers, as far as I could judge. However, over the past few years some ferret adrenal disease complex (FADC) and insulinoma have been recognized in Australian ferrets much to my personal dismay. Any idea of the percentage of ferret neoplasms in Australia is poor and I can only give the types of cancers I have seen in ferrets as in Table 13.9.

It is not noted in my list but my cases, whether treated by surgery or not, were given supportive treat-

Table 13.9 Selection of ferret tumours seen in my Perth practice, Western Australia 1971–2000

Ferret sex	Ferret age	Neoplasm	Clinical signs	Treatment	Outcome
Hob, sterilized	5 years	Squamous cell carcinoma	Eyelid cancer obvious	Surgical removal	18 months free of cancer
Entire jill	3½ months	Thymus lymphosarcoma	Sudden death		
Entire jill	4 years	Ovarian tumour	Alopecia, loss of condition	Surgical removal of ovaries	2 years free of cancer
Hob, sterilized	7 years	Axillary lymph node lymphoma		Not treated	
Jill, sterilized	6 years	Adrenal gland adenoma	Alopecia, loss of condition	Surgical removal of left adrenal gland	Died 6 months later of possible renal disease
Jill, sterilized	5 years	Splenic lymphosarcoma	Splenic enlargement, listlessness	Surgical removal of spleen	
Jill, sterilized	6 years	Tail tumour, no histology	None	Surgical removal	Jill became sick with pneumonia and died

ment that included fluid therapy, prednisolone and some herbal medication. I have not used chemotherapy, which is routine in the USA. It must be remembered that treating a ferret patient using the protocols 1 and 2 might well be an expensive exercise for some ferret-owning clients. One must weigh this up against the additional lifespan obtained for the animal and whether it should be carried out, with a guarded prognosis, and reference to possible toxic side-effects of the drugs. It is hoped that improved protocols will be developed, but the best way to alleviate the cancer problem is to consider the causes and whether by better husbandry they can be avoided (see Aetiology discussion, Ch. 14).

Lymphoma in Australian ferrets

I have seen a splenic lymphosarcoma in a 7-year-old sable hob, Sammy, and a gross splenic lymphosarcoma in a 5-year-old sable jill, Nipper. The latter ferret was found to have lost weight and on examination had a grossly enlarged spleen. I decided to perform a direct splenectomy under ketamine/halothane anaesthesia. As a result, a 50 g spleen was removed from a 670 g ferret. I had no experience with the Brown/Rosenthal protocols, so opted to use the holistic postoperative treatment suggested by Susan Brown.

Nipper recovered well from the operation, was given postoperative cover of clavulanic acid/amoxicillin (Clavulox drops, Pfizer) and started on the suggested regimen of vitamin C and Pau d'Arco extract. Vitamin C is a powerful anti-cancer agent, increasing interferon production and stimulating T-effector cell activity. It is also a powerful antioxidant that protects the body against free radicals. The dosage is 100–1000 mg vitamin C p.o. b.i.d. I used a 500 mg chewable tablet dissolved in 10 mL water in a white plastic recycled tablet container (to protect it from light). I gave 1 mL of the solution twice daily. One has to work up to the higher dosage over several weeks providing the ferret does not get diarrhoea. Pau d'Arco extract is from a Brazilian tree bark, which contains a natural antibiotic and also supports the immune system. Similarly, a 500 mg capsule, the only size available, of Pau d'Arco extract was broken into 10 mL of water in another plastic container and shaken into suspension. I gave 0.2 mL p.o. b.i.d. The outcome was that Nipper improved in activity and her weight, compared with two companion jills before and after the splenectomy, is shown in Table 13.10. (Variation of ferret weight does occur sometimes monthly and with the seasons.)

Unfortunately, Nipper died 6 months post-operation and the possibility of an extension of lifespan using chemotherapy protocols was not investigated.

Reproductive system neoplasia in Australian ferrets

I have seen ovarian tumours[25] and other reproductive tract cancers could be present but are as yet not recorded. American ferret owners do not usually see ovarian cancers, as their ferrets are sterilized often at 6 weeks of age and definitely at 6 months of age unless they are breeding ferrets. Older breeding ferrets can get ovarian cancers after years of producing litters and then apparently becoming sterile.[25] Some ferret owners insist that their jills get over post-oestrous anaemia, then the jills eventually get ovarian cancers. Ferret jills treated for post-oestrous anaemia with megestrol acetate (Ovarid, Jurox Pty.) repeatedly, were prone to later getting ovarian cancer. The incidence is small, however, as this treatment is rarely used now. Cotchin surveyed the incidence of smooth muscle hyperplasia and neoplasia in domesticated ferrets.[39]

Author's clinical example

Ferret ovarian tumour

My 6-year-old albino jill, Juno, became sterile and developed alopecia, without signs of possible post-oestrous anaemia. On laparotomy under ketamine/halothane anaesthesia, the left ovary was found to be normal (10 × 2 mm) but the right ovary was enlarged (35 × 25 mm). However, within 4 days of the ovariohysterectomy operation, with post-operative antibiotic cover, the hair around the jill's neck was seen to be regrowing and in 3 months she showed a thick white coat. She had a new lease of life for a further 2 years.[25]

Table 13.10 Comparison of jills' weights with reference to Nipper's cancer treatment

Jills	2/1/1998	29/1/1998 (Nipper's operation)	17/4/1998
Lucky (5 year)	680 g	700 g	650 g
Pandy (4 year)	620 g	620 g	590 g
Nipper (5 year)	720 g	670 g	670 g

CHAPTER THIRTEEN
General neoplasia

The signs of reproductive tract cancers are variable. Alopecia and a swollen vulva, presumably caused by excessive oestrogen production by the ovary, are seen in cases of ovarian cancer. Regarding my jill, Juno, she had only the alopecia and unfortunately no histology was done on the swollen ovary. Ovarian tumours possibly include thecoma, fibromyoma, carcinoma, leiomyoma or arrhenoblastoma. An ovarian teratoma has also been reported.[3] In one survey, 20 ovarian leiomyoma were recorded in just one group of 21 ferrets.[39] The extended range of reproductive system neoplasms has been recorded in the USA[2] as affecting the ovary, uterus and mammary gland in the jill and testicles, preputial gland and prostate in the hob. There are some undetermined tumours picked up in the reproductive system of the ferret; the various tumours have been described in all ages of ferrets from 1 year on.

Ovarian leiomyoma are evidently common in ferrets, do not appear to interfere with ovulation and pregnancy and are incidental findings at post mortem.[24] Most of the signs of reproductive tract cancers are related to fertility reduction as in my jill, Juno. When mated as an older jill, she had just two kittens and the next season failed to conceive and went into lethargy and alopecia, with weight loss and hair loss.

A 6-year-old unsterilized jill, Foxy, showed complete alopecia (Fig. 13.17). This had been happening on and off for years. The owner did not want the jill spayed and she had been having proligestone (Covinan) injections to suppress heat. It was not sick and lived to 9 years of age. I was suspicious that the cause of alopecia was an ovarian tumour but no surgery was possible.

Retained testicle in the male ferret may be the site of a testicular neoplasia and might be seen more if testicle retention becomes a genetic feature of breeding (Ch. 5). Prostate cancer is seen in the sterilized male ferret and associated with FADC with dysuria and haematuria.[40] In the entire hob, prostate cancers are rare.

Clinical examples

1. A 1-year-old de-sexed mitt hob, Burt, showed lethargy, ascites, some inappetence, loose scats and raised temperature, although the hob was reasonably bright and alert at first. The attending veterinarian treated him with antibiotics and steroids for greenish diarrhoea. Burt improved somewhat, with some reduction in ascites. A blood check was not successful under xylazine sedation, as it was found difficult to get blood from the jugular vein of the thick-necked entire male ferret (Chs 7, 20). However, a radiograph indicated the presence of ascites and a possible liver mass. It was decided to operate on Burt. A liver adenosarcoma was found plus a prostate tumour so euthanasia was carried out. The ferret, incidentally, as regards the green diarrhoea, had been fed on a dry cat food diet. The above example illustrates that there can be a complexity of symptoms in ferret cases. Work-up can be difficult when not seeing large enough numbers of ferrets to gain experience in taking blood samples. (From Dr R. Alito, Mosman Park Vet Hosp, Perth, WA, pers. comm. 1998.)

2. A hepatic haemangiosarcoma was recorded in a 5-year-old spayed sable jill, Jemma, which had suddenly become very sick and developed green urine and lassitude, went downhill rapidly and died in 2 days. Post mortem showed a discreet, blood-filled tumour attached to the mesentery of the liver. The liver was enlarged and pale brown/orange in colour, with dark mottling indicating liver involvement. The spleen was normal. Haemangiosarcoma has been recorded in the USA as a prominent tumour of the liver, 18 being listed in a survey of 48 primary neoplasms of the cardiovascular system.[2] Affected ferrets would die unexpectedly from this tumour.

From Edleston, Goonoo-Goonoo Vet Hosp, Tamworth, NSW, pers. comm. 1998.

Hepatic cancers

The liver can be the site of various types of lymphoma of which an adenosarcoma and a haemangiosarcoma have been described in Australian ferrets. Liver diseases are discussed in Chapter 9.

An interesting condition of hepatic portal dysplasia was seen in a 2-year-old de-sexed Australian male ferret, Oliver (B. Donneley, pers. comm. 2005). The ferret had presented with abdominal distention, reduced appetite and ascites, so fluid was tapped by abdominocentesis. Ultrasound suggested a smaller liver with increased density. Laparoscopy found multiple nodules in the right side of the liver with sharp liver margins. The histology found liver capsular changes and the ascites was associated with portal hypertension. Aspirate from the mass in the right hepatic lobe revealed possible neoplastic

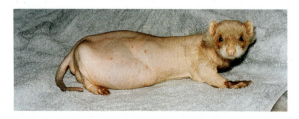

Figure 13.17 Ferret, Foxy, with complete alopecia.

cells. *Note*: the type of scenario may be attributed to enlarged adrenal neoplasia growing in or pressing on the vena cava or cardiomyopathy (V. Jeki, Czech Republic, pers. comm. 2005). Thus biliary cysts or portal dysplasia are not the real cause of the ascites and therapy must be directed to the primary disease with supportive liver therapy (vitamins B and C, amino acids, etc.). Surgical excision of any biliary cysts is possible.

On surgery, Oliver had the affected liver lobe removed completely and two small masses were found attached to the peritoneum. Histopathology found the liver mass to be a bile duct carcinoma and the two masses were mesotheliomas. The oncologist felt that the mesotheliomas were carcinoma originating from the bile duct carcinoma. The ascites was probably an effusion from the two masses rather than of hepatic origin. *Note*: mesotheliomas and carcinoma are difficult to separate histopathologically. Oliver was started on intraperitoneal carboplatin with a very guarded prognosis.

A Canadian survey of 60 ferrets in a housed situation in the Department of Biology, University of Saskatchewan, revealed the presence of eight cases of haemangiosarcoma in 13 ferrets over a period of 22 months.[41] The 60 ferrets were used for breeding and reproductive studies. The colony was managed in a manner similar to mink farms (Ch. 4). Ferrets that were autopsied were from 2–5 years. Ten of the 13 were males. Eleven of the 13 were in good nutritional condition but had died unexpectedly.

Haemoperitoneum was found in 9 of the 13 ferrets and in each case, rupture of the tumour masses was evident. In five of the animals, cavernous haemangiomas were found as dark 2–20 mm nodules raised above the surface of the livers. On histology, they consisted of large lakes of blood bounded by single layers of flattened endothelium.

The haemangiosarcomas found in eight ferrets were primary tumours of 2–3 cm, large red lobulated masses, some containing blood-filled caverns, confined to one liver lobe. Having as many as 13 uncommon tumours being picked up in a ferret colony situation within 22 months was noteworthy. The cause of the 13 tumours in the ferrets was speculative as there had been no known exposure to agents such as cause vascular tumours in humans, e.g. vinyl chloride, radiation, bracken fern in the diet or nitrosamine-contaminated foods (Ch. 4). If the cause was genetic, it was considered the cancers should be occurring in the ferret offspring. The colony did later register one splenic haemangiosarcoma and three mesotheliomas. (Further reference to hepatic tumours is seen in Chapter 9.)

A Canadian case from Ontario involving a 4-year-old de-sexed male sable ferret was unusual. It was presented with chronic serous drainage from the perineum and right inguinal region over 3 months.[42] Though the ferret was bright and alert it was not in top condition. The drainage tract was adjacent to the rectum and was passing serous fluid. A contrast medium, diatrizoate meglumine, was used with radiography and was seen to occupy the left inguinal region and flow 1 cm down the right side of the tail. Exploratory surgery on the left inguinal region revealed a 1 mm red/brown mass, which was later confirmed as a locally invasive haemangiosarcoma. Other similar but larger masses were found adjacent to the rectal wall on the right side and at the base of the tail. There were small 1 mm masses along the path of the contrast medium from the perineum to the left inguinal region. Also on post mortem, 1 mm masses were found in the omentum and the sacral lymph node had a mass of neoplastic tissue. *Note*: in the ferret the cranial and caudal mesenteric, left colic, sacral and internal iliac lymph nodes receive lymphatic drainage from the large intestine, rectum and anal glands.[42] The ferret was put to sleep as treatment was deemed unworkable.

Cutaneous haemangiosarcoma may be multicentric and locally invasive but metastasis is rare. This ferret case shows how contrast media can aid diagnosis of neoplasia associated with serous tracts from primary neoplastic sources.

Bone tumours

In one American survey, four osteomas, three chondromas and three unspecified bone tumours were recorded between 1968 and 1997.[43] Osteosarcoma was diagnosed for the first time on the rib and maxilla of two adult ferrets by Wilber and Williams.[44] A humerus sarcoma was diagnosed in a 6-year-old male ferret, which was euthanized (G. Rich, pers. comm. 2005) (Fig. 13.18).

A 4-year-old male ferret was presented with acute onset of leg lameness. There was no palpable tumour on legs or hip but severe pain on spinal palpation. An osteosarcoma of the thoracic vertebrae was found on X-ray (Fig. 13.19) (G. Rich pers. comm. 2005). Mark Burgess found an extensive osteosarcoma of a ferret's hind leg (Fig. 13.20).

One 3-year-old 1200 g neutered male silver mitt was presented with a pharyngeal mass.[45] The mass occupied 60% of the left oropharyngeal area and had not been there on examination of the ferret a month earlier. The owner had noted it 3 weeks later. The tongue base was deviated to the right but the mass was not painful. The mucosa covering appeared normal and there were no difficulties in swallowing or dyspnoea. Radiography and CT imaging were used in the examination of this osteoma. After taking numerous biopsies, the ferret became acutely lethargic and the owner required it be put down.

CHAPTER THIRTEEN
General neoplasia

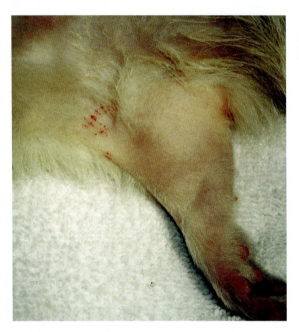

Figure 13.18 Femoral swelling: sarcoma. (Courtesy of G. Rich.)

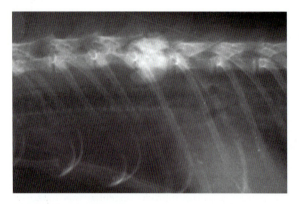

Figure 13.10 Osteosarcoma of thoracic vertebrae. (Courtesy of G. Rich.)

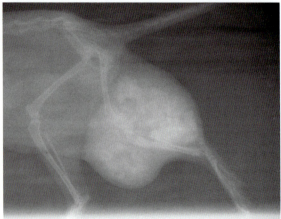

Figure 13.20 Hind leg osteosarcoma. (Courtesy of M. Burgess.)

etc. Even with removal, the neoplasia can recur. *Note*: it is difficult, even impossible, to differentiate between true neoplasia and an inflammatory overgrowth and bone lesions of a hypertrophic nature.[46]

Comparative spinal damage in an American pet ferret

A T-cell lymphoma was diagnosed in the USA by Hanley et al. in 2004. The lymphoma was on the ferret spinal cord at the position of L5 as a soft tissue mass.[47] The 22-month-old sterilized male had developed acute pelvic paresis when presented, but the owner insisted that the animal had been okay 5 hours earlier (a similar comment to the Casper case). There was no history of trauma. The ferret lived indoors and was fed commercial ferret food.

On examination, the ferret was paraparetic, the right hind leg more affected but both limbs lacked postural reactions, also reduced withdrawal reflexes were noted. The damage appeared to focus around the L4 to S3 spinal cord segments. Differential diagnosis appears in appendix Table A.8.

The ferret's blood picture appeared normal. It was treated overnight with cage rest after an injection of 1 mg/kg ketoprofen i.m. It did not improve during the next 12 hours and it lost bowel control. A blood cell count then showed a leukocytosis and lymphocytosis but little more. Radiology showed on lateral and ventrodorsal views a lysis of the left lateral aspect of L5 (Fig. 13.23). The end plate appeared normal. Consideration was given to either a tumour or trauma.

Treatment was attempted with 2 mg/kg of prednisolone orally b.i.d. and 1 mL/kg bismuth subsalicylate

It is considered that osteomas are benign bony growths of the intramembranous bone of the skull and vertebral column. On X-ray the osteoma is fairly well defined. They are usually progressively growing with a possible quiescence stage, which can be lengthy. The tumour is rare, mostly in horses or cattle, but also in dogs, pigs, birds mice and ferrets. Aetiology is unclear but interestingly a retrovirus has produced osteomas in mice.

The growing mass affects the surrounding tissues and this is dangerous at jaw angles, invading nasal cavities,

Bone tumours

Author's clinical example

A 4-year-old albino ferret, Casper, was seen by its owner to be dragging his hind limbs but found to have some use of the legs when presented. It had been walking normally 24 hours previously. It was not incontinent, was mentally bright and alert and was drinking and eating normally. There was a swelling in the midlumbar spine, which was firm and painful (Figs 13.21, 13.22). Casper was able to move his legs but had a reduced pain reflex when pinch-tested. The tail response to pinch test was good. No abnormalities were detected on abdominal palpation. Casper lived with three placid jills and there was nothing in the cage where he could have suffered an injury. The X-rays showed a bony tumour in the midlumbar region. Measurements of the lumbar vertebrae involved put them at one and a half length with about 0.5 cm between the vertebrae taken up by the tumour. The osteoma had a 2.5 cm diameter encroachment from its centre between the lumbar vertebrae. Considering the assumed slow growth of these types of tumours the osteoma could have been developing for some time and reached a critical point which affected the lower spinal nerves. Casper had to be euthanized. He was frozen and post mortem and histology carried out later at my request.

Histopathology found an extensive area of necrosis and haemorrhage with an attempted encapsulation evident at the periphery. The architecture of the lesion suggested a mass composed of trabeculae of woven bone interspersed with some loose connective tissue and showing a peripheral response of reactive fibroplasia. A small portion of the periphery of the lesion appeared to be intact but this might have reflected portions of the vertebrae, as the orientation of the specimen was uncertain. There was reactive woven bone at the periphery of the lesion with evidence of overt anaplasia. Occasional islands of chondroid tissue could be seen but the majority of the tissue was composed of bone with no evidence of significant inflammation.

The pathological comment on this case was an unusual proliferative lesion, which appears to have undergone secondary necrosis. The primary lesion appeared to be a proliferative reaction of relatively well differentiated woven bone interspersed with some fibroblasts and some bone marrow elements. The features were suggestive of a benign osteoma. The lesion showed some secondary reactive woven bone as well as some remodelling. No unequivocal evidence of any osteomyelitis was noted and no clear indication of any anaplastic process was seen. The possibility of a lesion such as an osteochondromatosis could not be entirely ruled out.

From Dr W. Hobley, Railway Avenue Veterinary Hospital, Armadale, WA; Dr J. Jardine, Vetpath Laboratory Services, Perth, WA 2005.

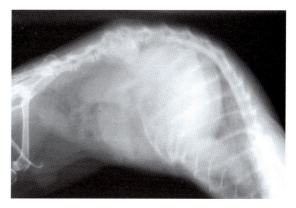

Figure 13.21 Ferret male, Casper's, spine tumour lateral. (Courtesy of W. Hobley, Railway Avenue Veterinary Hospital, Armadale, WA).

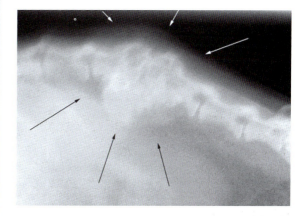

Figure 13.22 Ferret male, Casper's spine tumour (see arrows). (Courtesy of W. Hobley, Railway Avenue Veterinary Hospital, Armadale, WA.)

t.i.d. for diarrhoea. The bladder was atonic and had to be expressed t.i.d. The ferret's weight and appetite were checked. It did not improve after 5 days and had lost weight, though it was eating.

A CBC showed:
- Persistent leucocytosis (12.6×10^9/L)
- Early left shift (0.38×10^9/L) ref range 0 to 0.972×10^9/L
- Absolute lymphocytosis (6.05×10^9/L).

Due to possible immunosuppression of the prednisolone (plus the diarrhoea), treatment with 12.5 mg/kg Clavulox orally b.i.d. was added.

Interestingly, the ferret was set up for a computed tomography (scan) by the following routine (see also Ch. 16). Premed 0.01 mg/kg glycopyrrolate i.m., 0.2 mg/kg

CHAPTER THIRTEEN

General neoplasia

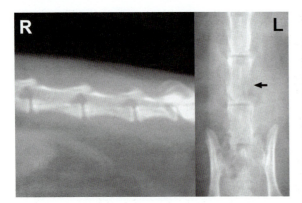

Figure 13.23 Lateral and ventrodorsal views of ferret showing lysis of the left lateral aspect of L5, seen from the midbody through the caudal portion, visible only on the ventrodorsal view (black arrow). (Courtesy of C. Hanley.)

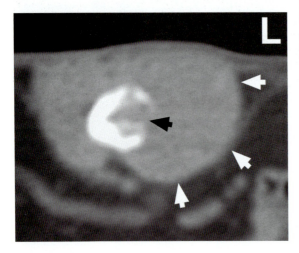

Figure 13.24 Computed tomography section at the L5 vertebral midbody of the ferret; there is a complete lack of vertebral bone on the left side (black arrow) and a large, soft tissue mass (white arrows). (Courtesy of C. Hanley.)

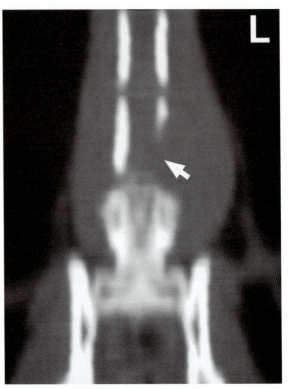

Figure 13.25 Computed tomography (CT) reconstruction of the ferret from vertebra L4 caudally: there is marked bone lysis (white arrow), especially compared with that visible on the ventrodorsal radiograph (see Fig. 13.23). (Courtesy of C. Hanley.)

butorphanol i.m., plus acepromazine 0.1 mg/kg i.m. Then it was anaesthetized with 4 mg/kg propofol i.v. and tubed to be on oxygen and isoflurane while under the scan.

Scan results showed bony lysis of the dorsal lamina, left lateral pedicle, lateral aspect of the body and transverse process of L5 from the midbody to the caudal side but with minimal periosteal proliferation. There was a striking large mass associated with the soft tissues of the lumbar spine (Figs 13.24, 13.25).

In addition, an ultrasound indicated a mass within the left lumbar hypaxial muscles. The mass had spread into the vertebral canal with bony lysis of the dorsal and lateral aspects of the L5 vertebra.

It was not possible to palpate the mass so aspirates were taken for cell examination, which were medium to large cells with a round nucleus having prominent nucleoli and basophilic cytoplasm, which appeared to be lymphoblasts. With a few small lymphocytes present, a suggested diagnosis was put at spinal lymphoma. It was considered that the pressure of the lymphoma compressing or destroying the spinal cord caused the neurological dysfunction. The prednisolone was not working so to have any chance of return of function a radiation therapy course was suggested to the owner to destroy the aggressive lymphoma.

The ferret was sent home, 7 days after admittance, with the treatments indicated previously while the owner considered the radiation aspect. However, when they did agree, in 2 days the ferret went into severe lethargy with a low temperature, tachypnoea and dyspnoea with harsh rales. It had lost more weight. Now the lumbar mass was palpable, probably due to emaciation and

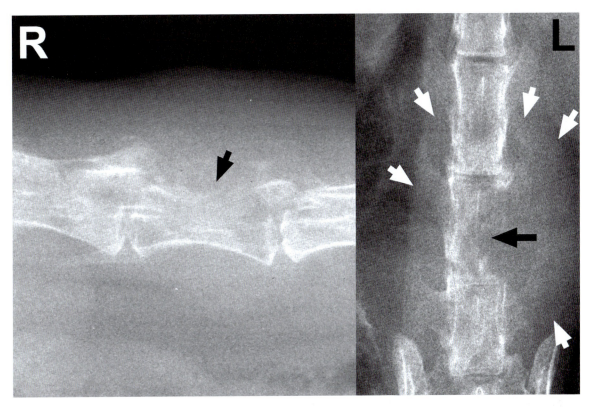

Figure 13.26 Lateral and ventrodorsal views of the ferret taken 13 days after the onset of clinical signs; bone lysis is clearly evident in both views (black arrows), and a soft tissue mass is visible on the ventrodorsal view (white arrows). (Courtesy of C. Hanley.)

growth of the neoplasm. Radiology showed the lysis now evident on lateral and ventrodorsal views (Fig. 13.26). The next morning the ferret was dull and dyspnoeic and was given oxygen but was finally put to sleep.

Note: A check on the lymphoma tissue samples did not reveal any sign of retroviral or like viruses. An interesting point of this case was that the 22-month-old ferret had such an acute onset and rapid progression more characteristic of diseased ferrets under 1 year but shows it can happen in the 1–2 year range. Lymphoma also occurs less often in the central nervous system than other parts of the body and T-cell lymphoma is the most common type seen in young ferrets up to 18 months old, with an average age of 6–9 months. However, ferrets of this age with T-cell lymphoma have a mediastinal mass (Fig. 13.2). This ferret did not, thus it is possibly the first record of T-cell lymphoma in a ferret spine.

This ferret lymphoma was unresponsive to prednisolone even in high doses unlike lymphoma in other regions of the body (see Dr J. Mayer's protocol). Other treatments for the ferret could have been by intravenous chemotherapy as described earlier but would involve toxic drugs which might have worsened the case. Overall, this spinal condition would have been difficult to overcome.

Nervous system neoplasia

Fox tabulates known nervous tissue neoplasia between the central nervous system (CNS) and the peripheral nervous system (PNS).[2] In the CNS a single granular cell tumour, meningioma, astrocytoma, and glioma have been recorded and in the PNS seven schwannomas/neurofibromas have been described on the skin and adrenal glands while two neurofibrosarcomas have occurred in eyelid and para-adrenal. In addition, two ganglioneuromas have been identified in ferret abdomen and thorax situations. Invasion of the CNS by tumour cells results in nerve disruption while tumours growing in the PNS cause space-occupying problems. A second meningioma has been recorded by Garner.[16]

CNS granular cell tumour

This tumour's cellular origin is not known. It is sometimes called a myoblastoma.

In one 4-year-old sterilized hob, it caused progressive right head tilt (Ch.12) with circling right, ataxia, seizure and torticollis.[48] On presentation, it showed pain in the dorsal cranial cervical region and was dehydrated. Diazepam at 1 mg/kg was tried to control seizures while the ferret was treated with i.v. 0.45% saline/2.5% dextrose b.i.d. plus 20 mg/kg amoxicillin t.i.d. s.v. No progress was made as the seizures increased so the ferret was euthanized. On post mortem, it was found that the tumour occupied part of the middle right forebrain.

PNS schwannomas

This tumour is of the Schwann cells or related perineural cells of peripheral nervous sheaths. In one ferret, a schwannoma in the vagus nerve interrupted vagal neural transmissions while a subcutaneous schwannoma in a 4-year-old ferret was multinodular and partly polycystic. A neurofibrosarcoma (malignant) was detected in the eyelid of one ferret and in the para-adrenal area of another. *Note:* Schwann cells of schwannomas have basement membranes and can be differentiated from cells of fibroma, fibrosarcoma, leiomyoma and spindle cell tumours of the adrenal gland by electron microscopy.[2]

PNS ganglioneuromas

These tumours are rare and benign and possibly derived from surviving primitive neuroepithelial cells, which differentiate towards post-mitotic neurons. One 5-month-old ferret was found to have a multilobular 4–5 mm diameter mass situated 2 cm cranial to the right adrenal gland.[2] In another ferret's mediastinum, a 3 mm dark brown ganglioneuroma was found. Both tumours histologically had predominantly neurons within the neuropil or fibrous glia stroma. Oval or pyramidal neuronal cells could be seen with a large amount of Nissl substance. There were large and often eccentric nuclei present. In one ferret's adrenal medulla, a few clusters of large neuron-like cells were seen. With the second ferret, the neuron-like bodies had extensive intracytoplasmic deposits of lipofuscin while both ferrets had epithelial tubules or acini in the tumourous nodules.

Neoplasia aetiology

There are various theories regarding neoplasia in ferrets and these are discussed in detail in relation to lymphoma, adrenal gland complex and insulinoma in Chapter 14.

References

1. Dillberger JE, Altman NH. Neoplasia in ferrets: eleven cases with a review. J Comp Path 1989; 100:161–176.
2. Xiantang L, Fox JG. Neoplastic diseases. In: Fox JG, ed. Biology and diseases of the ferret, 2nd edn. Baltimore: Williams & Wilkins; 1998:405–447.
3. Brown S. Neoplasia. In: Hillyer EV, Quesenberry KE, eds. Ferrets, rabbits and rodents: Clinical medicine and surgery. Philadelphia: Saunders; 1997:99–114.
4. Beach JE, Greenwood B. Spontaneous neoplasia in the ferret (*Mustela putorius furo*). J Comp Path 1993; 108:133–147.
5. Carpenter JW, Finnegan MV. A ferret with a midventral cervical mass. Vet Med 2003:May.
6. Erdman SE, Reinmann KA, Moore FM, et al. Transmission of a chronic lymphoproliferative syndrome in ferrets. Lab Invest 1995; 72:539–546.
7. Erdman SE. Malignant lymphoma in ferrets. Proc North Am Vet Conf 1993:734.
8. Erdman SE, Kanki P, Moore FM, et al. Clusters of lymphoma in ferrets. Cancer Invest 1996; 14:225–230.
9. Batchelder MA, Erdman SE, Xiantang L, et al. A cluster of cases of juvenile mediastinal lymphoma in a ferret colony. Lab Anim Sci 1996; 46:271–274.
10. Erdman SE, Brown SA, Kawasaki TA, et al. Clinical and pathologic findings in ferrets with lymphoma: 60 cases (1982–1994). J Am Vet Med Assoc 1996; 208:1285–1289.
11. Taylor TG, Carpenter JL. Thyoma in two ferrets. Lab Anim Sci 1995; 45:363–365.
12. Lewington JH. Splenic lymphosarcoma in the ferret. Control and therapy. University of Sydney: Postgraduate Foundation 1998; 203:1016–1017.
13. Brown S. Clinical management of malignant lymphoma in the ferret. Proc North Am Vet Conf 1993:730–732.
14. Rassnick KM, Gould W III, Flanders J. Use of vascular access system for administration of chemotherapeutic agents to a ferret with lymphoma. J Am Vet Med Assoc 1995; 206:500–504.
15. Hamilton TA, Morrison WB. Bleomycin chemotherapy for metastatic squamous cell carcinoma in a ferret. J Am Vet Med Assoc 1991; 198:107–108.
16. Williams BH, Weiss CA. Neoplasia. In: Quesenberry KE, Carpenter JW, eds. Ferrets, rabbits and rodents: Clinical medicine and surgery. Philadelphia: Saunders; 2003:91–106.
17. Li X, Fox JG, Erdman SE, Aspros DG. Cutaneous lymphoma in a ferret (*Mustela putorius furo*). Vet Pathol 1995; 32:55–56.
18. Fox JG, Dangler CA, Snyder SB, Richard MJ, Thilsted JP. C-cell carcinoma (medullary thyroid carcinoma) associated with multiple endocrine neoplasia in a ferret (*Mustela putorius*). Vet Pathol 2000; 37:278–282.
19. Williams BH, Yantis LD, Craig SL, Geske RS, Li X, Nye R. Adrenal teratoma in four domestic ferrets (*Mustela putorius furo*). Vet Pathol 2001; 38:328–331.
20. Li X, Fox J, Erdman G. Multiple splenic myelolipomas in a ferret. Lab Anim Sci 1996; 46:101–103.
21. Williams BH. Pathology of the domestic ferret (*Mustela putorius furo*) Pathology of non-traditional pets. Am Coll Vet Pract Symp; 2004.
22. Bell RC, Moeller RB. Transitional cell carcinoma of the renal pelvis in a ferret. Lab Anim Sci 1990; 40:537–538.
23. Labelle P, Cock HEV De. Metastatic tumours to the adrenal glands. Vet Pathol 2005; 42:52–58.
24. Ryland LM, Bernard SL, Gorham JR. A clinical guide to the pet ferret. Comp Contin Edu Pract Vet 1993; 5:25–32.

25. Lewington JH. Ferrets. Vade Mecum Series. University of Sydney: Postgraduate Foundation; 1988:C10.
26. Rosenbaum MR, Affolter VK, Usborne AL, et al. Cutaneous epitheliotropic lymphoma in a ferret. J Am Vet Med Assoc 1996; 209:1441–1444.
27. Parker GA, Picut CA. Histopathologic features and post-surgical sequelae of 57 cutaneous neoplasms in ferrets (*Mustela putorius furo*). Vet Pathol 1993; 30:499–504.
28. Brunnert SB, Heron AJ, Altman NH. Leiomyosarcoma in a domestic ferret: morphologic and immunocytochemical diagnosis. Lab Anim Sci 1990; 40:208–210.
29. Rickman BH, Craig LE, Goldschmidt MH. Piloleiomyosarcoma in seven ferrets. Vet Pathol 2001; 38:710–711.
30. Graham JF, Roberts RE, Wilson GH, et al. Perianal apocrine gland adenocarcinoma in a ferret. Compend Cont Edu Pract Vet 2001; 23:359–362.
31. Williams B. Squamous cell carcinoma arising from the anal sac in the ferret. Exot DVM 2002; 4:8.
32. Dunn DG, Harris RK, Meis JM, et al. A histomorphologic and immunohistochemical study of chordoma in twenty ferrets (*Mustela putorius furo*). Vet Pathol 1991; 28:467–473.
33. Roth L, Takata I. Cytological diagnosis of chordoma of the tail in a ferret. Vet Clin Path 1993; 21:119–121.
34. Allison N, Rakich P. Chordoma in two ferrets. J Comp Pathol 1988; 98:371–374.
35. Henrick MJ, Goldschmidt MH. Chondrosarcoma of the tail of ferrets (*Mustela putorius furo*) Vet Pathol 1987; 24:272–273.
36. Williams BH, Eighmy JJ, Berbert MH, et al. Cervical chordoma in two ferrets (*Mustela putorius furo*). Vet Pathol 1993; 30:204–206.
37. Sakai H, Maruyama M, Hirata A, et al. Rhabomyosarcoma in a ferret (*Mustela putorius furo*). J Vet Med Sci 2004; 66:95–96.
38. Nakanishi M, Kawamura M, Yamate J, et al. Gastric adenocarcinoma with ossification in a ferret (*Mustela putorius furo*). J Vet Med Sci 2005; 67:939–941.
39. Cotchin E. Smooth muscle hyperplasia and neoplasia in the ovaries of domestic ferrets (*Mustela putorius furo*). J Path 1980; 130.
40. Jenkins JR, Brown SA, eds. Ferrets. In: A practitioners guide to rabbits and ferrets. Lakewood: American Animal Hospital Association; 1993.
41. Cross BM. Hepatic vascular neoplasm in a colony of ferrets. Vet Pathol 1987; 24:94–96.
42. Vannevel J. Unusual presentation of haemangiosarcoma in a ferret. Can Vet J 1999; 40.
43. Li X, Fox JG, Padrid PA. Neoplastic disease in ferrets: 57 cases (1968–1997). J Am Vet Med Assoc 1998; 212:1402–1406.
44. Wilber J, Williams B. Osteosarcoma in two domestic ferrets (*Mustela putorius furo*). Vet Pathol 1997; 34:487.
45. Voe RS De, Pack L, Greenacre CB. Radiographic and CT imaging of a skull associated osteoma in a ferret. Vet Radiol Ultrasound 2000; 43:364–348.
46. Davies GO. Veterinary pathology and bacteriology. London: Balliere Tindall Cox; 1962.
47. Hanley CS, Wilson GH, Frank P, et al. T cell lymphoma in the lumbar spine of a domestic ferret. (*Mustela putorius furo*). Vet Rec 2004; 155:329–332.
48. Sleeman JM, Clyde VL, Brenneman KA. Granular cell tumour in the central nervous system of a ferret (*Mustela putorius furo*). Vet Rec 1996; 138:65–66.

CHAPTER 14

Endocrine diseases

'Adrenal gland neoplasia and insulinoma, the terrible twins of disease.'

John H. Lewington, 2000

Ferret endocrinopathy is a major worry with pet ferrets, as the ferret seems to have become prone to two endocrine-based diseases, adrenal disease and pancreatic insulinoma. They have been seen in alarming numbers in pet ferrets in the USA and can occur together.[1] Tables 13.6 and 13.7 indicate the 1990–1997 survey. It is suggested that nearly every older ferret gets adrenal disease but not every ferret shows clear symptoms. Some ferrets over 6 years old are skinny with thin fur and sleep a lot. In one UK practice, an increase in incidence to five adrenal cases in 4 weeks has been recorded (J. Chitty, pers. comm. 2005). Adrenal gland disease has also been recorded in Australia.[2]

Insulinoma has been recorded in the Netherlands since 1998 (Sabine van Voorne, pers. comm. 1998). Sometimes, lesions are seen in the pancreas without clinical symptoms, (Moorman-Roest, pers. comm. 2004). Insulinoma is seen in 3–8 year olds, especially if they are on poor quality food with high carbohydrate.

I have seen only one adrenal disease case and it was my own jill, Josie. There have been more seen in Australia since 2000 (R. Malik, pers. comm. 2005). In addition, there can be a tendency for ferrets treated by surgery for insulinoma to develop diabetes mellitus, which is otherwise a rare condition in ferrets,[3] but has been found, however, in the American black-footed ferret.[4] Looking from an Australian and New Zealand viewpoint, the major differences in environment seem to be that American ferrets are mostly kept as indoor pets and fed commercial ferret dry foods, while ferrets 'down under' have traditionally been outdoor animals, whether pets or workers, and fed fresh meat. This is also the case in the UK and continental Europe. Whether ferret accommodation, feeding or other factors affect the incidence of any neoplasia is a hotly debated topic. With the increase in popularity of ferrets as pets, especially as household pets, in Australia and elsewhere, the factors affecting American ferrets will possibly produce disease in ferrets elsewhere. Indeed, beside my own experience, these diseases have started to be seen sporadically outside the USA.

Ferret adrenal disease complex (FADC)

Note: adrenal gland malfunction in the ferret has been described as adrenal gland disease (AGD), adrenal gland neoplasia (AGN), adrenal cortical disease (ACD) or adrenal associated endocrinopathy (AAE). The general term of adrenal disease is used as it is considered we do not yet know if it is hyperplasia, adenoma or adenocarcinoma when it starts and because sometimes all three are present. It is due to a high production of sex hormones by the adrenals. The term ferret adrenal disease complex (FADC) is thought suitable as it actually involves behaviour and other clinical issues, including prostate involvement in males, so this term is used here (Cathy Johnson-Delaney (C J-D), pers. comm. 2005).

FADC is manifested by a pathological rise in blood levels of certain oestrogen precursors: androstenedione (50–60%), oestradiol (90%) and 17-hydroxyprogesterone (50–60%) (Table 14.1). This work was done by

Table. 14.1 Oestrogen precursor values in normal and AGN affected ferrets

Steroid[a]	Normal ferrets[b]	AGN ferrets[c]
Androstenedione (nmol/L)	6.6	50–60% rise
Oestradiol (pmol/L)	106	90% rise
17-Hydroxyprogesterone (nmol/L)	0.4	50–60% rise

[a]Only three steroids deemed of significance. [b]Normal ferret readings under review.
[c]The steroid rises from over 3000 adrenal ferret panels run in confirmed cases.
Data according to Oliver and Johnson-Delaney, pers. comm. 2005.

Dr Jack Oliver (University of Tennessee Clinical Endocrinology Service) and the tests prove that cortisol measurement at 7.5% is not a diagnostic tool for FADC evaluation.[5] *Note* that about 8% of adrenal cases have no hormone elevation. Also that adenocarcinomas tend to be more active biologically and may show high elevation of sex hormone values. A number of biosynthetic enzymes in ferrets are affected but adrenal disease does not affect thyroid hormone levels.[6]

It was noted that in some cases, oestradiol was normal with one or both of the other two elevated so that there is a need to measure all three hormones. Tennessee University has produced a validated sex steroid serum panel for diagnosing and monitoring the three hormones as a commercial unit. Data were collected as part of a controlled hormone study by C J-D and Oliver. It was decided that dehydroepiandrosterone (DHEAS) was not really helpful in evaluating adrenal disease and no longer important so it is not shown. The adrenal serum panel kits devised by Oliver are readily available and affordable. They provide the practitioner with the tools needed to evaluate ferret hormone levels. One should be aware that there is an ongoing investigation of ferret endocrine regulation.

The adrenal panel now needs to be interpreted with regard to the time of year. It is found for instance that neutered ferrets have seasonal hormonal cycles even though you think they should not. Thought is now given to using FADC signs along with ultrasound readings and/or biopsy of the glands plus attention to the time of year (northern hemisphere; none of this work has been done in the southern hemisphere).

With the three hormones, androstenedione, oestradiol and 17-hydroxyprogesterone as adrenal activity markers under review, once all the study values are analysed the normal values may be changed. Considering a spayed jill ferret during Feb–April; in the experience of C J-D, the oestradiol could be up to 210 pmol/L and for the male ferret in Dec–March, the androstenedione may be up to 25 nmol/L (Table 14.1). In the female in Feb–April with an oestradiol of

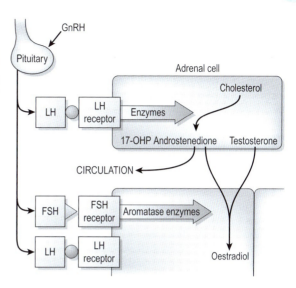

Figure 14.1 Hypothesized neuroendocrine pathway for adrenal stimulation in the ferret. The adrenal cells can be a site of sex steroid steroidogenesis. Test of the hypothesis: GnRH agonist (leuprolide acetate) initially causes an increase in LH, FSH, and metabolism of cholesterol to sex steroids. Sustained high levels of GnRH agonist decrease LH, FSH, and thereby block sex steroidogenesis.

210 pmol/L, 17-hydroxyprogesterone of 24 nmol/L and androstenedione of 40 nmol/L, she is classified adrenal (FADC). If the 17-hydroxyprogesterone and/or androstenedione fall within the published normals, she is probably fine. Thus, the interpretation of FADC is not going to be black and white, at least in American cases.

The basic working of the neuroendocrine pathway for adrenal gland stimulation can be given in a diagrammatic form as in Figure 14.1.

The normal theorized hormonal pathway involves the hormones gonadotropin-releasing hormone (GnRH), luteinizing hormone (LH) and follicle-stimulating hormone (FSH). Under extended light stimulation, GnRH from the hypothalamus stimulates the secretion of LH and FSH by the pituitary gland. If there is no LH to signal the progression of the sexual cycle, the stimulation would remain on. Thus, the adrenal tissue can become hyperplastic and progress into an adenoma or even adenocarcinoma neoplasia.

The disease treatment requires switching on the pituitary control to block LH and FSH release and thus stop sex steroidogenesis within the adrenal gland.[7] The drug leuprolide acetate (see below) is a GnRH agonist, having an affinity for the cellular receptors for GnRH. Initially it causes an increase in LH and FSH with the metabolism of cholesterol to sex steroids (Fig. 14.1) but sustained high levels decrease LH and FSH and block sex steroidogenesis.

FADC is considered a definite adrenal gland disease, which does not involve stimulation from pituitary gland tumours. It is theorized that in the embryonic stage, the ovaries and adrenal gland develop in the same embryonic region and possibly some ovarian cells are taken by the adrenal gland and become part of the outer cortex.[3] This introduces the possibility of early sterilization of the jill stimulating those ovarian cells in the adrenal glands to act irrationally. Investigations have been carried out on the level of serum oestradiol in ferrets.[8] A total of 17 ferrets with progressive non-pruritic alopecia were studied and it was concluded that high serum oestradiol levels could be used to show adrenocortical neoplasia in ferrets. In a later study in 1996, 32 ferrets with hyperadrenocorticism with associated adrenocortical neoplasia or nodular hyperplasia were compared with 26 clinically normal ferrets.[9] The results showed that median plasma levels of 17-hydroxyprogesterone plus androstenedione and dehydroepiandrosterone sulphate were significantly higher in diseased than in normal ferrets.

Most generalized alopecia cases in neutered ferrets over 3 years old are caused by FADC; it is considered to be in 30% of pet ferrets over 3 years of age in one American practice.[1] Evidently neoplasia conditions led to a rise of one or more oestrogen precursors as in Table 14.1. The neoplasia factor has been studied.

An American survey (1987–1991) recognized adrenocortical adenoma, nodular hyperplasia or adenocarcinoma in 50 ferrets comprising 35 sterilized females and 15 sterilized males.[10] All pet ferrets at the time came from Marshall Farms, New York and were sterilized at 6 weeks of age. The mean age when clinical signs occurred was 3.4 years (range 1–7 years). A total of 39 ferrets were treated by adrenalectomy, 34 by unilateral and 5 by bilateral operations. *Note*: five died postoperatively. The remaining ferrets were checked at 1 month and 34 months post-operation.

Clinical signs

The common sign of impending FADC is alopecia in neutered ferrets of either sex, over 3 years of age in 82% of cases.[6] The degree of alopecia bears no relationship to the pathogenicity of the tumour. There can be pruritus in 8% of cases and sterilized jills show vulval swelling in 50% of cases with possible vaginitis.

American ferrets had shown sexual behaviour in desexed adults; this can appear as aggression to other males by males. The ferrets might lick each other or the owner and resort to hob marking behaviour with urine (Ch. 5). Mounting might be seen in the sterilized jill

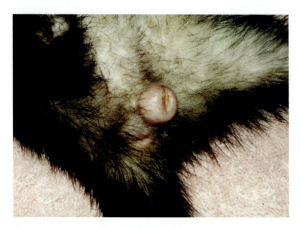

Figure 14.2 American female ferret showing alopecia and vulval swelling. (Courtesy of G. Rich.)

but never occurred in my Josie. *Note*: real aggression is not a feature of pet ferrets unless associated with the hormonal imbalances of adrenal endocrinopathies (D. Whiteside, Calgary, Canada, pers. comm. 2005).

Some FADC ferrets have been seen to drink their own urine. (I have seen this happen often with healthy jills in my old ferret colony, more as a habit.)

Consider symptoms in this American ferret (Fig. 14.2). A 5-year-old sterilized female had hair loss, pruritus and hyperplasia (swollen vulva).

The FADC alopecia I have seen usually started from the tail and extended forward over the body in a bilateral fashion. *Note* that other bilateral coat losses in ferrets can occur because of seasonal changes, usually confined to the tail in hobs, hyperoestrogenism in jills (POA), and possibly due to mast cell tumours (see Fig. 13.7). The progressive adrenal disease hair loss is said to occur in late winter or early spring (northern hemisphere) and continues until the ferret is completely bald.[3] In the case of my ferret, she started losing hair in 1994 (southern hemisphere summer) and was completely bald by late January. Josie, as she was in 1990, is shown with a normal coat in Figure 14.3.

In America, cases of hair loss can re-grow in the autumn but alopecia can recur the next winter or spring with the effect repeating for 2–3 years. Finally, the hair does not re-grow and the disease is stable.[11] *Note*: intact male ferrets may lose hair partially on tail and rump in October/November (northern hemisphere) and hair does not regrow at end of breeding seasons.

FADC has not been seen in ferrets in Australia less than 5 years old to my knowledge. One older case was recorded as possibly FADC and insulinoma (Alderton, Sydney, pers. comm. 1998).

As indicated earlier, spayed American ferrets with FADC have a history of an enlarged vulva and perhaps

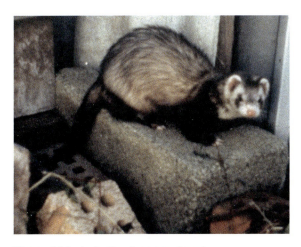

Figure 14.3 Josie showing normal coat.

vulval discharge.[3] The possibility of retained ovarian tissue from an early (6 weeks) or later (6 months) sterilization cannot be discounted.

My sterilized jill, Josie, showed hair loss sign at 6 years of age. She had been sterilized at 6 months and had been an outdoor ferret in the ferretarium and garden and became a resident 'in-house' ferret as she got older. She did not show an enlarged vulva. I had spayed her and checked for complete removal of ovaries. She was also non-pruritic, unlike the one third of American cases that show an acute pruritus. The latter condition has been seen in pet ferrets with hair loss but some, without showing hair loss, are found to be FADC cases. The area between the shoulder blades is the usual pruritus site and erythema is seen.[3] With male ferrets under investigation as well as jills, they have been found to be prone to dysuria and stranguria secondary to cystic prostatic enlargement and bacterial prostatitis as part of FADC.[11] I have not seen FADC in male ferrets. The sebaceous glands in the skin can be activated in FADC and cause the ferrets to smell, which did not occur in my jill.[1]

One Australian veterinarian reports 10 FADC cases (five sterilized males, five females) of which the females had no swollen vulva or pruritus (B. Alderton, pers. comm. 2005). Another has seen swollen vulva and pruritus but not every time and not always together (M. Simpson, pers. comm. 2005). A UK veterinarian has seen a swollen vulva as a consistent finding with pruritus variable. He has seen two ovarian remnants but the majority of cases have been hyperadrenocorticism (HAC) (J. Chitty, pers. comm. 2005).

Diagnosis

Complete alopecia of the sterilized jill is characteristic, with weight loss, which makes the ferret look 'skeletal'. The skin, as indicated previously, can become dry and mildly, to intensely pruritic but can also become thin and soft, which happened to Josie, with a typical atrophy of the abdominal and hind leg musculature leading to a classic pot-bellied appearance. Josie was relatively heavy for a jill, weighing 960 g at the beginning of her illness, which was reduced to 900 g at her operation for FADC.

Adrenal disease cannot be diagnosed reliably using the dexamethasone suppression test (DST) or the ACTH stimulation test and one author suggests that cortisol excess is not involved in FADC, so DST is not a suitable test.[3,8] Similarly, ferrets do not register a change of cortisol levels with an ACTH challenge.[11] Clinically, the blood picture is normal in FADC cases though rarely anaemia may be present, if there has been retention of some ovarian tissue during sterilization. As with postoestrous anaemia (POA), a PCV <15% indicates a grave prognosis. The enlarged vulva in some ferrets with FADC may respond to proligestone (Covinan, Intervet) as for POA to give a reduction of vulva size. Polydipsia and polyuria may be present in the disease[1] but neither was seen in my ferret. A dangerous complication occurs where there is concurrent insulinoma with hypoglycaemia; this is seen unfortunately in some American FADC cases but, again, did not occur with Josie. *Note*: in FADC, as cortisol is not increased, there is no cortisol delay in wound healing in these cases.[12]

Gould et al. described the evaluation of urinary cortisol:creatine (UC:CR) ratios as a possible diagnosis of hyperadrenocortism associated with adrenal gland tumours in ferrets.[13] They found that the UC:CR ratio was elevated in 12 ferrets diagnosed as FADC cases when compared with a collection of 51 clinically normal ferrets. Two of the 12 were sterilized males. The ferrets showed the classic signs of FADC alopecia. However, the UC:CR ratio idea was discounted as inaccurate (S. Brown, pers. comm. 1999), although it appears sensitive at least in the dog.

However, urinalysis can be overlooked in adrenal disease diagnosis where in the male, cornified squamous cells often show up in significant numbers with expressed urine samples due to squamous metaplasia of the prostate. In the female cornified squamous cells derive from the vaginal canal. In both cases, these are good indicators of oestrogen influence (M. Burgess, pers. comm. 2005).

In 1993, I had two *unsterilized* hobs, Tuppy and Sammy, who alarmed me by having extreme thinning of body hair not just on the tail. This occurred in February (southern hemisphere summer) and they had spontaneous re-growth of the whole body hair by June (winter). The phenomenon did not happen again and was unexplainable. The two hob ferrets did not go on to become FADC cases as did the sterilized male ferrets in the USA.

CHAPTER FOURTEEN
Endocrine diseases

Table 14.2 Adrenal gland and ovary weights in the ferret

Group	Left adrenal (mg)	Right adrenal (mg)	Paired adrenals (mg)	Paired ovaries (mg)	Jill body weight (g)
1. 36 anoestrous ferrets	51.3	55.5	107.1	67.7	653.0
2. 11 ferrets in anoestrus or early pro-oestrus	37.7	41.0	79.1	111.1	741.0
3. 9 ferrets in late pro-oestrus or full oestrus	53.0	57.5	111.0	121.0	747.0

Physical palpation of enlarged diseased adrenal glands is sometimes possible.[3] It is the left adrenal gland that is enlarged in 90% of FADC cases. The adrenal glands are found embedded in fat adjacent to the upper medial borders of the left and right kidneys but their exact position varies with individual animals.[14] Some idea of the size of ferret adrenal glands and ovaries in relation to jill body weight is given by Holmes in Table 14.2 (see also Figs 2.23, 2.24 and Figs 18.4, 18.5).

The spleen may be found enlarged on palpation of the left side of the ferret abdomen but enlargement does occur in older ferrets. A needle biopsy can be used to detect neoplastic changes.[1] However, as older ferrets have a high percentage risk of lymphoma, the removal of a suspect spleen at the time of adrenalectomy might be wise. Radiographs are useful and ultrasonographic detection has been demonstrated with adrenal tumours in two ferrets[15] and is detailed by Barthez et al.[16]

Treatment and study cases

Lawrence et al. have described treatment of adrenocortical tumours in five ferrets between 1990 and 1992 by unilateral adrenalectomy.[17] The ferrets were spayed adults ranging from 4.75 to 6.75 years with a mean of 5.4 years when clinical signs were first noticed (one ferret's age was unknown but believed to be between 1 and 5 years). The mean body weight was 0.75 kg (range 0.6–0.84), i.e. all under 1000 g. They were fed on commercial dry or canned cat food. The symptoms shown were basic symmetrical alopecia, which was noticed between 1 and 6 months before a vet check. All had vulval swellings; one jill had a haemorrhagic vaginal discharge. They were basically alert and eating with good attitude and activity.

Further diagnosis was carried out by ultrasound and showed an enlarged adrenal gland, in three ferrets, the left, which is more usual, and in two ferrets, the right gland. The sizes ranged from $8 \times 7 \times 7$ mm to $18 \times 6 \times 6$ mm. The uterine stumps were identified. Other clinical findings show the presence of stump pyometra with purulent vaginal discharge possibly brought about by high levels of oestrogen precursors. An example of a stump pyometra is shown in Figure 14.4. The stump pyometra condition in sterilized jills led to consideration of sterilization by hysterectomy rather than ovariohysterectomy. However, hormonal injections would be required to stop heats and may have ongoing consequences. It is considered best to spay jills after sexual maturity to prevent both diseases of POA and FADC (A. Melillo, pers. comm. 2005).

Under general anaesthesia, the neoplastic adrenal glands of the five ferrets were removed via a midline celiotomy. Difficulty in removing the right adrenal glands was admitted in one case with damage to the caudal vena cava which was repaired. The unaffected adrenal glands were considered to be in danger of going into atrophy so to prevent hypoadrenocorticism secondary to the atrophy the ferrets were given, while under G/A, either dexamethasone sodium phosphate at 0.014 mg/kg of body weight up to 0.3 mg/kg i.v. or dexamethasone at 0.08–0.1 mg/kg i.v. or 0.2 mg/kg i.m. as directed by the surgeon. *Note*: four ferrets had a second dose 3–6 hours later. Further, a course of prednisone was given to all ferrets with dosages ranging from 1 mg/kg per day tapering to 0.5 mg/kg every other day over 3 weeks, or 1 mg/kg per day tapering to 0.25 mg/kg every other day over

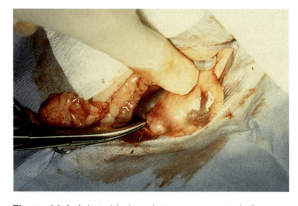

Figure 14.4 Adrenal-induced stump pyometra in ferret. (Courtesy of G. Rich.)

3 months, to 0.25 mg/kg per day tapered to 0.1 mg/kg every other day over 3 weeks.

The rationale of the postoperative treatment was that the tumours might be secreting excessive amounts of cortisol, so one might expect a contralateral gland atrophy secondary to negative feedback effects of the pituitary gland and decreased ACTH secretion. If the tumours were oestrogen-secreting rather than cortisol-secreting there would be no adrenocortical suppression to the contralateral gland and thus no supplementation would be required. In two of the five ferrets, the contralateral gland was not easy to identify, suggesting atopy of the adrenal gland. In fact, none of the ferrets had hypoadrenocorticism signs after surgery. (Mary Van Dahm, ferret breeder, discusses the reduction of cortisol postoperatively later in this chapter.)

The histology found adrenocortical adenomas in four ferrets and the last had an adrenocortical adenocarcinoma. The overall results with the five ferrets were the regression of vulval swelling and complete hair re-growth in 1–2 months. Four ferrets were clinically normal 5–8 months after surgery, while one ferret developed cardiomyopathy (Ch. 11) and was put to sleep. No recurrence of adrenal neoplasia was found on post mortem. No further follow-up after 8 months is indicated but the likelihood of the remaining adrenal gland becoming cancerous is highly possible (see below).

Weiss et al. have described further surgical treatment and results with 56 ferrets affected by FADC between 1994 and 1997.[18] The mean age of sickness in these ferrets was 4.4 years (range 2.2–7.5). It was considered that the treatment of choice for ferrets with adrenal disease is surgical intervention by adrenalectomy. The ferrets either had a bilateral adrenalectomy immediately or unilateral adrenalectomy, which was followed by removal of the other adrenal once the disease affected the remaining gland. This operation method is detailed in Chapter 18. Concerning the symptoms shown in the 56 ferrets, 46 showed classic alopecia, 38 lethargy, 28 muscle atrophy, 14 jills with enlarged vulva, 12 pruritic, 5 males sexual behaviour and 5 males with stranguria.

Note: clinical signs disappeared within 2–4 weeks postoperatively in 48 ferrets; seven ferrets took up to 6 weeks. A few became worse 2–3 weeks after the operation but then had complete hair re-growth. However, in eight ferrets, the symptoms recurred 7–22 months after surgery. In three of them mitotane treatment was tried but only one responded well (see Medical treatments).

The study ferrets were observed over 18–39 months after the initial operation and it was interesting to see concurrent disease in these ferrets: one ferret died post-operation, 18 showed splenomegaly at some time, 12 insulinoma, 4 cardiomyopathy, 2 gastric hairballs, 1 renal failure and one splenic haematoma. *Note*: the 12 to suffer insulinoma were 21% of the total group in this study.

It is considered that, as long as an FADC case has no other major illness, surgery is the best option regardless of the ferret's age.[19] My jill, Josie, was operated on under ketamine/halothane anaesthesia using a tight facial mask plus giving Hartman's solution by slow i.v. drip. The anatomy involved with this operation is reviewed in Chapter 2. The technique of this delicate operation for one or both adrenal glands is illustrated in Chapter 18. The progress of Josie's (1996) operation can be seen in Figures 14.5–14.8.

I removed only the left adrenal gland and postoperatively, Josie was given dexamethasone i.m. at 1 mg/kg body weight and after 24 hours started a course of oral prednisolone at a dose rate of 0.10 mg/kg once daily for 5 days. This was then given every other day for

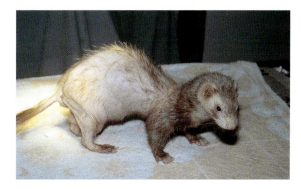

Figure 14.5 Josie showing alopecia due to FADC.

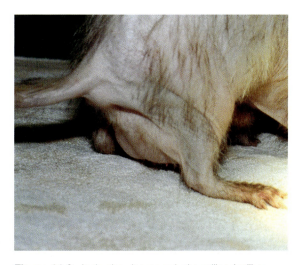

Figure 14.6 Josie showing no vulval swelling (unlike FADC cases seen in America.)

CHAPTER FOURTEEN
Endocrine diseases

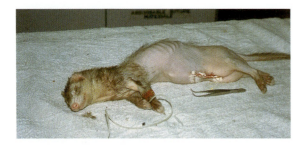

Figure 14.7 Josie on operating table.

Author's clinical example

A large adrenal gland adenocarcinoma was removed from an American sterilized jill (Fig. 14.9) where the jill showed a swollen vulva (Fig. 14.2) and further hair loss on the dorsum and tail head (Fig. 14.10) indicating FADC.

G. Rich, pers. comm. 2005.

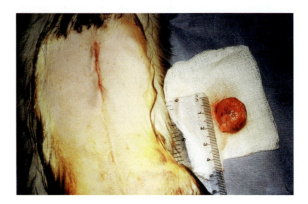

Figure 14.9 Adrenal gland carcinoma. (Courtesy of G. Rich.)

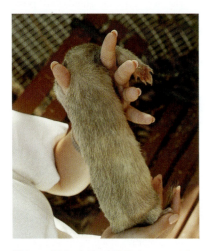

Figure 14.8 Josie with hair re-growth.

three doses. It was considered best to use corticosteroids for short periods.[1] One author suggests not giving postoperative corticosteroids as a study showed that ferrets are able to respond to ACTH challenge after an adrenalectomy with a cortisol release.[3] Steroids are only to be used if the ferret is lethargic postoperatively or has had both adrenal glands removed. With my ferret case, except for a slight relapse, Josie improved with signs of coat re-growth in 1 month and with a full body coat in 2 months.[2] However, perhaps the corticosteroids are unnecessary and just an added stress to the kidneys? One author states the administration of glucocorticoids seems to improve postoperative recovery. If a bilateral adrenalectomy is performed, the therapy will be required for a longer period (A. Bennett, pers. comm. 1999).

If only one adrenal gland is affected and removed, there is a strong possibility that the other gland will be affected in 1 year. My jill died 7 months after the adrenal gland operation from suspected kidney failure.

In early cases it was considered that the left adrenal gland was the cause of 90% of FADC; because the right adrenal gland was not easy to identify and remove.

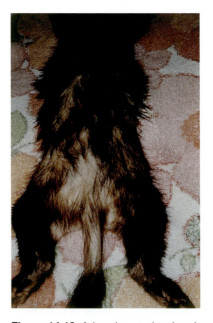

Figure 14.10 Adrenal case showing dorsal alopecia. (Courtesy of M. Finkler.)

Ferret adrenal disease complex (FADC)

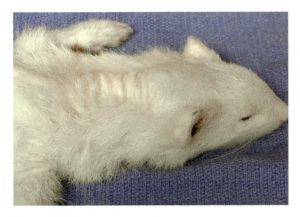

Figure 14.11 Adrenal case alopecia on dorsal aspect of neck. (Courtesy of G. Rich.)

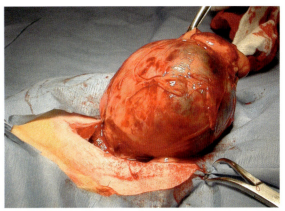

Figure 14.13 Neoplastic adrenal gland exteriorized. (Courtesy G. Rich.)

The disease can occur equally on either side (S. Brown, pers. comm. 1998). She pointed out that you have to consider the dorsal surface of the right adrenal gland as the cancer focus; it is not often visible or barely so. Both adrenal glands are usually embedded in fat, the extent of which depends on the condition of the ferret.

There are now microsurgery techniques available for bilateral adrenalectomy as illustrated in Chapter 18. It has become clear, in the light of veterinary practice experience in America, that prevention of this disease, along with insulinoma, should be of major concern.

Alopecia can occur in focal areas such as the dorsal aspect of the neck.[20] This is illustrated in Figure 14.11. In this ferret, the head was most obvious but the rest of the coat was thinning.

This adrenal gland operation (Figs 14.12–14.14) shows the exteriorization of a tumorous gland and comparison

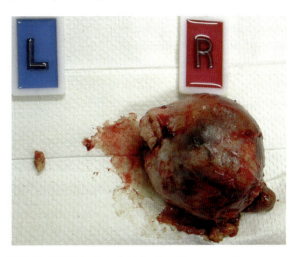

Figure 14.14 Left and right adrenals compared. (Courtesy G. Rich.)

with the normal adrenal gland; the neoplastic adrenal gland was 2.5 cm wide.

Adrenal disease problems in the male ferret

Male ferrets with FADC can have the added painful problem of stricture due to prostatic/para-urethral enlargement secondary to the elevation of androgens produced by the neoplastic tissue. The fact that male ferrets can be de-sexed at the early age of 6 weeks may well contribute to the male urethra being underdeveloped in internal diameter.

Constriction of the urethra at the prostate level (see Fig. 2.29) was recorded in four ferrets.[21] A surgical

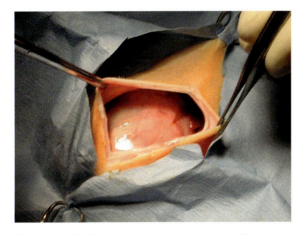

Figure 14.12 Start of adrenal gland operation. (Courtesy of G. Rich.)

technique for relief has been suggested in the form of temporary tube cystostomy. The four ferrets had alopecia and an even more dangerous common complaint, painful stranguria and dysuria with turgid bladders. The ferrets were put under isoflurane anaesthesia, a midline exploratory was done and the neoplastic adrenals removed. *Note*: complete adrenalectomy was done on the unilaterally-affected adrenal masses of ferrets 1, 2 and 3, while ferret 4, with bilateral disease, had the large right adrenal removed but only part of the left gland was taken. Two ferrets were diagnosed as having prostatic cysts.

Because of the swollen non-expressible bladders, adrenal tumours, prostate problems and history of urinary obstruction, tube cystostomy was done on three ferrets. The catheterization worked but obstruction occurred when they were removed. (The fourth ferret had to have a cystocentesis performed.) The tube cystostomy technique required a stab hole to be made through the ventral body wall, (using no. 15 blade) during the exploratory celiotomy. The cystotomy tube, a 5 or 8 French Foley catheter, is passed. The bladder is exteriorized and a purse string suture is placed in the avascular ventral portion of the bladder with a 3.0 polydioxanone suture. A stab incision is made in the centre of the purse string suture entering the bladder lumen so that the Foley catheter is able to pass into the bladder through the stab incision. Once in the balloon is inflated with sterile saline. The purse string suture is then tightened around the catheter and tied. Then the catheter is used to bring the bladder close to the body wall and simple interrupted tacking sutures between the body wall and the anchored bladder are placed for added security. Finally, the stab incision in the skin is closed with another purse string suture that continues as a Chinese finger trap suture around the Foley catheter. In addition, the Foley catheter is capped with a catheter adapter and intermittent injection cap. The whole is enclosed in a light body wrap and an Elizabethan collar applied (Ch. 20).

The ferrets recovered well from surgery but one ferret was put to sleep later as it was diagnosed with a metastatic carcinoma. Postoperatively, the ferrets were given i.v. fluids and cystotomy tube aspirations every 2–3 hours. They received prednisolone or antibiotic cover and wore body stockinettes. Voluntary urination occurred 6–120 hours postoperatively and the three stable ferrets were discharged 2–4 days post-surgery. The owners had the job of draining the ferrets' bladder every 4–6 hours with a syringe as instructed. The ferrets were under amoxicillin cover at 22 mg/kg p.o. b.i.d.

The outcome was that the cystotomy tubes remained in place for 5–14 days with one having to be removed at 5 days because of self trauma. However, all three ferrets were urinating normally at the time of tube removal. Long-term observation found that urinary obstruction occurred in one ferret (adenocarcinoma case) at 6 months while the other two (adrenal adenoma cases) were put to sleep for other reasons at 8 and 24 months, respectively.

Note. It is controversial now to use antibiotic therapy postoperatively as it may decrease infection risk but can select for resistant bacteria. In the case of these three ferrets, antibiotics were used due to the presence of inflammatory urinary sediment and difficulty in having an aseptic environment for the animals. All urine should be cultured for pathogens and sensitivity.

Medical therapies for FADC

Medical treatments without recourse to surgery have been carried out in the USA. Mitotane or (o, p'-DDD) (Lysodren, Bristol Meyer Squibb Oncology, Princetown, New Jersey) has previously been the drug of choice.[3] It has shown variable success with cortical adenomas but not with adrenocortical adenocarcinoma.[1] It works by chemical debulking of the affected adrenal gland but not by any direct anti-hormone action.

Furthermore, if the ferret has a concurrent insulinoma, as very often happens, the condition is worsened by mitotane reducing corticosteroid levels, causing a hypoglycaemic attack or coma. The response to mitotane therapy is growth of hair and reduction of vulval size but one author considers that the clinical signs of FADC return as soon the mitotane treatment is stopped.[3] It is suggested that the drug be used only on older ferrets, which are a surgical risk, have bilateral adrenal disease or have owners not able to afford expensive surgery. One author maintains that there has been some success in decreasing adrenal tissue mass by using mitotane at 50 mg/kg p.o. q. 24 h, given at once or twice a week. Evidently, pulsing the therapy is better tolerated by the ferret and less likely to trigger a hypoglycaemic attack (C J-D, pers. comm. 2005).

Mitotane dosage: The drug was given to ferrets with primary FADC at a basic dose rate of 50 mg daily p.o. for 1 week. The maintenance dose thereafter is 50 mg every 3 days for up to 8 weeks. The drug has low toxicity in ferrets and does not affect the bone marrow, so serial CBC counts are not required but there may be some rare gastrointestinal upsets.[1] However, as noted above, if there were a concurrent insulinoma, a traumatic hypoglycaemia could occur a few days into therapy, in which case the drug would be stopped and the ferret treated (see Insulinoma section).[3] A major problem of mitotane, like a lot of drugs for ferrets, is its expense, also, coming in tablet form, it needs to be changed to a suspension or added to a gel substance for administration. The tablet is not easy to divide accurately but is broken into roughly 50 mg portions and these can be then mixed with cornstarch filler and placed in very small gelatin capsules.[1] This can be done by a chemist and the capsules must be given whole – not easy to do with a ferret! The gel capsules can be coated with olive oil and given. As the suspensions are compounded, it is thought that the potency varies with the bioavailability for oral absorption; thus the adrenal tissues do not get enough of the drug. The client would have to be keen to keep the medication going for 8 weeks.

Mitotane can be given as an adjunct to Lupron (see below) to decrease the adrenal tissue mass at 50 mg/kg p.o., given consecutively for up to 4 days a week (depending on the ferret's condition) then off for 3 days. The powder is mixed with a 'treat' and given immediately (C J-D pers. comm. 2005).

It is possible to monitor the use of mitotane with an ACTH stimulation test for the effects of adrenal cortisol production.[3] The drug cosyntropin is given at 1 µg/kg i.v. or i.m. and the plasma cortisols are measured at immediate administration and then 60 min later. The plasma cortisol levels are increased four-fold in normal ferrets from the resting level (resting levels shown in Table 14.4 below). The actual efficiency of mitotane cannot be judged by the ACTH test; it is only to assess if the drug loading was adequate. Most information on treatment progress comes from the high number of FADC cases seen in the USA.

Deslorelin: A synthetic GnRH analogue (deslorelin, USA) is the new drug implant for reduction of testosterone levels in the entire dog as a contraceptive process. Finkler has recorded drugs, human or otherwise, which are possible treatments for FADC.[6] Deslorelin is the American equivalent of the Australian drug suprelorin (PEPTECH Animal Health) registered only for use in trials for chemical castration of dogs. Each implant contains 4.7 mg deslorelin acetate. It is similar to the drug Zoladex, used for prostate cancer treatment, as an active agonist of LH-RH, causing the desensitization of the pituitary, thus stopping the release of gonadotropins.

A project to assess the use of deslorelin acetate for ferrets was carried out by Wagner at Pittsburgh University. Using slow-release 3 mg deslorelin acetate implants, he found that the clinical signs and steroid hormone concentrations could be reduced over the short term.[22] Using 15 FADC ferrets, within 2 weeks of the implant, vulval swelling, pruritus, sexual behaviours and any aggression disappeared or were reduced. In 4 weeks, the steroid plasma hormone levels decreased until clinical relapse which ensued on average at 13.7 ± 3.5 months, with a range of 8.5–20.5 months. *Note*: in five ferrets, large adrenal tumours were palpable in about 2 months of the clinical relapse or shortly thereafter. Adrenal tumours did metastasize to the liver. However, four ferrets had a second deslorelin implant and Wagner maintained in 2003 that the four were clear of FADC symptoms for over 2.5 years since the original treatments.

They were checked by palpation and use of ultrasonography (Ch. 17). Laboratory details were recorded.[22] The overall conclusion was that deslorelin implants may be useful in the long-term management of FACD from hormone-induced causes. Ferrets thought to be surgical risk cases might benefit from such medication on a long term basis.

Deslorelin implants have been used for prevention of oestrus/suppression of ovulation in jills by Angella Prohaczik in Hungary (2005). The implants were administered in February, before the breeding season. Ovarian function was monitored with progesterone metabolite ELISA from serially-collected faecal samples until the end of the year. Simultaneously, other females were treated with synthetic gestagens, or received hCG at their oestrus. Deslorelin suppressed the ovarian function for about 1.5 years while the other treatments were followed by oestrus some weeks or months later.

Prohaczik has had successful treatment of three cases of nodular adrenocortical hyperplasia (NAH). Oestrogen levels were determined in pairs of samples taken before and 3–4 weeks after treatment from one previously ovariectomized female and one castrated male. Before treatment, about 100 pmol/l oestradiol levels were detected in both animals. *Note*: 3–4 weeks after deslorelin treatment the oestradiol levels were undetectable and both ferrets had a full clinical recovery (Dr A. Prohaczik and Professor G. Huszenicza, Szent Isten University, Budapest, pers. comm. 2005).

Deslorelin (from Ovuplant, Fort Dodge) has been used in mares as an implantable substance-released GnRH to induce ovulation. Though not long-acting like Lupron Depot, see below, Finkler has seen clinical results lasting up to 3 months.[23] However, the overall success rate is around 60%. The 2.1 mg pellet is given s.c. It can be ground into a suspension and given at half dose rate. *Note*: the result in one spayed female ferret was mammary hyperplasia 2 weeks after injection.

Leuprolide acetate (Lupron Depot: TP Pharmaceuticals Inc. USA) is a human drug which has been trialed by various veterinarians. It is a slow-release injectable[24] labelled to treat testicular cancer in men and endometriosis in women. It is not ferret-registered but has been used since September 1996.[6] It is also an analog of the natural GnRH or LH-RH. Animal and human studies show that the drug causes an initial surge of LH (stimulation effect), however, prolonged administration causes a suppression of ovarian and testicular steroidogenesis.

One survey of leuprolide acetate was to examine the use of the drug as a 30-day depot affecting hormone levels and comparing it to the effects of a unilateral adrenalectomy.[5] There was a worry about a steroidogenic 'rebound' in ferrets undergoing the partial operation where hormonal levels are higher 6 months postoperatively than at the initial diagnosis (C J-D, pers. comm. 2005). It is theorized that ferrets are programmed for reproduction and have a hormonal setup tapered to the event. With domestication and the seasonal copulation-stimulated breeder ferret becoming a house pet and highly inbred, it has become a smaller more immature adult type with less sexual dimorphism. Factors contributing to this trend are discussed at the end of this chapter.

Criteria for ferrets undergoing Lupron treatment survey were that they should have elevated hormones and no concurrent insulinoma or lymphoma and the left adrenal gland should be enlarged, as judged by ultrasound or laparotomy.

The results attained indicated that loss of hair or hair growth was not a good indicator of the degree of the disease. It was found that female ferrets apparently tolerate higher hormone levels for longer than males before the tumours develop more and metastasize. In addition, males move on to getting prostate involvement and metastasis. It is thought that partial adrenalectomy should be accompanied by the preoperative use of Lupron. The Lupron dosage should be adjusted to the individual ferret and season of the year.

Note: Lupron is effective in taking a jill out of oestrus and chemically sterilizing a hob for 30–60 days. What affect it could have on yearly use is not stated (see ovarian tumour discussion in Ch. 13). Leuprolide was trialed on 20 ferrets with adrenal disease.[25] The ferrets were treated with leuprolide (100 μg i.m. once only), while they were under isoflurane anaesthesia for a complete physical examination. The plasma hormone concentrations were measured before treatment and then at 3 and 6 weeks after the injection. Results showed a great reduction in the plasma oestradiol, 17-hydroxyprogesterone (17-OHP), androstenedione and dehydroepiandrosterone (DHEA). This removed signs of vulval swelling, pruritus and aggressive plus abnormal sexual behaviour in the sterilized ferrets

The outcome was elimination or at least reduction in clinical signs with the effects lasting from 6 weeks to 8 months. *Note*: none of the ferrets died before the clinical signs recurred. There were no reports of any adverse reaction to the drugs but it is interesting to note the concurrent diseases that occurred in the group: two ferrets had heart disease, two had insulinoma, one had renal disease while another developed an inoperable adenocarcinoma of the right adrenal gland. This seems to be the overall clinical picture of American pet ferrets. The authors commented on the high incidence of FADC in pet ferrets possibly associated with sterilization at an early age and abnormally long photo-periods, which are discussed later. It was noted by Wagner that ferret adrenal gland tumours have LH receptors and that LH is known to cause adrenal cortical tumour development in mice, which have also been known to develop adrenal gland tumours after castration.

Leuprolide acetate (Lupron) acts on the hormone pathways as seen in Figure 14.1, shutting down the FSH and LH secretions. It appears to 'buy time' even with ferrets with adrenal adenocarcinoma and has actually shrunk some adrenal tumours. Though not curative it is safe, especially with older patients.

Note: a USA sable male ferret, Robbie, had a left adrenalectomy at $2^{1}/_{2}$ years of age with removal of insulinoma tumours. At $4^{1}/_{2}$ years, after treatments and lots of TLC, he had prostate enlargement and complete urethral blockage. Robbie was the first ferret with FADC to be treated with Lupron, which worked. He finally died of insulinoma.

Finkler (USA) advises a dose rate of 100 μg per ferret i.m. (after Wagner). The results seen generally include decreases in vulval swelling, pruritus and undesirable sexual behaviour and aggression within 14 days of treatment, with hair growth by 4 weeks.[6]

Other dose rates include 2.0 mg/ferret s.c. of a 4-month repositol form (Weiss) and a lower dose of 100 μg/kg, which equals 0.1 mg/kg i.m., q. 4 weeks of a 1-month repositol form (C J-D). In all cases, the treatment would have to be repeated after 4–8 months. *Note*: Lupron Depot could be kept for 4–6 months in a deep freeze.

With cases of sterilized ferrets in the USA, Finkler[23] is using the following protective plan:

a. *Indoor pet ferrets exposed to unnatural photo-periods*: give 1 mg Lupron Depot 4-month product s.c. every 6–8 months, beginning around 4–8 months of age.
b. *Outdoor pet ferrets exposed to natural photo-periods*: give 1 mg Lupron Depot 4-month product s.c. annually in February or March (northern hemisphere), beginning around 4–8 months of age.

In one Australian practice, they use leuprorelin acetate (Lucrin Depot, Abbot) after the C. Johnson-Delaney protocol, giving 100 μg/kg once every 4–8 weeks. They have had no adverse reaction with this drug.[26]

Drug administration technique: The Lucrin depot drug costs $450 per vial and can deliver about 75 doses. Under sterile conditions, the 7.50 mg vial is made up according to instructions and mixed well. The solution is drawn into a 10 mL syringe (usually about 2.2 mL) and topped up with sterile water to 7.50 mL. This is then injected into a sterile vial and gives 1000 μg/mL of leuprorelin. This is then drawn up into 0.10 mL (or 100 μg) aliquots, which can be frozen. Sick ferrets less than 1000 g are given one dose while heavier ferrets are given two doses, which works well. This procedure is cost-effective to the client but what a palaver to keep pet ferrets in modern times! *Note*: The Lucrin depot cost in the exotic practice can be justified when considering it is also useful in treating avian problems.

Other USA drugs suggested by Finkler and C J-D for consideration in the future include:

Viadur: (Alza Corp). A 1-year leuprolide implant scheduled to come on line. It would be possible to give with a yearly distemper vaccination.

Goserelin: (the Zoladex mentioned above). Used for dogs to lower oestradiol levels and treat certain mammary cancers. The drug is expensive, with a dose rate of 60 µg/kg s.c. q. 21 days. The goserelin acetate implant of 10.8 mg is supposed to last 3 months in humans. No ferret evaluation as yet.

Bicalutamide: (Casodex). This drug blocks androgen receptors; it leads to increased testosterone and oestradiol levels if used alone. It comes as a 50 mg tablet, which must be compounded. The dose rate is 5 mg/kg p.o. s.i.d. until clinical signs cease. At the time of writing, it is on clinical trials only. However, the client must continue using the drug with the ferret on a week on, week off basis to maintain remission for the animal's life. C J-D asserts it could be used in severe prostate cases in conjunction with Lupron. It can result in a return to male sexual behavior in 1–2 weeks. The drug can be used for short periods against prostatitis and aggression along with Lupron according to Wagner.[27]

Anastrozole: (Arimidex). A drug which inhibits the production of oestradiol and oestrogen, i.e. blocks adrenally-generated androstenedione to oestrone to oestradiol in peripheral tissues. Some trials are current. Again, the 1 mg tablet must be compounded and the dose rate is 0.1 mg/kg. p.o. s.i.d. (not as effective as Lupron Depot or Casodex). C J-D has noted some correlation with elevated androstenedione and aggression. Anastrozole can help to shrink enlarged prostates more quickly while Lupron starts to work. *Note*: Casodex should not be used with Arimidex as they cancel each other's effects.

The drugs above are not registered for ferrets but appear safe in the short term. However, pregnant women should not handle bicalutamide and anastrozole. The drugs after compounding should be kept in a fridge and shaken before administration.

Finasteride: (Proscar). This drug is a 5-alpha reductase inhibitor which prevents the formation of dihydrotestosterone. The tablets are 5 mg and dog dosage is 5 mg p.o. q. 24 h. Dosage is tolerated by ferrets. It can be used as an adjunct to Lupron.

Flutamide: (Eulexin). This drug is an androgen blocker and is used in humans with leuprolide acetate for prostate cancer. Toxicity trials have been done on rats, dogs and rabbits but it needs further investigation for ferret use.

Tamoxifen: (Nolvadex). An anti-oestrogen agent like anastrozole, being an oestrogen receptor blocker. It has had minimal success in dogs and ferrets but with high incidence of toxicity. If the uterine stump remains, there may be discharges.

Aminoglutethimide: (Cytadren O). This drug inhibits adrenocortical steroid synthase enzymes, blocking conversion of cholesterol into pregnenolone. Adrenal steroid synthesis is suppressed and also other pathways including synthesis of thyroid hormones and cortisol. The decreased cortisol leads to increased ACTH output with diminished drug effect according to C J-D. The drug lacks desirable specificity of action as it may need concurrent treatment with cortisol.

Deprenyl: (Anipryl O). A drug which decreases elevated ACTH. Shown by Schoemaker et al. to be ineffective in ferrets, as animals with hyperadrenocortism did not have detectable abnormalities in plasma concentration of ACTH or alpha-MSH.[28]

Melatonin: The pineal gland produces melatonin which is concerned with the ferret sexual cycles (Ch. 5). Dr J. Paul-Murphy has researched melatonin supplementation as a means of treating FADC. The affected ferrets were given melatonin implants, whereby a temporary response was attained but the tumour growths resumed in 2–3 months.[29] Melatonin implants were first used in mink and given in autumn to cause the winter coat to come in for pelting (C J-D, pers. comm. 2005). The toxicology work was done on ferrets by the Food and Drug Administration (FDA). It was known that 30–34% was eluted from the capsules each month for the first 3 months – considered an effective dose for the coat change, caused in mustelids by depressing prolactin and progesterone primarily. The capsules continued to elute a little melatonin out for 273 days. However, repeated administration and administration at other times of the year may have had little effect on the coat. *Note*: melatonin capsules were designed for mink over 800 g.

The controlled study by Dr J. Paul-Murphy showed that melatonin was good in suppressing prolactin and progesterone, and there was some remission of outward clinical signs. The ferrets were given 0.5 mg melatonin p.o. daily and were checked every 4 months over 1 year. There was an ultrasound examination of the adrenal glands and assessment of sex hormone levels (including prolactin). In nine ferrets the clinical signs of vulva swelling, prostate involvement and hair loss were reversed with oestradiol, 17-hydroxyprogesterone and DHEAS levels decreased for the first 4 months; but then by 8–12 months after treatment started, the hormone levels became higher than initially seen. The androstenedione level gradually increased in each ferret at the

CHAPTER FOURTEEN
Endocrine diseases

4-week intervals. However, the melatonin had no effect on tumour growth.[29]

Dr J. Murray used subcutaneous implants on ferrets with FADC in a study with C J-D. Male mink melatonin implants (5.4 mg) gave a depot release of melatonin over a 3–4 month period.[30] He considered the implant might supercede the daily tablet and eliminate the administration of drug at a specific time, being 7–8 hours after sunrise. As there were no blood level determinations of melatonin in mink or ferrets (an expensive exercise) just the effects of the melatonin on sick ferrets was observed. He used 38 male and 32 female ferrets which had clinical signs of FADC. They were given the male mink melatonin implant s.c. in the intrascapular region.

Results post-injection were that in 1–2 weeks, the vulva size diminished to normal; in 6–8 weeks, there was hair re-growth with thick 'winter coats'; ferret activity increased and weight increased with appetite return. No increase in size of adrenals was palpable but no ultrasound was performed. Lethargy was the only side-effect which occurred in the first 3–5 days post-injection. One female ferret registered the presence of a right adrenal carcinoma and concurrent lymphoma and was taken out of the study.

The change in adrenal hormone levels was shown in one ferret:

17-hydroxyprogesterone	0.27 to 0.0 nmol/L (100% down)
Androstenedione	14.0 to 6.6 nmol/L (51% down)
Oestradiol	159.0 to 187 pmol/L (18% increase)

The oestradiol increase is the opposite to that which happened with the Paul-Murphy study (see above). *Note* the reduction of androstenedione was not seen with oral melatonin but occurred with one ferret in the implant study. The hormonal levels increased after 8 months in the Paul-Murphy study, so that additional hormone panels are advised to monitor the ongoing effects of mink melatonin implants. The implants appeared safe in ferrets and toxicity trials were done on mink to get FDA approval of the drug. Of course, in mink the melatonin implant was to be a once-only injection. Trials done at the University of Saskatchewan and in New Zealand showed no adverse reactions.

It is considered that further long-term studies are required on the use of melatonin implants with ferrets. There should also be more monthly panels and adrenal gland measurements using ultrasound on a monthly basis. The treatment of FADC becomes ongoing and time-consuming. Moreover, specific testing for melatonin receptors on ferret adrenal glands, prostate and bone marrow is required for a full picture of disease treatment.

Melatonin does profit FADC cases by its action as an antioxidant, appetite stimulant and bone density protector according to Murray.[30] He suggests that melatonin can be used in FADC cases with the other drugs in the following cases:

- For prostatic neoplasia: with leuprolide acetate or finasteride or bicalutamide
- For oestrogen-induced anaemia: with leuprolide acetate or anastrozole or epoetin alfa
- For oestrogen-induced cytopenia and/or mammary gland hyperplasia: with leuprolide acetate or anastrozole.

As with mitotane there is a potential problem with commercial oral formulation with a lack of standardization of melatonin as the over the counter products are not FDA-regulated drugs but classified as 'supplements'.

Cathy Johnson-Delaney (C J-D) considers that a study of intact ferrets using melatonin is required to show the drug is delivered by oral or subcutaneous implants and will function to suppress sex steroid production for a certain duration. *Note* the commercially available melatonin implant for mink is still the 5.4 mg form.

C J-D says of her controlled study in 2004 that she placed melatonin implants in intact male ferrets in season (January northern winter) and measured the hormone panels monthly.[31] Four male ferrets, Nick, control, with just a placebo microchip, while Crais, Husky and Bubba had 5.4 mg melatonin implants inserted under ketamine/acepromazine sedation. The ferrets had hormonal assay at 30, 60 and 90 days post-implant. They were checked for behaviour and testicle size. Results seem to suggest that the melatonin did not suppress sex steroid production as the levels of oestrodiol, progesterone and androstenedione did not decrease. It was noted that the three ferrets with the implants were not as active as usual in play.

In addition, a fourth implant was used on one of two female ferrets, Zoe, in a Lupron versus adrenalectomy trial. The other ferret Bonnie, had a microchip placebo. The females had been stable on Lupron for over 2 years showing both had just slightly enlarged adrenals (using ultrasound) just before the melatonin implant.

It was noted that the drug appeared to be similarly effective to the 30-day Lupron, which was administered monthly. However, Zoe never had a second implantation at 90 days and the experiment was terminated. This was because she showed an adverse reaction to the drug by being sleepy and having to be roused daily to eat. It was of concern because it was not her usual behaviour and no other physical or medical reason could be given for the effect seen. There was no statistical difference between Zoe and Bonnie though Zoe showed an increased hormonal level which was different to her previous hormone panel on Lupron. Her activity slowly came back to normal 4 months after the melatonin implant.

C J-D considers melatonin should not be used on ferrets below 600 g weight because of the 'sleep' factor as the dose might be too high. Larger ferrets over 1000 g do not seem to show the effect so it might be a dose factor.

The study indicated that the implants did not significantly suppress sex steroid production in intact males although there was some individual suppression primarily at 60 days. C J-D admits the trials involved small numbers of ferrets. C J-D considers that melatonin implants designed for mink have not been proven effective in the long term nor beneficial, other than at some times of the year promoting hair growth. She could not get suppression of adult intact males in season but she could get suppression using Lupron. Thus, she is reluctant to use melatonin. Furthermore, ferrets get refractory to the drug with repeated administration and there may be toxic effects in small ferrets. There have been reports of ferrets with melatonin implants, put in every 3 months for a year, which have died of kidney disease. The effect of any major drug treatment is a worry for future renal disease in my opinion.

Considering mink, the melatonin implants reach a refractory period where the drug fails to deliver its effects. Ferrets may become refractory to the effects of melatonin as a result of the time of year, reaction to the implant exogenous material or the stage of the FADC. In other words, with melatonin, the ferrets' coats may look good but it does nothing for the adrenal tumour crisis. C J-D has data on the same ferrets in 2002 when they were used for a 30-day trial of Lupron Depot as well as the 3-month Lupron trials. In addition, she has an intact control running, so that she has 4 years of hormone panels.

It is thought that more studies should be done on commercial implants but they do seem to promote hair growth and control clinical symptoms. It is up to practitioners to monitor adrenal size and growth, any metastasis problems and prostate health, regardless of the methods used in treatment of FADC. According to C J-D she would not use melatonin implants without close monitoring and even additional medications. The affected ferrets should have 3-monthly check ups for progress. With many FADC ferrets being geriatric, conditions may change radically over a short time.

C J-D is adamant that veterinarians should look closely at the effects of hormone suppression on intact male and female ferrets throughout the year to gauge how well it is working and if repeated administration is as effective. Research into melatonin in the laboratory for hormone studies shows that it works somewhat but was not the same the year round, and that the ferret (and other seasonally reproducing animals) will develop tolerance or break through, going into season eventually but out of sync with the calendar.

It was decided that melatonin implants are a useful adjunctive therapy; any suppression is helpful in buying the ferret time and hopefully allowing the ferret its 5-7 year lifespan. C J-D considers a hormone panel check once yearly for unaffected ferrets and always at the beginning of therapy. Considering the appearance of the ferret must tie in with the use of ultrasound to watch the adrenal size and metastasis. She considers January (northern winter) the best month to check male ferrets and early February to early March for females. This corresponds with the normal time of the year for highest hormone levels in spayed/castrated ferrets (and intact ones too). Controlling the hormones at this time gives the best chance to slow tumour growth.

The other 'key' time is what should be the lowest time of the year, if it is not controlled then there will be problems. This is possibly the best time of the year to initially diagnose the ferrets as well with hormone panels and again, this should be low. August/early September (northern summer/autumn) for male ferrets, late September through October for female ferrets.

Regarding the overall treatment of FADC cases, C J-D states debulking is very useful along with suppression of hormone production. She is against risking the ferret's life by doing adrenal surgery. Interestingly her data shows that the ferret lifespan does not differ using surgery vs Lupron Depot. Vets should be practising a level of medicine on FADC ferrets that warrants the diagnostic work. (Practitioners complain about cost of hormonal panel outlay and ultrasound repeats.) The whole thing should involve the client's baseline of costs.

Cost: The melatonin implant (Ferretonin Implant, Melatek, LLC, Fort Collins, CO) is 5.4 mg and costs US$19.95 each plus postage. Total cost of single implant US$23. The implant is more expensive than Lupron (at US$5.50/100 μg assuming ferret receives 100 μg per month of 7.5 mg Lupron). C J-D reckons US$16.50 for 3 months or, for ferrets receiving 200 μg Lupron per month, it would be US$33 for 3 months' treatment.

There is ongoing work on the ferret genome by Dr M. Hawkins at UC Davis California. In January 2005, the team started to collect normal (asymptomatic) young ferret tissue. Once the full ferret genome is worked out, it is anticipated the team would be able to hunt for the tumour suppression genes, which are at the root of the problem. Then there can be an assay for genes and hopefully there will no longer be ferrets on lifetime anti-tumour medication.

Again, Finkler[23] has a practitioner's idea for using melatonin:

a. *Indoor pet ferrets exposed to unnatural photo-periods*; give the oral product at 1.0 mg/kg for life or s.c. implant of 2.7 mg in September (northern hemisphere) and repeat every 2–3 months. (Note: Some dogs on this drug develop sterile abscesses and granulomas at the injection site.)
b. *Outdoor pet ferrets exposed to natural photo-periods* should get the same as above though only during the long days (i.e. April though September, northern hemisphere).

In the meantime, nothing is a cure for this disease but several drugs may help. It is considered by the above USA sources that FADC management in the long term should be tailored to the individual affected ferret. Sound diagnostic approach, examination and evaluation with ongoing 3-monthly check-ups should be routine

Unusual American ferret cases

The female

The possibility of leaving ovarian material when only partially de-sexing a jill ferret can be a nightmare when the jill unexpectedly comes into heat or, more alarming, goes into post-oestrous anaemia. Some authors have described two de-sexed jill ferrets with FADC, where adrenal cell tissue tumours have been found located caudolaterally to the caudal pole of the right kidney at the site of the ovarian pedicle.[32] The adrenal glands themselves were normal. Finding of ectopic adrenal tissues in the perirenal fat associated with the renal artery or in other sites close to the adrenal gland have been reported before. The findings with the two female ferrets promoted an investigation to see if the steroidogenic tumours originated from gonadal or adrenal cells.

Ferret A was 2 years old having shown progressive alopecia over the preceding 6 months. It had been sterilized plus musk gland removal at 6 months of age. It was a house companion to another sterilized ferret, which was of normal coat. When examined Ferret A was bright and alert with a normal size vulva. It showed sparse hair on the dorsal region of the body and some signs of pruritic scratching. Other clinical features were normal and blood samples were taken for sex hormone study. An exploratory operation found a $3 \times 2 \times 2$ cm cystic mass caudolateral to the caudal pole of the right kidney. The adrenal glands were normal and the mass was excised for histology. The result was good with the ferret coat growing back in 2 months. The ferret was seen to be normal 2 years after surgery.

Ferret B, a 5-year-old jill, had a similar history. It was a laboratory ferret at MIT. At 3 years of age it had been sterilized to stop persistent oestrus. It had begun to show alopecia but with a small vulva in the months before euthanasia. Again a cystic mass $5 \times 3 \times 3$ cm was found caudolateral to the right kidney.

Steroid assay: (Table 14.3). With ferret A, adrenal gland disease was suspected pretreatment from alopecia signs and from the steroid levels, e.g. high 17-hydroxyprogesterone and androstenedione, though the oestradiol was practically normal. After surgery for the tumour mass the high steroids decreased, initiating hair growth to a new coat. The hormone values for ferret B were similar to those of ferret A before its operation, high androstenedione and 17-hydroxyprogesterone concentrations, but oestradiol levels close to normal.

Histological features: defined mixed tumours of ectopic adrenal origin affecting the two jills from an ovarian pedicle source, a case of ectopic adrenal gland material and cause of the alopecia. The anatomical site of the ovarian pedicle of two previously sterilized ferrets were the sites of sex steroid producing tumours.

The authors noted the hypothesis of adrenal tumours frequently producing sex hormones because embryonic gonadal cells lie alongside adrenal cells in the embryonic neural crest and they are more likely to migrate together to the adrenal site in the embryo and develop in later life in the ferret.

Table 14.3 Sex steroid assay results: ferrets A and B compared with reference range

Can use serum or plasma for assay	Oestradiol (pmol/L)	17-hydroxyprogesterone (pmol/L)	Androstenedione (pmol/L)
Ferret A			
Before surgery	185	13	219
After surgery	140	0.39	20.5
Ferret B	133	9.04	257
Reference range[a] for neutered ferret	3–180	0–0.8	0.15

[a]Clinical Endocrinology Service, University of Tennessee. (Courtesy of Cathy Johnson-Delaney, 2005.)

Immunohistochemical analysis, using a polyclonal antibody against Mullerian-inhibiting substance (MIS) (anti-Mullerian hormone used in human cancer work) failed to be specific as it labelled not only ferret granulosa and thecal cells but also normal adrenal cortical cells. This may be due to different cross-reactivity of steroids and/or other molecules in ferret endocrine and epithelial cells. Ferrets may produce MIS-like substances in a broader array of cell and tissue types than do humans. The authors advised further studies of this type of condition.

The male

As stated previously, in the USA, male ferrets have suffered from adrenal disease as well as females. Rich has recorded a 6-year-old male ferret with FADC, which had the unusual presentation of a mammary teat swelling (Fig. 14.15) (G. Rich, pers. comm. 2005).

Mammary involvement with FADC in the male had been recorded earlier in a 5-year-old white castrate ferret, which had back alopecia for 3 months before examination at Oklahoma State University.[33] The ferret body was abnormally large and there were two bilateral large lobulated mammary masses. (A similar mass had been removed previously and considered a mammary gland hyperplasia.) On examination, the ferret was otherwise normal; it had been fed on pelleted ferret food but not vaccinated. Similarly, a BCC and serum chemistry were normal but its urine had a low SG of 1.013 and contained pus. Radiography showed a moderate abdominal peritoneal effusion. The ferret was operated on under isoflurane anaesthesia and a 4 × 3 × 3 cm firm smooth mass was found at the cranial aspect of the right kidney and on histology found to be an adrenocortical carcinoma. Mammary masses of about 1 × 1 × 1 cm from the right gland and 3 × 1.5 × 1 cm from the left, were removed and found to be of multilobular hyperplastic nodules which contained much duct tissue. *Note*: an increase in ductular tissue in the jill is the normal physiological feature of early pregnancy and is due to a response of the mammary gland to progesterone. Thus the ferret had a concurrent mammary hyperplasia associated with the effects of FADC. It died 7 days after surgery (see Fig. 14.20 below, for another case).

This condition in the male ferret may parallel mammary hyperplasia and hyperprogesteronism in cats. It has been seen that a sterilized cat with dermatitis and eosinophilic granuloma, under treatment with progesterone develops hyperplasia of the mammary glands.[34]

An interesting skin condition involving a castrated adult ferret with adrenal disease has been reported.[35] A BEW had severe bilateral symmetrical alopecia over the trunk region. It had severe pruritus for 6 months and showed a complex of cutaneous erythematous macules over the head and extremities. It was suggested by the owner that the red blotches had been there before the ferret had developed alopecia. On examination the ferret appeared to be in good health otherwise, the blood picture was normal, but a cranial mass was found in the abdomen on palpation. Surgery found a 5 × 3 cm neoplasm involving the right adrenal gland. The tumour mass was found to be a poorly differentiated adrenal cortical cell mass that invaded the whole gland, an adrenocortical carcinoma. Skin sample biopsies were taken of the erythematous areas and the condition of cutaneous telangiectasia was diagnosed; this is an uncommon veterinary finding seen only in dogs as a clinical feature of canine Cushing's disease. The ferret regained its coat by 6 weeks post operation but the cutaneous telangiectasia had not changed in character or distribution. The lesions were not determined as malignant.

Adrenal cortical carcinoma with myxoid differentiation was established in 15 ferrets, from sample biopsy and necropsy submissions in the period 1992–2002.[36] The mean age of ferrets checked was 5.38 years (range 3–9). Some ferrets showed metastases to the liver, lungs and lymph nodes. The tumours were thus highly malignant. This is a variant of the adrenocortical carcinoma showing prominent mucin production and interpreted as myxoid differentiation. Histology and immunohistochemical methods were used in the survey. A common feature of ferret adrenocortical carcinoma is the presence of spindle cells associated with the neoplastic cells. The cells were shown by immunohistochemical staining to express smooth muscle action and may arise either from smooth muscle cells within or beneath the capsule or are a morphologically distinct type of cells. There is debate as to whether the cell population is

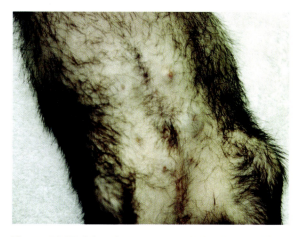

Figure 14.15 Adrenal tumour case sterilized male with male teat swelling. (Courtesy of G. Rich.)

CHAPTER FOURTEEN
Endocrine diseases

neoplastic, metaplastic or just reactive hyperplasia but the spindle cells can invade adjacent adrenal tissue and have been mistaken for leiosarcomas. The report features this myxoid variant of adrenal cortical carcinomas which is not present in cases of adrenocortical nodular hyperplasia or adenoma. Interestingly, the neoplastic adrenocortical cells with myxoid features are shown by histopathological, histological and immunohistopathological tests to be remarkably similar to myxoid adrenocortical carcinoma in humans.

The risk of ferret adrenal disease complex (FADC) outside the USA

In one Canadian practice, FADC and insulinoma top the list of commonly seen ferret conditions with many ferrets derived from the USA Marshall Farms line (Vannevel, Ontario, pers. comm. 2005). Even back in 1989, a pet ferret was recorded at the University of Montreal with hyperadrenocorticism in association with an adrenocortical adenoma.[20] The case was a 4-year-old spayed house jill which interestingly had a 2 cm area of alopecia on the dorsal aspect of the neck which had been present for 8 months. A 1.5 × 2.5 cm area of alopecia had occurred on the tail base and lumbosacral region. The ferret weighed 650 g and was active, being fed on commercial dry cat food. No conclusions could be reached on the diagnosis of the alopecia but when seen 4 weeks later the ferret had polyuria and polydipsia. It had lost weight in spite of good diet and the alopecia had increased.

Blood checks showed normal BCC and serum biochemical factors and again the ferret went home. However, 2 weeks later the ferret had a synoptic episode and was seen in emergency weak and anorexic. It weighed only 500 g, being dehydrated and was given s.c. fluids. It underwent an exploratory operation under halothane anaesthesia and an enlarged left adrenal gland (6 × 7 × 9 mm) was removed. After intensive care with fluids and a course of ampicillin and dexamethasone the ferret regained its appetite, the polyuria and polydipsia stopped, and the hair grew back in a few weeks. The ferret was last seen well at 7 months post-operation. It would be interesting to wonder if the synoptic episode, possibly based on low blood glucose, might also have been a forerunner of a later insulinoma because of the cat food diet?

Ferrets are popular in the UK, Europe, Russia and Australia and were so in New Zealand until the recent ban. It seems that only Russia is free of FADC. Ferrets are house pets in Japan and FADC, insulinoma and lymphoma, which were quite unknown to residents, have followed on in imported ferrets.

Adrenal gland neoplasia has been seen now in Australia and one case is said to have developed later with possible concurrent insulinoma. Cases occur in European countries now. In the Netherlands a survey reported 50 ferrets with hyperadrenocorticism out of a collection of 1267 animals.[37] Spain has recorded cases of FADC, insulinoma and heart disease from imported ferrets (Montesinos, pers. comm. 2005). Large numbers of *Helicobacter*-type diseases also occur (Ch. 9).

In the Netherlands, a 1500 g 5-year-old sterilized male, Macho, became sexual in spring, mounting other ferrets, etc.[38] The owner had noted the trend for several springs but it usually wore off. In this case, he started to leave urine marks as if marking territory (Ch. 5). Then he was found apparently paralysed lying in the 'flattening' position (Ch. 7). The position implies the ferret is in pain and in this case, he had a swollen bladder which could only be relieved by emergency catheterization (Ch. 20). An enlarged prostate was suspected and underlying FADC was confirmed by an operation to remove an enlarged right adrenal gland. Macho went home a few days later as the prostate had decreased in size and he could urinate normally. Once back with his fellow pet ferrets he had lost his sexually aggressive tendencies.

In Japan, a 1300 g 4½-year-old castrated male ferret, Mystic, was presented with dysuria and abdominal swelling. Radiographs and ultrasound revealed images of a multicystic structure in the caudal abdomen. Prostatomegaly from possible FADC was suspected and CT images revealed the urinary bladder was displaced with both ureters identified by contrast medium in the upper right side of the CT scan (Figs 14.16–14.20). Surgery was carried out with debulking of the cystic structures and omentalization for the enlarged prostate plus a left side adrenalectomy was performed. As a result, the enlarged prostate began to shrink and the ferret was

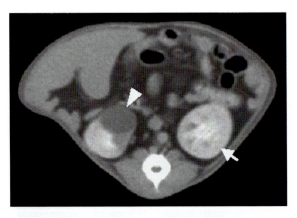

Figure 14.16 CT kidney cyst. The enhanced CT image after administration of contrast medium shows the renal cyst (arrowhead) within the enhanced right kidney. Compare the left kidney (arrow), which is enhanced entirely. (Courtesy of Yasutsugu Miwa.)

Insulinoma

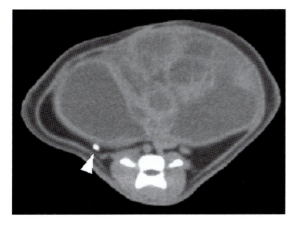

Figure 14.17 Enhanced CT image showing multi-cystic structures and enhanced right ureter (arrowhead) but the bladder could not be detected. (Courtesy of Yasutsugu Miwa.)

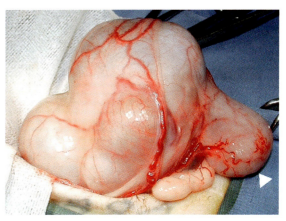

Figure 14.19 Operation site showing appearance of the cystic structures and urinary bladder (arrowhead). (Courtesy of Yasutsugu Miwa.)

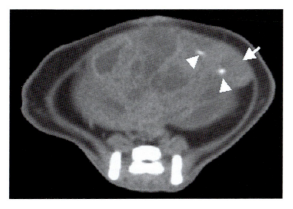

Figure 14.18 Enhanced CT image showing multicystic structures and enhanced both ureters (arrowheads). Dislocated urinary bladder (arrow) was detected. (Courtesy of Yasutsugu Miwa.)

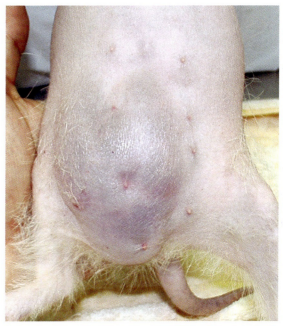

Figure 14.20 BEW ferret jill showing mammary duct ectasia. (Courtesy of Yasutsugu Miwa.)

able to urinate freely (Yasutsugu Miwa, pers. comm. 2005).

Incidentally, Miwa has seen a case of mammary duct ectasia in pet ferret. A 5-year-old BEW sterilized jill was presented because of systemic alopecia of over 2 years duration plus unilateral caudal mammary swelling of the right side. Clinical examination including measurements for serum hormone levels suggested FADC. On surgery, the swollen left side adrenal gland was removed along with the affected mammary gland. A diagnosis of adrenocortical carcinoma and mammary gland ectasia (hyperplasia, not neoplastic) was made. The pre-operation hormone value for estradiol was 1513.0 pmol/l and for 17-hydroxyprogesterone was 8.8 nmol/l; by 3 days post-operation, these had fallen to 37 nmol/l and 6.4 nmol/l, respectively. It was theorized that long exposure of the mammary gland to sex hormone levels led to the mammary hyperplasia, which is shown in Figure 14.20.

The ferret died some months after the operation but no post mortem was possible. It was considered that the large right adrenal tumour, which had not been removed because of its size and association with the vena cava, was the cause.

Conclusion

Ferret adrenal disease complex is a slow progressive disease, which may allow the ferret to live 2–3 years without treatment, but the owner would have to accept a bald ferret. It can also be complicated by insulinoma. *Note* that untreated ferrets with adrenal gland disease need to have special skin ointments and be kept on soft beds.[1] Such a ferret would benefit from anabolic steroids and vitamin additions to the diet, but would be in a sorry state for any ferret.

The prevention of adrenal disease should be the aim in preference to having sick ferrets on constant medication. The reason why FADC occurs is debatable and the spectrum of possible aetiology of neoplasia of all kinds is discussed at the end of this chapter after considering the other ferret killer, insulinoma.

Insulinoma

Whereas adrenal disease can be 'cured' to some extent by surgery, insulinoma cannot and becomes an ongoing medical problem for ferrets and a source of extreme anxiety and stress for their owners. I have not diagnosed it in Australia. Insulinoma can be seen in ferrets of both sexes 3 years and over and which, like most ferrets in the USA, are usually indoor pets. In the USA Ehrhart et al. have recorded 20 cases of pancreatic beta cell tumours over the period 1986–1994.[39] The median age of ferrets with pancreatic disease was 5 years (range 2–6 years). The median time of clinical signs before diagnosis was 90.5 days. A total of 17 ferrets had an exploratory operation and 12 of the 20 had multiple pancreatic nodes seen on surgery or post mortem.

Endocrine dysfunction procedure

Small tumours of the pancreatic islet cells will produce a high blood level of insulin, which can be fatal in producing hypoglycaemia due to blood sugar depression. The normal feedback mechanism to stabilize the animal with low blood sugar is compromised by the neoplastic cells. In early cases, there is some stimulation of liver glucogenesis and glycogenolysis but the process becomes inefficient. The blood sugar depletion affects the brain function, with deprivation of energy source and resulting dullness and confusion.[40]

Clinical signs

There are signs of hind leg weakness, the ferret appears to stare blankly into space and shows excessive drooling. In early attacks, there may be some body response with increased blood glucose and the owner may not recognize the condition. The body will initially respond to the crisis and a mechanism for increasing blood glucose occurs, so that the animal may recover quickly without the owner realizing it has had an attack.[3] Salivation with possible pawing at the mouth may indicate nausea. The disease may start as brief attacks but is progressive, with longer periods of weakness and lethargy until the ferret goes into seizures, coma and death. Due to the intermittent nature of the disease, the ferret might be presented after some time with just a history of weight loss but having a normal appetite. The ataxia and weakness in the hindquarters must be differentiated from trauma, toxicity or other metabolic disease.

Diagnosis

The clinical signs of a ferret with staring eyes and blank expression, if caught at the right time, could be a presumptive diagnosis. However, blood tests for fasting low blood sugar are the basis for insulinoma confirmation. To do this, the ferret is fasted no longer than 4–6 hours before the blood test, as in the event of insulinoma being active the animal could go into hypoglycaemic shock.[1] Multiple blood samples may be required to confirm a ferret's hypoglycaemic state. American authorities were so concerned about ferret insulinoma that they advised blood sampling annually for all ferrets over 3 years old, which is the seemingly geriatric age for their ferrets (Brown, pers. comm. 1998).

The normal fasting blood glucose level is 90–120 mg/dL (5–6.7 mmol/L). Non-fasting may go has high as 200 mg/dL (11.1 mmol/L). A diagnosis of insulinoma is given as being below 70 mg/dL (3.9 mmol/L) or lower; an insulin level above 20 U/mL in the presence of hypoglycaemia strengthens the diagnosis. In contrast to the ferret, the dog with insulinoma has normal serum insulin values and this is the case for ferrets where the blood glucose level is 65 mg/dL (4.7 mmol/L) or lower.[1] Insulin values for the normal ferret are given in Table 14.4. A study by Marini et al. of six ferrets, aged 5.5–7.5 years, (one male, five female), with functional islet tumours showed mean glucose and insulin concentrations of 44 mg/dL (2.4 mmol/L) and 58 µU/mL, respectively.[41]

The glucose/insulin, insulin/glucose and amended insulin/glucose ratios are helpful in distinguishing diseased animals. The amended insulin/glucose ratio is most used and gives less false positives in insulinoma-free ferrets than when done in similar conditions in dogs.[40] A formula has been given by one author[42] for the diagnosis of insulinoma in ferrets using the following ratios: glucose:insulin <2.5 mg/μU, insulin:glucose >0.3 μU/mg and amended insulin:glucose ratio >30. The amended insulin:glucose ratio is calculated as follows:

$$\frac{\text{Insulin in } \mu U/mL \times 100}{\text{Glucose (mg/dL)} - 30}$$

It may be necessary to multitest the suspect ferret if blood levels remain high in the insulinoma condition, and at different times of day to detect low blood glucose levels. The glucose manometers used for human diabetic cases are useful and easy to use for blood checks.[40] Blood checks should be read immediately to prevent any interference of the test by artefacts. A complete blood test is useful with possible findings of elevated ALT and AST indicating liver involvement, with lipidosis secondary to dangerously low blood sugar concentrations. There is a possibility of rare metastasis in the liver, which can be indicated by these raised values. The blood picture can be of leukocytosis, neutrophilia and monocytosis.[40] Unlike in FADC, ultrasonography is not applicable to insulinoma nodule diagnosis, as the nodules are too small. It can, however, be useful for prognosis with regard to pancreatic metastasis.[43] One author is of the opinion that the best prognosis in this disease results with the lack of metastasis in younger ferrets with a very early diagnosis. However, the outlook is not good in older ferrets where metastasis may have occurred and the diagnosis is too late (Brown, pers. comm. 1998).

A reference table of values for tests of the endocrine system in ferrets is given in Table 14.4.

Treatment

Melo and Caplan have discussed surgical and medical treatment of insulinoma in the dog, cat and ferret together.[44] They put a median age for the disease at 5 years with a range from 2–7 years.

The treatment of choice is surgery, followed by a stabilization of the ferret metabolism with attention to diet. Surgery can involve removing the pancreatic nodules or a partial pancreatectomy.[1] (Bennett and Pye in Chapter 18 describe the surgical procedure in detail.) In a retrospective study of 66 ferret insulinoma cases, the partial pancreatectomy on a first surgery proved the value of this technique.[45] During any insulinoma surgery, the abdomen should be fully explored and liver/spleen biopsies performed to screen for other cancers and possible metastasis. The histology of removed pancreatic tissue can show hyperplasia, adenoma or adenocarcinoma and insulin immunoreactivity is marked.[43]

It is considered that surgery will never cure the problem, as by the time the ferret is admitted for treatment or an operation, microscopic metastatic invasion of other parts of the pancreas and other organs has occurred (Brown, pers. comm. 1998). Only a complete pancreatectomy would be disease-limiting but has not been attempted. Surgery for removal of the visible white masses of insulinoma really only buys time so that the disease can be delayed or depressed by further medication.

Postoperative treatment of insulinoma cases

This requires the ferret to be fasted for 24 hours, during which 2.5% or 5% dextrose in half-strength saline at 10% of the body weight can be given via an i.v. catheter.

Table 14.4 Values for the endocrine system of the domestic ferret

Hormone	Sex	Values
Insulin[a]		35–250 pmol/L (4.9–34.8 μU/mL)
Cortisol[b] (nmol/L)		25.9–235 (mean ± SEM: 73.8 ± 7)
Thyroxine[c] (μg/dL)	Hob	1.01–8.29 (mean 4.5)
	Jill	0.71–2.54 (mean 1.38))
Tri-iodothyronine[c] (ng/mL)	Hob	0.45–0.78 (mean 0.61)
	Jill	0.29–0.73 (mean 0.53)
Mean thyroxine[d] (μg/dL)	Hob	2.53 at 0 h, 3.37 at 2 h, 3.97 at 4 h, 3.45 at 6 h

[a]Reference range for Vet Research Laboratories, Farmingdale, NY. [b]Administration of cosyntropin, 1 μg/kg intramuscularly, generally caused a 3–4-fold increase in plasma cortisol concentration in this study.[5] [c]Data from Garibaldi BA, Pequet-Goad ME, Fox JG. Serum thyroxine (T_4) and tri-iodothyronine (T_3) radioimmunoassay values in the normal ferret. Lab Anim Sci 1987; 37:544–547. [d]Mean T_4 at baseline (0 h) and 2, 4 and 6 h after administration of thyroid-stimulating hormone, 1 IU i.v. ($n = 8$ intact males). Data from Heard DJ, Collins B, Chen DL, Coniglario J. Thyroid and adrenal function tests in adult male ferrets. Am J Vet Res 1990; 51:32–35. (After Quesenberry, 1997, with permission.)[40]

CHAPTER FOURTEEN
Endocrine diseases

The 2.5% dextrose can be given s.c. if catheterization is not done.[1] After the initial 24-hour period, the patient is given a bland strained meat baby food at small frequent meals. Fluid therapy is continued s.c. but using Ringer's solution, which should also have been given pre-op, at 10% of the body weight for a further 24 hours. The ferret is returned to normal food 3 days after the operation. *Note* that according to one author, the patient should require no further medication and can be sent home. If, however, the ferret has been on corticosteroids before surgery they should be continued but gradually reduced in dose over the following weeks.[1]

In addition, the ferret, showing glucosuria and elevated blood glucose, might experience a short diabetic condition. This is caused by the atrophy of the pancreatic beta cells and it is advisable to check urine glucose twice daily for 2–3 days after the operation. The situation usually resolves itself in a few days. The fasting blood glucose should be rechecked 2 weeks after the operation. It is advisable to do 1–2-monthly blood checks from then on, as insulinoma is known to have a high incidence of recurrence. There could be multiple surgeries on insulinoma tumours that recur but this is not recommended as it is stressful to the ferret. Instead, emphasis should be on control of the condition with diet and medication (S. Brown, pers. comm. 1998). (At the present time in Australia, few ferret owners would go to the expense of multiple operations for insulinoma.)

If the insulinoma tumours have spread to the liver, it is more difficult to control the blood sugar and thus it is important to do a liver biopsy at the time of surgery. In the USA recently cases of CNS signs such as those affecting the pupil are more prevalent. It is not clear whether the problems are separate, such as diseases of the optic nerve/brain or related to low glucose levels in insulinoma cases affecting brain function locally or generally. Diet is important for maintenance of the insulinoma-prone American ferret. The possibility that American processed ferret foods are a factor in insulinoma is still not clear. The nutritional approach to avoiding insulinoma in American ferrets has been commented on.[46] The author maintains that excessive carbohydrate intake stimulates excessive insulin production from the pancreas leading to hyperplasia and finally neoplasia. It is proposed that pathogenesis involves the additive stimulation of pancreatic cells by the potent insulin secretogogues. These are amino acids (protein) and simple carbohydrates (simple sugars and rapidly-digested starches) while free fatty acids (FFAs) may play a similar stimulatory role. The author compares the feeding of high carbohydrates in the cat species where insulinoma is rare to that of feeding high carbohydrate to ferrets where insulinoma is common, at least in the USA. Cats are said to be prone to the 'opposite' endocrinopathy when fed on high carbohydrate, i.e. diabetes mellitus (DM).

It could be argued that cats on a high carbohydrate diet initially reach a hyperinsulinaemic state, followed by an eventual exhaustion atrophy of the islet cells, resulting in DM. On the other hand, the islet cells of the ferret seem to 'rise to the challenge' and become hyperplastic rather than atrophic. It may also be that American ferrets have a genetic predisposition to insulinoma formation (see Ch. 4). Comparisons with cat endocrinology are discussed later in aetiology of ferret neoplasia conditions.

In other countries like Australia, New Zealand and UK, ferrets are traditionally fed on fresh meat and do not appear candidates for insulinoma. They do not usually get 'sweet treats' as their American counterparts frequently do, or perhaps did, as there is some change of thought on their diet. Ferrets suffering insulinoma or postoperatively should be fed frequent meals of a high-quality animal protein.[46] Foods can include high quality cat or ferret foods but not canine or feline semi-moist diets. It is considered by one author that cat food is not high enough in fats.[1] Brown suggests cooked meat or egg and also cottage cheese or yogurt to stimulate anorexic patients. Foods that can be given per os by syringe include baby foods and Hill's Prescription Diet a/d.

Increased fibre is of no use for ferrets in a diabetic condition, unlike in humans, as ferrets cannot digest fibre easily and it might add to the problem (S. Brown, pers. comm. 1998). Sweet treats like honey or any sugar-based foods are forbidden as they can cause an insulin increase and dangerous hypoglycaemia. Honey should be available however to help in any subsequent hypoglycaemic attack in the insulinoma patient. In that event, honey/water mixture is rubbed onto the ferret's gums and it should recover within 30 minutes.

The ferret is given a protein meal directly to forestall another acute hypoglycaemic event.[1] Suggestions of helpful supplementation for insulinoma cases include use of brewers' yeast, which contains chromium, the glucose tolerance factor (GTF), which has helped to stabilize blood glucose in humans. Thus, the insulinoma ferret needs constant monitoring. Dieting will not control the signs of insulinoma when the fasting blood sugar falls below 50 mg/dL. Prednisolone medication, to stimulate hepatic function, is given at a dose rate of 0.25 mg/kg body weight orally and used for the life of the ferret.

The prednisolone is given 2–3 times daily initially and can be increased to 2 or even 4 mg/kg body weight. The lowest dose to keep the ferret stable should be aimed for and kept to.[1] The insulin blocking agent, diazoxide, can be used in severe insulinoma cases in combination with prednisolone at a dose rate of 10–20 mg/kg body weight by mouth. It was an expensive drug at $85 per 1 oz. bottle in 1998 but at the time of writing this had risen to $120 per 1 oz bottle.[47]

To wean insulinoma ferrets off prednisone, ferret breeder Mary van Dahm of Ferret Advice & Information

Resource, Chicago (FAIR) came up with an insulinoma elixir. She has used the mixture on dozens of sick ferrets. (The recipe is in the Appendix.) She asserts that as insulinoma beta cell cancers can be pinhead size, surgery is not always a viable option. Long-term use of steroids instead may agitate the adrenal glands causing thinning of the skin, fat deposit formation in the abdomen and a loss of muscle mass. The elixir formula helps stabilize the blood sugars, so that little or no prednisone needs to be used, giving the ferret a long drug-free period if surgery is not an option. The sick ferret should get regular vet check-ups. She also asserts that having used the mixture on ferrets with insulinoma over several years (Chicago Ferret Shelter), she has noticed that ferrets with concurrent cancers, such as lymphosarcoma, also benefit from the mixture. *Note*: even juvenile lymphoma ferrets, where death is usually within 3 months after contraction, were living 2–3 years of quality life on the elixir. Other ferrets that were started on the mixture while still healthy (usually at 2 years of age) stayed cancer-free for longer periods of time than their counterparts that did not receive the mixture. She maintains that ~50% of all USA ferrets start developing cancer by 3 years of age. Most ferrets on the elixir, however, did not show signs till 5–6 years of age. She cannot say which particular elements of the mixture are most effective; the shark cartilage is presumed to have anti-cancer properties; the milk thistle is presumed to help the liver and kidneys and the echinacea is said to promote overall good health.

Medical treatment

If surgery is not an option due to expense or the insulinoma being microscopic as discussed above, medical methods can be tried.[47] Symptomatic therapy is aimed at controlling the hyopglycaemia but will not affect or stop the development of pancreatic cancer. Glucocorticoids are used, with prednisone the drug of choice as it was in post-surgical recovery (see above). The drug dosage for ferrets is given at 0.5–2 mg/kg p.o. q. 12 h. An oral suspension is available as Pediapred (Celltech Pharmaceuticals, Inc. Rochester, NY). Ferrets with clinical signs or postoperative patients can take this treatment. *Note*: prednisone can be compounded for higher concentrations. However, prednisone formulations with alcohol will cause sedative effects which would confuse the clinical signs.

It is seen that over time, the actions of prednisone will become less effective even at increased dosage but it is considered side-effects with ferrets are rare. This view is not shared by others, e.g. Mary van Dahm of FAIR. As suggested by Brown, the minimum dose should be found and adhered to and other authors have quoted the use of 1 mg/kg p.o. q. 12 h to control clinical signs.[47] The rationale for the use of corticosteroids in general small animal practice is discussed by Sturgess.[48]

The action of the prednisone is to inhibit glucose uptake by peripheral tissues, by increasing both liver gluconeogenesis and peripheral glucose concentration in the blood. Glucocorticoids also have the action of inhibiting insulin binding to the insulin receptors and thus inhibiting the postreceptor effects of insulin.

Diazoxide (Proglycem, Baker Norton Pharmaceuticals, Miami, FL) has been used with prednisone as seen above or alone. The drug is a non-diuretic benzothiadiazide which can decrease insulin secretion, promote gluconeogenesis and stop the cellular uptake of glucose. It is available in liquid or tablet form. Dosage is from 5 mg/kg p.o. b.i.d. up to a maximum of 30 mg/kg. *Note*: Brown used 10–20 mg/kg b.i.d. As with prednisolone, this drug can be increased, from the starting low dose, according to the severity of symptoms.

Side-effects include anorexia, vomiting and diarrhoea which can be avoided to a great extent by putting the drug in food.[44] Once a ferret becomes anorexic, further treatment is not helpful. Side-effects also include the possibility of hyperglycaemia, bone marrow suppression and sodium retention, so the drug should be used with caution in ferrets with cardiomyopathies. As diazoxide is degenerated in the liver, if the ferret has liver dysfunction, then lower doses of the drug may cause side-effects.

Additional drugs have been indicated.[47] These have been used in either dogs or humans with pancreatic endocrine tumours. Somatostatin (Sandostatin, Novartis Corporation, NY) is only used for small numbers of clinical cases, with doubtful results. It has a synthetic long-acting analogue called Octreotide which inhibits the synthesis and secretion of insulin from the normal and neoplastic pancreas beta cells. (*Note*: it also inhibits glycogen, secretin, gastrin and motilin.) The drug is used in dogs with insulinoma and shows no adverse reactions. This drug has not been evaluated in ferrets though a dose has been calculated at 1–2 µg/kg s.c., b.i.d.–t.i.d.[44]

Specific chemotherapy for ferret neoplastic pancreas cells is limited and drug toxicity to the ferret is a factor. Streptozotocin (Zanosar, Pharmacia & Upjohn Co, Kalamazoo, MI) is okay for use in humans and dogs. In dogs, the use of the drug with an agent for diuresis is recommended. The drug is potentially nephrotoxic and would not be safe for ferrets. Doxorubicin (Adriamycin, Pharmacia Inc, Kalamazoo, MI) is effective in humans and thought to be safe and well-tolerated for ferret use. A dose of 1 mg/kg i.v. q. 21 days has been calculated but has not yet (2004) been used for ferrets.

Prognosis

American insulinoma cases can live for 1–3 years after diagnosis on a combination of surgery, dietary control and constant medication. It requires a lot of owner patience

CHAPTER FOURTEEN
Endocrine diseases

Dutch clinical example

In September 1996, a 3-year-old sable sterilized ferret, Siegfret, had a left adrenal gland tumour removed. He recovered from the surgery but became listless a month later, sleeping longer and a poor appetite. He had to be carried back from walks. This continued and in January 1997, his glucose level was found to be low, using diabetic blood check apparatus. Siegfret was fed on high protein food, Totally Ferret, as routine and through his illness. The local vet suspected insuloma and advised an operation once Siegfret was strong enough. However, he became weaker and his owner insisted on an operation in February 1997. He had been put on prednisolone at 2.5 mg/day with decreasing dosage. The exploratory operation revealed only three cancer foci and postoperatively he was put on prednisolone again. He was mostly an outpatient and the owner checked his blood. His health improved on medication and much tender loving care!

A few months later he was on 0.625 mg prednisolone per day and eating but only with owner encouragement. In June 1997, Siegfret had a second pancreatic cancer operation by a different vet for more suspect cancer foci. None were seen on the gland surface but a partial pancreatectomy was done on a suspect area. This is considered to improve survival rates.[44] He was hospitalized for 3 days but not put on prednisolone. His owner took him home but a day later the ferret nearly went into a coma with low blood sugar and had to be put back on prednisolone and kept on it. His health gradually improved on medication. His owner was not encouraged by the results and declined any more operations on Siegfret.

In November 1997, he developed cataracts when his sugar level was too low. His owner had heard of ferrets getting glaucoma after cataracts. She contacted Dr Susan Brown, who advised medication with additionally diazoxide (dose rate 10–20 mg/kg p.o. once daily with prednisolone). The suggested prednisolone or prednisone dose from Brown was 0.30 mg/kg b.i.d. increasing it by 0.10 mg/kg with each dose as needed to control signs. She advised not having any sugar in the diet except for emergency situations. His owner's routine was then to give medicines twice daily and Siegfret's condition became more stable between January and April of 1998. An hour after the prednisolone he was given the diazoxide. In December 1997, Siegfret started to lose hair from the tail and the condition covered the rest of the body, indicating right adrenal gland involvement. In the last few months before he died (in August 1998) some hair grew back. The drug dosage was increased at the end of April 1998 and again in June, July and August. In July 1998, Brown suggested prednisolone up to 1.5 mg/kg b.i.d.

Thus, increases of 0.05 mg (0.05 mL) were given daily until the effective dose was reached, as shown in Table 14.5. The maximum given in 1 day was 1.5 mL a.m. and 1.5 mL p.m.

Brown suggested the diazoxide be increased to 1 mL b.i.d. if needed but warned that if Siegfret got more sluggish it should be withdrawn as the drug is a hypotensive, decreasing blood pressure. A fasting blood sugar needed to be done periodically. She also advised that Siegfret should be taken off the diazoxide sometimes for a few days to see if prednisolone was the more indicated drug. Siegfret was only awake for a short time, 5–10 min, 6–7 times a day. When he ate, the owner gave him a small bit of butter, which he liked; it is recommended for sick insuloma patients.

Siegfret had a seizure in March 1998 and again in June. He lost coordination, falling to his side all the time. In July, he was so bad with one seizure he could not walk all day. In late August, he was very sick and could not keep medicine down. He went into a light coma and died. Siegfret's illness is given in some detail for the purpose of making those like myself, who have never yet diagnosed the condition, aware of what a terrible disease it is for ferrets. It is a twin tragedy when it is combined with adrenal gland neoplasia. It shows that any treatment is long and requires a devoted owner to carry it out. (This ferret case example is put in to emphasize prevention is better than treatment.)

Siegfret's weight varied throughout the illness. In November and December 1996 and January 1997 it was around 550 g (19.4 oz) and at the end of February, increased to 600 g (21.1 oz). In April 1997, his weight went to 800 g (28.2 oz). At the time of the second surgery, he was over 700 g (24.7 oz). The surgery made him feel worse and his weight decreased to 500 g (17.6 oz). His weight increased very slowly and at the end of 1997, it was more than 650 g (22.9 oz) and stayed between 650 g (22.9 oz) and 700 g (24.7 oz) until he died.

Sabine van Voorne, World Ferret Union, The Netherlands, pers. comm. 1998.

Table 14.5 Prednisolone dosages for insulinoma

Day	Morning dose (mL)	Evening dose (mL)
1	0.80	0.75
2	0.80	0.80
3	0.85	0.80

and love to work on the sick ferret. The Malik insulinoma case seen in 1998 had an immediate partial pancreatectomy for the neoplastic nodes and as of 5 July 1999 was known to be maintaining itself without treatment until contact with owner was lost.

Note that ferrets with insulinoma should be fed good quality protein and fat. It would be best to make up a formula of raw beef liver, raw eggs and goats' milk or whole cow's milk in equal parts and mixed in the blender to a creamy consistency. More milk can be added and the mixture frozen in ice cube trays and used daily once thawed, e.g. one cube (5–10 mL) per day. This is a good rich protein/fat mixture for sick ferrets (S. Brown, pers. comm. 1998).

Other pancreatic tumour cases

In the USA, 57 cases of pancreatic islet cell tumours were registered from various veterinary hospitals between 1986 and 1994.[49] Interestingly, the ferret ages ranged from 2 to 7 years, with a median of 5 years. In all cases lethargy, weakness and collapse were major signs and hypoglycaemia and hyperinsulinaemia were present. These features indicate insulinoma but differentials were put as neoplasia, diffuse liver disease, starvation, sepsis, hypoadrenocorticism and even sample mishandling. Ptyalism was observed in 10 ferrets and could be a sign of nausea.

Note: splenic enlargement was common in 40 ferrets but it is also possible with old ferrets as seen in Chapter 13. Conditions such as lymphosarcoma, haemangioma, haemangiosarcoma, Aleutian disease, cardiac disease, fungal disease and hyperadrenocorticism can show splenomegaly. Surgery was done in 50 cases, consisting of a nodulectomy where possible, or partial pancreatectomy for multiple nodes. Ultrasound was used to pinpoint pancreatic nodules in 5 of 23 ferrets.[49] In many cases of insulinoma the reacting cells may be small or microscopic, making them unresponsive to ultrasound.[47] During surgery, a single pancreatic nodule was found in 13 ferrets, while 37 showed multiple nodules.[49] In 34 ferrets there was primary pancreatic carcinoma alone while in 23 ferrets a complication of carcinoma and either hyperplasia or adenoma was present. Metastasis had occurred to the regional lymph nodes or liver in four cases. Three ferrets had just medical treatment and four were untreated.

In 26 ferrets hypoglycaemia was still present post-surgery and required lifelong treatment on prednisone or diazoxide or both as seen in the Sabine van Voorne case illustrated before. *Note*: 16 ferrets acquired a hypoglycaemia from 1–2 years post-surgery and only seven ferrets were normal post-operation. The treated group was given a poor prognosis on the whole due to the malignant nature of the tumours.

Disturbing cases seen in the UK

In the UK, similar experiences of FADC and insulinoma occurred.

In April 2000, a 3½-year-old 760 g jill developed a swollen vulva.[50] It had been spayed at 6 months of age and had a tail amputation for chondrosarcoma in 1999 (Ch. 13). The swollen vulva had been noticed for 2 days and the jill had been observed mounting and excessively grooming cage mates and itself. *Note*: the ferret was housed in a garden shed and also came indoors. The group of nine ferrets were fed on a commercial complete ferret food (Ch. 4).

After examination, radiology, ultrasound and blood sampling (under isoflurane G/A) initial findings were negative for adrenal gland or abdominal abnormalities. The ferret's weight had dropped to 720 g. Blood sampling was from the cranial vena cava (Chs 7, 20). The ferret underwent a midline exploratory operation 4 days later as it weighed 706 g (starved prior to surgery). Interestingly, the right adrenal gland was much larger than the left. Usually the left adrenal gland is the first affected in FADC. Careful dissection removed the right adrenal gland which proved to be a cortical adenoma. *Note*: as the right adrenal gland is dangerously close to the caudal vena cava, delicate surgery is required. Cryosurgery can be used[27] but was not available in this case. At 7 days postoperatively, the ferret weighed 7900 g and the wound had healed by 15 days; 26 days postoperatively, the vulval swelling went down but the ferret dropped some weight, down to 777 g. The jill ferret had not shown classic alopecia of the body hair but hair did regrow on the operation site. Eight months after the initial inspection, the ferret was healthy but at 720 g. Seen in May 2001, the ferret weighed 730 g but was having occasional fitting attacks with collapse, salivation and disorientation. It presented a classic 'glassy-eyed' look. The owner felt that feeding the ferret helped the situation.

The ferret was prepared by starving for blood collection from the jugular vein under isoflurane anaesthesia. It weighed 715 g. The blood sugar picture showed 2–4 mmol/L (normal is 5–6.7 mmol/L resting value). A diagnosis of insulinoma is given at 3.9 mmol/L.

On recovery from the G/A the ferret had 10 mL of 0.9% sodium chloride and 5% glucose s.c., then was fed a liquid meal of Hill's a/d diet. Therapy for insulinoma was started with prednisolone at 0.5 mg b.i.d. The insulinoma symptoms were overcome. On checking in August 2001, the ferret weighed 740 g. It did have 'wobbles' but no salivation, and was eating. The prednisolone was increased to 1 mg/day but by December 2001, collapsing episodes had occurred with salivation and characteristic pawing at the mouth. The weight dropped to 685 g.

CHAPTER FOURTEEN

Endocrine diseases

Diazoxide was started as in the Sabine van Voorne case at a dose rate of 12.5 mg/day. However, the ferret went into a severe hypoglycaemic attack the next day with collapse, screaming, disorientation and ptyalism. Using isoflurane anaesthesia again, a blood sample was obtained. Fluids were giving using an intraosseous infusion catheter (Ch. 20). Fluids used were 40% dextrose solution and 0.5 mL dexamethasone, initially followed by 0.5 mL dexamethasone, 10 mL, 0.9% NaCl but given over an 8-hour period. The blood glucose was at 6.7 mmol/L later in the evening. The ferret continued with the collapsing episodes and 1 mg diazepam was tried as an anticonvulsant without effect. The next day, the symptoms were the same and again the ferret was anaesthetized for another blood sample. The blood glucose was at 20.4 mmol/L. From a blood calcium check at 1.8 mmol/L (Vet Test: Idex normal range 1.99–2.94 mmol/L) a problem of hypocalcaemia was suspected. Again using the intraosseous technique, the ferret was given 70 mg calcium borogluconate and 0.9 mg magnesium hypophosphite 5%.

Another exploratory laparotomy under G/A and the pancreas was examined with a mass being found on the tip of the right lobe. Suspecting neoplasia a partial pancreatectomy was performed (Ch. 18) and the histology of the mass confirmed two islet cell tumours. The ferret was again hospitalized after the operation with a repeat of fluids by interosseous infusion. The ferret stabilized regarding the fits but was left vacant and disorientated, so reluctantly, with knowledge of the neoplasia effects, euthanasia was decided upon as the kindest thing. This case shows the difficulty in treating the combination of adrenal disease and insulinoma.

Surgery for both types of neoplasia is required with follow-up medication, which, if there is a good response from the patient, is long term and difficult for both ferret and owner.

It is well known that the male ferret is not immune to FADC or insulinoma in the USA. The presence of pancreatic neoplasia has been recorded in two male polecat-coloured ferrets in the UK.[51] The first 6-year-old 1000 g ferret had been sterilized at 7 months and presented with weight loss of 2 weeks, periodic weakness and hind leg ataxia. It was an indoor ferret fed on Ferrets' Choice 3 times daily. The ferret was in good body condition so a jugular blood sample was taken for analysis and fluids given s.c.

The blood results suggested dehydration with a mildly elevated urea, albumin and PCV. The WBC count was normal. Using a Vet test machine (Idex labs), other elevated values were:

- alkaline phosphatase: 273 U/L (range 0–134)
- aspartate aminotransferase: 180 U/L (range 47–99)
- alanine aminotransferase: 479 U/L (range 0–60).

As is characteristic in insulinoma, the blood glucose was low: 3.21 mmol/L (range 4.07–7.70).

An exploratory operation under 5% isoflurane anaesthesia found a solitary 5 mm diameter nodular white mass in the right pancreatic lobe, which was excised and formalinized for histology. The other internal organs were normal. The ferret was given fluid therapy plus s.c. injection of 10 mg enrofloxacin and 0.02 mg buprenorphine postoperatively.

The blood glucose rose in 12 hours to 4.79 mmol/L, with the patient beginning to eat. The ferret was kept in for a further 24 hours and then sent home with oral enrofloxacin, 10 mg s.i.d. over 5 days. It was fed every 4 hours and the owners were advised about treating any hypoglycaemic crisis with honey by mouth. The histology confirmed a carcinoma of the pancreas. The ferret improved over the next fortnight with weight increase to 1100 g and the blood sugar at 28 days and 38 days stood at 10.32 and 5.21 mmol/L, respectively. However, the ferret went into a collapse and shock at 139 days with a blood sugar finding of 2.2 mmol/L and was put to sleep.

The second ferret, also a 6-year-old, had been desexed at 9 months of age and was collapsed when examined. It was a non-worker and was fed on Whiskas feline diet twice daily. It was hypothermic (rectal temp 36.5°C) and non-responsive to stimuli. At 1200 g the body weight was good. On palpation, cranial and caudal abdominal masses were found. Externally the ferret had no lesions. Being in an emergency situation the ferret was given s.c. injections of 20 mL of compound sodium lactate (Isolec) and 1 mg dexamethasone (Dexadreson). It was wrapped in towels and put on a heat mat in a warm room. It made a complete recovery in 20 minutes.

Ultrasound was used to demonstrate a single multicavitated mass of some 4.5 × 3.5 cm in the cranial abdomen. An object in the caudal abdomen was possibly fat. Under 5% isoflurane anaesthesia, the cranial mass was found to be a cholangiocellular adenoma (biliary cyst adenoma) as part of the left medial liver lobe. The tumour was removed by resection of the liver lobe (Ch. 18). *Note* the pancreas was not examined at the time. Postoperatively, the ferret was given by s.c. injection 6 mg carprofen (Rimadyl) and 12 mg enrofloxacin. It was hospitalized and sent home the next day with 12 mg enrofloxacin b.i.d.

The ferret was seen 5 weeks later again collapsed. Injections s.c. of 2 mg of dexamethasone and 40 mL of 4% sodium chloride (Vetivex 18) were immediately given. It recovered in 15 minutes. A jugular blood sample was taken and tested using a QBC analyzer and Vet test machine. Significantly, the blood glucose was low at 1.5 mmol/L (range 6.5–7.9 mmol/L) while other parameters were normal. In addition, an insulin assay

(Axiom Labs) was done where insulin stood at 1023.97 pmol/L (range 35.04–250.15 pmol/L).

Because of the ferret's age, conservative oral medical treatment was suggested, using 1.2 mg prednisolone (Prednicare) s.i.d. and 24 mg amoxicillin/clavulanate (Synulox palatable drops) b.i.d. In this case, the prednisone helped for 4 weeks but then the ferret deteriorated and was euthanized. Post mortem results showed a 5×5 mm nodular mass in the pancreas, which histologically was an islet cell adenoma.

Drs Lloyd and Lewis concluded that working UK and European ferrets are less likely to be victims of endocrine neoplasia but inbreeding in American ferrets, for the more docile pet ferret, has led to their predisposition to this type of disease. Dr Eatwell comments in her conclusion that neoplasia in the UK is not being picked up, because fewer ferrets are taken to vets and fewer are sterilized.[50] The UK ferret population appears to have sterilizations at an older age where necessary and a larger gene pool results in an greater heterozygosity. I wonder if these two cases might not have occurred if the two ferrets had been fed on a natural diet (Ch. 4)?

In my opinion, circumstances indicate a healthy ferret population with regards to adrenal disease and insulinoma risk in the UK. If notice is taken of the points in the following aetiology of the two deadly diseases, perhaps the UK will not go the way of the USA ferrets with further cases. Treating ferrets for adrenal disease and insulinoma can be a costly business for the client. The diazoxide would cost the client around $28 for a month's course.[47]

Aetiology of general and endocrine neoplasia in the ferret

Controversy surrounds the reason why ferrets get lymphoma and other neoplasms including FADC and pancreatic cancers. As mentioned in Chapter 13, the list of possibilities includes genetics, early sterilization and effect of photo-period, diet and possible viral factors. The list could grow to include chemicals stimulating cancers and other environmental causes.

Genetics

The possibility of genetic predisposition to neoplasia in ferrets is still under investigation. It can be reasoned that the genetic make-up of a confined colony of animals will in time, produce genetic defects. However, the incidence might be small. Marshall Farms, New York had some birth defects such as spina bifida but the ferrets were destroyed at birth (J. Bell, pers. comm. 1993). They also had cranial abnormalities, bent necks and cleft palates. (Ch. 5). Few congenital cataracts occur and the jills concerned are eliminated from the ferret colony. However, as there may be a need to carry out foster-mothering of kittens, from large litters to small, the actual mother of the defective kittens sometimes cannot be traced when the defect is noticed. Considering that Marshall Farms were dealing with colonies of ferrets around 27 000 strong, the percentage of any genetic defect is considered very low (J. Bell, pers. comm. 1993). Marshall Farms have exported ferrets to Canada and Japan so any genetic traits will be in their ferrets. In the USA, some small-scale ferret breeders have maintained that their ferret lines are not prone to FADC but the claim has not yet been scientifically proved.[23]

General ferret genetics is discussed in Chapter 5, while the genetic possibility of ferret cataracts is considered in Chapter 12. Australia has had no new ferret blood lines since 1920. Ferrets kept for laboratory purposes (human influenza trials) are not available to the common stock. Ferrets are bred by private breeders and inbreeding must have occurred. Ferrets can be exchanged between Australian states and I have had jills from Canberra. Ferrets have also been exported to the USA. Some Western Australian ferrets exported in 1998 have shown one deaf kitten and two kittens with supernumerary incisors as possible genetic faults (Amy Flemming, pers. comm. 1999). New Zealand has commercial organizations, Southland Ferrets and Mystic Ferrets, which can export but not receive stock. NZ feral ferrets were used as a gene pool by ferreters and these ferrets were easily tamed. The UK and continental Europe have a greater gene pool than Australia. The genetic diversity within any pet ferret gene pool with no possibility of new blood is of concern.

Tumour suppression genes

In many species, including mice, rabbits, dogs and man, the continuing stimulation of a secretory gland to cause it to progress from hyperplasia to possible adenoma and then adenocarcinoma is controlled by tumour suppression genes.[5] These genes are considered 'guardians of the genome' with the job of preventing normal cells mutating to cancerous cells, e.g. the well-documented p53 gene is a primary tumour suppressor and is highly conserved across species. Two human genes of this type are the multiple endocrine neoplasia genes (MEN); MEN 1 and MEN 2. C J-D and Michelle Hawkins (MH) have recognized the phenomenon in man running parallel to the condition in the pet ferret. They are

CHAPTER FOURTEEN
Endocrine diseases

seeking the homologue of the MEN gene in ferrets. MEN is a dominant gene whereas the p53 suppressor gene is recessive. In humans who have suffered traumatic pre-pubertal neutering by some accident, it has been found that in later life, over 40 years of age, the victims get thyroid neoplasia, lymphoma, mast cell tumours or adrenal neoplasia i.e. the development of tumours is guaranteed with an early neutering accident. Setting that feedback loop at puberty is important to delay the phenotype being expressed. How does this place the ferret condition of neoplasia etc. after early sterilization? They hope to find out by trials. C J-D and MH have a ferret at UC Davis with thyroid carcinoma, adrenal gland and islet cell disease to work on. They consider they will find a homologue MEN and a possible defective p53 suppressor gene too and that early spay/neuter guarantees the phenotype will be expressed. Their model fits too perfectly for any other mechanism to explain why some ferrets have a very high tumour rate, evidently higher than a p53 knockout mouse (C J-D, pers. comm. 2005).

The tumour suppressor genes would protect ferrets. It is considered the underlying reason for the prevalence of FADC, islet cell and mast cell tumours and lymphoma in relatively high numbers could be due to the absence of such genes in the Mustelidae.

Early sterilization

The ferret can be sterilized when it is immature like any other animal, but the effects on the juvenile endocrine system may be such that neoplastic conditions can occur in later life. With Marshall Farms, their ferrets are sterilized at 6 weeks of age to standardize the animal for laboratory work. The operation would prevent POA in the jill and reduce body odour in males and females. Sterilization at such an early age, when the endocrine system has not fully developed, is a controversial point in relation to any future hormonal problems. Many private breeders in the USA objected to the early sterilization of ferrets and get their own stock done at 5–6 months of age (A. Flemming, pers. comm. 1998). Ferrets that should have a life expectancy of 6–10 years seem to get cancer problems sooner if they have been sterilized young. Early-sterilized ferrets, as has been stated, in the USA are considered almost geriatric at 3 years of age! It is interesting that prominent American veterinarians I know do not get their own pet ferrets sterilized very young and I would never do it.

Note: Schoemaker et al. carried out a survey in the Netherlands to try and correlate the age of neutering and age of hyperadrenocorticism in ferrets.[37] (The authors point out that the early sterilization theory is supported by studies done on certain mice strains, which developed nodular adrenocortical hyperplasia or even adrenocortical tumours after early sterilization.) The survey was done on 1274 pet ferrets and an associated retrospective study with 43 known FADC cases. Of the total ferrets surveyed, 694 were male and 580 female. Median age of the ferrets surveyed was 3 years. Median age of sterilized ferrets was 3 years. Most ferrets (91% males, 82% females) had been sterilized between 6–18 months, 108 ferrets after 18 months of age. *Note*: 87 ferrets (25 males and 62 females) were unsterilized; of these 27 ferrets (11 males, 16 females) were over 18 months old. The median age of the unsterilized ferrets was 1 year.

Of the 1274 ferrets surveyed, there were seven cases of hyperadrenocorticism (confirmed by adrenalectomy). There were seven other suspects, on which the owners disallowed further study. Thus, cases of hyperadrenocorticism in the survey population were confirmed as 0.55%. Of a total of 50 ferrets with hyperadrenocorticism (seven from the survey, 43 from university and private practice sources), 46 had been confirmed by histology of adrenal glands post-adrenalectomy. In the other four ferrets, macroscopic appearance of the adrenal glands and improvement after adrenalectomy were taken as diagnosis confirmation.

Note: all 50 ferrets (33 male, 17 female) had been sterilized. However, a significant difference in frequency distribution by sex between ferrets with FADC and ferrets in study without FADC was not detected.

The median age at time of sterilization was 1 year (range 0.5–6 years) and the median age of diagnosis of FADC was 5 years (range 1–10 years) (Fig. 14.21). Also, the median time between sterilization and diagnosis of FADC was 3.5 years (range 0.5–8 years). In addition, there was a good correlation between age at sterilization and age at diagnosis.

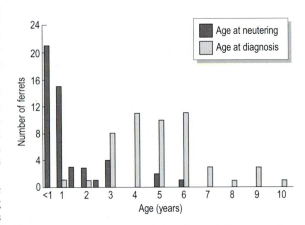

Figure 14.21 Age at neutering and age at diagnosis of hyperadrenocorticism in 50 ferrets. (Courtesy of Hanneke Moorman.)

Conclusions of this study: The authors were aware that in one USA practice, 20–25% of client's ferrets had FADC, but did not consider this a reliable outline of disease prevalence as it was a selected population.[52] They consider their results in the Dutch study of a prevalence of 0.55% FADC high for pet ferrets in that country. They are sure the correlation between age of sterilization and time of FADC indicates that neutering may influence the disease to occur in pet ferrets. *Note*: FADC has been reported in seven unsterilized ferrets. It is surmised that other cases in entire ferrets may not have been noticed as a common sign of the disease is sexual behaviour. In an entire ferret it would not be regarded as abnormal, in the sterilized ferret it is immediately noticeable.

The ratio of male to female ferrets with FADC has been described as 50:50.[52] In the Dutch survey it was considered that, although two thirds of FADC cases were male, the differences in male/female proportions with ferrets with and without FADC was not significant. Thus, gender did not affect the issue. The authors put the mean age of ferrets developing FADC as 5.1 years, being older than the recorded age of 3.4 years in USA ferrets.[53] The interval between age of sterilization and presence of disease in Dutch ferrets is put at 3.5 years, similar to USA ferret studies.[10] (This assumes USA ferrets were sterilized at 6 weeks of age.) The actual reason for the time gap has not been explained by any studies.

Schoemaker et al. have also examined the morphology of the pituitary gland in ferrets with hyperadrenocortism.[53] The latter can be caused by pituitary tumours in other animals but what function the pituitary has in the hyperadrenocortism in ferrets is not known. The histology of four healthy ferrets, intact or neutered, alongside 10 neutered ferrets with hyperadrenocortism, was studied using immunohistochemistry of various hormones. The authors concluded that an initially high concentration of gonadotrophins in the pituitary pars intermedia resulting from castration, may initiate hyperactivity of the adrenal cortex. The 10 hyperadrenocortical ferrets had unilateral or bilateral changes in their adrenal glands and only two of this group had pituitary tumours. Low incidence of the latter tumours and the low density of gonadotropin-positive cells in non-affected pituitary tissues studied suggested that the persistent hyperadrenocortism was not dependent on persistent gonadotropic stimulation.

The embryonic disturbance of early sterilization has been explained at the beginning of this chapter. *Note* the use of leuprolide (Lupron Depot) as a GnRH antagonist shown in the medical control of FADC supports the idea that neutering does play a role in the development of the deadly disease (C J-D, pers. comm. 2005).

Note: There is now a European law that all pets need to be fully grown before they can be sterilized, also removal of scent glands, shortening of ears or tails and extraction of teeth or nails are all banned, unless there is a medical indication (Stephanie Baas, The Netherlands, pers. comm. 2005).

D. Kemmerer-Contrell (pers. comm. 2005) relates that she de-sexed a group of 100 English ferrets, which had been imported to Florida at 6 months of age. She maintains that the group did get adrenal disease in later life and wonders if the alteration of photo-period might be a bigger factor in FADC. With the ferrets being exported from a northern temperate zone to Florida, a subtropical zone, there might well have been photo-period increases by keeping ferrets in an indoor semi-constant light environment of the average American home. (This could indicate a similar situation in Australia?)

Effect of photo-period manipulation

The normal effect of day length is described in Chapter 5 in relation to the ferret sexual cycle and for commercial interests this can be interfered with by manipulating the light and dark periods in large ferret breeding sheds so that the breeding of jills can be extended. No clinical signs of ovarian/adrenal dysfunction, should it occur, are observed as there is usually no alopecia in the jills while they are constantly mated. Alopecia could occur, however, with some jills coming into heat while still nursing a litter and they are immediately taken out of heat with GnRH or HCG injection. Forced continuous breeding in jills by light manipulation may have other destructive effects on the hormone system. Ferrets living indoors under continuous long light periods may be at risk of adrenal disease as shown earlier. It is established that in the USA where ferrets are mostly kept indoors as pets they are liable to be FADC cases, whereas ferrets kept outside as pets or working animals in Australia and elsewhere are not. Why?

With my jill ferret, Josie, described earlier as an FADC case, the aetiology of one ferret in a colony of several, caused me a lot of worry. At the time, my ferrets were living under the following conditions:

- In the garden and ferretarium overnight (Ch. 3)
- At the veterinary hospital daily and under artificial light on dull days
- Travelled in the car to and from the veterinary hospital, subject to daylight and from light glare at night
- Played in the garden in the evening under artificial light. (I now half-light the garden when I go out to the ferrets and I use a torch!)
- Came into the house in the evening and played in artificial light.

Does this combination of environments endanger the ferret to a light-stimulated adrenal gland neoplasia? It

CHAPTER FOURTEEN
Endocrine diseases

can be seen that having one's own pet ferret affected can cause almost paranoid awareness of the ferrets being subjected to extended photo-periods! On the other hand, Josie was a ferret sterilized at 6 months of age and fed only fresh meat. However, as a rescue ferret, no genetic history was known.

Ferrets coming indoors now sleep in a closed sleeping box with a small entry hole to the exercise and feeding area. There is an 8×2 cm airhole near the top at one end and the box is dark inside and the room light mostly kept off (see Fig. 3.27). Ferrets staying in all day should have the exercise run covered to keep it dark. Overnight, the cover can be removed or left with the far end uncovered so that urine vapour is not trapped.

In the veterinary hospital, possible problems became apparent. In winter and on dull days the lights in the kennels had been left on all day so we had a situation similar to laboratory and/or refuge home ferrets. A notice went up to make sure lights were turned off when ferrets were in the kennels during the day. Summer evenings are short here so artificial lighting in the garden is used all the year round and of course indoors. In my case, only one out of eight ferrets developed adrenal disease, but she was the 'in-house' pet ferret.

Some practical points on keeping ferrets indoors would be to simply cover the usual ferret cage with a blanket most of the day! This might be unsightly but if ferrets are not being played with indoors, they go to sleep. They quickly awake when roused. The equivalent of a 'bolthole', a closed sleeping box with perhaps a pipe entrance cutting down light entry placed in one corner of a room would suffice along with only putting lights on when necessary.

With my hob, Pip (who died recently, 2006, see Ch. 12), I tended to feed and play with him in the evening and then, as a trial, let him sleep in the indoor sleeping box overnight with a blanket over the exercise run (see Fig. 3.27). He slept overnight with no problems. In the morning, I gave him a run in the garden and then he came back into the indoor sleeping box to be fed and sleep with the blanket again over the exercise run. After lunch, I found him asleep and transferred him to the bolthole in ferretarium 2. Other than going to the toilet in the aboveground scats tray, he settled in to sleep again. He never wandered the garden in the afternoon. He stirred at about 6.30 p.m. and came to be let into the house. He was then fed and played with as before. He could be placed in the indoor box with the blanket in place while we had dinner.

The point is, he maintained an evening/morning activity. If I had had the time, I could have kept him awake all day playing etc. indoors or out. But, would I have put him at risk in an extended photo-period? I think so. Though the pet ferret would play till tired and hungry, a morning/evening short period of play suffices. The effects of manipulation of the photo-period are summarized by Finkler.[23]

Female ferrets, jills: Jills will not come into heat if light periods are kept at 8–12 hours. They can be induced into first oestrus at $4\frac{1}{2}$ months by increasing light to 16–18 hours. A 14-hour light period prolongs the breeding season. A successful breeding programme needs fluctuating photo-periods, short followed by long to induce breeding behaviour and a consistent photo-period during the actual breeding season. For adequate lactation, jills with litters should get 14 hours of light.

Male ferrets, hobs: Spermatogenesis is known to be influenced by the photo-period. Thus with 14-hour photo-periods, hobs are potent for 9 months and then will 'cycle off'. Hob libido may decrease with decreasing photo-periods to 8 hours.

The circadian rhythms are not fully understood in animals, but photo-periods probably play an important role. It is interesting that prolactin in mink is affected by photo-periods; production increases in the spring as day length increases, the opposite of melatonin production.

On the whole, ferrets in countries outside the USA/Canada are kept outside in natural light periods. The trend of ferret gardens and ferretariums, which are floodlit in the evening, has only recently begun (Ch. 3). Lighting can be reduced or not left on unless humans are in the garden. Ferret owners are beginning to keep ferrets indoors as pets and there are reports of more than one ferret breeder having the breeding stock in one room of the house. A lot of this is for convenience of handling, less disturbance of jills and perhaps for security reasons. Ferret owners should be advised about the possibility of problems with extended photo-periods.

Working ferrets and ferrets with breeding stock outside in cages, yards, courts or sheds have shown no cases of FADC in sterilized ferrets. No other jill ferret of mine kept indoors since Josie has shown any signs of FADC, so perhaps there is another undiscovered causative factor.

A study was carried out in 1997 into the effect of light cycles on ferret endocrinology.[54] The researcher, Mary van Dahm, realized that most mustelids are nocturnal by nature and active in the early morning or late evening. Many spend their daytime underground to avoid the heat as my ferrets do. Thus, the actual time spent in the light is just a few hours a day and that light is often subdued. Mary took 30 ferrets aged 3 months–$2\frac{1}{2}$ years old and separated them into six groups. Each group contained one or two ferrets that were early neuters, two ferrets that had been sterilized at 6–9 months and one or two ferrets that were de-sexed between $1\frac{1}{2}$–$2\frac{1}{2}$ years of age. The late-altered ferrets (juveniles and adults) had all come to the Chicago shelter from different parts of the country as random pickups. They had been bred in the areas of Illinois, Indiana, Iowa, Kentucky, Michigan, Missouri and Wisconsin, and possibly had different bloodlines. The ferrets were set up so that they had a sleeping room with no windows at all in it and the lights were only turned on for a short time to clean the cages. Three playrooms were set up so that each shift could have about 12 hours of playtime (see Fig. 3.34).

The ferrets received light for short periods, about 6 hours each day. A combination of indirect fluorescent light and indirect light from a north window were used. The ferrets were fed on Totally Ferret, IAMS kitten food, Eukanuba cat food, Marshall's ferret food and an occasional scoop of Purina Kitten Chow or Cat Chow as a treat. They were 'free-fed' and were also offered a 'ferret gruel' daily, which was a mixture of whatever crumbs were left in the bowls from the day before moistened with water and a dash of Ferretone brewers' yeast, pro-balance and shark cartilage added.

Results at almost 5 years after the start of the programme were promising. Only three ferrets showed signs of possible adrenal disease with thinning hair of the tail. One of these ferrets had a very low blood glucose level and was put on a high dose of prednisolone, which may have aggravated the adrenal glands. The other two ferrets had somewhat bad coats to begin with, even as juveniles, so there is a possibility that their hair loss was an hereditary condition and not FADC causing their poor coats, as they were sisters. Six ferrets experienced non-adrenal related surgeries such as hairballs, cystic spleens and insulinoma. The ferret ages ranged from $3\frac{1}{2}$ to $6\frac{1}{2}$ years at the time of surgeries. They all had completely normal adrenal glands and two were sterilized early. Some ferrets died during the period of 5 years under observation: one from lymphoma, two cardiomyopathy, one nephritis and one hepatic disease. These ferrets were not ones sterilized at 6 weeks of age and had healthy adrenal glands observed at post mortem.

In 2001, the rest of the group were going strong, although a few had developed insulinoma. The oldest ferret was $7\frac{1}{2}$ years old and had been sterilized later than 6 weeks of age, while the older jill was $6\frac{1}{2}$ years old and was an early alter. Mary felt from the results that light does play an important part in FADC. In the usual run of events in ferret shelters, increased light photo-periods would be caused by the volunteers working with the ferrets.

In an update for 2005, Mary asserted that most of the ferrets never developed adrenal disease. They died fully furred or else lost their hair during the last month or two of their lives. Those that did develop FADC late in life and after 5–6 years of age, as was evident from post mortems, did not show clinical symptoms. One old ferret remaining is 10 years old, his hair is thin on his tail and he has a possible mass in his abdomen. (It would be interesting to see how many insulinoma cases would have occurred if the ferrets were being fed fresh meaty bones rather than commercial diets (Ch. 4)).

Problems of ferret diet

There is a possibility that ferrets fed on processed foods are more likely to suffer neoplasia than those fed on a natural diet. Ferrets are obligate carnivores and their diet should reflect that (Ch. 4). Ferrets do not digest fibre well at levels over 2%.[55] Is the fibre content of commercial food really guaranteed? Could pelleted dry foods with high fibre content cause gastric irritation and possible induced cancer of the bowel? It is noticeable that ferrets on dry foods have been the ones that show a 'green diarrhoea' and provoke ideas of a possible viral infection.

Finkler compared the endocrinology situation in the ferret with research on diabetes mellitus in the cat.[46] To understand the hyperinsulinaemic state in the ferret, one can consider the common form of feline diabetes being Type 2. (Type 1 is more common in dogs.) The exact aetiology of Type 2 diabetes is unknown but the decreased insulin secretion (in response to glucose load) and insulin resistance are two characteristics. With insulin resistance, more insulin is required for the same glucose-lowering effect, compared with the normal state. Thus, hyperinsulinaemia is an early feature of Type 2 diabetes in humans and occurs in cats with impaired glucose tolerance. It suggests that insulin resistance may be the initial defect in the pathogenesis of Type 2 diabetes.

Pancreatic islet amyloid deposition is associated with type 2 diabetes in felines. The amyloid fibrils are synthesized from islet amyloid polypeptide (IAPP), which is produced in pancreatic beta cells, stored in secretory granules along with insulin, and co-secreted with insulin. The role of IAPP in Type 2 diabetes is thought to be multifactorial, through its direct effect on amyloid deposition, inhibition of insulin secretion, and induction of insulin resistance. Dogs with insulinoma do not develop amyloid deposits and neither do ferrets.

Abnormal beta cell function is another proposed mechanism of feline diabetes development. With this, increased insulin levels indicate beta cell dysfunction with hypersecretion of insulin being the primary abnormality, inducing insulin resistance and finally beta cell exhaustion. Thus, feeding cats a diet rich in highly digestible carbohydrates may induce a lifelong high insulin demand, contributing to beta cell failure. So perhaps ferret beta cells, following chronic stimulation by a high carbohydrate diet, undergo compensatory hyperplasia, rather than becoming exhausted, as in cats.

CHAPTER FOURTEEN
Endocrine diseases

Finkler hypothesizes that ferrets develop a hyperinsulinaemic ('pre-insulinoma') state due to the additive effects of various insulin secretogogues in their diet. This theory presumes that insulin secretion in the ferret is similar to that of the cat, dog, human and rodent. Glucose and other simple carbohydrates are strong stimuli and elicit a rapid and marked rise in insulin levels.[46] Insulin release in cats is biphasic as with other species; glucose increases first phase secretion more than amino acids do. However, amino acids are equally potent in the second phase release of insulin. Glucose and amino acids are additive stimuli in cats. Free fatty acids (FFAs) can induce insulin secretion. *Note* the additive effects of simple sugars, amino acids and FFAs may indeed cause a chronic hyperinsulinaemic state in ferrets, thus triggering beta cell hyperplasia in response to the increased demand for insulin.

Could it be that a high glucose load is more detrimental to cats (and ferrets?) than dogs or humans? Cats are less efficient in lowering blood glucose levels as they have a minimal glucokinase activity compared to dogs and humans. Cats rely on the enzyme hexokinase to help clear glucose from the blood, which acts more slowly than glucokinase. Glucose tolerance tests in dogs take 60 minutes, while cats take 2 hours.

Note: the consumption of the cat's natural diet, protein, generates a smaller and delayed insulin response compared with carbohydrate consumption. Ferrets are obligate carnivores like cats and if on a high carbohydrate diet they would be undergoing a prolonged stimulatory effect for insulin secretion. (Their lack of enzymes for galactose assimilation and cataracts is described in Ch. 12.)

The conclusion drawn from the foregoing is that both cats and ferrets have evolved to consume a high protein diet and both in some way can be affected by high carbohydrate foods. *Note*: proteins do not stimulate secretion of as much insulin as carbohydrates so the latter can be dangerous, especially to ferrets. Finkler suggests there is no published data as yet on glucose tolerance curves, glucokinase levels or hexokinase levels in ferrets.

With insulinoma in mind, he suggests it is possible to feed some canned kitten foods which have high protein but low carbohydrate. Most USA ferret owners prefer to feed dry kibble such as Purina DM Feline Formula™ (for diabetic cats) which however has 15% carbohydrate to the 8% in tinned food. There is also Hill's Prescription Diet m/d (for obesity in cats) which has 15.5% carbohydrate but an alarming 5.5% fibre compared with Purina fibre content at 3.6%. Remember that no feline diets have been tested on ferrets over the long term (Ch. 4).

Ferrets require a low carbohydrate diet, as they can obtain energy better from fat. It may need to be asked whether we are really improving, in the long term, the lives of the ferret by departing from the 'natural' fresh meat diet? (This has also been raised regarding feeding dogs and cats, in Ch. 4.) One has only to look at a well-maintained group of working ferrets, in Australia at least, kept on a natural meat diet, from rabbit to kangaroo, to see that they are active and healthy. Rarely are cancers recorded, if at all, in ferrets over 7 years. The working ferrets' teeth that I have examined have been cleaner than even my own ferrets! Many American veterinarians are considering fresh meat diets as an improvement for ferret health. One major hospital has switched to feeding their ferrets on a carnivore diet made up of organs, muscle and bone and the ferrets are reported to be looking good on it. It is evidently hoped that the diet will also decrease the incidence of eosinophilic gastroenteritis (EG), which is apparently on the increase in American pet ferrets (Ch. 9).

The virus factor

The possibility of specific ferret viruses was considered in the study of retrovirus.[56] It is known that lymphoma and leukaemia in humans, cattle, cats and other species can be caused by transmissible viruses. The features of lymphoma in ferrets, for instance, suggest an infectious cause but the actual viral agent has not yet been identified. With regard to adrenal disease, present work with cats has produced an experimental vaccine that blocks the LH receptors on cat ovaries.[57] The immunized cats did not come into normal heat as the LH receptor antibodies produced inhibited the binding of the LH and chorionic gonadotropin to ovarian receptors. Other work has been done on non-primates.[20] In different species of mammals, the LH appears to be similar, so presumably are the LH receptors. Thus there is a cross species non-specificity of antibodies against the LH receptors. It is considered that as LH receptors occur in ferret adrenal gland cancers a possible LH receptor vaccine could be produced for this species.

Diabetes mellitus

This is a condition that can arise after surgery for pancreatic beta cell tumours but is otherwise very rare in ferrets.[3] It has been recorded in older ferrets in association with insulinoma, but occurred in young and old ferrets, which were fed on a diet high in refined sugar some years ago. The condition was regulated with insulin (Brown, pers. comm. 1999).

The affected ferret shows typical symptoms with polydipsia and polyuria in association with a persistently high blood sugar (>300 mg/L) and low blood insulin. If there is a history of a recent pancreatic surgery, the hyperglycaemia is highly likely to return to normal

1–2 weeks after surgery. If tests other than blood glucose levels are required, the glucogen and insulin concentrations can be tested.

Treatment is similar to that in other animals, with one author suggesting the use of neutral protamine Hagedorn (NPH) insulin with a proposed starting dose of 0.1 units per ferret.[3] For satisfactory results the aim is to obtain negative ketone levels in the urine and only a small amount of urine glucose, as it is considered difficult to really regulate diabetic ferrets. The prognosis can be good with post-surgery cases if caught early enough but grave with any other cases, which are fortunately rare.

Pseudohypoparathyroidism

Seizures in ferrets can be alarming and of various causes. In the normal animal, the parathyroid regulates blood calcium and phosphorus levels. Pseudohypoparathyroidism (PHP) recorded by Wilson et al.[58] is an hereditary condition caused by a lack of response to high circulating concentrations of parathyroid hormone, rather than deficiency as in normal hypoparathyroidism (HP) i.e. low serum calcium, high serum phosphate and high serum parathyroid concentrations.

A fully-vaccinated 17-month-old 1460 g sterilized male had intermittent seizures over 6 hours before examination. It lived with three other normal house ferrets but was congenitally deaf. The ferrets were on heartworm prevention and a balanced ferret chow. The sick ferret was lethargic between seizures but alert and eating and otherwise normal. Clinically, the ferret had no fever and respiratory and heart rates were normal out of seizures. Blood tests showed low glucose at 65 mg/dL (normal range 94–207 mg/dL). (Possible causes of seizures are given in Table A.8.)

Overnight treatment included i.v. prednisolone sodium succinate at 20 mg/kg and 70 mL/kg of electrolyte with 5% dextrose i.v. The ferret was still lethargic the next day and urine and blood samples taken were normal except for low serum total calcium at 4.9 mg/dL (normal range 8.0–10.5 mg/dL) and high serum phosphate at 8.4 mg/dL (normal range 6.4–7.0 mg/dL) and a high urine SG of 1.042.

Calcium carbonate supplementation at 50 mg. p.o. q. 12 h made no difference, even when increased to 100 mg. The parathyroid hormone (PTH) was checked on day 6 and found to be extremely high at 75.3 pmol/L (healthy control ferret 13 pmol/L).

Serum ionized calcium was low at 0.54 mmol/L (control ferret was 13 pmol/L). The serum total calcium had decreased to 4.6 mg/dL while the serum phosphorus had risen to 9.1 mg/dL. The ferret did improve over 9 days from days 6–15 but then the serum calcium increased to only 5.3 mg/dL while the phosphorus increased to 9.4 mg/dL.

Note: there is no published data on serum magnesium in ferrets. The sick ferret had a concentration of 2.1 mg/dL but four healthy ferrets of the same age, as controls, showed magnesium levels 2.1–2.9 mg/dL.

A dramatic improvement occurred when using vitamin D analogue, dihydrotachysterol (DHT) given at 0.02 mg/kg p.o. q. 24 h. The demeanour and appetite were good from days 15–25. Then there was a relapse to inappetence and lethargy. On day 27, the blood and serum tests were found to be within normal limits (phosphorus 5.7 mg/dL, calcium 10.1 mg/dL). There were no radiological signs related to DHT overuse and the latter was discontinued. The calcium carbonate was continued at 100 mg twice daily. The ferret regained stability between days 27–43 when the serum calcium was found low at 6.3 mg/dL and phosphorus at 6.0 mg/dL. The serum vitamin D was slightly high at 144 nmol/L (control ferret 128 nmol/L). DHT was given again at a longer dosing interval of 0.02 mg/kg p.o. q. 7 days plus the calcium. The ferret was stable over the next 9 months and an eye examination found no evidence of cataract or other abnormalities (Ch. 12). At 345 days, serum calcium was normal at 9.9 mg/dL with serum phosphorus at a low 5.6 mg/dL. Serum PTH was well down at 2.3 pmol/L. There was some concern over the serum urea nitrogen at 47 mg/dL (normal range 12–43 mg/dL), creatinine at 1.0 mg/dL (normal range 0.2–0.6 mg/dL) and urine SG was low, 1.018 with concern about possible nephrocalcinosis with reduced renal function.

However, trying to change the treatment to a different calcium salt brought the clinical signs back again. In fact the calcium:phosphorus ratio on day 354 was calcium 5.7 mg/dL:phosphorus 10.5 mg/dL. Almost a complete reverse!

Treatment with DHT at 0.01 mg/kg p.o. twice weekly with the same calcium dose brought the ferret back to stability between days 354–373. It remained normal till checked at 849 days when the serum calcium was normal but the serum urea nitrogen, creatinine and phosphorus were increasing despite the ferret drinking more. Alarmingly, the ferret had a ravenous appetite and increased its body weight to 1800 g to become obese!

Note: serum thyroxine levels were normal at 2.6 µg/dL (range 1.01–8.29 µg/dL). The ferret was last checked at 3½ years and found to be obese but healthy and stayed on the treatment for life.

Hyperthyroidism and hypothyroidism

These conditions of thyroid malfunction are as yet not recognized in pet ferrets. (C J-D, pers. comm. 2005). Normal reference values have been given.

CHAPTER FOURTEEN
Endocrine diseases

References

1. Brown SA, Jenkins JR, eds. Ferrets. In: A practitioner's guide to rabbits and ferrets. Lakewood: American Animal Hospital Association; 1993.
2. Lewington JH. Adrenal gland neoplasia. Control and therapy. Sydney University: Postgraduate Foundation 1995; 185:800.
3. Rosenthal KL. Adrenal gland disease. In: Hillyer EV, Quesenberry KE, eds. Ferrets, rabbits, and rodents. Clinical medicine and surgery. Philadelphia: WB Saunders; 1997:91–98.
4. Carpenter JW, Meliton NN. Diabetes mellitus in a black-footed ferret. J Am Vet Med Assoc 1977; 171:890–893.
5. Johnson-Delaney C. Update on ferret adrenal research. Exot DVM 2002; 4:61–64.
6. Finkler MR. Practical ferret medicine and surgery. Roanoak, VA: Roanoak Animal Hospital; 2002.
7. Johnson-Delaney C. Ferret adrenal disease: alternatives to surgery. Exot DVM 1999; 1:19–22.
8. Wagner RA, Dorn DP. Evaluation of serum oestradiol concentrations in alopecic ferrets with adrenal gland tumours. J Am Vet Med Assoc 1994; 205:703–707.
9. Rosenthal KL, Peterson ME. Evaulation of plasma androgen and estrogen concentrations in ferret with hyperadrenocorticism. J Am Vet Med Assoc 1996; 209:1097–1102.
10. Rosenthal KL, Peterson ME, Quesenberry KE, et al. Hyperadrenocorticism associated with adrenocortical tumour or nodular hyperplasia of the adrenal gland in ferrets: 50 cases (1987–1991). J Am Vet Med Assoc 1993; 203:271–275.
11. Rosenthal KL. Adrenal gland disease in ferrets. Vet Clin N Am Small Anim Pr 1997; 27:401–418.
12. Pilny AA, Hess L. Ferrets: wound healing and therapy. Vet Clin N Am Exot Anim Pr 7:105–121.
13. Gould WJ, Reimers TJ, Bell JA, et al. Evaluation of urinary cortisol: creatinine ratios for the diagnosis of hyperadrenocorticism associated with adrenal gland tumors in ferrets. J Am Vet Med Assoc 1995; 206:42–46.
14. Holmes RL. The adrenal glands of the ferret *Mustela putorius*. J Anat 1961; 95:325–336.
15. Ackermann J, Carpenter JW, Godshalk CP, et al. Ultrasonographic detection of adrenal gland tumors in two ferrets. J Am Vet Med Assoc 1994; 205:1001–1003.
16. Barthez PY, Nyland TG, Feldman EG. Ultrasonograph of the adrenal glands in the dog, cat and ferret. Vet Clin N Am Small Anim Pract 1998; 28:869–885.
17. Lawrence HJ, Gould WJ, Flanders JA, et al. Unilateral adrenalectomy as a treatment for adrenocortical tumors in ferrets: five cases (1990–1992). J Am Vet Med Assoc 1993; 203:267–270.
18. Weiss CA, Williams BH, Scott JB, et al. Surgical treatment and long-term outcome of ferrets with bilateral adrenal tumors or adrenal hyperplasia: 56 cases (1994–1997). J Am Vet Med Assoc 1999; 215:820–823.
19. Finkler M. Practical ferret medicine and surgery for the private practitioner. Roanoke, VA: Roanoke Animal Hospital; 1999.
20. Paradis M, Bonneau NH, Morin M, et al. Hyperadrenocorticism in association with an adrenocortical adenoma in a pet ferret. Can Vet J 1989; 30:60–62.
21. Nolte DM, Carberry CA, Gannon KM, et al. Temporary tube cystostomy as a treatment for urinary obstruction secondary to adrenal disease in four ferrets. J Am Anim Hosp Assoc 2002; 38:527–532.
22. Wagner RA, et al. Clinical and endocrine response to treatment with deslorelin acetate implants in ferrets with adrenocortical disease. Am J Vet Res 2005; 66:910–914.
23. Finkler MR. Prevention strategies: adrenal gland disease, insulinoma. Am Ferret Assoc Vet Symp Proc 2003; 3:59–74.
24. Johnson-Delaney CA. Medical therapies for ferret adrenal disease. Sem Avian Exot Pet Med 2004; 13:3–7.
25. Wagner RA, Bailey EM, Schneider JF, et al. Leuprolide acetate treatment of adrenocortical disease in ferrets. J Am Vet Med Assoc 2001; 218:1272–1274.
26. Simpson M. Common problems in rabbits and ferrets. Veterinarian 2004; December:26–29.
27. Wagner RA. Adrenal cortical disease in ferrets: medical or surgical treatment? Am Ferret Assoc Vet Symp Proc 2003; 3:44–53.
28. Schoemaker NJ, Mol JA, Lumeij JT, et al. Plasma concentrations of adrenocorticotrophic hormones and a-melanocyte-stimulating hormone in ferrets (*Mustela putorius furo*) with hyperadrenocorticism. Am J Vet Res 2002; 63:1395–1399.
29. Paul-Murphy J, O'Brien R, Ramer J. Melatonin use in ferret adrenal gland disease. Proc North Am Vet Conf 2001; 15:897.
30. Murray J. Melatonin implants: an option for use in the treatment of adrenal disease in ferrets. Exot Mammal Med Surg 2005; 3:1–6.
31. Johnson-Delaney CA. Melatonin study with 4 intact adult male ferrets and 2 adrenal disease ferrets. Exot Mammal Med Surg 2005; 3:7–10.
32. Patterson MM, Rogers AB, et al. Alopecia attributed to neoplastic ovarian tissue in two ferrets. Comp Med 2003; 53:213–217.
33. Mor N, Qualls CW, Hoover JP. Concurrent mammary gland hyperplasia and adrenocortical carcinoma in a domestic ferret. J Am Vet Med Assoc 1992; 201:1911–1912.
34. Dorn AS, Legendre AM, McGavin MD. Mammary hyperplasia in a male cat receiving progesterone. J Am Vet Med Assoc 1983; 182:621–622.
35. William BH, Fisher PG, Johnson TL. Diffuse cutaneous telangiectasis in a ferret with adrenal-associated endocrinopathy. Exot DVM 2002; 4.2:8–9.
36. Peterson RA, Kiupel M, Capen CC. Adrenal cortical carcinoma with myxoid differentiation in the domestic ferret (*Mustela putorius furo*). Vet Pathol 2003; 40:136–142.
37. Schoemaker NJ, Schuurmans M, Moorman H, et al. Correlation between age at neutering and age at onset of hyperadrenocorticism in ferrets. J Am Vet Med Assoc 2000; 216:195–197.
38. Moorman H. Macho the 'paralytic' ferret. S Aust Ferret Assoc News 2005; 17:9–10.
39. Erhart N, Withrow SJ, Ehrhart EJ, et al. Pancreatic beta cell tumor in ferrets: 20 cases (1986–1994) J Am Vet Med Assoc 1996; 209:1737–1740.
40. Quesenberry KE. Insuloma. In: Hillyer EV, Quesenberry KE, eds. Ferrets, rabbits, and rodents: Clinical medicine and surgery. Philadelphia: WB Saunders; 1997:85–90.
41. Marini RP, Ryden EB, Rosenblad WD, et al. Functional islet cell tumor in six ferrets. J Am Vet Med Assoc 1993; 202:430–433.
42. Carpenter J. Biology and medicine of the domestic ferret, an overview. J Small Exot Anim Med 1994; 2:151–162.
43. Rosenthal K. Ferrets. Vet Clin North Am Small Anim Pract 1994; 24:1–23.
44. Melo K, Caplan ER. Treatment of insulinoma in the dog, cat and ferret. In: Bonagura JD, ed. Kirk's current veterinary

therapy XIII. Small animal practice. Philadelphia: Saunders; 2000:357–361.
45. Weiss C, Williams B, Scott M. Insulinoma in the ferret: clinical findings and treatment comparison of 66 cases. J Am Anim Hosp Assoc 1998; 34:471–475.
46. Finkler MA. Nutritional approach to the prevention of insulinoma in the ferret. Lecture talk; 2004.
47. Pilny AA, Chen S. Ferret insulinoma: diagnosis and treatment. Compend Contin Edu Vet Pract 2004; 26:722–728.
48. Sturgess K. Rational use of corticosteriods in small animals. Practice 2002; July/August:368–375.
49. Caplan ER, Peterson ME, Mullen HS, et al. Diagnosis and treatment of insulin-secreting pancreatic islet cell tumors in ferrets: 57 cases (1986–1994). J Am Vet Med Assoc 1996; 209:1741–1745.
50. Eatwell K. Two unusual tumours in a ferret. (*Mustela putorius furo*). J Small Anim Pract 2004; 45:454–459.
51. Lloyd CG, Lewis WGV. Two cases of pancreatic neoplasia in British ferrets (*Mustela putorius furo*). J Small Anim Pract 2004; 45:558–562.
52. Weiss CA, Scott MV. Clinical aspects and surgical treatment of hyperadrenocorticism in the domestic ferret: 94 cases (1994–1996). J Am Anim Hosp Assoc 1997; 33:487–493.
53. Schoemaker NJ, Hage MH van der, Flik G, et al. Morphology of the pituitary gland in ferrets (*Mustela putorius furo*) with hyperadrenocorticism. J Comp Pathol 2004; 130:255–265.
54. Dahm M Van. Update on our ferret photo-sensitivity study. Ferret Advice Information Resource Society. FAIR Rep 2001; XI(5):1–4.
55. Willard T. Performance Foods review. Int Ferret Newsl 1998; 15:3–9.
56. Pearson R, Gorham JR. Viral disease models. In: Fox JG, ed. Biology and diseases of the ferret, 2nd edn. Baltimore: Williams & Wilkins; 1998:487–497.
57. Saxena FF, Clavio A, Singh M, et al. Effect of immunization with bovine luteinizing hormone receptor on ovarian function in cats. Am J Vet Res 2003; 64:292–298.
58. Wilson GH, Greene CE, Greenacre CB. Suspected pseudohypoparathyroidism in a domestic ferret. J Am Vet Med Assoc 2003; 222:1093–1096.

15

Managing ferret toxicoses

Jill Richardson

'Knowledge is of two kinds. We know a subject ourselves, or we know where we can find information on it.'

Richard Feynman, 1918–1988

Ferrets are extremely curious and are very adept at accessing areas where baits, cleaners, chemicals and medications are stored. Ferrets can even pry caps from child-resistant bottles or chew through heavy plastic containers. Products such as flavoured medications or pest control baits have an appealing taste and, because the average weight of the adult ferret is <2 kg, even small amounts can be dangerous. Therefore, proper and prompt treatment of toxicoses, including stabilization and de-contamination, is essential. The purpose of this chapter is to discuss management of toxicoses in ferrets.

The US ASPCA Animal Poison Control Center in Urbana, Illinois, sees a number of house pet ferrets for poisoning of various kinds. From January to December 2004, they recorded 170 ferret cases, which was 0.2% of the total pet animals. In 2003, the figure was 193 cases, still 0.2% of total. (ASPCA unpublished data, courtesy of Dr S.L. Welch.) Some clinical examples are given later in this chapter.

Assessment of the animal's condition

Assessing the condition of the ferret is the initial step in managing a potential toxicosis. The assessment should be performed quickly and include the following: an examination of the respiratory rate, capillary refill time, mucous membrane colour, heart rate and core body temperature.

If the ferret is stable, a comprehensive history of the ferret and the exposure should be taken, and then a thorough physical examination should be performed. Examination of a ferret that is unconscious, in shock, seizing, or in cardiovascular or respiratory distress, must be conducted simultaneously with stabilization measures.

Signalment and history are crucial when dealing with a toxicosis and often affects the manner in which the animal is treated. The physical examination of a ferret is similar to that of any small mammal.[1] Most ferrets are docile and can be examined easily. The critically ill ferret may be listless and require minimal restraint.[2] Energetic ferrets can be restrained by 'scruffing' the loose skin on the back of the neck and suspending it with all four legs off the table. With this hold, most ferrets become relaxed and will allow a thorough examination. Treats can be used as a distraction for the ferret during the examination.[1]

Stabilization of vital functions

Stabilizing the ferret is a priority. A patent airway should be established and artificial respiration given if the animal is dyspnoeic or cyanotic. Artificial respiration can be given with a 2.5–3.5 mm endotracheal tube.[3] The cardiovascular system should be monitored closely, preferably with a constant ECG monitor, and any cardiovascular abnormality should be corrected.[2] The normal adult ferret heart rate is 180–250 bpm, but can vary with normal sinus arrhythmia. If cardiac arrest occurs, cardiopulmonary resuscitation should be instituted. Anticonvulsant therapy, such as diazepam at 1–2 mg/kg i.m., should be given if the animal is tremoring or seizing.[4]

The placement of an indwelling intravenous catheter may be necessary for the administration of medications and intravenous fluids. Catheter placement is performed with the ferret under anaesthesia. Isoflurane provides the safest means of anaesthesia in the critically ill ferret, and an induction chamber is recommended because ferrets often resist face-mask usage.[2,5] A 22–24 gauge peripheral catheter can be placed in the lateral saphenous or the cephalic vein.[2] Jugular vein catheters are more difficult to place and are used less frequently.[5,6]

De-contamination

Preventing absorption of the substance through appropriate de-contamination measures is an important step in treating a toxicosis. Following dermal exposure to a toxicant, the ferret should be bathed with a mild liquid hand dish detergent or a non-insecticidal pet shampoo. The skin should be monitored for redness, swelling, or pain. For ocular exposures, a minimum of 20–30 minutes irrigation with tepid tap water or physiological saline is recommended. If the substance is corrosive, the eye should be examined for evidence of corneal ulceration. Follow-up examinations or consultations with a veterinary ophthalmologist may be needed with cases involving corneal damage.[7]

Emesis, gastric lavage and activated charcoal may be required with oral exposures. Inducing emesis may be considered for recent ingestions. Ferrets do have the ability to vomit; however, the length of time since ingestion, the ferret's age, its previous medical history, and the type of poison can affect the decision to induce emesis. Any ferret who has a history of cardiovascular abnormalities, epilepsy, recent abdominal surgery, or severe debilitation is not a candidate for emesis induction.[7]

Emesis should not be induced in any animal that is severely depressed or in a coma, as it could lead to aspiration, while inducing vomiting on a hyperactive animal could trigger a seizure. Additionally, inducing vomiting on a ferret that has already vomited is not recommended.

Another factor affecting the decision to induce emesis is the nature of the substance ingested. Emesis is contraindicated for corrosive materials such as cationic detergents, acids, and alkali. Induction of vomiting is not recommended with corrosives because of re-exposure of the oesophageal tissues to the corrosive material. For corrosives, dilution with milk or water is the recommended initial treatment. In addition, emesis is contraindicated when a hydrocarbon has been ingested, the main concern being possible aspiration during emesis. Some examples of hydrocarbon-containing products are tar, lubrication oils, fuel oil, kerosene, mineral spirits and gasoline.[7]

Establishing the time of exposure is important because the ferret has a short gastrointestinal transit time (3–4 hours in the adult) and emesis will be useful only if induced soon after the exposure.[7] Emesis is more likely to be productive if the animal is fed a small moist meal, such as canned cat food, before inducing vomiting. Three-percent hydrogen peroxide solution, which can be purchased over the counter, can be given orally at a dose of 1 mL/lb, and has been shown to be an effective emetic for ferrets.[7] Hydrogen peroxide can be administered with an eyedropper or a syringe. Hydrogen peroxide causes mild gastric mucosal irritation, resulting in emesis. Typically, vomiting occurs within 15 minutes. If not, 3% hydrogen peroxide can be repeated one additional time at the same dose. In cases when emesis is contraindicated but emptying stomach contents is essential, a gastric lavage under general anaesthesia and using a cuffed endotracheal tube should be considered.

Activated charcoal is a non-specific adsorbent that binds to many substances through weak chemical forces, and prevents their absorption. It is ineffective and generally not indicated for corrosive substances, hydrocarbons or heavy metals such as iron, lead, mercury or arsenic. Activated charcoal is available in liquid, powder and granular forms. The granular or powder form of activated charcoal can be mixed with water to facilitate administration. Activated charcoal can be administered orally with a syringe or via gastric tube at a dose of 1–2 g/kg.[7]

Cathartics increase the clearing of intestinal contents. Cathartics are used to enhance the elimination of activated charcoal and adsorbed toxicant. Pre-mixed products that contain both activated charcoal and a cathartic are available commercially or cathartics can be added to solutions of activated charcoal. Unless the animal has diarrhoea or is dehydrated, administer activated charcoal with a cathartic to facilitate removal of the charcoal-bound substance.[7] This will decrease the chances that the bonds between the charcoal and poison can weaken and allow the poison to be released. Caution should be used when administering magnesium sulfate as a cathartic when the animal has renal compromise.[8] Magnesium sulfate is excreted by the kidneys and an overdose can occur with renal impairment. Excess magnesium can cause drowsiness or CNS depression, muscular weakness, bradycardia, hypotension and respiratory depression.[8]

Supportive care

Supportive care involving the evaluation of vital signs and any parameters likely to be affected by the toxicants is an important step in treating toxicoses.

CHAPTER FIFTEEN
Managing ferret toxicoses

Monitoring of the acid–base balance, chemistry profile, hydration or electrolytes may be necessary. Preventive measures such as the use of gastric protectants or antibiotics may be needed. For example, ingestion of alkaline agents such as sodium or potassium hydroxide, which is found in some drain cleaners, can cause corrosive damage to the mouth, tongue and stomach. Supportive care in this case would include several days of gastric protection and antibiotics. Hydration can be assessed in the ferret by checking skin turgor, capillary refill time and the moisture of the oral mucous membranes.[1,2,5] The animal's body temperature should also be monitored closely. The normal body temperature of the ferret is reported to be 100–104°F, with the average being 101.0°F.[1,2]

Blood samples may be needed to perform CBCs, chemistry panels or clotting profiles to monitor the effects of the poison. Some toxicants, such as iron, copper, acetaminophen and arsenic, are hepatotoxic, while others, such as oestrogen, lead and anti-neoplastic medications can cause anaemia.

To obtain small samples of blood (less than 0.5 mL), use an insulin syringe with a 28-gauge needle to retrieve blood from the lateral saphenous or cephalic vein.[1,2] A quarter-inch Penrose drain can be utilized as a tourniquet to aid in vein visualization. For larger volumes of blood, the jugular vein or anterior vena cava are preferred sites of venipuncture.[1,2] The PCV and hydration level should be established before attempting to withdraw substantial amounts of blood.

The ferret's clinical signs should be treated according to signs. The appropriate antidote or antagonist should be administered; however, very few poisons actually have specific antidotes. Therefore, most cases are handled by monitoring the patient and treating the symptoms as they arise.

Daily fluid requirements for ferrets have not been determined. However, the use of 75–100 mL/kg per day appears to be adequate for maintenance. Compensation should be made for excessive fluid loss or to correct dehydration. Debilitated animals may require additional supplementation with dextrose, vitamin B or potassium.[1,2] An infusion pump should be used to prevent overhydration.[2,6] The ferret should be monitored for wet lung sounds or the development of a heart murmur, which could indicate over-hydration. Ferrets with cardiovascular disease are at a higher risk for over-hydration. Closely monitor ferrets with indwelling catheters to prevent entanglement in the line or chewing. Subcutaneous fluids may be used, but the intravenous route is preferred. Subcutaneous fluids can be administered in the loose skin along the back and dorsal cervical area.[6]

Diuresis may be beneficial for exposures to nephrotoxic agents or to enhance elimination of the poison. Examples of nephrotoxic agents that could benefit from diuresis include ethylene glycol, zinc, mercury, oxalic acids, nonsteroidal anti-inflammatory drugs, diquat herbicide and aminoglycoside antibiotics. Adverse effects associated with diuresis include pulmonary oedema, cerebral oedema, metabolic acidosis or alkalosis or water intoxication, therefore close monitoring is necessary.[6]

Ancillary procedures

Ancillary measures, such as nutritional support, are key components for complete recovery for the ferret. Anorectic ferrets are at risk of developing hepatic lipidosis and hypoglycaemia, therefore, it is extremely important to maintain the ferret's nutritional requirements. Hypoglycaemic ferrets may appear weak, lethargic, or dazed.[2] Previously undiagnosed insulinomas (pancreatic islet cell neoplasm) occur frequently in ferrets and can predispose the animal to develop hypoglycaemia.[1,2] A pharyngostomy tube may be necessary to provide adequate nutrition to the animal. The technique is identical to that described for cats and utilizes an 8–10 French paediatric feeding tube.[2] Diazepam at 1 mg/kg i.m. or less could be used to stimulate appetite.[4] Adult ferrets can be force-fed paste supplements or liquid soy-based or meat-based diets at 2–5 mL 3–4 times daily.[2,6] A more complete diet should be used if forced feeding continues more than one day.[1] Hospitalized ferrets eating voluntarily can be fed their normal diet or a premium ferret, cat or kitten food.

Good nursing care should be continued until the ferret completely recovers. The ferret should be hospitalized in a quiet area, separate from dogs and cats. Ferrets are agile escape artists and can squeeze through extremely small openings, so only use cages with very narrow spacing between vertical bars.[1]

Hospital personnel with flu symptoms should avoid contact with ferrets.[2] Several strains of the human influenza virus can infect and mainly cause upper respiratory disease.[2,9] The severity of signs varies with the virus strain.[9]

Common household hazards

Ant baits

Ant and roach baits are common objects found in households. They are also referred to as hotels, traps or stations. The insecticides used most commonly in these baits are chlorpyrifos, sulfluramid, fipronil, avermectin, boric acid and hydramethylnon. The baits usually contain inert ingredients such as peanut butter, breadcrumbs, sugar and vegetable or animal, which could be attracting to ferrets. Exposures to these types of ant baits usually do not require de-contamination or treatment. Most often, if signs are seen at all, they are mild in nature and self-limiting and are usually attributed to the inert ingredients instead of the active ingredient.

Silica gel packets

Silica gel is used as a desiccant and often comes in paper packets or plastic cylinders. They are used to absorb moisture with leather, medication and in some food packaging. Silica is considered 'chemically and biologically inert' upon ingestion. However, with ingestion, it is possible to see signs of gastrointestinal (GI) upset, such as nausea, vomiting and inappetence. Additional problems could occur if the silica gel was used as a desiccant in medication, since silica could possibly absorb qualities of the medication.

Liquid potpourri

Liquid potpourri may contain essential oils and cationic detergents, both of which can be harmful. Because product labels may not list ingredients, it is wise to assume any liquid potpourri contains both ingredients. Essential oils can cause mucous membrane and gastrointestinal irritation, central nervous system depression, and dermal hypersensitivity and irritation. Severe clinical signs can be seen with potpourri products that contain cationic detergents. Dermal exposure to cationic detergents can result in erythema, oedema, intense pain and ulceration. Ingestion of cationic detergents can lead to tissue necrosis and inflammation of the mouth, oesophagus and stomach. Cationic detergents can also be found in some household cleaners, disinfectants, sanitizers and fabric softeners.

Chocolate

Chocolate contains theobromine and caffeine, which are both methylxanthines. The amount of methylxanthines present depends on the type of chocolate. In general, the less sweet the chocolate, the more toxic it could be. Unsweetened baking chocolate contains almost seven times more theobromine than milk chocolate.

Methylxanthines cause CNS stimulation, tachycardia and tremors. Signs seen with chocolate toxicosis include vomiting, diarrhoea, hyperactivity, polyuria, polydipsia, lethargy, tachycardia, cardiac arrhythmias, seizures and death. Ferret response levels have not been evaluated, however, moderate effects would be expected in dogs at doses of 40–60 mg/kg and severe effects would be expected at doses over 60 mg/kg (Table 15.1).

Table 15.1 The chocolate problem

Type of chocolate	Caffeine (mg/oz)	Theobromine (mg/oz)
Milk chocolate	6	44–56
Semi-sweet	22	138
Baking chocolate	33–47	393

Table 15.2 Nicotine content of common source of drug

Nicotine product	Nicotine content
Cigarettes	3–30 mg per 1 whole cigarette
Cigarette butts	5–7 mg
Cigars	15–40 mg
Moist snuff	4.6–32 mg/g
Dry snuff	12.4–15.6 mg/g
Chewing tobacco	2.5–8 mg/g
Nicotine gum	2–4 mg per piece
Transdermal patches	15–114 mg per patch
Nicotine nasal sprays	10 mg/mL
Nicotine inhaler rods	10 mg per cartridge

Cigarettes

Tobacco products contain varying amounts of nicotine with cigarettes containing 13–30 mg and cigars containing 15–40 mg. Butts contain about 25% of the total nicotine content. The lethal dose in ferrets is not known, however the oral LD50 in dogs is 9.2 mg/kg. Signs often develop quickly (usually within 15–45 min) and include excitation, tachypnoea, salivation, emesis and diarrhoea. Muscle weakness, twitching, depression, tachycardia, shallow respiration, collapse, coma and cardiac arrest can follow the period of excitation. Death occurs secondary to respiratory paralysis (Table 15.2).

Pennies

US pennies minted after 1982 are composed of copper plating around a zinc core. One penny contains approximately 2440 mg of zinc. Zinc toxicosis has been reported as a result of ingestion of even 1 penny. Other sources of zinc include zinc hardware and galvanized objects. Zinc can affect the renal, hepatic and the haematopoietic tissues. Zinc can cause haemolytic anaemia, which could lead to haemoglobinaemia and/or haemoglobinuria. Treatment guidelines established in dogs include antiacids, zinc object removal and supportive care (fluids, blood transfusion, GI protection). The use of chelating agents with zinc is not commonly recommended.

Bread dough

When bread dough is ingested, the animal's body heat causes the dough to rise in the stomach. Alcohol is produced during the rising process and the dough expands. Signs seen with bread dough ingestion include abdominal pain, bloat, vomiting, ataxia and depression. Bread dough toxicosis has only been reported in dogs, however, the risk is a potential for other household pets as well.

Mothballs

Naphthalene is the most dangerous type of mothball. Mothballs contain approximately 100% naphthalene and weigh 2.7 g. Toxicity has been reported with the ingestion of one mothball. Most common signs seen with mothball ingestion include vomiting, methaemoglobinaemia, Heinz body anaemia, haemolysis, haemoglobinuria, lethargy and seizures. Hepatitis is a rare effect and if seen would occur 3–5 days post-exposure. Acute renal failure is possible, secondary to haemolysis. Seizures and coma could develop in severe cases.

Rodenticides

Anticoagulants

- *Short acting*: warfarin
- *Long-acting*: pindone, diphacinone, difethialone, chlorophacinone, brodifacoum and bromadiolone.

The anticoagulant rodenticides act by competitive inhibition of vitamin K epoxide reductase, thus halting the re-cycling of vitamin K. Factor VII is the first parameter affected. It is located in the extrinsic pathway and can be measured with prothrombin time (PT). In early cases of toxicoses, the PT when checked between 36–72 hours will be elevated, but the animal will still appear clinically normal. Beyond 72 hours, factor IX becomes depleted and shuts down the intrinsic pathway, at which time haemorrhage is a possible effect. The presence of circulating clotting factors in normal animals is the reason for the delay in the development of signs. Haemorrhage, pale mucous membranes, weakness, exercise intolerance, lameness, dyspnoea, coughing and swollen joints are possible clinical signs. Often, the animal is not presented to the veterinarian until the signs are severe. For diagnostics, PT tests the extrinsic and common pathways. It will be elevated with any deficiency of factor VII and is the best test for early detection (due to the short half-life of factor VII) of a vitamin K-impaired coagulopathy.

Treatment tips
Stabilize the ferret if clinical. Transfusions with whole blood or plasma may be necessary to replace clotting factors and then initiate vitamin K_1 therapy. Decontamination is only effective with recent exposures. Induce emesis if ingestion occurred within 2 hours. Activated charcoal can be given 1–2 times within 24 hours of ingestion. Potentially, any dose of anticoagulant would be a dangerous dose with a ferret, given their size. Vitamin K_1 should be given prophylactically with any anticoagulant rodenticide exposure in a ferret. Vitamin K_1 should not be given intravenously and it is possible to have an anaphylactic reaction when it is given subcutaneously. The dose of vitamin K_1 is 3–5 mg/kg per day orally. This dose should be divided b.i.d. or t.i.d. and should be given with a fatty meal to enhance absorption. With small animals like ferrets, the injectable solution can be administered orally. To enhance the flavour and also to enhance absorption, the solution can be mixed with peanut butter or canned cat food (fatty meals help to enhance the absorption of vitamin K_1). Also, it is advisable to check a PT at 48 hours post the last dose of vitamin K_1. Vitamin K_1 should be continued if the PT is still increased. Try to avoid the use of other highly protein-bound drugs during the treatment and instruct the owner to restrict activity of the ferret during this time (Table 15.3).

Bromethalin

Bromethalin is an uncoupler of oxidative phosphorylation. Bromethalin causes a reduction of ATP. ATP is necessary to sustain the sodium/potassium ion channel pumps. When the pump mechanism is inhibited, fluid build-up occurs, which results in fluid-filled vacuoles between myelin sheaths. This leads to decreased nerve impulse conduction. Clinical signs could occur within 24 hours up to 2 weeks and include: muscle tremors, seizures, hyperexcitability, forelimb extensor rigidity, ataxia, CNS depression, loss of vocalization, paresis, paralysis and death. Most common post mortem lesions

Table 15.3 Anticoagulants and therapy

Type of anticoagulant	Minimum duration of therapy
Warfarin	14 days
Bromadiolone	21 days
Brodifacoum and others	30 days

include cerebral and spinal cord oedema and a spongy appearance to the cerebellum.

Treatment tips
Aggressive de-contamination is most important. Induce emesis with recent ingestion. Repeated doses of activated charcoal (every 8–12 hours) and a cathartic are recommended. There is no antidote, so de-contamination is extremely important. Supportive care should be given for clinical signs. Agents such as mannitol, furosemide and corticosteroids may reduce the cerebral oedema. Unfortunately, these drugs are of little benefit in reducing the severity of signs in experimental animals. The prognosis is poor for animals showing severe signs. Animals exposed at lower dose end exhibiting paralysis may recover.

Cholecalciferol

Cholecalciferol (vitamin D_3) is metabolized in the liver to calcifediol (25-hydroxycholecalciferol). Calcifediol is then metabolized by the kidney to calcitriol (1,25-dihydroxycholecalciferol). Cholecalciferol increases intestinal absorption of calcium, stimulates bone resorption and enhances renal tubular reabsorption of calcium. This results in a serum calcium increase. This can lead to acute renal failure, cardiovascular abnormalities and tissue mineralization. The minimum toxic dose ranges from 0.5 mg/kg to 3.0 mg/kg in dogs; the minimum toxic dose in ferrets is not known. Clinical signs usually have a delay in onset and usually occur 18–36 hours post-ingestion. The most common signs seen with cholecalciferol toxicosis include vomiting, diarrhoea, inappetence, depression, polyuria, polydipsia and cardiac arrhythmia. Renal failure arises from the deposition of calcium in the kidney. Post mortem lesions seen with cholecalciferol toxicoses include elevated total kidney calcium concentrations and diffuse haemorrhages of the gastrointestinal tract. Mineralization and necrosis of gastrointestinal, cardiac and renal tissues may be seen histologically.

Treatment tips
Aggressive de-contamination is key. Emesis and repeated activated charcoal is important. Obtain a baseline serum calcium and BUN immediately post-exposure. Monitor serum calcium and BUN every 12–24 hours each day, for 3 days post-exposure. If the calcium level remains normal for 96 hours, no further treatment would be needed. Treat renal effects with supportive care including fluid diuresis twice maintenance using 0.9% saline. Normal saline fluids help to decrease tubular reabsorption of calcium. Pamidronate inhibits osteoclastic bone resorption and has been successfully used in dogs and cats to treat cholecalciferol toxicosis. The dose used in dogs is 1.3–2.0 mg/kg as a slow (over 2 hours) i.v. infusion. This dose may need to be repeated in 5–7 days. Data are lacking for its usefulness in treating ferrets.

Human medications

Acetaminophen

Acetaminophen is a synthetic non-opiate derivative of p-aminophenol. Acetaminophen toxicity can result from a single toxic dose or repeated cumulative dosages, which lead to methaemoglobinaemia and hepatotoxicity. In dogs, acetaminophen is used therapeutically for analgesia at a dose of 10 mg/kg q. 12 h.[8] Clinical signs of toxicity are not typically observed in dogs unless the dose exceeds 100 mg/kg, at which dose hepatotoxicity is possible. At 2000 mg/kg, methaemoglobinaemia is a possibility.[10] In cats, 10 mg/kg has produced signs of toxicity.[10] The level that would be toxic to a ferret is not known, however, given the ferret's similarity with cats, it can be assumed that ferrets are as intolerant to acetaminophen as cats.

Clinical signs of acetaminophen toxicity are related to methaemoglobinaemia and hepatotoxicity. Clinical signs include depression, weakness, tachypnoea, dyspnoea, cyanosis, icterus, vomiting, methaemoglobinaemia, hypothermia, facial or paw oedema, hepatic necrosis and death.

Treatment recommendations below have been used with success in treating dogs and cats with acetaminophen poisoning and may be used as guidelines for treatment of ferret poisoning. The objective of treatment in acetaminophen toxicity is to replenish glutathione, convert methaemoglobin back to haemoglobin and prevent or treat hepatic necrosis. N-acetylcysteine (NAC) directly binds with acetaminophen metabolites to enhance elimination and serves as a glutathione precursor. A 5% solution of NAC is given orally to dogs or cats at an initial loading dose of 140 mg/kg and then 70 mg/kg every q. 4 h for at least 3–5 treatments. Doses for treatment for ferrets have not been established. Again, it may be helpful to extrapolate the doses used for cats. The use of cimetidine in combination with NAC and ascorbic acid has been shown to be more effective than any of the agents alone in preventing acetaminophen-induced hepatotoxicity in animal studies. Ascorbic acid (vitamin C) provides a reserve system for the reduction of methaemoglobin back to haemoglobin. The effective dose of vitamin C in dogs and cats is 30 mg/kg q. 6–12 h orally or intravenously. Cimetidine can inhibit the cytochrome p-450 oxidation system in the liver and may be useful in reducing the metabolism of acetaminophen.

The dose of cimetidine is 5–10 mg/kg p.o., i.m. or i.v. q. 8 h in ferrets[11].

The patient should be monitored for the presence of methaemoglobinaemia. In cats, methaemoglobin values increase within 2–4 hours, followed by Heinz body formation. The liver enzymes should be monitored closely. Laboratory evidence of hepatotoxicity generally develops 24–36 hours post-ingestion.

Ibuprofen

Ibuprofen is a substituted phenylalkanoic acid with non-steroidal anti-inflammatory, antipyretic and analgesic properties. Ibuprofen has been used therapeutically in dogs at 5 mg/kg, but because it can cause gastric ulcers and perforations, it is generally not recommended.[8]

According to studies of acute ingestion of ibuprofen in dogs, vomiting, diarrhoea, nausea, anorexia, gastric ulceration and abdominal pain can be seen with doses of 50–125 mg/kg; these signs in combination with renal damage can be seen at doses at or above 175 mg/kg; and at doses at or above 400 mg/kg CNS effects such as seizure, ataxia and coma may occur. Cats are considered to be twice as sensitive as dogs because they have a limited glucuronyl-conjugating capacity. Ferrets appear to be even more sensitive to ibuprofen than cats and toxicity has been seen at doses as low as 18 mg/kg.

Most common signs of ibuprofen toxicosis include anorexia, nausea, vomiting, lethargy, diarrhea, melaena, ataxia, polyuria and polydipsia. Ferrets may go directly into a coma after ingestion of ibuprofen. Renal effects may not be as obvious in ferrets as they are in dogs and cats. Post mortem lesions associated with ibuprofen toxicosis include perforations, erosion, ulceration and haemorrhage of the gastrointestinal tract. A retrospective study (January 1995–March 2000) was conducted of ibuprofen ingestion in ferrets that was reported to the ASPCA Animal Poison Control Center. Data analysis included amount ingested and clinical effects. Of the cases with known exposure amounts, the ingested doses ranged from 18 mg/kg to 15 5000 mg/kg. Some 27 (93.1%) ferrets that had ingested ibuprofen developed neurologic signs, such as depression, coma, ataxia, recumbency, tremors and weakness. In addition, 16 cases (55.2%) had one or more GI effects including anorexia, vomiting, retching or gagging, diarrhoea and melaena. Polydipsia, polyuria, dysuria, renal failure, weight loss, shallow breathing, metabolic acidosis, dehydration and hypothermia were also reported. Death was reported in four cases. The lowest dose associated with death was 220 mg/kg.[12]

The primary goal of treatment is to prevent or treat gastric ulceration, renal failure, CNS effects and possibly hepatic effects. Prognosis is good if the animal is treated promptly and appropriately. Delay in treatment can decrease survival potential with large exposures.

Fluid diuresis for 24–48 hours is recommended with any ibuprofen exposure in a ferret. Peritoneal dialysis may be necessary if unresponsive oliguric or anuric renal failure develops.

Misoprostol (Cytotec®) may be helpful for treating or preventing gastric ulceration caused by ibuprofen. Misoprostol can be given at a dose of 1–5 μg/kg p.o. q. 8 h.[11] Sucralfate can be used to bind to erosions and ulcers, and protect them from exposure to gastric acid, bile acids and pepsin. Sucralfate is given at 0.25 g every 8–12 hours in ferrets.[11] H_2 blockers and/or proton pump inhibitors may also be helpful. Gastric protection is recommended for at least 5–7 days. When renal failure is a potential, BUN, creatinine and urine specific gravity should be monitored closely. A baseline level and then rechecks at 36, 48 and 72 hours is recommended. The animal should also be monitored for acidosis and electrolyte shifts during treatment. Symptomatic treatment for gastric signs and renal failure should be provided until the animal fully recovers.

Poisonous plants

Below is a list of potentially poisonous plants for ferrets. This list has been extrapolated from data involving dogs and cats. World libraries have lists of poisonous plants.

Cardiotoxic plants

- *Convallaria majalis*: Lily of the valley
- *Nerium oleander*: Oleander
- *Rhododendron* species: Rhododendron, azalea, rosebay
- *Taxus* species: American, Japanese, English and Western yew
- *Digitalis purpurea*: Foxglove
- *Kalanchoë* species: Kalanchoë
- *Kalmia* species: Mountain laurel, lambkill, calico bush
- *Leucothoë* species: Dog hobble, dog laurel, fetter bush
- *Lyonia* species: Fetter bush, male berry, stagger bush
- *Pernettya* species
- *Pieris* species: Fetterbush, lily-of-the-valley bush.

Plants that could cause kidney failure

- Certain species of lilies (clinical studies suggest this occurs in cats only)
- Rhubarb (*Rheum* species): leaves only.

Plants that could cause liver failure

- Cycads (*Cycad* species)
- *Amanita phalloides* – mushroom.

Plants that can cause multiple effects

- Autumn crocus (*Colchicum* species)
  - Can cause bloody vomiting and diarrhoea, shock, kidney failure, liver failure, bone marrow suppression
- Castor bean (*Ricinus* species)
  - Usually a lag period of 48 hours before signs appear
  - Castor beans are highly toxic; 2–4 beans can be lethal to adult humans!
  - Severe gastroenteritis, oral pain and irritation, increase in thirst, kidney failure, convulsions, death.

Mushrooms

ALWAYS assume that any ingested mushroom is highly toxic until that mushroom is identified by a mycologist. Toxic and non-toxic mushrooms can grow in same area.

Plants containing calcium oxalate crystals

- Peace lilies (*Spathiphyllum* species)
- Calla lily (*Zantedeschia aethiopiea*)
- Philodendron (*Philodendron* species)
- Dumb cane (*Dieffenbachia* species)
- Mother-in-law plant (*Monstera* species)
- Pothos (*Epipremnum* species).

Peace lilies, Calla lilies, Philodendrons, Dumb cane, Mother-in-law and Pothos plants contain insoluble calcium oxalate crystals. These crystals can cause mechanical irritation of the oral cavity and tongue of birds when plant material is ingested. Clinical signs usually include regurgitation, oral pain, dysphagia and anorexia. The signs are rarely severe and usually respond to supportive care.

Author's clinical examples

1. Suspected ibuprofen toxicosis

A case of poisoning after devouring parts of an ibuprofen (NSAID human drug) tablet was recorded in the USA.[13]

It was an interesting case, as the ferret, a 20-month-old house male castrate, was first suspected of having been affected the day before by a pyrethrin or perhaps pyrethrin/carbamate spray used by the owner. The ferret showed clinical signs of weakness but did respond to auditory and tactile stimulation, being wriggly on first examination. Using an oxygen mask over the ferret's nose, an examination concluded good clinical body signs except for an increasing depression. In fact, the ferret became recumbent and within 5 minutes was not responding to anything but deep pain stimulation.

A rapid support care regime was initiated with the ferret being given Lactated Ringer's solution i.v. via the cephalic vein with added 2.5% dextrose. Laboratory check on the blood found the glucose was 140 mg/dL (range 94–207 mg/dL).

A gastric tube was inserted and two doses of activated charcoal were given as toxin absorption material (2 hours apart). An emetic was not possible as the ferret was semi-comatosed. It was considered that with the normal ferret heart rate and pupillary function the idea of a pyrethrin or carbamate poisoning was in doubt.

Dexamethasone sodium phosphate was given i.v. and separately naloxone was given i.m., as with the sudden onset and severe lethargy of the condition, a narcotic toxicosis was suspect. There was no positive response. Blood analysis of the patient appeared normal. At this point, the team learned about chewed ibuprofen tablets. Evidently, the owner had found digested bits of the tablet in the ferret toilets that morning. Aware of this, a diagnosis of acute ibuprofen toxicity was made. The ferret stayed on i.v. fluids and was also on a warming pad and was turned frequently. Misoprostol was given i.m. to counteract the possible GI ulceration, which can be caused by NSAID drugs.

The ferret was semi-comatose for 8 hours. During this time the temperature, heart rate and respiratory rate had been steady. Then the ferret became unresponsive to stimuli, systolic and apnoeic and despite attempts to revive him using epinephrine i.v. and doxapram sublingual, he died. The patient had lasted approximately 12–14 hours after the suspected ibuprofen injection.

Post mortem revealed plastic-like orange material, which could have been the coating off the ibuprofen tablets.

Interestingly, serum, urine and liver toxicology revealed ibuprofen in the serum at 269 μg/mL (245 μg/mL in a pre-death serum sample), in the urine at 48 μg/mL and liver at 59.1 μg/mL. Levels were above those considered toxic in other species.

Evidently considering this case, NSAID toxicity reports can be as high as 50% with cats and dogs.[13] Thus, the indoor ferret having vomiting or signs of depression should be considered as a poison suspect if ibuprofen tables are missing and treated intensively for possible ibuprofen poisoning.

2. Possible acetaminophen toxicosis

Another possible case of a ferret ingesting a table of paracetamol (acetaminophen) has been recorded.[14] Paracetamol is the common non-steroidal anti-inflammatory; Panadol (Australia) or Tylenol (USA).

In this case, the owner had left two ferrets alone free in the house and returned to find one dead and 500 mg Panadol tablets on the floor with three missing and one partly chewed. The tablet foils of the missing tablets were not seen and presumably had been eaten. The remaining ferret was treated with Mucomyst and kept hospitalized for 5 days without clinical signs developing.

Toxicity signs for paracetamol have been recorded for dogs and cats. In cats, they succumb to decreased oxygenation of the blood and show cyanosis with higher respiratory and heart rates. Signs of hepatoxicity can occur. Post mortem on a poisoned ferret would reveal signs of liver and kidney damage but the stomach showed no signs of the paracetamol foil. It was however considered that the material had passed through the gut or had been vomited up. No signs were seen so the outcome was highly suspicious but not conclusive. Treatment of any cases would be as of the dog and cat.

Cases 1 and 2 illustrate the need to keep human and veterinary drugs well away from inquisitive ferrets!

3. Problems of heavy metals

Zinc poisoning has occurred in experimentally housed ferrets.[15] Some 20 of a total of 25 ferrets used for influenza virus investigation died of nephrosis, which was put down to the zinc contamination of the ferret meat from zinc powder coating the cage wires after weekly steam sterilization of the cage.

The symptoms shown by the sick ferrets were inappetence, muscular tremors, lethargy, coma and then death. Ferrets kept in cages, which did not have the same steam sterilization process, were unaffected.

Copper toxicosis was found in two unsterilized adult female ferrets with findings at post mortem of high copper levels and deposits of copper in the liver leading to chronic hepatic hepatopathy.[16] A 26-month-old ferret showed signs of CNS depression, lethargy and temperature depression. Though given oxygen and fluids at first examination, the ferret died within hours. A 32-month-old ferret showed CNS depression, icterus and temperature rise. Again, fluids, i.v. and oral were given but the ferret died.

Conclusion

Some of the guidelines discussed in this chapter can be used to aid in the management of toxicoses in ferrets. Assessing the condition of the ferret, stabilizing the animal, preventing absorption of the toxicant, controlling the signs and instituting ancillary measures are critical areas when dealing with toxicoses. The best way to avoid serious problems due to toxicosis is poison prevention. Being cautious with harmful substances by 'ferret proofing' the home environment is the only safe choice. The veterinary staff can educate ferret owners on ways to make their homes poison-safe. However, if a ferret is exposed to a toxicant, these steps and prompt action will be needed to avoid a potentially life-threatening problem.

References

1. Quesenberry KE. Basic approach to veterinary care. In: Hillyer EV, Quesenberry KE, eds. Ferrets, rabbits, and rodents: Clinical medicine and surgery. Philadelphia: WB Saunders; 1997:14–25.
2. Orcutt CJ. Emergency and critical care of ferrets. In: Rupley AE, Guest Editor. The Veterinary clinics of North America exotic animal practice, Vol. 1, No. 1. Philadelphia: WB Saunders; 1998:99–1250.
3. Mason DE. Anesthesia, analgesia, and sedation for small mammals. In: Hillyer EV, Quesenberry KE, eds. Ferrets, rabbits, and rodents: Clinical medicine and surgery. Philadelphia: WB Saunders; 1997:378–391.
4. Exotic Animal Formulary. A supplement to AAHA's practitioner guides to exotic animal medicine. Ferret drug dosages. Lakewood: The American Animal Hospital Association; 1995.
5. Mullen H. Soft tissue surgery. In: Hillyer EV, Quesenberry KE, eds. Ferrets, rabbits, and rodents: Clinical medicine and surgery. Philadelphia: WB Saunders; 1997:131–144.
6. Brown SA. Basic anatomy, physiology, and husbandry. In: Hillyer EV, Quesenberry KE, eds. Ferrets, rabbits, and rodents: Clinical medicine and surgery. Philadelphia: WB Saunders; 1997:3–13.
7. Richardson JA, Balabuszko RA. Management of toxicoses in ferrets. Exot DVM 2000; 2:23–26.
8. Plumb DC. Veterinary drug handbook, 3rd edn. Ames: Iowa State University Press; 1999.

References

9. Rosenthal KL. Respiratory diseases. In: Hillyer EV, Quesenberry KE, eds. Ferrets, rabbits, and rodents: Clinical medicine and surgery. Philadelphia: WB Saunders; 1997:77–84.
10. Richardson JA. Management of acetaminophen and ibuprofen toxicoses in dogs and cats. J Vet Emerg Crit Care 2001; 10(3).
11. Carpenter JW, Mahima, TY, Rupiper DJ. Exotic animal formulary, 2nd edn. Philadelphia: WB Saunders; 2001.
12. Richardson, JA, Balabuszko, RA. Ibuprofen and critical care. Ingestion in ferrets. J Vet Emerg 2001; 11(1).
13. Cathers TE, Isaza R, Oehme F. Acute ibuprofen toxicosis in a ferret. J Am Vet Med Assoc 2000; 216:1426–1428.
14. Lucas J. Paracetamol in the ferret. Internal medicine: small companion animal proceedings. University of Sydney: Post graduate Foundation 1998; 306:33–37.
15. Straube E, Walen N. Zinc poisoning in ferrets. Lab Anim 1981; 15:45–47.
16. Fox J, Zeman DH, Mortimer JD. Copper toxicosis in sibling ferrets. J Am Vet Med Assoc 1994; 205:1154–1156.

Part Three

Surgery

CHAPTERS

16 Anaesthesia and radiology 393
17 Ultrasonography in ferret practice by
Cathy A. Johnson-Delaney 417
18 General surgery by R. Avery Bennett and Geoffrey W. Pye . . 430
19 Ferret vasectomy, orthopaedics and cryosurgery 440
20 Ferret emergency techniques by Anthony Lucas 458

CHAPTER 16

Anaesthesia and radiology

'Given a fair chance, ferrets are tough healthy animals.'

Val Porter and Nicholas Brown, The Complete Book of Ferrets, 1997

Anaesthesia

The principles of anaesthesia and basic surgery apply equally as well to ferrets as to dogs and cats. My experience from the 1970s developed on a 'trial and error' basis. I never dealt with large numbers, as do present day specialist vets in busy ferret practices, especially so in the USA and Europe.

There are, however, specific points to consider if a veterinarian has had no experience with ferret anaesthesia. Ferrets, being of small size, 500–2000 g, require patience and skill in anaesthesia. They have a small body size with a high metabolic rate, which predisposes to the rapid removal and decreased duration of the effect of any anaesthetic given.[1] Thus an anaesthetic drug dose per unit of weight (mg/kg) usually increases as the animal size decreases. Using gas inhalation techniques with ferrets, the induction and recovery can be more rapid than with larger animals and one is dealing with only a small blood volume, small airways and thus small tidal volume.

The risk factor is always there but grades from healthy ferrets with slight risk, where there may be dental disease with asymptomatic characters, to moderate risk cases where anaemia, dehydration or physical fractures may be involved and the necessary precautions are taken to reduce risk.

Important considerations

1. The ferret should not be stressed before an operation. If ferrets are not sick, they can be hyperactive. I used to have them in overnight and settle them in, away from other animals (Ch. 3). The ferret could also come in first thing in the morning and if possible, be allowed to settle down and be operated on in the afternoon. Being single-handed when in practice, I tried to get an undisturbed period in the day to operate on them. I found them usually asleep and relaxed before an afternoon operation. Ferrets coming in overnight can have a small meal in the cage at night and surgery may be scheduled for about 8 a.m. the next morning. Thus they could be fasted up to 12 hours before an operation. Some say 3–4 hours is enough (M. Finkler, pers. comm. 2005). Any sick ferrets due for an operation should be stabilized with fluids beforehand and intravenous catheterization may be required before or once the patient is anaesthetized (Chs 7, 20).

2. The ferret is accurately weighed on admission. The use of premedication should be avoided where it would prolong recovery. I have used very small numbers of accessory drugs with ferrets. Sedation with ketamine, etc. does lead to longer recovery times than using gas anaesthesia. Provided the animal is recovering steadily, the time factor is unimportant as long as it is not excessive. I rested ferrets overnight postoperatively as a precaution against postoperative shock. The slower recovery tided the patient over any immediate pain period and using ketamine or ketamine/xylazine the ketamine would have an analgesic effect for some time. Nowadays, analgesics such as butorphanol

CHAPTER SIXTEEN
Anaesthesia and radiology

are commonly used along with inhalation anaesthetics or reversible i.m. anaesthetics for quicker postoperative recovery.

The protocol for ferret operations in a modern USA hospital is discussed later in this chapter and involves a greater use of drugs. For major operations, e.g. adrenalectomy, pancreatic tumour neoplasia and orthopaedics, 24-hour hospitalization and use of analgesics should be mandatory for the ferret's comfort. The later cumulative toxic effects of numerous drugs might require investigation.

3. Hypothermia must be avoided with ferrets during and after surgery. As the glycogen reserves for ferrets can be small, like other small mammals, they can fall into hypothermia, which is also brought about by the large surface area:volume ratio and the relatively high body temperature they maintain.[1]

I used mobile oil-filled column heaters in the winter. Any hypothermia will cause a decrease in the requirement for anaesthesia, which could predispose to overdosing and also prolong recovery time. The problem in my part of Australia is to keep ferrets cool in the summer heat rather than warm in winter.

I confess to doing preparation and operation on the same table when in practice with ferrets. The cold stainless steel operating table was covered with newspaper and then a large towel; both assist in retaining heat. The anaesthetized ferret was laid, e.g. for a spay (Fig. 16.1), on a plastic support, itself covered by a warm flannel. Sterile drapes were then used as routine around the surgical site and a prep routine followed.

Care must be taken not to compress the ferret's chest as they rely more on diaphragmatic movement for ventilation under anaesthesia than costal movements. Heating pads can be used for operation sites and postoperative recovery but I found our set-up adequate. The surgical site was clipped and warm prep solutions applied. The ferret was placed postoperatively on a towel in a small cage, in the dark, to recover without external stimulation. A mobile heater was placed in the room if necessary just to warm the air.

4. Everything must be ready to give the ferret the initial anaesthesia and proceed with the operation. Delays may 'spook' the ferret and it may become uncooperative. The ferret has a keen sense of hearing and it is basically a nocturnal animal so it is quickly alert to loud noises. My approach to premedication of the ferret was to have the syringe with anaesthetic ready on the table. The assisting nurse stood ready with a suitable towel to wrap the ferret in. Towels are very useful assets with ferrets! I brought the ferret into the quiet operating room. If it was afternoon, the ferret had possibly been asleep and drowsy.

The ferret is placed in the towel and quickly wrapped up with a hind leg exposed. The injection is given quickly into the hind leg muscle and the ferret plus towel is placed in a cat basket on the floor and we wait. A ketamine injection can have an initial sting but I have seen no after-effects. The basket was covered by a towel. Usually, the ferret was sedated in 60 seconds and was lifted out like a limp doll and placed on the operating table. This procedure might seem too obvious to some practitioners experienced with ferrets but I was constantly asked how one gets the ferret to the operating table without getting bitten! The bottom line is that the ferret should not be unnecessarily stressed! Volatile anaesthetics can be given directly by facemask, using halothane or isoflurane. One author uses a gas chamber induction for ferrets, which I thought wasteful on the anaesthetic, especially as isoflurane was an expensive drug at the time.[2]

5. Ideally, a ferret should have a pre-anaesthetic check including thoracic auscultation, abdominal palpation and then laboratory blood screening on blood profile and liver/renal function. This is especially useful for older animals. The former checks would be routine when the ferret is admitted but other tests would depend on the

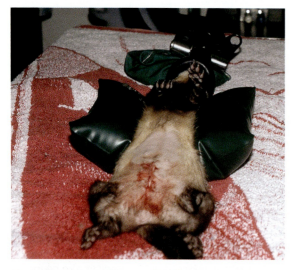

Figure 16.1 Spay operation. The jill is supported in a V-shaped plastic cradle and a clear facemask is useful while the drape is turned back to allow easy checking of respiration.

394

owner's agreement and are probably not needed for young active ferrets undergoing routine sterilization.

Incidentally, I never used surgical gloves and mask for neutering operations and I see from a recent questionnaire I am not alone, even now.[3]

Early anaesthetic protocols

I first anaesthetized ferrets with ether using a soaked ether swab in a jam jar placed over the ferret's head. Not perhaps high tech but quicker than a gas chamber! I progressed to ketamine i.m. first alone and then with halothane supplied by a Midget 3 System using a facemask as a step up.[4] On the whole ferrets are more easily, and safely, anaesthetized than other small mammals. There are now a number of new 'safe' anaesthetic drugs used on ferrets but giving an anaesthetic to any animal is not without risk.

It is assumed that new anaesthetics are safer but Clutton is of the opinion that, 'The reverse is often true, new allegedly safer anaesthetics may provoke a temptation to anaesthetize cases that would previously have been regarded as unacceptable risks'.[5] Thus it may be said that confidence in anaesthesia depends on the procedure being done regularly. I will now give details of my experience and give a review of the types of anaesthesia possible when dealing with ferrets.

I started with ketamine, on a cautious basis independently and recorded some experience with my own and other ferrets.[4] I found ketamine a good basic drug for ferrets despite new drugs coming onto the market. I advanced to using ketamine/xylazine in combination after seeing the Mooreland and Glaser article about a study that a combination of ketamine/xylazine was better than ketamine/diazepam or ketamine alone for i.m. sedation and anaesthesia in ferrets.[6] This now classic study illustrates the use of drug combinations. The use of two or more drugs has become more pre-

Table 16.1 Drugs and dosages used in study of intramuscular anaesthetic agents

Ferret group	Ketamine major drug (mg/kg)	Xylazine second drug (mg/kg)	Diazepam second drug (mg/kg)
Group 1	60		
Group 2	23	+2	
Group 3	35		+3

Table 16.2 Heart rate (bpm) of ferrets before and during anaesthesia

Time post-injection (min)	Group 1	Group 2	Group 3
0 (Unanaesthetized)	250 (160–320)	250 (160–320)	250 (160–320)
5	280 (240–340)	195 (120–240)	300 (280–360)
15	320 (260–320)	160 (160–200)	320 (300–360)
30	330 (280–360)	150 (120–180)	340 (280–400)
45	320 (280–400)	150 (100–200)	350 (320–400)
60	340 (280–400)	170 (110–200)	325 (320–330)

Note: normal ferret heart rate is considered between 200–400 beats per minute (bpm).

Table 16.3 Results of electrocardiograph examination of ferrets before and during anaesthesia

	Unanaesthetized	Group 1	Group 2	Group 3
Normal sinus rhythm	14/15	11/14	9/14	11/14
Ventricular premature contractions	1/15	3/14	5/14	3/14
Other conduction abnormalities (QRS notching)	0/15	2/14	1/14	2/14

14/15: illustrates 14, number showing indicated condition; 15, total population of ferret group, etc.

Anaesthesia and radiology

Table 16.4 Induction time and reflex responses of ferrets in the three groups

	Group 1	Group 2	Group 3
Induction time (min)	2.2	2.7	2.2
Loss palpebral reflex	0/15	12/15	0/15
Duration of loss (min)	–	33	–
Loss pain response toe	0/15	15/15	3/15
Duration of loss (min)	–	40	8
Loss of pain response pinch abdomen	13/15	15/15	12/15
Duration of loss (min)	23	47	21
Paddling	13/15	0/15	12/15
Duration of paddling (min)	33	–	24
Righting reflex regained (min)	55	69	41

Note: the eye 'stages of anaesthesia' are not exhibited as in i.v. Pentothal/gaseous anaesthesia.
Tables 16.1, 16.2, 16.3, 16.4 from Moreland and Glasser, 1985, with permission.[6]

valent with modern anaesthesia and is used in ferrets. Practitioners can consider the results, which included effects on heart rates, resulting ECG readings and indication of induction time and reflex responses as general parameters of ferrets under intramuscular types of anaesthetic agents. Fifteen sterilized hobs over 4 months of age were split into three groups and rotated for trials with the anaesthetics with rest periods between trials. The procedure and results can be seen in Tables 16.1–16.4.

In summary, the dosage of the three anaesthetics provided excellent immobilization and the induction time was within 3 minutes. Analgesia was superior in group 2 with respect to depth and duration but had a longer recovery time. For general surgery, this is no problem and the muscle relaxation was good in both groups 2 and 3. Heart arrhythmias occurred in all three groups but were brief and not unexpected. The ketamine/xylazine combination was considered superior to ketamine alone or ketamine/diazepam.

The ketamine/xylazine combination is frowned upon now by certain American ferret practices but I used it safely for some surgery, especially dental work. It was even used in 1982 by Ryland et al. on a jill ferret with post-oestrous anaemia to give repeated blood transfusions and the ferret survived as shown in Chapter 11. Note: most early anaesthesia investigations were done on laboratory ferrets using the ketamine/xylazine combination.[6] In the modern pet ferret world, the trend has been to go to gaseous anaesthesia using especially the good, but expensive, isoflurane but the older injectables still have their place when used with care.

D. Kemmerer-Cottrell (USA) agrees that ketamine/xylazine combination is still quite safe. She cites operating on 100 imported 6-month-old ferrets for sterilization using the combination. No ferrets died (DK-C, pers. comm. 2005).

Review of anaesthetic agents used for ferrets

Ketamine

Ketamine is my baseline injectable ferret anaesthetic. Ketamine hydrochloride use in ferrets can be evaluated by comparison with the pharmacological effects on cats. In that species the action is rapid with 'profound analgesia, normal pharyngeal reflexes, mild cardiac stimulation and respiratory depression'.[7] In the ferret, the use

Table 16.5 A selection of my operations using ketamine anaesthesia

Ferret name (sex)	Weight (g)	Operation	Ketamine dose rate	Recovery time
Paul (hob)	1000	Teeth scale	75 mg	30 min
Juno (jill)	900	Teeth scale	25 mg	30 min[a]
Juno (jill)	900	Teeth scale	75 mg	46 min
Jason (hob)	2000	Eye ulcer	50 mg	20 min
Walleye (hob)	1200	Castration	100 mg	140 min

[a]Used halothane supplement due to possible loss of ketamine dose during injection.

of ketamine also keeps intact the protective reflexes, coughing and swallowing. Salivation can occur and may be controlled by atropine as a premedication at 0.05 mg/kg i.m. or s.c. I have not had any problem with ferret salivation during operations, even without premedication. With ketamine as the sole anaesthetic agent, the muscle tone is variable, possibly normal, enhanced or diminished and thus the anaesthetic state does not fit into the conventional classification of stages of anaesthesia. Ketamine is said to produce a state of unconsciousness, which is termed dissociative anaesthesia in that it appears to selectively interrupt associated pathways to the brain before producing some sensory blockage.[7]

In cats, the degree of muscle tone is dependent on dose levels and variations of body temperature can occur, with low doses increasing muscle tone and body temperature and high doses resulting in lower muscle tone and reduced body temperature. Ferrets show a characteristic shivering that may be due to the same process.[4] The mild cardiac stimulation in the cat with increased cardiac output and slight increase in mean systolic pressure with hardly any change in total peripheral resistance possibly also happens in ferrets.

At higher doses, the respiratory rate in cats usually decreases. The assurance of a patent airway is greatly enhanced by virtue of maintaining pharyngeal-laryngeal reflexes and this is similar in ferrets. Ketamine at the right dosage in ferrets is a comfortable agent to use with that in mind. Other reflexes such as corneal and pedal are maintained during ketamine anaesthesia in cats and should not be used as criteria for judging depth of anaesthesia. The eyes usually remain open and the pupil dilated with cats and this is the same for ferrets. Following administration of recommended doses by intramuscular injection, cats become incoordinate in about 5 minutes and ferrets within 1–2 minutes. In cats, higher dosages of ketamine allow for internal abdominal surgery.[7] I have done ferret castrations with ketamine and one bone-pinning with high doses of it.[4] An operation for a malignant splenic lymphoma using ketamine anaesthesia at 20 mg/kg has been recorded.[8] It was an early drug with ferrets in the UK.[9] I have used a dose rate of 20–30 mg/kg and experimented with higher dose rates as indicated in Table 16.5.

Ketamine plus xylazine combination

Ketamine hydrochloride (100 mg/mL) is produced by five drug companies supplying the drug to Australia.[7] Only one company indicates its use in ferrets (Ketamil, Ilium Vet Products) which is odd as others indicate its use from horses to echidnas! Ilium give the dose for ferrets as 10–30 mg/kg i.m. or s.c.; xylazine hydrochloride (20 mg/kg small animal dosage) (Xylazine 20, Ilium Vet Products) is not registered for ferrets. However, both these drugs have been used in combination for ferrets and at a dose rate of 20–30 mg/kg ketamine plus 1–4 mg/kg xylazine i.m., as recommended by Moody et al.[10] Experience in the USA suggests that the combination should be 10–40 mg/kg ketamine but with xylazine at only 1–2 mg/kg (Table 16.6). Deaths have been observed with

Author's clinical example

Walleye (1-year-old hob); castration under ketamine. The following illustrates the use of ketamine and its effects on the ferret, with approximate timing to give a general idea.

10.40 a.m.	Walleye wrapped in towel and given 1 mL ketamine (100 mg) in divided dose into each leg. Some struggling but no musk gland release. Ferret plus towel placed in cat basket. Showed immediate collapse with shaking and licking lips.
10.42 a.m.	Walleye placed on operating table.
10.43 a.m.	He was licking his lips. Corneal and pedal withdrawal reflexes still present as expected. Jaw resistant to opening.
10.45 a.m.	Routine ear swab taken for ear mite check. Walleye had some hind leg movement and heart rate at 42/15 s (168/min).
10.47 a.m.	He was relaxed to skin pinch test. Castration operation commenced. No musk gland release during operation.
10.55 a.m.	Ferret castration over. Routine ear-cleaning and nail-clipping done.
11.00 a.m.	Walleye placed back in basket for initial observation. Prostrate with slight head shaking from ear treatment.
11.15 a.m.	Now placed in warm cage in cat kennels, still prostrate with slight head shaking.
11.20 a.m.	Walleye still prostrate with general shaking (shivering) of body.
11.50 a.m.	He was still shivering.
12.25 p.m.	Walleye still prostrate with muscle stiffening and tongue lying out of mouth but no excessive salivation.
1.00 p.m.	Still the same but raising head.
1.40 p.m.	Curled up in cage and licking lips but still shivering.

From then on Walleye made a full recovery from the anaesthetic and operation. This indicates the use of ketamine as a primary agent in minor surgery with the ferret and the safety margin appears to be wide for its use.

Anaesthesia and radiology

higher doses of xylazine due to serious bradycardia effects (S. Brown, pers. comm. 1997).

Note:
1. When using the combination, it is best to draw up the xylazine first in the syringe before the ketamine to avoid any acute immediate xylazine reaction.
2. Atropine will prevent heart arrhythmias due to tranquillizers and sedatives but will not completely reverse the xylazine effects on heart muscle.
3. Xylazine at the lower dose rate appears to work well with ketamine.

Use of tranquillizers

I did not use tranquillizers or premed atropine with plain ketamine/xylazine anaesthesia. I kept drugs to a minimum unless required but that is probably not universally 'correct' nowadays. Drugs that can be used for premed or sedation are shown in Table 16.7.

Comments: Diazepam at 2–3 mg/kg i.m. plus ketamine, 25–35 mg/kg, can be used for minor procedures giving good muscle relaxation and restraint but not sufficient for surgical operations.[11] Moreland and Glasser considered ketamine/xylazine superior to ketamine/diazepam (Tables 16.1–16.4).[6]

Acepromazine at 0.1–0.3 mg/kg i.m or s.c. can be used for sedation and also for induction. One author uses acepromazine at 0.1 mg/kg s.c. because of possible prolonged effect with hypertension being secondary to a marked peripheral vasodilatation.[1]

Midazolam at 5 mg/kg can be used with ketamine (5–10 mg/kg) and atropine (0.05 mg/kg) i.m. or s.c. as a premedication before gaseous anaesthesia. This combination is not sufficient for surgery on its own but only short-term sedation with relaxation.

Table 16.6 A selection of my ferret operations using a ketamine/xylazine combination

Ferret name	Weight (g)	Operation	Ketamine/xylazine dose (mL)	Recovery time, approx. (h)
Hector	1400	Radiograph	0.25/0.1	1
Snowy	1400	Teeth scale	0.5/0.05	2
Spike	1300	Castration	0.2/0.05	½
Boysie	1220	Radiograph	0.25/0.1	1
Hector	1200	Castration	0.3/0.3	3
Randy	1020	Castration	0.25/0.1	1
Penny	1000	Radiograph	0.2/0.1	1
Josie	1000	Teeth	0.2/0.1	1
Heidi	1000	Radiograph	0.2/0.1	1
Bandit	900	Teeth	0.2/0.05	1½
Tyke	800	Radiograph	0.25/0.1	1
Sasha	800	Facial abscess	0.25/0.05	¾
Paleface	760	Facial abscess	0.25/0.1	1
Penny	880	Ear tumour	0.2/0.1	½[a]
Tyke	1280	Teeth	0.25/0.1	2[b]

[a]Reversine used at 0.4 mL i.v. post-operation. [b]Reversine used at 0.2 mL i.v. post-operation.

Table 16.7 Drugs that can be used for premed or sedation

Commercial drugs for ferrets	Premedication effect (mg/kg)	Sedation (mg/kg)
Atropine	0.05 s.c. basically to dry oral and bronchial fluids	
Acepromazine		0.25–0.75 i.m., s.c.
Xylazine		0.5–2.0 i.m., s.c.
Diazepam	Muscle relaxation	i.m. (cannot be given s.c.)
Midazolam	Benzodiazepine compound related to diazepam	Water soluble so can be given s.c.
Glycopyrrolate	0.01 s.c. reduces gastric secretions and hypermotility	

Note: Yohimbine hydrochloride plus 4-aminopyridine (Reversine SA) is able to reverse xylazine; it is registered only for dogs and cats. It can be given to ferrets but only by intravenous injection. I have tended to use xylazine at the lower dose and mostly without recourse to reversine postoperatively.

Ketamine plus acepromazine combination

Ketamine hydrochloride and acepromazine mixed 9:1 by volume at dosage 35 mg/kg i.m. has been found good for 30–35 minute anaesthesia by Burke.[12] Ketamine 10–20 mg/kg plus 0.05 mL ACP 2 mg/mL can be used to sedate a ferret before masking down with halothane and intubating (B. Alderton, pers. comm. 2005).

The major gaseous anaesthetics are now halothane and isoflurane and the newer sevoflurane (in USA). Table 16.8 indicates features of halothane and isoflurane.

Ketamine plus halothane combination

The use of ketamine and a gaseous anaesthestic such as halothane makes for easier ferret surgery. Halothane is used on its own or in the ketamine/halothane combination commonly in Australian general practice though American sources would advise using the more expensive

Author's clinical example

Ketamine/halothane anaesthesia

Subject: Albino jill, Flash, 9 years old, weight 900 g. Early case, ex-working ferret in poor condition (1983) for euthanasia with permission to do practice spaying operation. Flash was held and given 0.5 mL ketamine i.m. and placed in a cat basket and immediately collapsed. Put on the operating table on her side, she was found incoordinate, unable to rise and had some resistance to jaw movement. Heart rate checked at 30/15 s, with irregular bursts up and down. Respiratory rate 9/15 s and very shallow. Flash was placed on her back, still resistant to jaw movement, and given oxygen (500 mL/min) and 0.5% halothane via Fluotec-3 and mask and showed signs of slight leg quivering. The ferret lay stretched out with steady breathing, forelegs in air, shivering slightly. She was found to have pedal reflex in hind legs. Halothane was increased to 1% and a spay operation was performed. Halothane was increased to 5% without killing the ferret and finally, she was euthanized. Time span to do this operation was 30 minutes approximately. *Note* the higher ketamine dose plus use of halothane made the spaying operation possible.

Table 16.8 Comparative features of halothane and isoflurane used as the major gaseous anaesthetics for ferrets

Halothane (potent inhalation agent) Induction 2–4% Maintenance 0.8–2%	Isoflurane (potent inhalation agent) Induction 3–4% Maintenance 1.5–3%
High concentrations at room temperature, delivery from precision vaporizer (Fluotec) recommended.	High concentrations at room temperature, delivery from precision vaporizer (Isotec) recommended.
Administer by mask or endotracheal tube.	Administer by mask or endotracheal tube.
Rapid induction and recovery.	Rapid induction and recovery; faster than halothane.
Can be used with or without premedication.	Can be used with or without premedication.
Atropine should be used although halothane is not so irritant to mucous membranes as isoflurane.	Atropine should be used, as isoflurane is irritant to mucous membranes.
Lower concentrations required for maintenance than isoflurane.	Higher concentrations required for maintenance than halothane.
Vapour concentration-dependent depression of blood pressure.	Vapour concentration-dependent depression of blood pressure.
Cardiac depression greater with halothane; depression of cardiac output and rate are dose-dependent. Catecholamine-induced dysrhythmias more likely.	Less cardiac depression than halothane. Cardiac output better maintained than with halothane. Heart rate shows little change. Cardiac dysrhythmias less likely.
Vapour concentration-dependent depression of respiratory function.	Vapour concentration-dependent depression of respiratory function. Depression slightly greater than with halothane.
About 20–25% metabolized.	Less than 1% metabolized.
Anaesthesia should be visually monitored.	Anaesthesia should be visually monitored.
A relatively cheap drug at the present time.	A relatively expensive drug at the present time.

Table compiled with major assistance from Dr L. Cullen, Senior Anaesthesiologist, Division of Veterinary and Biomedical Science, Murdoch University, Perth, Western Australia.

isoflurane. The combination of ketamine (20–40 mg/kg) plus either halothane or isoflurane by mask can be used on the pet skunk, the ferret's cousin.[1] There have been opinions given on the relative advantages and disadvantages of the two main gaseous anaesthetics for use for ferrets.[13–16] Essential for using gaseous anaesthesia would be a Fluotec-3 calibrated for halothane. *Note*: isoflurane cannot be used in the same Fluotec-3 without recalibrating it. Two units would be required which we had in series. The re-breathing bag should have the capacity of 5–6 times the animal's tidal volume.[17] In the ferret, a 0.5 L bag is suitable. A set of small clear plastic facemasks and series of endotracheal tubes from 2–3 mm are required.

The use of isoflurane anaesthesia on ferrets is now common-place in ferret practices. An assessment of the gas for inducing anaesthesia in ferrets and rats was done by Imai et al.[18] The reaction of the ferrets to four different dose rates of isoflurane are considered here. They used eight weighed healthy ferrets to determine the minimum alveolar concentration (MAC) of isoflurane at each of four MAC values of 0.8, 1.0 and 1.5 and 2.0. An assessment of anaesthesia depth from heart rate and other parameters was made as shown in Table 16.9.

Note, from Table 16.9, respiratory arrest was seen in three ferrets during the 2.0 MAC trials with conditions, which at the exact moment of arrest were not constant so the data were incomplete.

Table 16.9 shows the change of heart beat rate and respiratory rate across the four MAC values and, as anaesthetic dose increases, the systolic arterial blood pressure (SAP), mean arterial blood pressure (MAP) and diastolic blood pressure (DAP) decrease. Details shown in the table indicate the respiration frequency increased progressively from 25 ± 2 breaths/min at 0.8 MAC to peak at 38 ± 3 breaths/min at 1.5 MAC and then decreased to 18 ± 4 at 2.0 MAC in these cases.

With the haematology variables, as the anaesthetic dosage increased the arterial blood pH decreased. The $PaCO_2$ at 0.8 MAC was higher than that normally attributed to the resting conscious ferret at about 40 mmHg. However, it increased in small additions as a direct result of the isoflurane concentration. The $PasCO_2$ showed a greatly increased figure at 2.0 MAC to that at 0.8 MAC. The partial pressure of oxygen (PaO_2) however decreased slightly as the anaesthetic isoflurane increased to 2.0 MAC. The table shows that the PaO_2 at 2.0 MAC was greatly decreased compared to the value at 0.8 MAC.

Study of the eye movement is always one of the key factors when assessing a ferret, or any animal, under anaesthesia (see Ketamine). From the table, it is seen that eye aperture is related to the isoflurane dose rate and thus the eyelid aperture is significantly greater at 2.0 MAC than at the 0.8 MAC. However, the horizontal pupil diameter at each MAC stage was practically constant. Also, the vertical pupil diameter is not changed much at 1.5 or 2.0 MAC but was much greater than the values at 0.8 and 1.0 MAC. Globe rotation downwards was noted at 0.8 MAC in six ferrets but returned to the central position at all other three MAC points in the experiment. *Note*: palpebral and corneal reflexes were evident at 0.8 MAC in six ferrets but not detected at the other MAC values while neither lacrimation nor nystagmus were a feature of the isoflurane experiment. It was concluded by the authors that MAP and $PaCO_2$ changes in ferrets under isoflurane along with changes in the eyelid aperture are consistent guides to changes in depth of anaesthesia.

The basics of modern inhalant anaesthetics from halothane, methoxyflurane, enflurane, isoflurane, desflurane and sevoflurane has been assessed in dogs, cats, rabbits and rats, but not ferrets, by Keegan.[19] The point is made regarding MAC that 1 MAC is equivalent to 1 MAC sevoflurane (now used in ferrets), although the concentrations required to reach MAC (1.3% for isoflurane, 2.25 % for sevoflurane) are quite different. The potency of each inhalant is implicit in the MAC value and this value will vary between species. Johnson-Delaney (see below) advocates using sevoflurane with care and switching to isoflurane after induction with the inhalant gas.

Ketamine plus isoflurane combination

In the opinion of many, isoflurane is the drug of choice for anaesthesia in ferrets. Like halothane however, there are differing opinions on the advantages and disadvantages of isoflurane.[15–17] For the Australian practitioner, the high cost of isoflurane has been a factor but this has changed. Many practices that contact me about ferrets are using halothane. It also depends on the workload of operations on ferrets for its economic use and the American caseload with ferrets is very much higher at the moment than other countries. Isoflurane is less hepatotoxic than halothane. However, good vapour extraction from the operating theatre can diminish the risk with all gas anaesthetics. I would be doubtful of gas chamber anaesthesia of ferrets.

From the point of view of the expense of isoflurane, the switch to conserving gas by intubation of ferrets is essential. I have used isoflurane on ferret spays and castrations but still using a facemask. It is stated however that for very debilitated ferrets or those where work is done on the mouth or head they should be routinely intubated and isoflurane used (S. Brown, pers. comm. 1998).

Ferret intubation

One method of ferret intubation is to use a chamber induction, with isoflurane, until the ferret is recumbent

Table 16.9 Isoflurane assessment in ferrets

	Minimum alveolar concentration (MAC)			
	0.8	1.0	1.5	2.0
Number of ferrets	8	8	8	5[a]
Heart rate (bpm)	244	228	209	221
Arterial blood pressure (mmHg)				
Systolic	104.8	76.6	48.3	47.2
Mean	75.0	57.3	37.9	35.7
Diastolic	60.1	47.6	32.7	29.9
Respiration rate/min	25	30	38	18
Arterial pH	7.205	7.179	7.15	6.929
Arterial P_{CO_2} (mmHg)	71.4	78.1	82.7	158.5
Arterial P_{O_2} (mmHg)	469	443	429	315
Eye features				
Eyelid aperture (cm)	0.26	0.27	0.33	0.38
Pupil diameter (cm)				
Horizontal	0.32	0.32	0.39	0.46
Vertical	0.16	0.21	0.32	0.44
Eyeball position				
Down	In 6 ferrets	0	0	0
Up	0	0	0	0
Centre	In 2 ferrets	In 8 ferrets	In 8 ferrets	In 5 ferrets
Palpebral reflex				
+	In 6 ferrets	0	0	0
−	In 2 ferrets	In 8 ferrets	In 8 ferrets	In 5 ferrets
Corneal reflex				
+	In 6 ferrets	0	0	0
−	In 2 ferrets	In 8 ferrets	In 8 ferrets	In 5 ferrets
Lacrimation				
+	0	0	0	0
−	In 8 ferrets	In 8 ferrets	In 8 ferrets	In 5 ferrets
Nystagmus				
+	0	0	0	0
−	In 8 ferrets	In 8 ferrets	In 8 ferrets	In 5 ferrets
Light response				
+	In 7 ferrets	In 3 ferrets	0	0
−	In 1 ferret	In 5 ferrets	In 8 ferrets	In 5 ferrets
Haematology				
PCV (%)	37.2	35.0	36.0	43.4
Total protein (g/dL)	4.8	4.9	4.86	5.1

Modified from Imai et al.[18] *Note* simplification acknowledges the original data was presented as mean ± deviation and starts from time zero. [a]With MAC 2.0 the data were from only five ferrets as three died of respiratory arrest.

CHAPTER SIXTEEN
Anaesthesia and radiology

and transfer to mask to procure the necessary sedation to allow intubation. An indwelling catheter can be positioned so that, e.g. ketamine (6–10 mg/kg) could be used for i.v. induction. The cephalic saphenous or jugular veins are available and it might be necessary to make a small puncture by the side of the vein with a 15 scalpel or hypodermic needle so that the catheter needle can pass more easily through the skin and into the vein.[20]

Note: the 2.0 to 2.5 mm ID uncuffed endotracheal tube is used for ferrets under 800 g. For 1000 g ferrets and over, the size up to 3.5 mm ID uncuffed or even the 3.0 ID cuffed. In an emergency, the 2.0 mm ID tube can be used for most ferrets.

The larynx can be observed via a laryngoscope and the tubing is made easier if the assisting nurse holds the ferret's mouth open using shoelaces around the upper and lower canine teeth once a suitable anaesthetic depth is reached (Fig. 16.2). The tongue should be pulled forward and the ferret neck held extended. One author advises the use of 0.05 mL lidocaine (lignocaine) sprayed on the larynx to avoid laryngospasm during intubation[1] but it can be done without.[11]

Isoflurane has a pungent odour and causes tissue irritation, unlike halothane. Although halothane causes some salivation, the orthoprotective reflexes, while under induction avoid problems in the ferret which is not tubed. Thus atropine is required as a premedication with isoflurane more so than with halothane. *Note:* 0.1 mL of 0.65% atropine solution is taken and 1.2 mL of sterile water added to make 1.3 mL. Then 0.5 mL of this solution can be given s.c. before any gas anaesthesia (Cullen, pers. comm. 1996).

I used ketamine as a premedication before induction with isoflurane. Some authors suggest masking down with isoflurane only, using an oxygen flow rate of 1 L and

Author's clinical example
Ketamine/isoflurane anaesthesia for ovariohysterectomy operation

Subject: Sable jill, Pandy, 1 year old, weight 680 g. Pandy was given 0.15 mL ketamine i.m. plus 0.5 mL atropine (diluted) s.c., was placed in a cat basket, and showed sedation under the ketamine. She was then transferred to the operating table and the normal procedure for ferret spay set up. Pandy was masked and given a cautious 1% isoflurane with oxygen (1000 mL/min). The 1% isoflurane was given for 15 seconds and then reduced to 0.5% while she was prepared for operation with oxygen reduced to 500 mL/min. The oxygen flow was increased to 1000 mL/min and the isoflurane increased to 2.5% for the duration of the spay operation. Then the isoflurane was reduced to 0.5% as the skin sutures were done. The operation was finished in 38 minutes and the jill was placed in recovery cage. Pandy was walking around 1 hour later. This case illustrates a first time cautious approach to using ketamine plus isoflurane in respect to possible severe respiratory depression with the latter agent.

5% isoflurane. The ferret quickly relaxes and is usually anaesthetized in 1–3 minutes. A rate of 2–3% isoflurane is required for a surgical plane of anaesthesia. Recovery time is quicker than under halothane but as long as the ferret is recovering smoothly, this is academic. It is considered that 'probably the greatest drawback of isoflurane, like other volatile anaesthetic agents, is that it might produce appreciable cardiopulmonary depression particularly when high alveolar concentrations are attained. Cardiac output is depressed less by isoflurane than by equipotent concentrations of halothane but the respiratory depression is greater at least in the surgically unstimulated patient.'[15,16] In other words a severe apnoea in inducing anaesthesia can occur in isoflurane administration as for halothane administration. Thus, the slow cautious approach to induction with either agent is advisable in ferrets as in other animals. This applies to the new sevoflurane.

There is some discussion about the use of atropine in ferrets. There is an opinion that it should definitely be used for anaesthetics such as isoflurane, ketamine and tiletamine/zolazepam (Zoletil 20) at low dosage (Cullen, pers. comm. 1996). I have not used it with halothane but definitely with isoflurane, though American veterinarians doing cancer therapy on ferrets will mask down with isoflurane to catheterize ferrets without premedication.

Note: The new gaseous anaesthetic sevoflurane gives an extremely rapid induction. It is very sensitive and ferrets have to be extremely closely monitored. It can

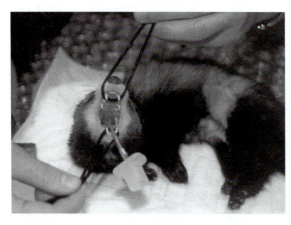

Figure 16.2 Intubating a ferret. *Note* the use of shoelaces to keep jaws open for placing endotracheal tube. (Courtesy of B. Alderton, Sydney, Australia.)

be used for induction, as the ferret will be anaesthetized in 10 seconds, and then revert to isoflurane for a safer anaesthetic time (D. Kemmerer-Cottrell, pers. comm. 2005). The effects of sevoflurane on blood haemodynamics and cardiac energetic parameters have been trialed in seven healthy domesticated ferrets.[21] The expired concentrations of sevoflurane at 1.25%, 2.5% and 3.75% were checked by blood sampling.

Used as a sole agent sevoflurane was found to cause minimal and predictable cardiovascular effects without increasing myocardial demands. Intra-abdominal surgery was required to permit instrumentation while under sevoflurane anaesthesia and the ferrets were finally euthanized.

Note: no adverse reaction was seen in the seven ferrets individually placed in an induction chamber with sevoflurane. They lost their 'rightening' reflex in about 2 minutes.

Sevoflurane is similar in action to isoflurane by inducing a stable heart rate and rhythm. It is known that all volatile inhalant anaesthetics can cause a certain amount of hypotension as well as a reduction in myocardial contractility. There is some concern about the use of sevoflurane in ferrets having cardiomyopathy as the gas may contribute to 'coronary steal' (coronary vasodilation causing redistribution of collateral blood flow away from ischaemic regions).

The authors noted that only partial examination has been made regarding the effect of sevoflurane on myocardial relaxation in normal and diseased hearts. It might be of interest to know that the ferret is still considered to be an excellent 'model' for cardiovascular research because of its small size and cheapness to house and care. Physically, the ferret heart has a well differentiated conduction system, like rats, a dominant left coronary artery, for surgical use, good heart mechanical and electrical stability, large energy reserve, plus slower basal heart rate and higher arterial pressure than rats. The ferret is unfortunately better suited for research into myocardial ischaemic injury than the rat.

Aspects of ferret anaesthesia involving ketamine

Some concerns have been raised about the use of ketamine with medetomidine, in that ketamine tends to increase heart rate and medetomidine may decrease blood pressure (Cathy Johnson-Delaney [C J-D], pers. comm. 2005). This combination is not good if the ferret has an underlying cardiomyopathy. The medetomidine can be reversed but the heart might not be able to cope with the ketamine effect and atropine may be no help. Dangerous low blood pressure might occur. The effect of vagal reflex during anaesthesia, intubation and response to various anaesthetics on the ferret cardiovascular function should be closely watched.

It has been suggested that ferrets and rabbits react in shock and anaesthesia just like cats but C J-D refutes this, finding that ferrets have a huge vagal response and can have massive histamine release, and apparently gastroenteritis problems which cats and rabbits do not get. It is thought that better surgical survival and lower stress are obtained by doing antihistamine protocols in addition to atropine and preoperative analgesia/sedation.

Cathy Johnson-Delaney (C J-D) protocol

It has been stressed that a ferret undergoing surgery should have a pre-operation physical examination which involves the cardiac and respiratory systems. Where available, all modern equipment, e.g. audio Doppler ultrasonic flow detector, should be used to check heart valve function. The ECG should be available to monitor any cardiac fluctuations.[22]

Note: in ferret cases where cardiomyopathy is suspected the use of echocardiography is useful. Blood pres-

Table 16.10 Cathy Johnson-Delaney's protocol for ferret operations (preoperative injections)

Drug	Dosage	Comment
Famotidine (10 mg/mL)	2.5 mg per ferret i.m. or slow i.v.	Decreases stomach acid production and oesophageal reflux
Diphendyramine HCL (10 or 50 mg/mL)	1.0–2.0 mg/kg i.v.	For anaphylaxis, vaccine reaction
s.c. fluids dextrose 50%	Use 1 mL added to 15–20 mL LRS or saline for s.c. fluids/kg	Pre- and postop 2–3 drops dextrose sublingual to aid hypoglycaemic recovery
Atropine (1/120 grains/mL 0.54 mg/mL)	0.1 mg/kg s.c. may be repeated by 0.05 mg/kg i.v. or s.c. as needed during surgery for stability	Pre-anaesthesia: treats bradycardia and hypermotility plus hypersecretions
Butorphanol (2 mg/mL)	0.2 mg/kg s.c.	Analgesic, sedative for pre-op.

CHAPTER SIXTEEN

Anaesthesia and radiology

Table 16.11 The use of Domitor/Vetelar/Antisedan combination

	Domitor 1 mg/mL i.m.	Vetelar[a] 50 mg/mL ½ normal strength i.m.	Antisedan 5 mg/mL i.m.
Dose rate	120 µg/kg Volume (mL)	10 mg/kg Volume (mL)	0.6 mg/kg Volume (mL)
Body weight of ferret (g)			
500	0.06	0.10	0.06
600	0.07	0.12	0.07
700	0.08	0.14	0.08
800	0.10	0.16	0.10
900	0.11	0.18	0.11
1000	0.12	0.20	0.12
1100	0.13	0.22	0.13
1200	0.14	0.24	0.14
1300	0.16	0.26	0.16
1400	0.17	0.28	0.17
1500	0.18	0.30	0.18
1600	0.19	0.32	0.19
1700	0.20	0.34	0.20
1800	0.22	0.36	0.22
1900	0.23	0.38	0.23
2000	0.24	0.40	0.24
2100	0.25	0.42	0.25
2200	0.26	0.44	0.26

[a]Vetelar (ketamine) UK 100 mg/mL
Note: dose rates can be halved if sedation only is needed. Table courtesy of M. Oxenham, pers. comm. 1997.

sure monitoring using the Doppler ultrasonic flow detector is achieved by connection to a cuffed limb.

Operative procedure

C J-D anaesthetizes the ferret with isoflurane via a facemask and intubation is done after the larynx is sprayed with topical cetacaine. Having indwelling venous catheters for giving fluids during operation over a long period is routine (Table 16.10).

Once set up on the gas machine, the ferret's vital signs should continue to be monitored, e.g. ECG and electronic rectal probe thermometer. The pulse oximeter has a use but C J-D maintains the SpO_2 may still be normal even after the ferret has died. Side stream capnography equipment for the measurement of metabolic changes requires ferret intubation and is expensive.

The ferret body heat must be maintained as discussed earlier and the use of water-heated blankets, etc. is necessary.

Possible irregularities in the general ferret operation

It has been known that some apparently normal ferrets, 3-year-old or less, under anaesthesia succumb to cardiac irregularities with isoflurane, which do not respond to atropine. The vagal reflex is set off by head and neck movement, pressure on the chest and some possibly unknown agents. Thus, heart rate can fall rapidly and can even stop. The re-use of atropine may be required to compensate and steady the heart rate.

Other factors that affect cardiac rhythm include histamine release in undetected gastrointestinal ulceration, pressure on major abdominal arteries and major haemorrhage. It might be noted in these cases that the ferret stays on a steady anaesthetic level but then suddenly the heart rate dives from 165 to 185 bpm to zero. There might be warning signs of minor arrhythmias and the decrease of the QRS complex. It is seen that handling of the gastrointestinal tract can give rise to ventricular premature contractions.

C J-D warns that the irregularities may occur *after* the gas anaesthetic agent is stopped. For that reason, she tends to keep the ECG linked up after the operation is finished. The preferred postoperative body temperature should be 37.7–38.8°C, with a systolic blood pressure above 90 mmHg.

C J-D asserts that with proper supportive care in the postoperative period and with the pre-operative, or perhaps postoperative, use of the drugs listed above, the likelihood of complications can be reduced.

Cardiac arrest during surgery

C J-D advises the ABC (airway, breathing, circulation) protocol swing into action with ferret cardiac arrest on the operating table or wherever. The gaseous anaesthetic is stopped, airway checked, oxygen administered by tube or face mask.

Gently squeeze the ferret chest in the region of the heart 15 times, aiming to generate a beat of at least 100 bpm. This carries on while the respiration is dealt with. Blowing over the ferret muzzle may be effective on the respiration as in mouth-to-mouth techniques.

These efforts will be monitored by the use of ECG, Doppler and stethoscope. However, if there is no heart response in 30–60 seconds, use epinephrine i.c., i.v. or i.os. at 0.2 mg/kg. With the heart started but showing bradycardia, give atropine i.v. at 0.05 mg/kg or via the trachea at 0.10 mg/kg.

Doxapram is good as a respiratory stimulant at 5–10 mg/kg i.v., i.c., intratracheally, intraperitoneally or sublingually.[22]

New anaesthetic drugs for possible use in ferrets

In recent times, new anaesthetic drugs marketed for intramuscular use in dogs and cats have been trialed on ferrets, though they are not registered for this species. I tried out medetomidine hydrochloride (Domitor) and atipamezole hydrochloride (Antisedan) in 1994 on my own and others' ferrets around the same time that Mike Oxenham (UK) was trialing these drugs with ketamine (Table 16.11). Domitor has the advantage over ketamine-xylazine anaesthesia in that Domitor can be reversed with Antisedan by the intramuscular route while xylazine needs to be reversed by intravenous yohimbine (Reversine), which might be difficult in some ferret cases.

Medetomidine hydrochloride (Domitor), is a sedative and analgesic registered for dogs and cats. This drug is a potent selective and specific α^2-adrenoreceptor antagonist. The α^2-adrenoreceptor activation by medetomidine induces a dose-dependent decrease in release and turnover of noradrenaline in the CNS, which manifests itself as sedation, analgesia and bradycardia.[11,23] Vasoconstriction occurs in the peripheral blood vessels by the activation of post-synaptic α^2-adrenoreceptors in the vascular smooth muscle with the rest of the initial blood pressure increase after the drug's injection. The pressure reverts to normal, or slightly below, within 1–2 hours. The respiratory frequency may be temporarily lowered. The duration and degree of sedation and analgesia with Domitor use is of course dose-related. Typically, during the maximal effect the animal is relaxed, will lie down and is not reactive to external stimuli.[23] *Note*: there is a marked synergistic effect between medetomidine and cyclohexamine compounds such as ketamine and also between medetomidine and drugs such as fentanyl, producing deep anaesthesia. Medetomidine also has the potent ability to reduce the dose requirements of volatile anaesthetics like halothane. Thus, the drug has potential use with ferret anaesthesia. Medetomidine is rapidly absorbed from intramuscular injections, well-distributed in the CNS and also readily metabolized and excreted in the urine and faeces. The peak concentration of the drug is reached within 15–20 minutes and eliminated from the body after 1 hour or so.

Domitor is not recommended for use in pregnant animals and is to be used with care in cats and dogs with cardiovascular, respiratory, liver or kidney disease or poor general health; the same applies no doubt to ferrets. The concomitant use of other CNS depressants would naturally potentiate either drug so cautious dose adjustments should be made. Domitor decreases the heart rate and body temperature and sedated animals should be kept warm in an even temperature for 12 hours, postoperatively. Dogs and cats on Domitor may vomit but this has not been a problem with ferrets. Muscle-jerking, as observed in the dog and cat, has been seen in ferrets but with no adverse effects. *Note* the use of atropine or glycopyrrolate to correct the bradycardia effect is dangerous because it can cause severe hypertension.[24]

Atipamezole hydrochloride (Antisedan)

This drug is the reversal agent for medetomidine and acts s.c. or i.m. with rapid onset being more than 200–300 times greater in affinity for α^2-adrenoreceptors than yohimbine or idazoxan.[24]

CHAPTER SIXTEEN
Anaesthesia and radiology

Author's clinical examples

Domitor use in ferrets

1. A 1400 g hob ferret, Snowy, for vasectomy stitches to be removed. If a working/breeding stock ferret hob they might be difficult to handle. Snowy was wrapped in towel and given 0.05 mL Domitor i.m., placed in cat basket and quickly sedated. He was placed on the table and the stitches were easily removed. He was then given 0.1 mL Antisedan i.m. for complete reversal in minutes. *Note*: the dosage of Antisedan for cats is half the Domitor volume but it is impossible to measure dosage with ferrets and 0.05 or 0.1 mL worked with no adverse reactions.

2. Treatment of a 1600 g hob ferret, Alby, with facial fight wound abscess. *Time sequence*: 2 p.m., Alby was given 0.1 mL Domitor i.m. with immediate sedation. Then it was possible to lance the abscess and treat with antibiotics. At 2.10 p.m., he was given 0.1 mL Antisedan i.m. and was fully recovered by 2.25 p.m. There were no adverse reactions.

3. A 960 g jill, Heidi, for radiograph. *Time sequence*: 9.43 a.m., Heidi given 0.1 mL Domitor i.m. and at 9.46 a.m. she was relaxed enough to be placed in dorsal recumbency on the X-ray table and radiographed. At 9.48 a.m., Heidi was placed on the operating table for an ear check and nail trimming. At 9.54 a.m., she was given 0.1 mL Antisedan i.m. and placed in a warm cage to recover. By 9.58 a.m., Heidi moving and attempting to walk and went on to complete recovery. There were no adverse reactions.

4. A 1000 g hob ferret, Tyke, for blood sampling from jugular vein and tail artery. *Time sequence*: 9.00 a.m., he was given 0.06 mL Domitor i.m. At 9.02 a.m., Tyke was relaxed for blood taking. At 9.12 a.m., he was given 0.06 mL Antisedan i.m. and put in a recovery cage and was walking at 9.22 a.m. There were no adverse reactions.

Domitor plus Antisedan combination in ferrets

A dosage of medetomidine hydrochloride has been given for the ferret as 100 μg/kg s.c to give light-to-moderate sedation in 1997.[24] I used the drug in 1994 scaling down the dose from the cat and using it cautiously.[25] For cats the Domitor moderate sedation dose is 50–100 μg/kg which equates to 0.25–0.5 mL/ 5 kg animal. For deep sedation, Domitor needs to be 100–150 μg/kg which equates to 0.5–0.75 mL/5 kg animal. *Note*: the Antisedan needs only to be half the dose (volume) of the Domitor to reverse its action. Ferrets weigh 500–1600 g (hobs possibly to 2000 g) and using a low cat dose (0.25 mL/5 kg), I scaled down to 0.050 mL/1.25 kg (1250 g ferret). The dose was given in the usual tuberculin/insulin syringes.

Domitor plus ketamine plus Antisedan combination

This combination has been described by Oxenham in the UK – I tried it out independently in 1994.

Domitor and ketamine given separately

Author's clinical examples

1. Castration of 900g hob, Tuppy

I decided to use a dose of 0.05 mL Domitor plus 0.25 mL ketamine. Unlike Oxenham, I did not mix the drugs but gave the Domitor first.

Time sequence:

2.16 p.m.	Tuppy was given 0.05 mL Domitor i.m. and placed in cat basket where he collapsed with licking lips and yawns; moved slightly but looked sedated in a couple of minutes and was placed on operating table.
2.20 p.m.	He was placed on his back and rolled over. After 1 minute he was placed again on his back and he stayed in position. He allowed examination without interference.
2.25 p.m.	Tuppy was given 0.25 mL ketamine i.m. in other leg muscle.
2.26 p.m.	He was relaxed and breathing steadily with loss of sensation to allow castration operation.
2.30 p.m.	Castration operation completed.
2.34 p.m.	Tuppy was given 0.1 mL Antisedan i.m. and was left on the operating table (respiratory rate 48/min). Decreased to 40/min and stabilized.
2.42 p.m.	He was given 0.25 mL chloramphenicol i.m.
2.45 p.m.	Tuppy's jaw was tight and his body quivering. Eye reflex was present. Possibly the effects of ketamine, as the medetomidine would be the quicker drug eliminated from the body.
2.47 p.m.	He was placed on his left side on a towel in a recovery cage in a warm room.
3.00 p.m.	Then turned onto his right side. Now shows jaw muscle tone and tongue extended.
3.10 p.m.	Repeated turning of Tuppy to other side.
3.30 p.m.	Now legs moving and also lip licking.
3.45 p.m.	He was now paddling with legs, licking lips and head arched back as seen in ketamine anaesthesia. He continued in this manner until 6.15 p.m. when Tuppy was fully recovered and then taken home. There were no adverse reactions.

2. Teeth scale of 1300g hob, Snowy

Time sequence:

12.10 p.m.	He was given 0.20 mL Domitor i.m., placed in a cat basket on the floor and collapsed in 2 minutes.
12.15 p.m.	Snowy was given 0.25 mL ketamine in other leg muscle.
12.20 p.m.	He was breathing easily and relaxed on the operating table and it was easy to do the teeth scale.
12.25 p.m.	Teeth scale now finished, Snowy was given 0.2 mL Antisedan i.m. and then placed in a recovery cage in a warm room.
12.35 p.m.	Snowy showed head movements and proceeded to slowly recover.
5.00 p.m.	Snowy only then really mobile and taken home. There were no adverse reactions.

It is stated by the manufacturer of Domitor (Ciba Geigy) that any medetomidine-induced bradycardia is counteracted by ketamine-induced cardiac stimulation. *Note* the above two cases show a slow recovery to Domitor plus ketamine anaesthesia, where the two drugs are given apart. The recovery is somewhat quicker in the Oxenham method of giving the two drugs together. However, if the patients can be kept overnight to recover and rest, the former process seems to have no adverse effects.

Domitor and ketamine given together

This combination was used by Oxenham in the UK and recorded in chart form (June 1994). The drugs have been used in combination on zoo short-clawed otters. Oxenham recommended the drugs for all general surgery in the ferret which in his experience covers spaying, castration, vasectomy, laparotomy, leg amputation, tumour removal, wound repair, abscesses, blood sampling and radiology. He stated that some ferrets had been very ill and debilitated but no fatalities were experienced with the combined drugs. He had been concerned about possible respiratory depression when using the ketamine plus xylazine combination (Oxenham, pers. comm. 1994). It is suggested that once the anaesthesia is induced, respiration for the Domitor plus ketamine combination has been noticed to be shallow for about 5 minutes but oxygen can be supplemented with a facemask. The ferrets are not intubated. An accurate ferret body weight is required as usual for anaesthesia, to the nearest 20 g using a good quality spring balance and canvas ferret-carrying bag with purse string cord. Accurate kitchen scales can also be used. The drugs are given in 1 mL tuberculin syringes and using 22–25 gauge needles, as is standard for ferrets. *Note*: as the quantity of keta-

Author's clinical example

Teeth scale of 720g jill, Nipper

Time sequence:

2.50 p.m.	She was held and given 0.08 mL Domitor, plus 0.14 mL (50/50 solution) ketamine (Table 16.10) in the same tuberculin syringe via quadriceps muscle and placed in a cat basket. She collapsed in 2 minutes. Nipper was then placed on the operating table and the teeth scale easily done.
3.00 p.m.	She was given 0.08 mL Antisedan i.m. in opposite leg, then placed into a cage in a warm room and observed for reaction.
3.16 p.m.	Nipper was seen still in lateral recumbency but shaking and with jaw tensed on checking.
3.29 p.m.	She was moving unsteadily around the cage and had a sneezing fit.
3.55 p.m.	She was now moving around the cage but was still unsteady.
6.00 p.m.	Nipper curled up in natural position, sleeping. There were no adverse reactions.

mine to be used is so small, it is advised that a 50/50 solution of the 100 mg/mL stock bottle be used. This gives a 50 mg/mL strength (see detailed Table 16.11). Unlike my first method, the drugs are mixed together in the same syringe and given by intramuscular injection into the quadriceps muscle. In this way, the onset of anaesthesia is about 2 minutes, which I have also found using this technique. At the finish, the Antisedan is given the same as Domitor dose to reverse. I have found the reversal effect occurring from 6 to 12 minutes, with the ferret recovering slowly. It is also suggested by Oxenham that because of the pharmacological action of Domitor, it is unnecessary to premedicate with atropine but the drug should be used with all other anaesthetics.

The use of Domitor plus Antisedan or Domitor plus ketamine plus Antisedan appears acceptable for sedation and anaesthesia. I still use Domitor/50/50 ketamine for any dental work on my own ferrets. Dose rates of these two combinations for sedation and anaesthesia in laboratory ferrets have been given[24] and are shown in Table 16.12.

Note: no reversal agent exists for ketamine but it is a very safe drug for ferrets.

While Mike Oxenham, UK and I were trialing medetomidine and ketamine, an evaluation had been carried out on the two drugs plus butorphanol (analgesic) on ferrets by the University of Florida.[26]

CHAPTER SIXTEEN
Anaesthesia and radiology

Table 16.12 Use of Domitor alone or with ketamine for ferrets

	Use of drug
Domitor plus Antisedan	
Domitor at 100 µg/kg s.c.	Light to moderate anaesthesia
Antisedan at 1 mg/kg s.c., i.p. or i.v.	Reversal of Domitor
Domitor plus ketamine plus Antisedan	
Domitor at 100 µg/kg plus ketamine at 8 mg/kg	Surgical anaesthesia
Antisedan at 1 mg/kg s.c., i.p. or i.v.	Reversal of Domitor

Table 16.13 Domitor (medetomidine) and drug combinations anaesthesia trial

	Group A	Group B	Group C	Group D
Body weight (kg)	1.5	1.6	1.7	1.5
Trial drugs	M	M + B	M + K	M + B + K
Injection to recumbency time (min)	3.4	3.5	2.2	2.4
Loss of palpebral reflex (duration, min)	63.3	92.5	45.0	94.2
Loss of corneal reflex (duration, min)	1.7	13.3	25.0	80.8
Toe pinch analgesia (duration, min)	10.8	90.8	48.3	93.3
Skin pinch analgesia (duration, min)	20.8	92.5	61.7	91.7
Tail pinch analgesia (duration, min)	16.7	91.7	60.8	95.0
Time between injection and intubation (min)	NA	19.2	9.2	7.5
Duration of intubation (min)	NA	80.8	45.8	92.5
Atipamezole injection time to reverse medetomidine (min)	7.2	8.0	5.7	7.5
Quality score of induction	2.5	2.8	2.8	3.0
Quality score of recovery	3.0	3.0	3.0	3.0

M, medetomidine (Domitor) alone; M + B, medetomidine with butorphanol, M + K, medetomidine with ketamine; M + B + K, medetomidine, butorphanol and ketamine. Adapted from Ko et al.[26] to Table 16.4 style. Bear in mind simplification acknowledges that original data were presented as mean ± deviation and recorded from time zero. NA, not applicable. With group A, sedation was not adequate for procedure.

The project used 10 ferrets which were 1-year-old hobs weighing 1500–2200 g – heavy animals. Each ferret was its own control for the study. The ferrets were fed a commercial ferret food and housed individually. Evaluation of medetomidine (Domitor) alone (M), medetomidine with butorphanol (M + B), medetomidine with ketamine (M + K), and medetomidine, butorphanol and ketamine (M + B + K) together were assessed.

Considering ferret groups as A, B, C, D, and drug combinations as M, M + B, M + K, M + B + K, the effects were as shown in Table 16.13.

In all set cases, the ferrets went into lateral recumbency within 4 minutes and stayed prone for 100 minutes. *Note* the drug uses were extrapolated from the use in cats and the author's experience.

Medetomidine (Domitor) was used i.m. at 80 µg/kg body weight, butorphanol at 0.1 mg/kg and ketamine at 5 mg/kg. In addition, atipamezole (Antisedan) was used i.m. as a reversal of Domitor in some cases. The drugs in combinations were taken up separately and then mixed in a primary syringe. The trial doses were injected into the semitendinosus/semimembranosus muscle of the hind leg. Medetomidine sedation will outlast its analgesic effects and the ferret stays sedated for 3 hours unless reversed by atipamezole. However, the use of butorphanol (80 µg/kg) or ketamine (5 mg/kg) were shown to increase the duration of analgesia.

It was noted that respiratory depression occurred with the medetomidine, butorphanol, ketamine used in combination. Also medetomidine has some analgesic effect with good sedative and muscle relaxation properties. However, prior to the study, a ferret under medetomidine at 80 µg/kg and with ketamine at 100 mg/kg collapsed in 3 minutes and experienced apnoea for more than 80 seconds. Intubation was rapidly done to oxygenate the ferret. When the assisted ventilation was stopped, the ferret became hypoxic rapidly and showed purple membranes. A pulse oximeter read 60% and recovery took over 4 hours.

Oxenham noticed shallow respiration with Domitor/ketamine as indicated previously but only gave extra oxygen by facemask. I found no trouble with prolonged 'scary' apnoeas using the Oxenham protocol (Table 16.11).

Another ferret before the study, given medetomidine (80 µg/kg body weight) and butorphanol (0.2 mg/kg body weight) had extreme respiratory depression as calculated by high exhaled CO_2 concentration. When a dosage of 0.2 mg/kg butorphanol was used with the Domitor/ketamine combination there was another worrying apnoea. Therefore, a dose rate of 0.1 mg/kg butorphanol was thought more prudent.

To evaluate quality of sedation and anaesthesia recovery with ferrets using the three drugs, scoring from 3 (best) to 1 was set up.[26] Note the results in Table 16.13.

Scoring for sedation quality characteristics

3: No outward sign of excitement, ferret rapidly assumes lateral recumbency with good muscle relaxation.
2: Mild signs of excitement, continuous movement, numerous attempts to rise immediately after assuming recumbency, poor muscular relaxation.
1: Hyperkinesis, obvious signs of excitement, does not become recumbent or assumes recumbency briefly, poor muscular relaxation.

Check for above signs in patient post-injection.

Scoring for anaesthesia recovery characteristics

3: Assumes sternal recumbency with little or no struggling, attempts to stand and walk with little or no difficulty.
2: Some struggling, requires assistance to stand, very responsive to external stimuli, becomes quiet in sternal recumbency.
1: Prolonged struggling, unable to assume sternal recumbency or difficulty in maintaining sternal or standing position, becomes hyperkinetic when assisted, prolonged paddling and swimming motion.

Check for above signs in patient post-operation.

The effect of anaesthesia on pulse rate, oxyhaemoglobin saturation, systolic blood pressure, respiration rate and carbon dioxide (CO_2) are considered by the authors. Some conclusions on heart rate are shown in Table 16.14 (as Table 16.2 for ketamine alone).

The pulse rates decreased from the baseline in all four groups with the lowest in A, thought to be due to medetomidine which acts that way in cats and dogs.

Table 16.14 Heart rate (bpm) of ferrets before and during anaesthesia

	Group A	Group B	Group C	Group D
Drugs	M	M + B	M + K	M + B + K
Time post-injection (min)				
0 (unanaesthetized)	225 (197–253)	238 (199–277)	233 (207–259)	235 (215–255)
5	160 (150–170)	156 (143–169)	182 (165–199)	168 (157–179)
10	152 (137–167)	143 (132–154)	173 (157–189)	174 (158–190)
15	137 (125–149)	134 (120–148)	173 (151–195)	171 (156–186)
20	139 (120–158)	130 (116–144)	155 (137–173)	159 (146–172)
30	119 (107–131)	116 (108–124)	148 (130–166)	142 (122–162)
40	114 (100–128)	112 (105–119)	142 (118–166)	129 (113–145)
50	109 (91–127)	108 (100–116)	135 (121–149)	121 9106–136)
60	108 (95–121)	106 (92–120)	130 (110–150)	115 (103–127)
5 min post-Antisedan i.m. after 100 min[a]	130 (114–146)	143 (90–196)	176 (132–220)	163 (110–216)

M, medetomidine (Domitor) alone; M + B, medetomidine with butorphanol, M + K, medetomidine with ketamine; M + B + K, medetomidine, butorphanol and ketamine. Ferrets checked till 100 min. Note pulse rate increase 5 min post-Antisedan i.m. Adapted from Ko et al.[26] to Table 16.2 style. Bear in mind simplification acknowledges that original data were present as mean ± deviation and recorded from time zero.

From 5–50 minutes after injection, the mean pulse rates were higher in the M + K and M + B + K groups than the M and M + B groups. This was due to ketamine as it can stimulate heart rate by direct CNS stimulation.

The SpO_2 reduced in all four groups following drug administration, seen between 10 and 40 minutes post-treatment; the M + B + K group has the lowest at 73.2% . Oxyhaemoglobin saturation above 90% for the anaesthetized ferret is acceptable but hypoxia develops quickly when the SpO_2 falls below 90% and cell death can occur when the SpO_2 is less than 85% for 1–2 minutes. The anaesthetized ferrets were breathing room air. Thus using <90% indicated that M + B + K ferrets could develop hypoxia and thus mask-administered oxygen was suggested with ferrets under this combination.

Cardiac features showed respiratory sinus type arrhythmias, before and after injection of drugs in all groups, ventricular premature contractions (VPCs) and second degree heart blocks occasionally in all groups except M + K.

Respiration was depressed in all groups but importantly more in the M and M + B groups. Though depressed from the baseline in M + K and M + B + K groups, the respiration drop was not significant. The high CO_2 exhaled indicated respiration was more depressed in the M + B and M + B + K groups when compared with the M and M + K groups (at 30–100 minutes). It is considered important by the authors that gaseous oxygen be given to the ferrets anaesthetized by all four methods. The use of Antisedan at five times the dose of Domitor is effective at reversing the sedation 100 minutes following injection of the Domitor i.m. It gives rapid recovery as I have experienced using the Domitor/ketamine/Antisedan combination.

Endotracheal intubation was easier with the M + K and M + B + K groups. With the M group, intubation was impossible and a time delay for the procedure in the M + B group was due possibly to the slow onset of butorphanol action.

The study was compared with anaesthesia using tiletamine/zolazepam, xylazine/ketamine, and tiletamine/zolazepam/ketamine/xylazine groups where there can be moderate to severe salivation and sneezing. When using ketamine alone and xylazine/ketamine, I never found it a problem. It is stated that with medetomidine groups, salivation is minimal.

Note: Finkler records using ketamine, medetomidine and butorphanol i.m. or s.c. for ferret spays, castrations and musk gland removal but using an oxygen mask only for additional isoflurane. He suggests that a ferret can become somewhat hypoxic on all three injectable drugs but not if butorphanol is omitted (M. Finkler, pers. comm. 2005).

Other drugs suggested for use with ferrets

Alphaxalone

At 8–12 mg/kg can be used to give 10–15 minutes surgical anaesthesia but needs to be given i.v. which can be difficult with a possibly wriggling ferret. Most i.v. work on ferrets requires them to be somewhat sedated.

Pentobarbitone

An old anaesthetic drug which at 25–30 mg/kg can give 30–120 minutes anaesthesia but must be given i.v. or i.p. in accurate dose. Adams in 1979 used halothane/oxygen on 72 ranch mink and 20 ferrets with great success and remarked it offered a distinct advantage over pentobarbitone sodium![27] Now pentobarbitone is mostly used for euthanasia of ferrets by i.v. or i.p. routes. *Note*: for ferret euthanasia, the use of meloxicam and acetylpromazine followed by isoflurane overdose is favoured (C J-D, pers. comm. 2005). The Tributame Euthanasia Solution (Embutramide: chloroquine phosphate USP and lidocaine USP. Phoenix Scientific, USA) has been approved for euthanasia by i.v. in dogs and no doubt will be used for ferrets.

Tiletamine/zolazepam (Zoletil 20)

This drug is a combination of the phencyclidine drug tiletamine and the benzodiazepine drug zolazepam, which together in equal proportions give an effective general anaesthetic with quick induction, good muscle relaxation, analgesia and the retention of the laryngeal, pharyngeal, palpebral and corneal reflexes during light or deep anaesthesia. It is a safe drug but relatively expensive and once made up has a short shelf life, which could only be 2 weeks. Zoletil 20 has been used successfully in the wild and zoo animals and is used in the USA. Now only Zoletil 50 and 100 injectable are available in Australia. Use of Zoletil (Virbac Australia Pty) in the Mustelidae is shown in Table 16.15.

The dosage for ferrets has proved to be insufficient and they require 22 mg/kg[28] or 25 mg/kg. Higher doses result in depression and a long recovery period. Alderton finds the drug effects variable and it may need gaseous supplementation.[11] I used 0.4 mL on a 1400 g hob ferret, Sammy, for bite wound surgery and he took 6 hours to recover. One veterinarian used Zoletil 20 on British bulldogs (high anaesthetic risk) and ferrets. He maintained safe results in both species with the ferret being

Table 16.15 Use of Zoletil 20 in Mustelidae

Mustela putorius (Ferret, European polecat)	5.0 mg/kg i.m.
Mustela vison (Mink)	8.0 mg/kg i.m.
Meles meles (Eurasian badger)	9.8 mg/kg i.m.
Mellivoa capensis (Honey badger)	2.2 mg/kg i.m.
Taxiidea taxus (American badger)	4.4 mg/kg i.m.
Mephitis mephitis (Striped skunk)	8.3 mg/kg i.m.

given 12 mg/kg. He had used it on a number of ferrets with body weights from 300–1800 g with anaesthetic times of 30–40 minutes (Dipold, Nowra, NSW, pers. comm. 1997).

Finkler advocates the use of the combination Telazol 3.0 mg/kg (tiletamine–zolazepam) with ketamine 2.4 mg/kg plus xylazine 0.6 mL/kg i.m. with glycopyrrolate 0.01 mg/kg to produce lateral recumbency within 2 minutes, 40 minutes of sedation for endotracheal intubation, and analgesia for 25 to 35 minutes (M. Finkler, pers. comm. 2005). The combination does not cause hypotension but there can be short periods of hypoxia (pulse oximeter reading SpO_2 <90%). Once intubated the combination could be supplemented with isoflurane (1–2%) and on recovery in 90–110 minutes the ferret would be completely mobile.

The time factor for preparation before the first incision varies with the drug numbers used and complications of setting up ancillary equipment and mask or intubation gas anaesthesia. As an example, a ferret with adrenal disease was premedicated with 0.04 mg medetomidine (Domitor) and 4 mg ketamine s.c. Ten minutes later the ferret, weighing 706 g, was masked with 100% oxygen with 3% isoflurane. Once anaesthetized, the ferret was intubated with a modified 14 gauge French urinary catheter and attached to a ventilator (Vetronic Systems). Finally a 24 G intraosseous needle (Cook, UK) was placed into the left tibial tuberosity using sterile technique. The ferret then had preoperatively 2.5 mL Harman's solution, 2.5 mL plasma expander and 2 mg carprofen (Rimadyl) using the intraosseous needle. The site was prepped. A clear surgical drape was used to maintain a sterile field and was fixed in place with clear adhesive dressing (K. Eatwell, UK FADC/insulinoma case, Ch. 14). In conclusion, the use of anaesthetics of any kind on ferrets requires careful thought and application.

Radiology diagnosis in ferrets

Ferrets on the whole require some form of sedation or anaesthesia for radiological investigations.

Radiograph film should be of the rare earth screen system and high detail film if possible (Orthochromatic DuPont, USA). Other choices would include mammography film, dental film and non-screen film (R. Nye, Mid-West Bird & Exotic Animal Hospital, Westchester, IL, USA, pers. comm. 1999). Basic criteria are set down in Table 16.16.

Use of contrast media: An interesting use of contrast medium was seen when a 2-year-old 570 g hob ferret was attacked by a dog and presented with an acute traumatic soft tissue swelling.[29] Iopamidol (Isovue, 1 mL/kg) was given to the sedated patient via i.p. injection. The ferret was held in two hands and gently tipped from

Table 16.16 Criteria for ferret radiography

Essential requirement	Comment
X-ray machine with capability of producing 300 ma. (Mine was an Atomscope 903A (0.02–10 s).	Should have minimum exposure time of 1/120(0.008) s.
KVP for small patients often in 50–60 range.	*Note*: should be able to vary KVP in the range by small amounts as for changes in higher KVP range.
Tube stand adjustable for horizontal as well as vertical beam exposures.	I only did vertical beam exposures with ferrets.
Possible to adjust the focal length.	Possible to select distance between tube and film.
Technique for ferrets less than 10 cm thick.	Radiology on ordinary table (ours has lead sheets attached to underside of table).
Technique for ferrets greater than 10 cm thick.	Use of grid suggested. (Not used with our table.)
Use of high resolution screen combinations requiring low radiographic exposure desirable.	Interpretation of films modified with ferret's small body size, anatomical variation, and rapid respiratory rate. Require knowledge of normal anatomy and to be aware of radiological pattern changes due to disease process.

CHAPTER SIXTEEN
Anaesthesia and radiology

Table 16.17 The features of ferret anatomy compared with rabbit and guinea pig

	Ferret	Rabbit	Guinea pig
Relative size of thorax	Large	Small	Intermediate
Location of heart	Mid-thorax	Cranial thorax	Mid-thorax
Size of retrosternal lucency	Very large	Very small	Intermediate
Size of accessory lung node	Large	Small	Small

side to side to disperse the contrast medium. On radiology, after stabilization of the ferret with fluids, etc., it was found that there was leakage from the peritoneal cavity into the subcutaneous space and a small bowel entrapment had occurred. This transverse abdominal hernia was attended to under general anaesthesia with the ferret being given butorphanol, 0.1 mg/kg i.v. and antibiotic cover cefazolin sodium 20 mg/kg. After cage rest, it made a full recovery.

Note: with this type of contrast medium, some radiologists feel that there can be some irritation of the peritoneal lining giving a possible low grade peritonitis. However, contrast medium can show abdominal, diaphragmatic or pleural-pericardial herniation if ultrasound is not available or nondiagnostic.

There have been some criteria for radiology of ferrets and other small pets as set down by Silverman.[30] The long lithe form of the adult ferret compared with the stocky heavier adult rabbit and the small stubby guinea

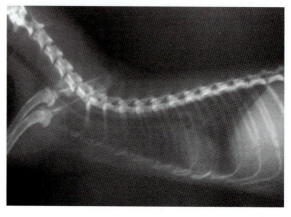

Figure 16.3 Ferret-normal chest. *Note* size of air; filled trachea in relation to the anterior chest cavity, where a gland or tumour obstruction at chest cavity apex can easily be fatal. (Courtesy of J. Chitty, UK.)

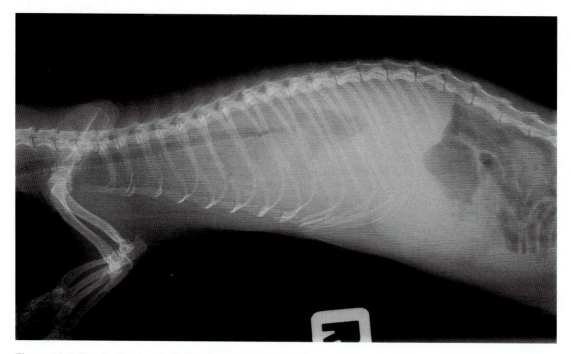

Figure 16.4 Ferret with pleural effusion due to massive heartworm infection recorded in WA for first time, 1999.

Radiology diagnosis in ferrets

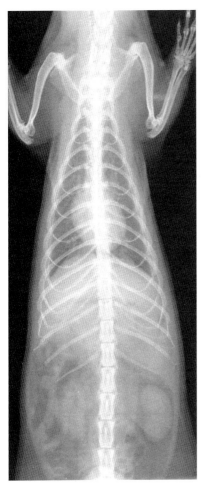

Figure 16.5 Thorax and abdomen; dorsoventral view. *Note* clear right kidney. (Courtesy of C. Bernard.)

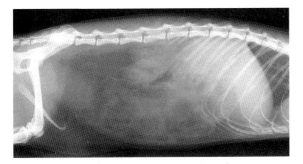

Figure 16.6 Lateral thorax/abdomen: male ferret showing penis baculum. Bladder and kidneys distinct, heart/diaphragm space normal. (Courtesy of C. Bernard.)

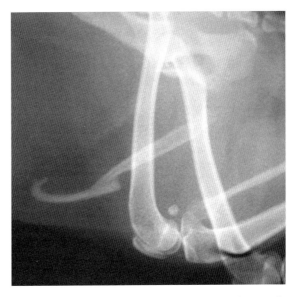

Figure 16.7 Lateral view of ferret pelvis shows fractured baculum. Ferret presented with anorexia, dehydration and pain. Owner thought it had eaten foam pillow material. Fracture considered an old wound with no idea of cause. (Courtesy of C. Johnson-Delaney.)

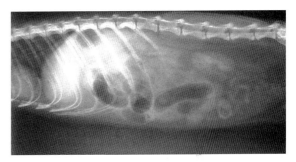

Figure 16.8 Lateral chest abdomen – cherry pip foreign body. This is an *atypical* f/b with ferrets as they usually ingest soft rubbery toys, etc. The pip was lodged in the mid-jejunum: note the gas dilation of the proximal small bowel typical of obstructive disease. (Courtesy of M. Burgess.)

pig can be kept in mind as in Table 16.17. The ferret skeleton (see Fig. 2.10) gives the idea of form for a lateral X-ray showing a tubular body with a narrow thoracic inlet opening into the chest cavity in a funnel shape.

The ferret chest is large and long. The chest gives an unobscured view of the chest contents unlike the rabbit and guinea pig with small chest cavities and superimposition of the forelegs on the cranial aspect of the chest. The ferret heart is situated normally between the

413

CHAPTER SIXTEEN
Anaesthesia and radiology

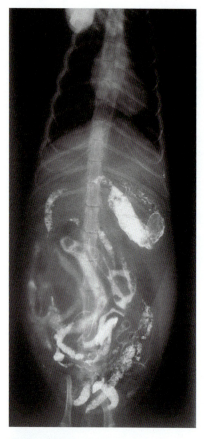

Figure 16.9 Ferret with intestinal trichobezoar (hair) 1 hour after barium meal. The barium is in the stomach and small bowel. No f/b visualized as yet. (Courtesy of M. Burgess.)

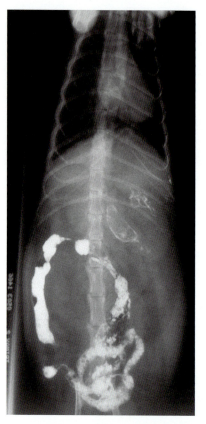

Figure 16.10 Ferret with intestinal trichobezoar (hair) 3 hours after barium meal. The second X-ray shows most of the contrast material has left the stomach but traces of barium have outlined a kidney-shaped trichobezoar in the gastric lumen. (Courtesy of M. Burgess.)

sixth and eighth rib in the central thorax area. Conditions such as pneumonia and bronchitis are more easily diagnosed accurately in the ferret, with its large thoracic cavity, than in the rabbit or guinea pig. Similarly, cardiomyopathy is more observable, though ECE is required for a complete diagnosis. Remembering both dilated and hypertrophic types of cardiomyopathy, note that the two forms may have similar outline silhouettes on X-ray.

In the ferret chest cranial mediastinal area mass lesions can be lymphosarcoma tumours as shown in dissections case (see Fig. 13.2) or fibrosarcoma case (see Fig. 13.3).

Ferret normal and abnormal abdominal interpretations comparisons

The ferret abdomen is relatively expansive with good serosal detail under normal radiography when compared with the screening results with rabbit and guinea pig. The ferret spleen can be large compared with other similar sized animals. It can be a site of neoplasia. *Note*: insulinoma cannot be seen on plain radiograph. Diagnostic interpretation of the ferret abdomen in disease follows on from methods associated with cat medi-

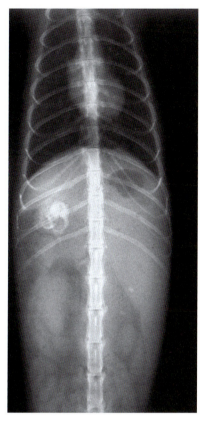

Figure 16.11 Ferret with mineralized duodenal adenocarcinoma. They are somewhat prone to neoplasia in the proximal duodenum adjacent to the pylorus. This mass is atypical in that it had mineralized, becoming radiodense enough to be visualized in the cranial abdomen. (Courtesy of M. Burgess.)

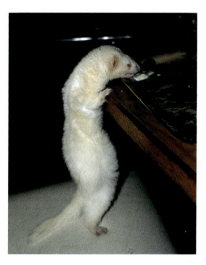

Figure 16.12 Juno sipping milk.

cine. Examples of ferret radiographs are given in Figures 16.3–16.11.

Finally, my ferret jill, Juno. recovered well from anaesthesia and surgery on a massive ovarian tumour (Ch. 13) and was soon sneaking spilt milk from the table (Fig. 16.12).

References

1. Heard DJ. Principles and techniques of anaesthesia and analgesia for exotic practice. Vet Clin North Am Small Anim Pract 1993; 23:1301–1327.
2. Mullens H. Soft tissue surgery. In: Hillyer EV, Quesenberry KE, eds. Ferrets, rabbits and rodents: Clinical medicine and surgery. Philadelphia: WB Saunders; 1997:131–144.
3. Tivers MS, Travis TRD, Windsor RV, et al. Questionnaire study of canine neutering techniques taught in UK veterinary schools and those used in practice. J Small Anim Pract 2005; 46:430–435.
4. Lewington JH. Ferrets: A compendium. Vade Mecum Series. University of Sydney: Postgraduate Foundation; 1988:C10.
5. Clutton RE. New drugs in companion animal anaesthesia. Waltham Focus 1998; 8:9–16.
6. Moreland AF, Glasser C. Evaluation of ketamine, ketamine-xylazine and ketamine-diazepam anaesthesia in the ferret. Lab Anim Sci 1985; 35:287–290.
7. Annual IVS. Information on ketamine. In: Alexander W, ed. Australia: MIMS; 1998:11–13.
8. Yanoff SR. Malignant lymphoma in the pet ferret. Vet Med 1984; 79.
9. Green CJ. Use of ketamine in the ferret. Vet Rec 1978; 102.
10. Moody KD, Bowman TA, Lang CM. Laboratory management of the ferret in biomedical research. Lab Anim Sci 1985; 35:272–279.
11. Alderton B. Anaesthesia in ferrets, rabbits and guinea pigs. In: Bryden I, ed. Proceedings of internal medicine small companion animals. University of Sydney: Postgraduate Foundation 1998; 306:241–259.
12. Burke TJ. Ferrets. Scientific proceedings, 48th AGM. Atlanta: American Animal Hospital Association; 1981.
13. Short CE. Advantages and guidelines for using halothane. Vet Clin North Am Small Anim Pract 1992; 22:321–322.
14. Gleed R. Precautions when using halothane. Vet Clin North Am Small Anim Pract 1992; 22:323–325.
15. Ludders JW. Advantages and guidelines for using isoflurane. Vet Clin North Am Small Anim Pract 1992; 22:328–331.
16. Dodman NH. Precautions when using isoflurane. Vet Clin North Am Small Anim Pract 1992; 22:332–334.
17. Muir WW, Hubbell JAE. Handbook of veterinary anaesthesia. St Louis: Mosby; 1989.
18. Imai A, Steffey EP, Farver TB, et al. Assessment of isoflurane-induced anaesthesia in ferrets and rats. Am J Vet Res 1999; 60:1577–1583.
19. Keegan RD. Inhalant anaesthetics: the basics. In: Gleed RD, Ludders JW, eds. Recent advances in veterinary anesthesia and analgesia: Companion animals. Ithaca: International Veterinary Information Service; 2005.

20. Rosenthal K. Ferrets. Vet Clin North Am Small Anim Pract 1994; 24:1–24.
21. McPhail CM, Monnet E, Gaynor JS, et al. Effect of sevoflurane on haemodynamics and cardiac energetic parameters in ferrets. Am J Vet Res 2004; 65:653–658.
22. Johnson-Delaney C. Ferret cardiopulmonary resuscitation. Semin Avian Exot Pet Med 2005; 14:135–142.
23. Annual IVS. Information on Domitor. In: Wroth O, ed. MIMS Australia 2004; 113.
24. Flecknell P. New drug available in US: potential use in ferrets, American Ferret Association. Am Ferret 1997; Jan/Feb:11–13.
25. Lewington JH. Medetomidine/atipamezole in ferrets. Control and therapy. University of Sydney: Postgraduate Foundation 1995; 183:761–762.
26. Ko JCH, Heaton-Jones TG, Nicklin CF. Evaluation of the sedative and cardiorespiratory effects of medetomidine, medetomidine-butorphanol, medetomidine-ketamine and medetomidine-butorphanol-ketamine in ferrets. Am Anim Hosp Assoc 1997; 33:438–448.
27. Adams CE. Anaesthesia of the ranch mink (*Mustela vison*) and ferret (*Mustela putorius furo*). Vet Rec 1979; 105.
28. Mason D. Anaesthesia, analgesia and sedation for small mammals. In: Hillyer EV, Quesenberry KE, eds. Ferrets, rabbits and rodents: Clinical medicine and surgery. Philadelphia: WB Saunders; 1997:378–391.
29. Clark B, Holland M. Acute traumatic soft swelling in a ferret. Vet Med August 2001; August:390–392.
30. Silverman S. Diagnostic imaging of exotic pets. Vet Clin North Am Small Anim Pract 1993; 23:1287–1299.

Ultrasonography in ferret practice

CHAPTER 17

Cathy A. Johnson-Delaney

'Science is nothing but trained and organised common sense.'

T. H. Huxley, 1825–1895

Ultrasonography is an extremely valuable tool for use in ferrets and should figure in routine examination, particularly as the ferret ages (Table 17.1).

Because the ferret is so flexible, abdominal organs can be easily isolated, manipulated and positioned readily for even novice ultrasonographers to identify and get measurements. This also aids in stabilization of an organ for guided biopsy or aspiration and drainage. Echocardiography is a primary tool to evaluate ferret heart health. Most ferrets will allow abdominal and even cardiac ultrasonography while awake with minimal restraint, often with just scruffing and a bribe of a treat held in front of their face to distract them (Fig. 17.1).

Occasionally, one will have a ticklish abdomen and will need mild sedation. Warming the acoustic gel prior to application will help to decrease contact sensitivity for the ferret. Any brand of water-soluble acoustic gel can be used. This should be wiped off when the examination is completed although it is not toxic if ingested. Ferrets tend to wipe it off all over their bedding and their holders, hence the advisability of cleaning it off first. The advantage of having the ferret awake and ingesting a treat such as a vitamin gel is that passage of the material through the gastrointestinal tract can be watched. This also aids in tissue identification between gut lumen fluid and blood vessels for those without colour Doppler.

Equipment

There are many manufacturers of ultrasound equipment for use in a veterinary practice. Features that are necessary to adequately assess organs and tissues in ferrets include a 7.5–12 MHz sector scanner (also called a transducer or probe) that has a fairly small footprint (<2 cm). These types of probes are ideal for other small mammals and birds. A 7.5 MHz curvilinear probe is used by the author (Fig. 17.2).

The frame rate should also be high to be able to image the heart for echocardiography. Machines should have the ability to digitally record both still images and movement such as during echocardiography. Many will interface with video recorders (VHS) or digital computer programs to record to hard drives, CD or DVD directly. Printers and other peripherals are fairly standard accessories. In choosing equipment, it is suggested that you try out the machine on a ferret prior to purchase. While a machine may give you an excellent picture for a dog or cat, it may not allow you to easily see ferret adrenals for instance, due to the shape and strength of the probe, or frame rate, or the ability of the machine to focus on various tissue depths. Colour Doppler with integrated electrocardiograms may be useful if the practitioner is experienced in cardiology or will be doing a large number of cardiac evaluations. A machine that can do split screen B and M mode, with guideline indicator, and built in measurement software will greatly aid in doing echocardiography. These features have become fairly standard on even portable units.

CHAPTER SEVENTEEN

Ultrasonography in ferret practice

Table 17.1 Routine use of ultrasound

Echocardiography, B and M modes
Thoracic mass evaluation
Liver mass evaluation, guided biopsy,
Vascular evaluation of liver as part of cardiac examination
Pylorus/gastric function-observation of ingesta passage, ulceration
Intestinal wall evaluation, motility, neoplasia
Lymph node measurements, evaluation, guided biopsy
Adrenal gland evaluation including vascularity
Compression of caudal vena cava
Pancreatic examination, neoplasia examination
Renal evaluation, guided biopsy, cyst drainage
Bladder and prostate assessment, guided drainage of cysts
Cystocentesis
Evaluation of urethra patency
Mass examination, guided biopsy

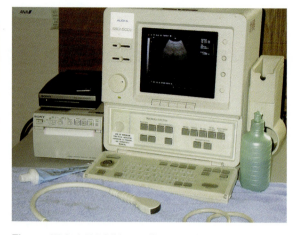

Figure 17.2 A 7.5 MHz curvilinear probe and equipment used by the author (digital image).

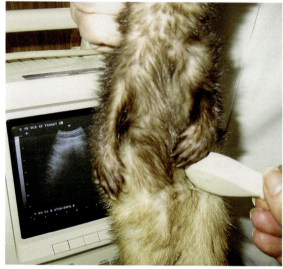

Figure 17.3 Probe placement for cardiac examination (digital image).

A basic understanding of the physics of ultrasound is essential to be able to adjust the machine to match the physiological and anatomic parameters needed to capture the best images. The author refers the reader to various ultrasound texts to describe in-depth the physics involved as this is beyond the scope of this chapter.

Basic guidelines

Air and hair cause many problems, artifacts and an inability to obtain a diagnostic image. This includes gas within the intestinal tract and trichobezoars in the stomach. Foreign bodies or barium within the gastrointestinal tract may also prevent proper imaging and create artifacts.

Bone or calcifications may interfere with imaging, particularly if the tissue to be examined is behind the bone or calcified material (such as a bladder stone). Ribs may interfere slightly with scans of the heart, but once identified, the ultrasonographer can determine which images are artifactual and obtain diagnostic images.

The heart can be well-imaged for echocardiographic measurements with the ferret on its back. It is not necessary to scan the heart in a sternal position as is

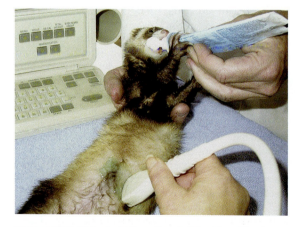

Figure 17.1 Demonstration of restraint and positioning for ultrasonography (digital image).

preferred in dogs and cats. The author has found that because of the chest's flexibility and the position of the heart against the sternum and ribs it is easily accessible (Fig. 17.3).

Formally, terms that are used to describe the appearance of ultrasound images relate to a tissue's echo intensity, attenuation and image texture. Areas of high echo intensity: echogenic, hyperechoic, high echo intensity or echo-rich. Areas of low echo intensity may be properly termed echo-poor or hypoechoic, whereas areas with no echoes are said to be anechoic or 'echo-free'. As urine and bile are the most anechoic, it is useful to use the bladder to adjust the screen to establish the baseline 'black'. The liver and spleen are normally in the mid-range of echogenicity and can be used to set the screen's contrast and brightness. Focus depth of the scan will depend on which organ you are imaging and may need to be changed during the examination.[1,2]

Tissue densities in ferrets are similar to those found in other animals (Table 17.2).

A comprehensive understanding of the anatomy of the ferret is required to locate structures. Variability in individual ferret anatomy, such as placement of the adrenal glands, may complicate initial scans, however due to the flexibility of the ferret abdomen, manual manipulation of key organs as landmarks will allow the practitioner to identify the structures.

Patient preparation

For a full abdominal scan, it may be necessary to shave the ferret from the pubic bone to the xiphoid process and approximately laterally to the margins of the palpable kidneys. If cardiac scanning is planned, the right and left areas of the chest from the midline to approximately half the distance to the spine at the level of the heart (palpable) should be clipped. If the ferret has a thin summer coat or alopecia due to other causes, smaller areas to none at all may be shaved.

The ferret may be restrained on its back and distracted with a treat. Alternatively, it can be 'scruffed' and held upright while being distracted (Ch. 7). Apply acoustic gel to the mid-abdomen. Begin the scan at the bladder to set the image contrast and brightness. If the ferret is cooperative, the entire examination may be done without sedation.

Scanning techniques

Knowledge of ferret anatomy is required.

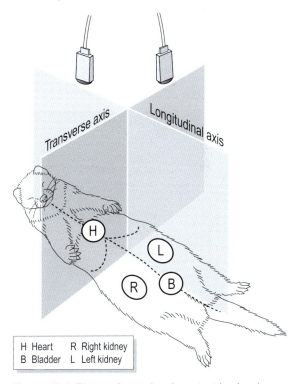

Figure 17.4 Planes of scanning. Important landmark organs for positioning. H, heart; R, right kidney; L, left kidney; B, bladder.

Table 17.2 Echogenicity of various tissues[1]

Order of increasing echogenicity
Urine, bile, transudates, serum
Renal medulla, fluid-filled cysts
Muscle
Renal cortex
Liver, lymph nodes
Storage fat, mesenteric fat
Spleen
Prostate, pancreas (normal tissue)
Renal sinus
Structural fat, vessel walls
Bone, gas, organ boundaries
Heavy metal, some calculi, surgical staples, hair, air
Variable echogenicity
Fluids and ingesta in the gastrointestinal tract
Exudates, granulomas, necrosis

CHAPTER SEVENTEEN
Ultrasonography in ferret practice

Figure 17.4 illustrates the planes used in scanning. A methodical routine should be practised so that no organs or tissues are missed. A suggested abdominal scan technique is provided:

Longitudinal: locate the bladder and adjust the machine according to your preference for contrast and brightness. This can and often is adjusted during the course of the examination depending on tissue densities.

1. *Longitudinal plane*: palpate the left kidney. Locate it with the beam. The normal left kidney is shown in Figure 17.5. Move medially at the level of the kidney and identify the caudal vena cava (cvc). Move laterally back to the kidney and position the beam so that you are at the cranial pole of the kidney. Move slowly medially. The left adrenal gland is in the area between the anterior left kidney and the caudal vena cava. It is usually at the depth of the renal vessels (Fig. 17.6).
2. *Transverse scan at the same level*. Use the kidney and cvc to locate the area of the left adrenal. The abdominal aorta will also be visible in cross-section.
    a. *Note*: if the spleen is enlarged, it may overlay much of the kidney and area of the left adrenal. Use the spleen as an imaging window.
    b. You can also do an examination of the spleen itself following both longitudinal and transverse movements as the spleen is curved through these directions. The medial side may be difficult to image if there is a lot of ingesta in the stomach or if there are adhesions to other organs (Fig. 17.7).
    c. Look for dilated vessels and variations in densities. Normally the spleen appears fairly homogeneous. *Note* that it will always be enlarged with any sedative or anaesthesia. Absolute size and architecture is best examined without sedation/anaesthesia. Enlarged vessels within the spleen are not considered normal.

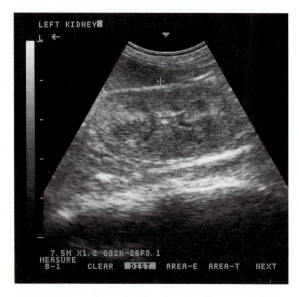

Figure 17.5 Normal left kidney, adult male, longitudinal axis.

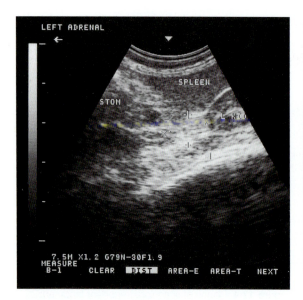

Figure 17.6 Normal left adrenal, adult male, longitudinal axis.

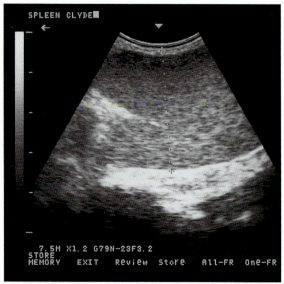

Figure 17.7 Spleen, normal density, isoflurane anaesthesia, adult male.

Scanning techniques

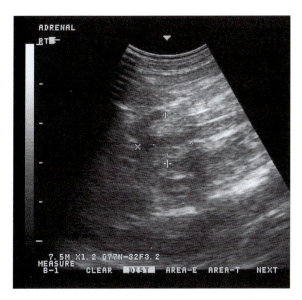

Figure 17.8 Normal right adrenal tissue surrounding caudal vena cava, adult female, longitudinal axis.

3. *Longitudinal plane*: palpate the right kidney. Locate with the beam. Move medially at the level of the kidney and identify the caudal vena cava. At the cranial pole of the right kidney there is usually liver overlapping the area where the right adrenal gland is located (Fig. 17.8).

Just dorsal (ventral on the image) to the liver lies the pyloric area of stomach and duodenum. If ingesta is moving through this, it is easy to differentiate the tissues. Vitamin gel or liquid does not interfere with the imaging and can be useful to see peristalsis, defects in the intestinal lining and rate of emptying. The right adrenal lies on the dorsal surface of the caudal vena cava, at the anterior pole of the kidney and in the fat between the kidney and the cvc. It may have separate vasculature.

Occasionally it will wrap around the cvc and, if enlarged, it may cause constriction of the cvc. It may also be on the left of the cvc and, if enlarged, push against the pyloric area of the stomach/duodenum. This constriction or alteration in the shape of the cvc is visible on longitudinal scan.

4. *Transverse scan at the same level*. Use the kidney, cvc and liver to locate the area of the right adrenal (Figs 17.9, 17.10).

The duodenum/pylorus and pancreas will also be surrounding the area where the gland is located. You can differentiate the GI tract by the motility, particularly if the ferret is awake and swallowing a vitamin gel.
   a. Just anterior to the area of the right adrenal will be the gall bladder, and the portal vein, although the portal vein is easier to locate on a longitudinal scan of the liver.

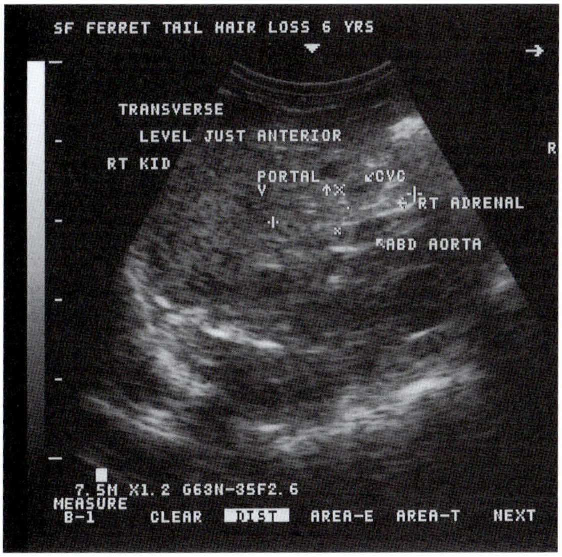

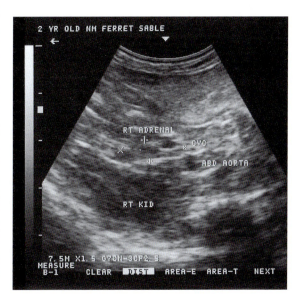

Figure 17.9 Transverse axis, just cranial to right kidney. *Note* compression of caudal vena cava by the slightly enlarged right adrenal tissue.

Figure 17.10 Transverse axis at cranial pole of right kidney.

CHAPTER SEVENTEEN
Ultrasonography in ferret practice

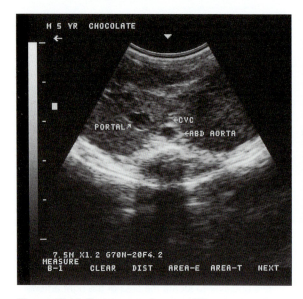

Figure 17.11 Transverse axis, normal liver.

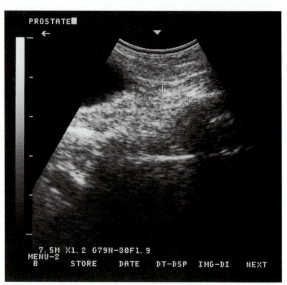

Figure 17.13 Longitudinal axis, bladder neck, urethra and prostate, 3-year-old neutered male.

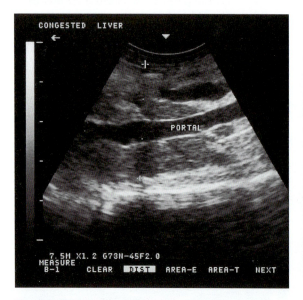

Figure 17.12 Longitudinal axis, congested liver. *Note* irregularity of diameter of portal vein.

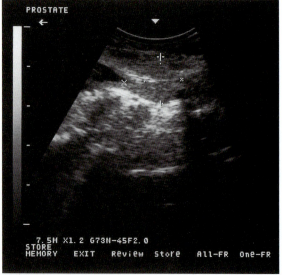

Figure 17.14 Longitudinal axis, bladder neck, urethra and prostate, 5-year-old neutered male.

b. If your picture is mostly liver, you are too anterior. Use the region between the anterior pole of the right kidney and the gallbladder to find the location of the adrenal tissue.

5. *Longitudinal scan of liver*: locate the gall bladder and portal vein. *Note* path of the portal vein and relative diameters of bile ducts, major vessels. Dilation of vessels in the liver is often seen with heart disease in the ferret. The liver may look almost 'cystic' in severe cases of congestion. Normal liver viewed in the transverse at the level of portal vein entry is shown in Figure 17.11. Figure 17.12 shows a congested liver with dilated vessels. The gall bladder is also visualized.

6. *Apical examination of the heart*: using the liver as a window, the heart can be scanned. This is done

Scanning techniques

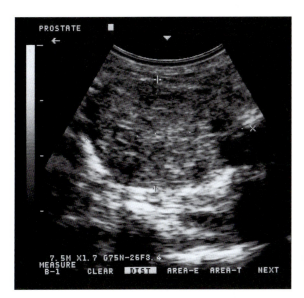

Figure 17.15 Longitudinal axis, enlarged prostate secondary to chronic adrenal disease, 6 months post-left adrenalectomy.

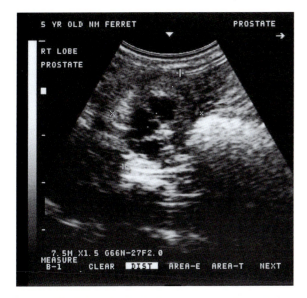

Figure 17.16 Longitudinal axis, enlarged cystic prostate secondary to adrenal disease.

from just right of the midline, approximating the right parasternal short axis view. *Note* movement, contractility, proportion of walls, pericardial condition. The most useful scans are both the right and left parasternal long axis 4-chamber view. M-mode can also be done, following the same parameters as used for dogs and cats.[1,2] Complete

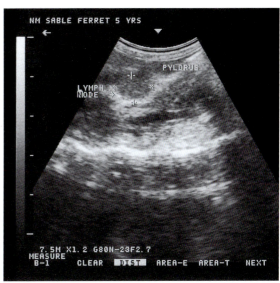

Figure 17.17 Transverse axis. Ingesta was observed from the stomach through the pylorus. Enlarged lymph node adjacent to the pylorus. History of pyloric ulcers.

the abdominal scan before proceeding to the cardiac examination and measurements.

7. *Bladder and prostate* (Figs 17.13, 17.14). Start with a longitudinal scan to image relative position of bladder and position of the urethra. The prostate lies at the pelvic brim and will appear as a dense mass. If enlarged and/or cystic, there may be urethral constriction, change in angle/positioning of the bladder, and some bowel displacement (Figs 17.15, 17.16).

8. Switch to transverse scanning to image the diameter of the urethra in cross-section. Spayed females with enlargements of the uterine stump can be imaged using essentially the same positioning as used to image the prostate in males. In intact females, the ovaries and uterine horns are easily imaged lying in a plane between the bladder and colon. The ovaries may be located laterally from the bladder, from approximately mid-bladder to just caudal to the level of the left kidneys. The location may depend on stage of the reproductive system and condition of the uterus. Ultrasound can be used to determine pregnancy and the gestational age.[3]

9. *GI tract and mesenteric lymph nodes*: Ingesta within the GI tract can cause artifacts. Gas, hair, obstructions, formed faecal material in the large bowel can be visualized particularly in contrast to liquid and/or gel moving through. Intestinal walls of individual bowel loops can be visualized particularly

CHAPTER SEVENTEEN

Ultrasonography in ferret practice

if there is significant body fat. Lining and wall thickness can be assessed. The mesenteric lymph nodes can be found usually by palpation and in the area of the mid- to caudal region of the left kidney, midline to slightly on the right. This depends a lot on fullness of the gut, amount of body fat and size of the lymph nodes. In the normal ferret, the nodes are quite small and homogenous. Imaging the pylorus transversely is useful to examine for motility and lining quality. In the transverse plane it may appear 'longitudinal' or may require probe manipulation to examine it in both longitudinal and transverse views. The stomach itself usually projects an artifact that streaks from the greater curvature (hence why it is better to approach the spleen from the caudolateral side). There is a lymph node that lies in the area of the lesser curvature of the stomach and frequently is closely associated with the pylorus. If this is enlarged or neoplastic, it may be easily visualized (Fig. 17.17).

Assessing abnormalities

If the ferret is cooperative or sedated, manual manipulation of the kidneys and other organs can also be done to isolate suspected masses and tissues seen in the scan. This is helpful to locate circumscribed masses and determine possible tissue of origin. In many cases, this can be difficult due to adhesions and inclusions of more recognizable organ tissues (Fig. 17.18).

Targeting the abnormal tissues for detailed examination is done at the conclusion of the full ultrasound examination. It is easy to focus in immediately on an obvious abnormality, but the entire ferret needs to be fully examined as other problems may exist that previously were unknown.

Frequent uses of ultrasonography

Ferrets frequently have renal cysts. These may be incidental or enlarge greatly to distend the abdomen. In many cases these cysts will not compress normal renal tissue, but enlarge outward and while they are uncomfortable for the ferret due to pressure and size, renal function will not be impaired. Perinephric pseudocysts may be the appearance of fluid pockets within the renal capsule.[4] Kidneys may have more than one cyst (polycystic) and frequently both kidneys are affected (Fig. 17.19).

Ultrasound-guided paracentesis can be performed under full anaesthesia with analgesic, aseptic technique to aspirate the accumulated fluid. The fluid should be analysed for infection or any abnormality from normal urine. The author has one ferret patient with severe left renal cysts that requires paracentesis 2–3 times a year,

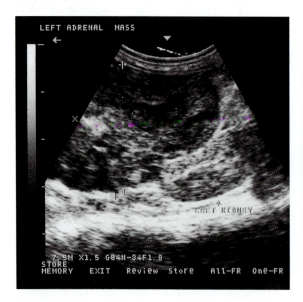

Figure 17.18 Longitudinal axis. Neoplastic mass, left adrenal gland.

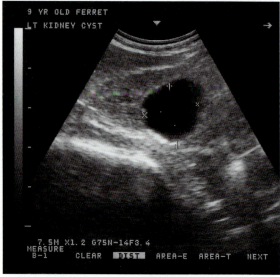

Figure 17.19 Renal cyst, incidental finding.

Frequent uses of ultrasonography

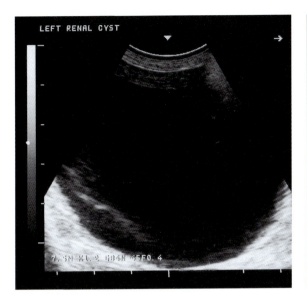

Figure 17.20 Large left renal cysts prior to ultrasound-guided drainage; 120 mL urine was aspirated.

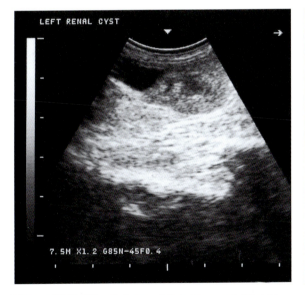

Figure 17.21 After drainage of the above cyst. Normal left kidney tissue is observed.

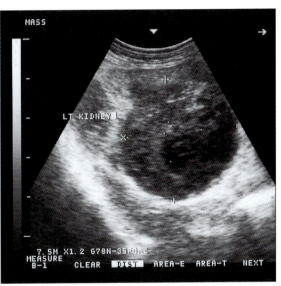

Figure 17.22 Longitudinal axis, adrenal neoplastic mass.

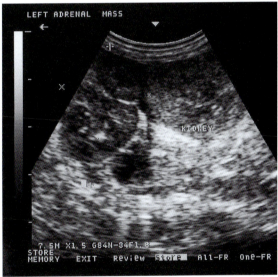

Figure 17.23 Longitudinal axis, left adrenal neoplastic mass.

with approximately 180 mL of urine aspirated. The condition has been treated for over 3 years with no complications (Figs 17.20, 17.21).

Fine needle aspirate of the mesenteric lymph node has been described.[5] The large mesenteric lymph node was typically round to ovoid and uniformly hyperechoic. The mean ultrasonographic dimensions of the node were 12.6 ± 2.6 mm by 7.6 ± 2.0 mm. Fine needle aspirate cytology compared well with samples obtained during laparotomy or necropsy.

By far the most common use in ferrets is to examine the abdomen for neoplasia. Well-described is the use to diagnose adrenal lesions.[6–8] While adrenal glands imaged may be enlarged, abnormally-shaped or highly vascularized,

CHAPTER SEVENTEEN
Ultrasonography in ferret practice

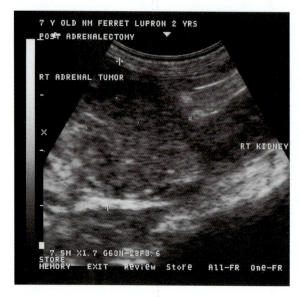

Figure 17.24 Longitudinal axis, right adrenal neoplastic mass.

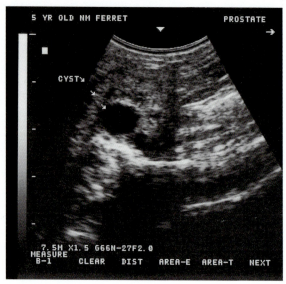

Figure 17.26 Cystic prostate gland secondary to adrenal disease. Urethra was occluded.

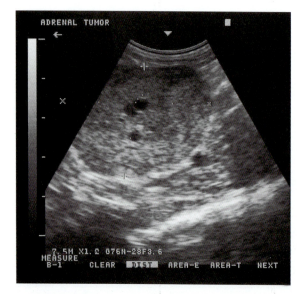

Figure 17.25 Transverse axis, just anterior to right kidney, right adrenal neoplastic mass.

the degree of adrenal disease or type of neoplasia cannot be determined by image and size alone. Size and shape has been found to be widely variable and not specific to any lesion type. Both benign and malignant adrenal tumours (adenomas, adenocarcinomas) appeared in one study more frequently as masses with increased thickness and a normal length and less frequently as larger masses or as nodules focally deforming the adrenal shape. Cortical cysts may be found that appear as a nodule. Hyperplastic glands as well as those of adenoma may appear normal in size and tissue density on ultrasound. Focal absence of periglandular fat between the adrenal gland and large vessels or liver, deviation or compression of the large vessels was found to correlate with malignancy (Figs 17.22–17.25).

In male ferrets, enlargement or cystic abnormalities of the prostate are extremely common and may result in life-limiting clinical signs such as complete blockage of the prostatic urethra. Large cysts can be aspirated to relieve pressure. Fluid should be cultured as well as have cytology performed. In most cases, as the sex steroid level is decreased in the treatment of the adrenal disease, and no secondary infection has taken place, the prostate regresses greatly and urethral constriction or obstruction is resolved (Fig. 17.26).

Thoracentesis may be performed using ultrasound to locate the fluid accumulations to be aspirated. This procedure should be done with appropriate anaesthesia and analgesic therapy with close monitoring of the heart and respirations as abrupt major changes of intrathoracic pressures can trigger vagal responses resulting in cardiopulmonary collapse.[9,10]

Echocardiography

Many older ferrets have some degree of cardiomyopathy which is not easily diagnosed or characterized as to type

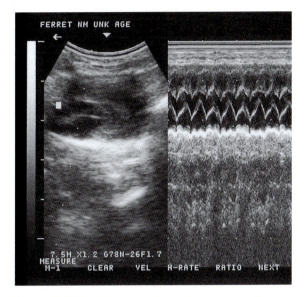

Figure 17.27 Split screen, left parasternal view with M-mode. This ferret had mild dilated cardiomyopathy, second degree heart block on ECG.

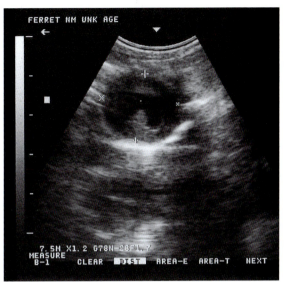

Figure 17.28 Short axis view showing right and left ventricles, papillary muscle.

of disease using radiographs, electrocardiography and auscultation. Echocardiography in the author's opinion is the best way to examine the ferret's heart. While B mode is excellent to look at the heart as a whole, check valves and function; M-mode is needed to determine actual contractility and size. Right parasternal long and short axis views can be used in using M-mode (Figs 17.27, 17.28).[2]

Two major studies have been published using two different types of anaesthesia during the measurements: ketamine hydrochloride (25 mg/kg) and midazolam (0.2 mg/kg) in one group; isoflurane in the other. Sur-

Table 17.3 Echocardiographic reference values in ferrets anaesthetized with isoflurane or a ketamine/midazolam combination[11,12]

Parameter	Isoflurane				Ket/midazolam			
	Mean	SD	Range	Median	Mean	SD	Range	Median
IVSd (mm)	3.4	0.4	2.5–4.4	3.4	3.6	0.7	2.0–5.0	3.3
IVSs (mm)	4.4	0.6	3.3–5.4	4.4	4.8	1.1	2.7–7.7	4.7
LVIDd (mm)	9.8	1.4	6.8–12.7	9.6	8.8	1.5	6.3–12.0	8.6
LVIDs (mm)	6.9	1.3	4.5–9.7	6.9	5.9	1.5	2.7–8.7	6.0
LVWd (mm)	2.7	0.5	1.8–3.7	2.7	4.2	1.1	3.0–7.0	4.0
LVWs (mm)	3.8	0.8	2.4–5.9	3.8	5.8	9.9	4.3–8.0	5.7
FS (%)	29.5	7.9	13.9–48.7	28.0	33.0	14.0	0–57.0	36.0
Ao (mm)	4.4	0.6	3.3–6.0	4.2	5.3	1.0	3.0–7.3	5.3
LA (mm)	5.8	0.9	3.2–7.3	5.7	7.1	1.8	4.7–12.0	6.7
LA:Ao (ratio)	1.3	0.2	1.0–1.8	1.3	1.3	2.7	0.8–2.0	1.4
HR (bpm)	238	20	225–244	234	273	31	240–330	300

IVSd, IVSs, thickness of interventricular septum in diastole and systole; LVIDd, LVIDs, left ventricular internal diameter in diastole and systole; LVWd, LVWs, thickness of left ventricular free wall in diastole and systole; FS, fractional shortening; Ao, aortic diameter; LA, left atrium diameter.

CHAPTER SEVENTEEN
Ultrasonography in ferret practice

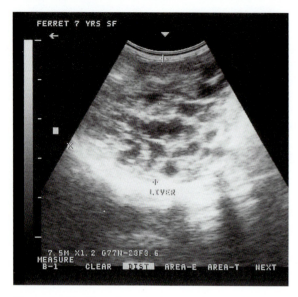

Figure 17.29 Cystic liver with increased tissue density between cystic structures. At necropsy: cystic biliary adenocarcinoma.

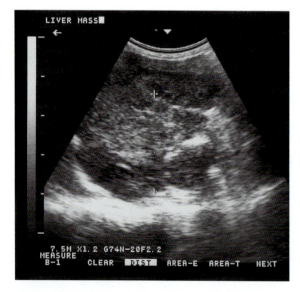

Figure 17.30 Cystic liver. At necropsy: cystic liver adenocarcinoma.

prisingly, the values were similar in many parameters (Table 17.3).

In both studies, there was no significant difference between male and female ferrets despite the difference in body weights. There was no significant correlation between body weight and any of the M-mode measurements.[11,12]

In many ferrets with cardiomyopathy, there will be some liver congestion, easily seen as dilation of the major vessels throughout the liver. This appears quite differently than if the liver has cysts such as seen with biliary adenocarcinoma (Figs 17.29, 17.30).

Dirofilariasis has been diagnosed using echocardiography in ferrets. Heartworms appear as hyperechoic densities within heart chambers and may extend into some of the great vessels through the valves.[13]

Special acknowledgements

Washington Ferret Rescue and Shelter, volunteers and ferrets; veterinarians and staff at both the Bird & Exotic Clinic of Seattle and the Exotic Pet & Bird Clinic of Kirkland, Aloka Ultrasound and George LaTorraca; Megan Ruether, Michael Delaney; Jack, Cinnamon, Buddy, Simon, Tichuk, Cyrano, the Farscape Kids and Robbie 'McFerret' Delaney, who taught me so much about understanding ferrets from the inside out.

References

1. Nyland TG, Mattoon JS, Wistner ER. Physical principles, instrumentation, and safety of diagnostic ultrasound. In: Nyland TG, Mattoon JS, eds. Veterinary diagnostic ultrasound. Philadelphia: WB Saunders; 1995:3–18.
2. Boon JA. Two dimensional and M-mode echocardiography for the small animal practitioner. Jackson, Wyoming: Teton NewMedia; 2002.
3. Peter AT, Bell JA, Manning DD, et al. Real-time ultrasonographic determination of pregnancy and gestational age in ferrets. Lab Anim Sci 1990; 40:91–92.
4. Puerto DA, Walker LM, Saunders HM. Bilateral perinephric pseudocysts and polycystic kidneys in a ferret. Vet Radiol Ultrasound 1998; 39:309–312.
5. Paul-Murphy J, O'Brien RT, Spaeth A, et al. Ultrasonography and fine needle aspirate cytology of the mesenteric lymph node in normal domestic ferrets (*Mustela putorius furo*). Vet Radiol Ultrasound 1999; 40:308–310.
6. Besso JG, Tidwell AS, Gliatto JM. Retrospective review of the ultrasonographic features of adrenal lesions in 21 ferrets. Vet Radiol Ultrasound 2000; 41:345–352.
7. Neuwirth L, Collins B, Calderwood-Mays M, Tran T. Adrenal ultrasonography correlated with histopathology in ferrets. Vet Radiol Ultrasound 1997; 38:69–74.
8. Ackermann J, Carpenter JW, Godshalk CP, et al. Ultrasonographic detection of adrenal gland tumors in two ferrets. J Am Vet Med Assoc 1994; 205:1001–1003.
9. Wyre NR, Hess L. Clinical technique: ferret thoracocentesis. Sem Avian Exot Pet Pract 2005; 14:22–25.
10. Johnson-Delaney CA. Ferret cardiopulmonary resuscitation. Sem Avian Exot Pet Pract 2005; 14:135–142.
11. Stepien RL, Benson KG, Wenholz BS. M-mode and Doppler echocardiographic findings in normal ferrets sedated with ketamine hydrochloride and midazolam. Vet Radiol Ultrasound 2000; 41:452–456.

12. Vastenburg MH, Boroffka SA, Schoemaker NJ. Echocardiographic measurements in clinically healthy ferrets anesthetized with isoflurane. Vet Radiol Ultrasound 2004; 45:228–232.

13. Sasai H, Kata K, Sasaki T, et al. Echocardiographic diagnosis of dirofilariasis in a ferret. J Small Anim Pr 2000; 41:172–174.

CHAPTER 18

General surgery

R. Avery Bennett and Geoffrey W. Pye

'A chance to cut is a chance to cure.'

Samuel Shem MD, The House of God, 1979

Ferrets are susceptible to a variety of diseases which are best managed surgically. Many procedures are analogous to those performed in other companion animal species. A knowledge of the anatomic and physiologic differences between ferrets and other species is important for a successful outcome.

Ovariohysterectomy

The indications for performing ovariohysterectomy in ferrets are similar to those for other companion animals. In addition, to prevent the dangerous state of hyperoestrogenism, female ferrets not intended for breeding should be spayed at 4–6 months of age or within 2 weeks of the onset of their first oestrus. The operation procedure is analogous to the procedure performed in cats. The incision is made midway between the umbilicus and pubis. The linea alba is generally easy to identify. The uterus is bicornuate, and the ovarian ligaments are loose and easily torn making it easy to exteriorize the ovaries.[1] The ovary may be surrounded by a large amount of fat and care should be taken to ensure complete removal (Fig. 18.1a).

The ferret uterus is bifurcated and could be considered a miniature of the cat (Fig. 18.1b).

Castration and vasectomy

The indications for castration in ferrets are similar to those for other species and include control of reproduction, behaviour modification to help control aggression and control of territorial marking behaviours. Additionally, castration significantly decreases the pungent odour of intact male ferrets.

There are two basic procedures for castration of ferrets, through a scrotal incision or a pre-scrotal incision. While most surgeons prefer an open technique, a closed technique may also be employed. Using the scrotal approach, an incision is made over the testicle through the scrotum. The tunic is opened and the testicle exteriorized. The spermatic cord is ligated in a standard manner. The scrotal incisions are allowed to heal by second intention.

A pre-scrotal castration is performed in a manner similar to castration of dogs. A testicle is pushed into the pre-scrotal region at the base of the penis. While holding the testicle in place, the skin, subcutaneous tissues, and tunic over the testicle are incised allowing the testicle to be exteriorized. The spermatic cord is ligated in a routine manner. The second testicle is removed in the same way. The subcutaneous tissues and skin are closed routinely. The advantage to this technique is that both testicles can be removed through a single incision and the incision is not made in the thin, sensitive scrotal skin.

Vasectomy is performed in ferrets to create sterile males which are used in breeding facilities to bring jills out of oestrus without using artificial means and without resulting in pregnancy and is described in Chapter 19.

430

Anal sacculectomy (descenting)

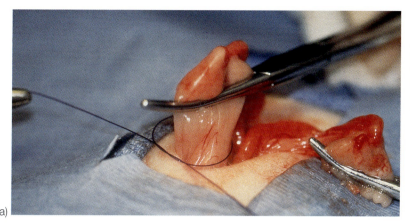

Figure 18.1
(a) Ovariohysterectomy in a ferret. *Note* the large amount of fat that may surround the ovary. Care must be taken to isolate the ovary to ensure complete removal.
(b) Ovariohysterectomy showing exposed bifurcation of uteri and ovary size. (Courtesy of G. Rich.)

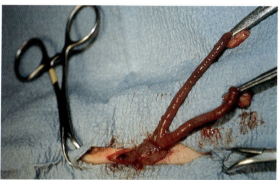

Vasectomy may be performed bilaterally, but some prefer to perform a unilateral castration along with a contralateral vasectomy as they feel castration is easier to perform than vasectomy. Leaving one testicle will provide enough testosterone that the ferret will have a normal reproductive drive and function.

Anal sacculectomy (descenting)

Anal sacculectomy is performed in ferrets to decrease their odour. It is important to realize that this procedure removes the anal sacs, but it is not possible to remove all of the anal glands or the glands in the skin which are also responsible for some of the natural odour of ferrets. Additionally, it appears that castration of hobs alone dramatically decreases the odour of the ferret to a level similar to that present in descented ferrets. Because of this, some feel anal sacculectomy is not necessary. Ferrets express their anal sacs when they are threatened emitting a foul odour to help keep predators at bay. If the anal sacs are not removed, ferrets will continue to express them when threatened. It is important to discuss the options with owners prior to performing this procedure.

Because the surgical site has a high potential for contamination, antibiotic therapy is indicated. There are various procedures described for performing anal sacculectomy in other companion animals. In ferrets, it is important not to allow the contents of the sacs to escape creating a seriously pungent odour in the room. The procedure described by Fowler accomplishes this best.[2] The duct of one sac is identified at either the 4 or 8 o'clock position on the anus. A fine mosquito haemostat is applied to the duct opening to prevent its con-

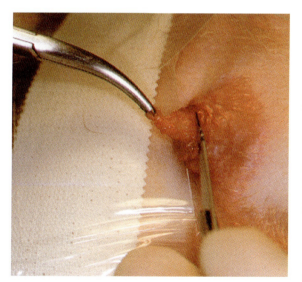

Figure 18.2 Anal sacculectomy in a ferret. The duct has been carefully dissected free and is being held closed with a microhaemostat. A No. 11 scalpel blade is being used to free the anal sac by scraping the surrounding anal sphicter muscle from its surface.

431

CHAPTER EIGHTEEN
General surgery

tents from escaping. The point of a No. 11 scalpel blade is used to make a circumferential incision in the anal mucosa around the clamped off duct opening. The anal sac and its duct are located within the anal sphincter muscle. The duct and sac are dissected from the muscle using the flat portion of the No. 11 blade in a careful scraping manner (Fig. 18.2).

The goal is to leave as much anal sphincter intact while removing the anal sac and duct without rupturing them. The wall of the sac and duct have a texture and colour different from those of the anal sphincter muscle. With the clamp on the opening of the duct to prevent leakage of the contents, carefully dissect the duct toward the bottom of the sac removing as much muscle from the sac as possible. Once the sac is completely removed, a relatively large defect will be present. The procedure is repeated on the other side. The wounds are left to heal by second intention.

Gastrointestinal foreign bodies

Because of their inquisitive nature, gastrointestinal foreign body obstruction occurs with some degree of frequency in ferrets less than 1 year of age. Young ferrets appear to be especially interested in soft rubber objects. Ferrets may also present with gastrointestinal obstruction caused by trichobezoars, so prophylaxis for hairballs is recommended.[3-6] Trichobezoars in ferrets are not hard balls of hair, but are more like a matted mass of hair capable of obstructing the flow of ingesta. Clinical signs associated with gastrointestinal obstruction include lethargy, depression, anorexia, melaena and dehydration. Vomiting is an inconsistent feature of this syndrome in ferrets. These clinical signs may persist for many days, however once a diagnosis is made, it should be considered an emergency and surgery should not be postponed.

The diagnosis of gastrointestinal foreign body obstruction is made based on history, clinical signs, physical examination, plain radiography and abdominal ultrasound. In most cases the object can be identified by abdominal palpation. Radiographically, a gas-distended stomach is consistent with a partial or complete gastric outflow obstruction, while an intestinal ileus pattern is consistent with an intestinal obstruction. Contrast radiography is not commonly necessary but may be used to confirm the presence and location of the object.[3]

Procedure

Prior to surgery, the patient is stabilized and any dehydration is corrected. A complete exploratory celiotomy should be performed and the entire gastrointestinal tract checked for foreign bodies. For gastric foreign bodies, a standard gastrotomy is performed in a relatively avascular portion of the fundic stomach. Use saline-moistened sponges to isolate the stomach from the other viscera and to prevent leakage of gastric contents into the abdominal cavity. Stay sutures may be placed to allow better control of the incision. A small portion of the border of the gastrotomy is collected for histopathologic examination to rule out gastric pathology like *Helicobacter*-induced gastritis. The foreign object or trichobezoar is removed and the stomach closed using a two-layer closure. For the first layer use a simple continuous appositional suture pattern and then oversew with a Cushing or Lembert pattern to invert the incision.

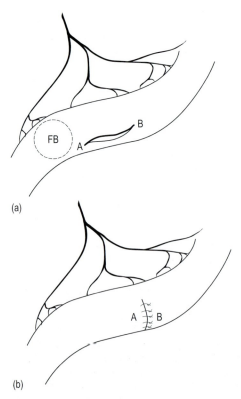

Figure 18.3 (a) Enterotomy in a ferret showing longitudinal incision (A to B) in the antimesenteric border of the bowel just aborad to the foreign body (FB). (b) Enterotomy in a ferret showing transverse closure of a longitudinal incision. The first suture is placed at the orad (A) and aborad (B) apices of the enterotomy incision. As this first suture is tightened, the longitudinal incision will be transformed into a transverse incision. Additional sutures are placed in a simple interrupted pattern to complete closure of the enterotomy. (Reprinted with permission from Comp Cont Edu Pract Vet 21(9,11):815–822, 1049–1057, 1999.)

If the object is in the intestine, it is best to make the enterotomy in the antimesenteric border of the healthier segment of intestine just aborad to the foreign body (Fig. 18.3a,b).[7]

The diameter of the intestine of ferrets is narrow and stricture following enterotomy has been reported.[1,6] Standard closure of the enterotomy results in narrowing of the lumen diameter, predisposing to stricture formation. It is, therefore, recommended that the enterotomy be closed in a transverse fashion to effectively enlarge the luminal diameter at the enterotomy (Fig. 18.3b).[8] The first suture is placed at the orad and aborad apices of the enterotomy incision. As this first suture is tightened, the longitudinal incision will be transformed into a transverse incision. Additional sutures are placed in a simple interrupted pattern to complete closure of the enterotomy. The closure can then be tested using saline or intestinal fluid to ensure no leaks are present.

After the object is removed, the abdomen is irrigated and contaminated instruments exchanged for sterile instruments. Antibiotics are used if indicated based on the level of contamination. The patient is fed the day of surgery and the owner must be educated on how to prevent recurrence.

Adrenalectomy

Adrenalectomy is indicated in ferrets with adrenal gland disease. Diagnosis of adrenal gland disease in ferrets is generally based on history and physical examination.

An adrenal steroid panel has been developed at the University of Tennessee evaluating the serum level of three of the most commonly elevated sex hormones in ferrets with adrenal disease (Clinical Endocrinology Laboratory, Department of Comparative Medicine, University of Tennessee, TN; see Table 14.1). If these values are normal, the patient may still have adrenal disease with the tumour producing a different hormone from those measured.

A variety of medical management therapies have been tried with inconsistent and poor results in ferrets, making surgery the treatment of choice for ferrets with adrenal gland disease.[9,10] The normal adrenal gland in female ferrets is roughly $7.5 \times 3 \times 4$ mm; in male ferrets it is roughly $9 \times 4 \times 3$ mm. Any evidence of discolouration, lumps, firm areas, cystic areas or gross enlargement would be indications of adrenal gland disease. The adrenal may be of normal size, but if there is a firm area or discoloured area, the gland should be removed.

Procedure

For left or right adrenalectomy, a ventral midline approach should be used. An 8–10 cm incision may be necessary to provide adequate exposure of the abdomen. A stay retractor (Lone Star Veterinary Retractor System, Jorgensen Laboratories, Inc., Loveland, CO, USA) will aid in exposing the contents of the abdomen and the hooks of the stays should be placed through the muscle of the body wall (see Fig. 18.6). The left adrenal gland is located cranially and medial to the cranial pole of the left kidney in the retroperitoneal fat (Fig. 18.4).[6,11]

The adrenolumbar vein courses from medial to lateral over the surface of the adrenal gland. Because of its retroperitoneal location within the fat, it is important to incise the peritoneum and explore around the adrenal gland to adequately visualize the entire gland prior to declaring it normal. Left adrenalectomy is significantly easier than right adrenalectomy because the right adrenal gland is intimately associated with the caudal vena cava. In order to remove the left adrenal gland, a ligature or haemostatic clip is placed on the adrenolumbar vein on each side of the adrenal gland to provide haemostasis. The adrenolumbar vein can then be transected and the adrenal gland dissected from the retroperitoneal fat. Large tumours may grow up into the caudal vena cava through the adrenolumbar vein or may invade adjacent structures such as the renal vessels and potentially the kidney.

The right adrenal gland is located by elevating the caudal pole of the caudate lobe of liver which lies

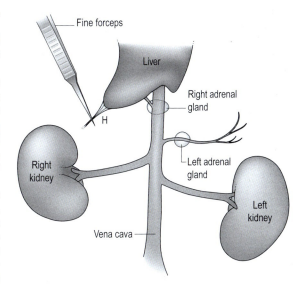

Figure 18.4 Anatomy of the ferret showing the left and right adrenal glands. The hepatorenal ligament (H) has been cut and held to elevate the caudate lobe of the liver, thereby exposing the right adrenal gland, positioned dorsally over the vena cava. The kidneys are shown for orientation. (Reprinted with permission from Comp Cont Edu Pract Vet 21(9,11):815–822, 1049–1057, 1999.)

over the cranial pole of the right kidney (Fig. 18.4).[1] The hepatorenal ligament is a transparent structure extending from the caudal point of the caudate liver lobe to the area of the kidney. This is incised, held with a microhemostat, and used to elevate the caudate lobe of the liver exposing the caudal vena cava and the right adrenal gland. In reality, the right adrenal gland lies more on the dorsal aspect of the caudal vena cava than specifically on the right side. It is also tightly adhered to the caudal vena cava. In order to adequately evaluate the right adrenal gland the peritoneum must be opened on both the right and left side of the caudal vena cava, and the retroperitoneal fat dissected to allow exposure and evaluation of the right adrenal gland (Fig. 18.5).

Because the right adrenal gland in ferrets is closely adhered to the caudal vena cava, right adrenalectomy is significantly more difficult. Vascular clamps are almost essential in performing a complete right adrenalectomy. These clamps occlude the vena cava without causing trauma to the vessel wall. They are placed on the caudal vena cava both cranial and caudal to the mass isolating the portion of the vena cava containing the adrenal tumour. Alternatively, a single neonatal Satinsky clamp may be placed as shown in Figure 18.6.

The right adrenal gland is dissected from the surrounding retroperitoneal fat as completely as possible on both the right and left sides of the vena cava to isolate the tumour prior to placing the vascular clamps. Additionally, the caudal vena cava cranial and caudal to the mass is isolated from the surrounding retroperitoneal fat. This will make suturing the vena cava more easily accomplished, should that become necessary. With the aid of magnifying loupes and microsurgical instruments, a plane of dissection between the adrenal gland and the caudal vena cava is identified. Dissection is continued along this plane until the adrenal gland is completely removed from the surface of the vena cava. With the aid of magnification, the wall of the vena cava is inspected for defects. Small holes are sutured with 8-0 to 10-0 nylon in a simple interrupted or mattress pattern. Larger defects may be sutured with the same material in a simple continuous pattern. Hemorrhage should be anticipated when the clamps are released. Before removing the clamp a piece of oxidized regenerated cellulose (Surgicel; Johnson & Johnson Medical, Inc., Arlington, Texas, USA) is wrapped around the vena cava where the mass was removed to aid in haemostasis. The clamp is removed and gentle digital pressure is applied for approximately 5 minutes to allow clots to form sealing the small holes. The oxidized regenerated cellulose is absorbable and left in place during abdominal closure. Blood pressure in the vena cava is generally low making postoperative hemorrhage less problematic.

Tumours of either the right or the left adrenal gland may invade the caudal vena cava (more likely with right adrenal tumour). These may be removed using a venotomy or by performing a resection and anastomosis of the caudal vena cava if the tumour is invading the vena cava wall. The caudal vena cava is occluded as described above and the venotomy is made as small as possible where the tumour invades the vena cava. Some adrenal tumours migrate up the lumen of the vena cava without adhering to the inside of the wall. These can just be pulled out of the lumen of the vena cava through the venotomy. Other tumours invade the wall of the vena cava and these require resection of more of the wall of the vena cava. If a venotomy is performed, it is best to close the longitudinal venotomy incision transversely to prevent attenuation of the lumen diameter. It is generally easiest to place several interrupted sutures to provide opposition prior to closing with a simple continuous pattern which will provide a better seal for the venotomy. In some cases, a portion of the vena cava must be removed to completely resect an adrenal tumour. The authors have removed up to 1 cm of

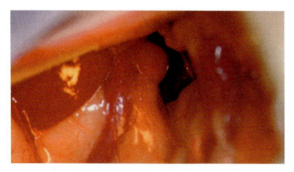

Figure 18.5 Enlarged right adrenal gland of a ferret. The hepatorenal ligament has been cut and the caudate lobe of the liver retracted to improve exposure of the gland and caudal vena cava. *Note* how the gland is positionally dorsal to the vein and has enlarged to the left.

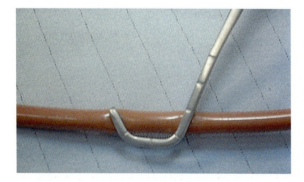

Figure 18.6 Using a red rubber tube, the correct placement for isolation of the portion of the caudal vena cava associated with a right adrenal gland tumour using a neonatal Satinsky clamp is depicted.

vena cava and have been able to create a tension-free anastomosis. Although some ferrets may survive caudal vena cava ligation, this procedure should not be recommended until its effects have been appropriately researched.

Partial adrenal gland resection may be indicated to debulk large tumours that cannot be resected based on availability of equipment for and the surgeon's familiarity with complete adrenalectomy. There are two basic procedures for debulking. One method involves removing as much of the adrenal tissue as possible without risking damaging the wall of the caudal vena cava. This technique is not appropriate for adrenal tumours that invade the vena cava and migrate up the lumen. The second technique involves using hemostatic clips, which are placed adjacent to the caudal vena cava, ideally between the caudal vena cava and the adrenal mass. Once the clips are applied, microsurgical scissors are used to cut along the hemostatic clips to allow removal of the adrenal tissue. The authors stress that these procedures are not recommended because complete removal of the gland and tumour is unlikely with those techniques, resulting in an increased risk of tumour regrowth.

Postoperative treatment is discussed in Chapter 14.

Prostatic disease

Prostatic disease in ferrets is usually secondary to the overproduction of male hormones from adrenal masses.[1,12] Prostatic enlargement, prostatitis, paraprostatic cysts and paraurethral cysts have been described (Fig. 18.7).

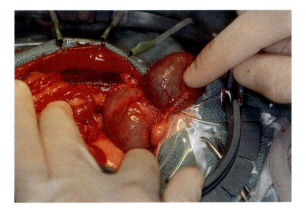

Figure 18.7 Prostatic cyst in a ferret. The large prostatic cyst can be seen dorsal to the reflected and elevated bladder. *Note* the use of a stay retractor to facilitate exposure of the abdomen. The hooks of the stays have been placed in the muscle of the body wall.

Cystic structures may be significantly larger than the urinary bladder and evident on abdominal palpation. The cysts generally contain a thick, tenacious, odouriferous, green fluid.[3] Treatment is directed at correcting the underlying problem (adrenal tumour). In most cases, once the adrenal tumour is removed the prostate rapidly reduces in size (1–2 days). Intraoperatively it is indicated to aspirate the contents of the cyst and submit these contents for culture and sensitivity. Biopsy of the affected prostate is also recommended to rule out primary prostatic disease. Marsupialization of the cystic structures is not usually necessary. Omentalization involves creating a defect in the cyst to which the omentum is sutured. The omentum will then function to absorb any fluid that the cyst continues to produce during the postoperative period. If there is a defect in the urethra, urine will leak into the abdomen. In such cases an indwelling urethral catheter is inserted and left in place for 2–4 days, allowing the urethra to heal around it.

Pancreatic beta cell tumours (insulinoma)

Hypoglycaemia in ferrets is usually due to overproduction of insulin by pancreatic beta cell tumours.[3,13–17] Presumptive diagnosis of pancreatic beta cell tumours is based on a fasting blood glucose level of <70 g/dL (90–100 g/dL is normal). A 4-hour fast prior to collecting the blood is recommended and it may be advisable to fast the ferret in the hospital in the event of a hypoglycaemic crisis. Most pancreatic beta cell tumours are too small to be imaged using ultrasound.

Surgery is considered the treatment of choice for ferrets with insulinoma.[16] However, it may be primarily a de-bulking and diagnostic procedure because insulinoma has high recurrence and metastatic potentials.[16,18] Though many ferrets show a temporary relief of the hypoglycaemia produced by pancreatic beta cell tumours following resection of identified masses, some continue to have hypoglycaemia even immediately postoperatively.

Procedure

Preoperatively an i.v. catheter is placed and 5% dextrose or 0.45% saline + 2.5% dextrose is administered during the operation.[1,3,16] A complete exploratory celiotomy is performed. Pancreatic beta cell tumours tend to metastasize to the liver, spleen, and regional lymph nodes making it important to biopsy these organs as part of the procedure.[14,16,18] These tumours range in size from microscopic and non-palpable to 2 cm in diameter. Most masses are 0.5–2.0 mm in diameter and can be visualized and palpated as firm masses within the pancreas (Fig. 18.8).[1,3]

Lumpectomy is generally performed for small single masses or where there are only a few masses. Blunt dissection is used to remove the mass from the parenchyma of the pancreas. Haemorrhage is generally minimal and a small piece of a haemostatic agent is placed in the defect and gently held in place to allow the ductules and capillaries to seal. Enzyme leakage does not generally cause a problem as the pancreatic enzymes have not been activated and will be absorbed by the omentum.[19]

If there are multiple masses in a distinct portion of the pancreas, partial pancreatectomy should be considered. Partial pancreatectomy has also been recommended when there is clinical pathologic evidence of insulinoma but no discrete mass can be found because of the potential for the presence of diffuse microscopic beta cell tumours.[3] There are basically two methods for performing a partial pancreatectomy; the suture fracture technique and the dissection/ligation of ductules and vessels technique.[19] The dissection/ligation technique involves gently dissecting between separate lobules of the pancreas until vessels and ducts or ductules are visualized. These are then ligated with a fine monofilament suture or hemostatic clips. The vessels and ductules are then transected between ligatures until the portion of pancreas to be removed is isolated. For the suture fracture technique, the portion of the pancreas to be removed is isolated by making a small opening into either the mesoduodenum for a right partial pancreatectomy or the omentum for a left partial pancreatectomy to allow a ligature to be passed circumferentially around that limb of the pancreas. As the suture is tightened, the parenchyma of the pancreas is crushed and the ducts, ductules and blood vessels are effectively ligated. That portion of the pancreas to be removed is then dissected from the adjacent mesentery or omentum. With either technique, the defect created in the omentum or mesentery is closed to prevent visceral entrapment.

During partial pancreatectomy, care must be taken not to compromise the pancreatic duct or the blood supply to other structures. The pancreatic duct is located near the apex of the two limbs of the pancreas (Fig. 18.9).

The pancreaticoduodenal blood vessels which supply the duodenum may be compromised during right partial pancreatectomy. The splenic vessels that supply a portion of the spleen may be compromised during a left partial pancreatectomy. These structures must be evaluated for vascular compromise prior to abdominal closure. Postoperative treatment is discussed in Chapter 14.

Surgery may be repeated when clinical signs recur, but it is usually more difficult to control the hypo-

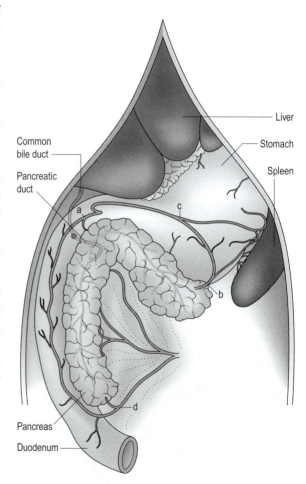

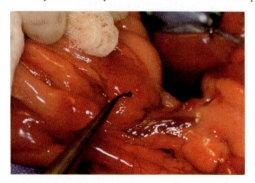

Figure 18.8 Insulinoma in a ferret. The ring tip microforceps are pointing at a 2 mm nodule typical of insulinoma.

Figure 18.9 Anatomy of the pancreas showing the close association of the spleen and duodenum. The common opening of the bile duct and pancreatic duct is also indicated. The cranial pancreaticoduodenal vessels (a), splenic vessels (b), gastroepiploic vessels (c), caudal pancreaticoduodenal vessels (d), liver, bile duct, stomach are also shown. (Reprinted with permission from Comp Cont Edu Pract Vet 21(9,11):815–822, 1049–1057, 1999.)

glycaemia with surgery at the second attempt. When clinical signs recur following the initial surgery, most patients are managed medically with medications and dietary management.

Liver, spleen and lymph node biopsy

It is not unusual for adrenal disease, insulinoma and lymphoma to occur in the one animal. In addition, insulinomas and adrenal adenocarcinomas may metastasize. Therefore, during abdominal surgery it is wise to consider taking biopsies of the liver, spleen and mesenteric lymph nodes.

There are two procedures generally used for liver biopsy in ferrets. If the liver has a lobe with a pointed aspect, then a ligature can be looped around the protruding section of the liver. As is done with the pancreatectomy, the loop of suture is tightened to cut through the liver parenchyma while ligating any blood vessels within. Two to four throws are placed on the suture material and scissors are used to transect the tissue 2–3 mm distal to the ligature. Alternatively, if the liver lobes have a rounded configuration, then a transfixation suture fracture technique can be used (Fig. 18.10).

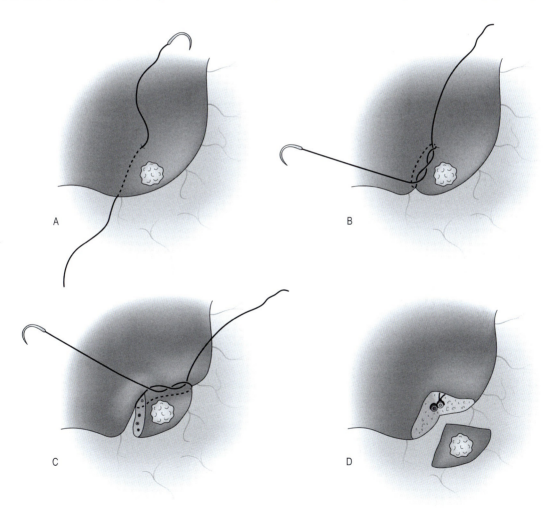

Figure 18.10 Transfixation suture fracture technique. The needle of the suture is passed through the liver parenchyma near the border of the liver (a) and tied to cut through the liver on one side (b). The suture is moved to the other side of the liver lobe and tied to cut through the parenchyma on the other side (c). The biopsy is cut 2–3 mm distal to the suture (d). (Reprinted with permission from Comp Cont Edu Pract Vet 21(9,11):815–822, 1049–1057, 1999.)

The needle of the suture is passed through the liver parenchyma near the border of the liver and tied to cut through the liver on one side. Two throws are placed on the suture material. After the knot has been created, the suture is moved to the other side of the liver lobe and another knot is thrown to cut through the parenchyma on the other side. The biopsy can then be cut 2–3 mm distal to the suture. With either procedure, if there is residual haemorrhage a piece of oxidized regenerated cellulose (Surgicel; Johnson & Johnson Medical, Inc.) can be placed over the site of biopsy collection and be left in place. Biopsy of the spleen can be done in a similar manner. For biopsy of a mesenteric lymph node, dissect the node from the surrounding fat taking care to not damage the vasculature of the surrounding bowel. Vascular clips can be used to ligate vessels to the node.

Cystotomy

Cystic calculi occur in male and female ferrets of any age; however, males are more likely to obstruct than females. Most calculi are composed of magnesium ammonium phosphate (struvite) and may be secondary to bacterial cystitis with *Staphylococcus* species.[20,21] More commonly crystals rather than distinct stones are formed. An improper diet containing a high quantity of vegetation or plant material has been implicated as predisposing ferrets to the development of cystic calculi.[3,20] In ferrets presenting with urethral obstruction, prostate disease must be considered as a differential (see section on adrenal disease). In ferrets with urethral obstruction, diagnosis is based on palpation of a large bladder, palpation of calculi, radiographs, ultrasound, or urinalysis with the presence of crystalluria. Clinical signs of dysuria or stranguria are present in males.

Male ferrets are difficult to catheterize but not impossible (Ch. 20). It is best to use a 3.0 Fr urinary catheter Slippery Sam Tomcat Catheter; SurgiVet, Waukesha, WI, USA. Tomcat catheters and red rubber catheters can be used, but the smallest available is 3.5 Fr which may be difficult to pass in a male ferret. The red rubber 3.5 Fr catheters are often easier to pass than Tomcat catheters as they bend along the ischial curvature more easily. Installation of lidocaine into the urethra and intravenous diazepam to relax the urethra smooth muscle may aid in passage of the catheter. An 18 gauge Teflon catheter may also be used as a urethral catheter in ferrets, but often these are too short and kink along the ischial curvature. Once the catheter is placed management of urolithiasis in ferrets is similar to domestic cats.

Cystotomy may be performed to remove cystic calculi as well as irrigate crystals out of the urethra. A standard ventral cystotomy is performed. When incising the skin and subcutaneous tissues in male ferrets, the caudal superficial epigastric blood vessels along the side of the prepuce should be identified and ligated prior to incision to prevent significant hemorrhage. It is important to inspect the apex of the bladder for a diverticulum, which can predispose to cystic calculi and has been reported in ferrets.[1] The calculi and wall of the bladder are cultured. Antibiotics are administered once the samples have been collected. The bladder is closed using a simple interrupted pattern with a monofilament absorbable material. Postoperatively the ferret is maintained on fluid diuresis and antibiotics pending culture results. Dietary management (placing the ferret on a diet free of plant material) is recommended.[3,22] Urine pH should be evaluated. Ferrets normally maintain an acidic pH in which case urine acidifiers are not indicated. In ferrets with a high urine pH, urine acidifiers may be beneficial in preventing recurrence.[23]

In ferrets with recurrent urolithiasis or where a urinary catheter may not be passed, a perineal urethrostomy may be performed. The procedure is analogous to that performed in cats, however, the use of magnifying loupes and microsurgical instruments is recommended.

Chordoma

Typically chordomas arise at the tip of the tail (41 of 44 reported cases), but can affect the cervical or thoracic spine.[24–26] Chordomas and chondrosarcomas can be difficult to differentiate histopathologically, but immunohistochemistry for cytokeratin will stain positively in cases of chordomas and not in cases of chondrosarcoma.[27] Chordomas on the tail are slow-growing and do not metastasize.[24] In one case of a cervical chordoma, a single metastasis formed following surgical debulking of the primary tumour (see also Ch. 13).[26]

Surgical amputation of the tail tip is recommended.[28] Amputate the tail at the second intervertebral space cranial to the tumour. Chordomas of the cervical and thoracic spine can compress the spinal cord causing ataxia that can progress to paralysis and loss of deep pain perception.[25,26] Magnetic resonance imaging is a useful diagnostic tool for demonstrating cord compression in cases of cervical and thoracic chordoma, and can be superior to myelography.[25] Chordomas of the thoracic and cervical spine can be surgically debulked and the spinal cord decompressed. Resolution of clinical signs following surgery is dependent on the length of time and severity of the compression. Early surgical intervention may result in a more favourable outcome.

Mast cell tumours

Mast cell tumours typically affect the skin in ferrets and are usually benign; however, there are reports of visceral mastocytosis.[29,30] They are most commonly found on the neck, shoulders and trunk as single or multiple hairless, raised, well-circumscribed nodules (see Fig. 13.9).[24,30] Cytologic examination of a needle aspirate may reveal mature mast cells.[30] Surgical removal is curative.[31] In dogs, mast cell tumours should be removed with a wide (3 cm) margin of normal tissue.[32] There are no recommendations published for ferrets, but a 0.5 cm margin appears adequate. Histopathologic examination is recommended to confirm the diagnosis and complete removal. Unlike dogs, pretreatment with histamine blockers does not appear to be necessary in ferrets.

Editor's comment: The possibility of ferrets interfering with surgical wounds is always considered. One case was reported on the 2005 Exotic DVM website, where after an adrenalectomy/pancreatectomy operation a ferret opened up the incision site and chewed its bowel. Using a simple interrupted suture method instead of the continuous method was advised.

References

1. Mullen H. Soft tissue surgery. In: Hillyer EV, Quesenberry KE, eds. Ferrets, rabbits, and rodents: Clinical medicine and surgery. Philadelphia: WB Saunders; 1997:131–144.
2. Fowler ME. Descenting carnivores. In: Fowler ME, ed. Zoo and wild animal medicine, 2nd edn. Philadelphia: WB Saunders; 1986:807–809.
3. Brown SA. A practitioner's guide to rabbits and ferrets. Denver: American Animal Hospital Association; 1993.
4. Brown SA. All those other diseases of the ferret. Proc North Am Vet Conf 1993:727–729.
5. Hoefer HL. Gastrointestinal diseases. In: Hillyer EV, Quesenberry KE, eds. Ferrets, rabbits, and rodents: Clinical medicine and surgery. Philadelphia: WB Saunders; 1997:26–36.
6. Mullen HS, Scavelli TD, Quesenberry KE, Hillyer E. Gastrointestinal foreign body in ferrets: 25 cases (1986 to 1990). J Am Anim Hosp Assoc 1992; 28:13–19.
7. Orsher RJ, Rosin E. Small intestine. In: Slatter D, ed. Textbook of small animal surgery. Philadelphia: WB Saunders; 1993:593–612.
8. Ellison GW. Enterotomy. In: Bojrab MJ, ed. Current techniques in small animal surgery. Philadelphia: Lea & Febiger; 1990:249–252.
9. Lawrence HJ, Gould WJ, Flanders JA, et al. Unilateral adrenalectomy as a treatment for adrenocortical tumors in ferrets: five cases (1990–1992). J Am Vet Med Assoc 1993; 203:267–270.
10. Rosenthal KL, Peterson ME, Quesenberry KE, et al. Hyperadrenocorticism associated with adrenocortical tumour or nodular hyperplasia of the adrenal gland in ferrets: 50 cases (1987–1991). J Am Vet Med Assoc 1993; 203:271–275.
11. Filion DL, Hoar RM. Adrenalectomy in the ferret. Lab Anim Sci 1985; 35:294–295.
12. Weiss CA, Scott MV. Clinical aspects and surgical treatment of hyperadrenocorticism in the domestic ferret: 94 cases (1994–1996). J Am Anim Hosp Assoc 1997; 33:487–493.
13. Brown SA. Adrenal and pancreatic neoplasia. Proc North Am Vet Conf 1993:725–727.
14. Caplan ER, Peterson ME, Mullen HS, et al. Diagnosis and treatment of insulin-secreting pancreatic islet cell tumours in ferrets: 57 cases (1986–1995). J Am Vet Med Assoc 1996; 209:1741–1745.
15. Ehrhart N, Withrow SJ, Erhart EJ, Wimsatt JH. Pancreatic beta cell tumours in ferrets: 20 cases (1986–1994). J Am Vet Med Assoc 1996; 209:1737–1740.
16. Elie MS, Zerbe CA. Pancreatic beta cell tumour in dogs, cats, and ferrets. Compend Cont Edu Pract Vet 1995; 17:51–59.
17. Hillyer EV, Quesenberry KE. Endocrine diseases. In: Hillyer EV, Quesenberry KE, eds. Ferrets, rabbits, and rodents: Clinical medicine and surgery. Philadelphia: WB Saunders; 1997:85–98.
18. Rosenthal KL. How we treat a pancreatic beta cell tumor in the ferret. Proc North Am Vet Conf 1994:822.
19. Harari J, Lincoln J. Surgery of the exocrine pancreas. In: Slatter D, ed. Textbook of small animal surgery. Philadelphia: WB Saunders; 1993:678–691.
20. Bell J. Management of urinary obstruction in the ferret. Proc North Am Vet Conf 1993:724.
21. Nguyen HT, Moreland AF, Shields RP. Urolithiasis in ferrets (*Mustela putorius*). Lab Anim Sci 1979; 29:243–245.
22. Hillyer EV. Urogenital diseases. In: Hillyer EV, Quesenberry KE, eds. Ferrets, rabbits, and rodents: Clinical medicine and surgery. Philadelphia: Saunders; 1997:44–52.
23. Edfors CH, Ullrey DE, Aulerich RJ. Prevention of urolithiasis in the ferret (*Mustela putorius furo*) with phosphoric acid. J Zoo Wildl Med 1989; 20:12–19.
24. Li X, Fox JG. Neoplastic diseases. In: Fox JG, ed. Biology and diseases of the ferret, 2nd edn. Baltimore: Williams & Wilkins; 1998:405–447.
25. Pye GW, Bennett RA, Roberts GD, Terrell SP. Thoracic vertebral chordoma in a domestic ferret (*Mustela putorius furo*). J Zoo Wildl Med 2000; 31:107–111.
26. Williams BH, Eighmy JJ, Berbert MH, Dunn DG. Cervical chordoma in two ferrets (*Mustela putorius furo*). Vet Pathol 1993; 30:204–206.
27. Dunn DG, Harris RK, Meis JM, Sweet DE. A histomorphologic and immunohistochemical study of chordoma in twenty ferrets (*Mustela putorius furo*). Vet Pathol 1991; 28:467–473.
28. Antinoff N. Musculoskeletal and neurologic diseases. In: Hillyer EV, Quesenberry KE, eds. Ferrets, rabbits and rodents: Clinical medicine and surgery. Philadelphia: WB Saunders; 1997:126–130.
29. Brown SA. Neoplasia. In: Hillyer EV, Quesenberry KE, eds. Ferrets, rabbits and rodents: Clinical medicine and surgery. Philadelphia: WB Saunders; 1997:99–114.
30. Orcutt C. Dermatologic diseases. In: Hillyer EV, Quesenberry KE, eds. Ferrets, rabbits, and rodents: Clinical medicine and surgery. Philadelphia: WB Saunders; 1997:115–125.
31. Parker GA, Picut CA. Histopathologic features and postsurgical sequelae of 57 cutaneous neoplasms in ferrets (*Mustela putorius furo*). Vet Pathol 1993; 30:499–504.
32. Vail DM. Mast cell tumours. In: Withrow SJ, MacEwen EG, eds. Small animal clinical oncology. Philadelphia: WB Saunders; 1996:192–210.

CHAPTER 19

Ferret vasectomy, orthopaedics and cryosurgery

'Ferrets can hit a high note … if you step on them.'

Klaus Bernard, Teddy's 'Dad', 2005

Vasectomy

Vasectomy of the hob ferret is an important operation for breeders concerned about resting their jills over a season without resorting to chemical means to prevent post-oestrous anaemia (POA).[1] Some ferret breeders are wary of hormonal treatment to take the jill off heat.

Anatomical detail

The male reproductive system has already been described[2] and essential drawings can be seen in Chapter 2 (see Fig. 2.30a,b). A review of the pertinent anatomical features will highlight the procedure in the operation. The ferret scrotum has two cavities which each house a testis and epididymis. Crouch has shown a detailed diagram of the male cat, which is comparable.[3] The epididymis is composed of a mass of convoluted spermatic duct, which is divided into head, body and tail on the dorsal aspect of the testis as it lies in the scrotal sac. The head of the epididymis receives the efferent ductules as they leave the testis at the cranial pole. The body of the epididymis has the main mass of convoluting spermatic duct, which passes to the tail of the epididymis at the caudal pole of the testis. The spermatic duct becomes apparent as a simple duct at the tail of the epididymis and passes cranially on the dorsal aspect of the testes as the ductus deferens (vas deferens). It is medial to the body of the epididymis.

The ductus deferens is accompanied by the deferent artery and vein and the main testicular artery and vein, which with nerve and lymphatic system vessels form the spermatic cord, which passes cranially to the inguinal passage into the abdomen. *Note* that in the ferret the ductus deferens lies medial to the testicular artery and vein in its passage as the spermatic cord. The testicular artery and vein part company with the ductus deferens inside the abdomen with the ductus deferens looping over the ureter of its respective side to join the urethra through the prostate gland (see Fig. 2.30).

Histologically, the testis, blood vessels, nerves, lymphatics and the ductus deferens are wrapped in a pouch of peritoneum called the vaginal sac. This sac extends through the inguinal canal in development prior to the descent of the testis. It is the common vaginal tunic of the spermatic cord which must, in the vasectomy operation, be delicately dissected open to expose the ductus deferens and to avoid injury to the main testicular artery and vein.

Vasectomy procedure

This operation may require the use of a magnifying head lupe lens. I have used ketamine (20–30 mg/kg) for anaesthesia, plus halothane via facemask for full anaesthesia as described in Chapter 16. A mature hob is the best candidate for this operation, no younger than 9 months. The ferret is set-up for surgery. The site of the vasectomy operation is shown in Figure 19.1.

Using the baculum as a guide, the caudal part of the penis is clipped and prepared for surgery. Using a size

Vasectomy

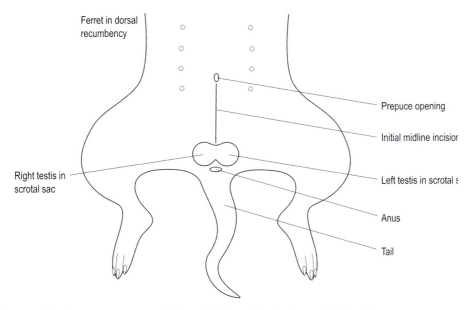

Figure 19.1 Diagrammatic external view of hob genitalia and vasectomy incision.

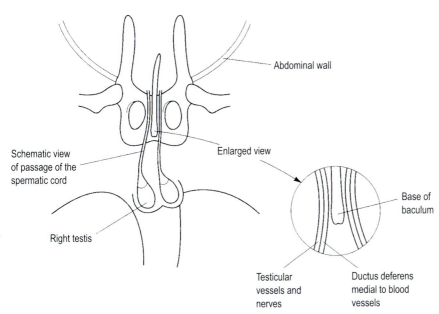

Figure 19.2 Ventral view of ferret pelvis based on radiograph image.

15 blade, an initial incision of some 2 cm or so exposes the fine tissue over the baculum of the penis. On either side of the baculum, the whitish structure of the tunica vaginalis (common vaginal tunica) can be identified. The ductus deferens are seen to arise from each side of the base of the penis on their passage to the cranial inguinal ring. The common vaginal tunica is opened delicately using a fresh size 15 surgical blade. Then, mostly by blunt dissection (ophthalmic forceps are excellent for this work) the separation of the ductus deferens from the testicular artery and vein proceeds. The ductus deferens is about the diameter of 4 metric chromic gut and is medial to the testicular vessels (Fig. 19.2).

The ductus deferens can be taken up from the cranial border of the testis where it is thicker; about 1 cm must be taken. *Note* that the ductus deferens can easily be

441

confused at first glance with a piece of the tunica vaginalis that has been tightly stretched. The tissue extracted can be checked by placing it under a coverslip on a microscope slide to confirm the ductus deferens has been taken and not possible tunica vaginalis tissue. The ductus deferens show a snake-like pattern of a tube with material within. Once satisfied with the tissue removed, the ductus deferens stumps on both sides are ligated with 2/0 chromic gut.

If it helps, it is possible to exteriorize a testicle cranially from the initial midline incision. When the operation is complete, the testicle can be returned to the scrotal sac without adverse effects (see also Ch. 18). No internal stitches are required on completion of the vas deferens severance and only simple interrupted 0.2 mm Vetafil sutures are required for the skin incision. Stitches are tolerated very well and can be removed 10 days post-operatively. If sedation is required medetomidine hydrochloride (Domitor) is useful for this procedure. Antibiotic cover using chloramphenicol i.m. is given and the ferret is allowed to recover in a warm quiet environment; I usually rested ferrets over one night. The vasectomized hob should not be used till 6 weeks after the operation, to allow for any spermatic cord semen to degenerate.

Ferret orthopaedics

The ferret sustains orthopaedic problems like the dog and cat and the same principles apply when attending cases. Some rabbit hunters prefer shooting to netting the rabbits. Working ferrets could be shot in the legs or back as they bound from the warren after the rabbits. Most ferreters are careful to avoid their workers! Though ferrets can get in the way of cars too!

The skeletal and muscle anatomy has been reviewed by Evans and An.[2] Palpation and use of radiology is required. Fractures will heal as in all mammals and with the ferret being light-limbed, the advantage of the weight-bearing forces being not so large may allow self-healing without interference in some cases or else basic use of bandages or splints.[4] Non-surgical techniques are often successful in small animals so these should be considered first. Ferrets however are active animals, though in my experience they will not interfere with sutures. Surgical repair is usually preferred if there is significant overlapping of the fracture segments or in the case of open fractures. An initial examination of the injured ferret will attain the amount of musculoskeletal trauma.

The four major areas of concern can be as listed:

1. Long bone fracture.
2. Chest injury with reference to signs of flail chest, lung trauma, pneumothorax, haemothorax diaphragmatic hernia or traumatic myocarditis.
3. Spinal injury with concern for multiple or unstable fractures. These should always be suspected with fractures involving the tail, sacrum or pelvis, as well as sacroiliac luxations.
4. Blunt abdominal injuries, which give trauma to the kidneys, urethra, spleen, liver or cause urinary bladder rupture.

Thus in many orthopaedic trauma cases, the life-threatening problems must be dealt with first. Fluid therapy and antibiotic administration especially in the case of open wounds is vital (Ch. 20). However, while the musculoskeletal injuries appear to be a low priority, their initial treatment might be critical to successful recovery. Effective early management will contribute greatly to maximum recovery to avoid complications. With the injured ferret stable, a more detailed physical examination is carried out with attention to the initial treatment of musculoskeletal injuries.

Getting the injured ferret to the hospital

Advise client to bring injured ferret in and to cover any open wounds if possible with a clean wet handkerchief to keep the wound from desiccation. The ferret would probably not tolerate an attempt to bandage a limb. Get the owner to wrap the whole ferret in a towel making a ferret 'pipe'. An agitated injured ferret might well bite, so cocooning it in a towel would be a safer move. A tight hold of each end of the 'pipe' would be required until the ferret arrived at the hospital. Once seen it might be advisable to give the ferret a pain killer or sedative. The latter has been described in Chapter 16. The range of suitable analgesics is given in Table 19.1.

A support of some kind for limb fractures is useful to avoid further displacement or damage to the surrounding soft tissue. This is important with spinal injuries and to avoid a closed fracture becoming an open fracture. Any fractures distal to the elbow or stifle should preferably be immobilized with a support dressing.

The fracture site is radiographed under sedation or G/A with the usual two standard views. As with other animals, the comparative radiology of the fractured limb with the good one helps in prognosis. Any palpation of affected limbs is best done under G/A with ferrets. Examining a ferret for possible fractures, the general principles of checking orthopaedic malfunction apply. Lameness or reduced limb function indicates injury, along with abnormal leg positioning and deformation or angular change of structure along any abnormal direction of motion of a limb.[4] *Note* swelling and oedema at the injury site and whether the ferret vocalizes with even gentle palpation. It may well hiss and fluff up its

Ferret orthopaedics

Table 19.1 Table of analgesic drugs suitable for ferrets

Drug name	Drug dose (mg/kg)	Comments
Butorphanol tartrate	0.05–0.5 i.m., s.c. q. 2–6 h	Synthetic opioid having excellent analgesic and antitussive properties
Buprenorphine	0.01–0.03 i.m., s.c. q.8–12 h	Good choice, effective and can be given b.i.d. Analgesic and opiate antagonist. Acts longer than butorphanol
Oxymorphine	0.05–0.20 s.c., i.m., i.v. q. 8–12 h	Potent synthetic narcotic particularly useful after orthopaedic surgery
Flunixin meglumine (Banamine)	1.0 i.m. only s.i.d.	Non-steroidal anti-inflammatory (NSAID) prostaglandin inhibitor, which must not be used with corticosteroids or other NSAIDs. Can cause gastric ulcers in long-term use and renal failure. Thus not used in gastritis, gastric ulcers, enteritis and renal disease
Medetomidine	30–60 µg/kg s.c., i.m. (0.03–0.06 mL Domitor)	Study in dogs shows it is a better analgesic (for soft tissue surgery) than butorphanol and buprenorphine. However, it may cause bradycardia
Aspirin	40–80 (up to 200?) p.o. q. 24–48 h	NSAID drug, so same precautions as flunixin
Carprofen	1.0 p.o. q. 12–24 h	NSAID drug, so same precautions as flunixin
Ketoprofen (Ketofen)	1.0 i.m. q. 24 h	NSAID drug, so same precautions as flunixin. *Note* drug approved in Canada for dogs/cats; USA only horses

Adapted from Finkler M. Practical ferret medicine and surgery for the private practitioner. Roanoak: Roanoak Animal Hospital; 2002.

tail in anger so beware. Try to check for increased or decreased motion of joints. With obvious injury to long bones, there can be open or closed fractures. With open fractures, the traumatized limb will expose the fracture site to possible wound contamination, further bone infection and non-union.

Initial wound treatment

This should involve removing any foreign material such as dirt, hair and dead tissues so as to establish wound drainage if necessary. The wound can be flushed with a suitable sterile fluid to remove potential contaminant organisms and foreign material. I use up partly-used Hartmann's solutions for initial cleaning out with the plastic tubing ideal for delving into ferret wounds. Solutions should be slightly warm so as not to chill the injured ferret. If possible, the fracture site should be stabilized by some means of temporary splinting to protect the blood supply around the site from further damage. Finally broad-spectrum antibiotic cover is given.

Common causes of bone fractures in ferrets:

1. Working ferrets can be back-kicked by a rabbit when in the confined space of a warren. Forelegs are at risk as the ferret goes for the rabbit.
2. Ferrets in outside cages can get into situations where a foot gets caught in wire and a bone broken.
3. House-dwelling ferrets in cages can get into a similar situation with multilevel wire cages and wire ladders. If one has to keep ferrets indoors in cages they should be on one level or use plastic corrugated pipes for gradual tunnels to another floor; these are more interesting to ferrets.
4. In-house pet ferrets can be trodden on, dropped, caught in swinging fly wire doors or get something dropped on them. Ferrets can get broken limbs by being trodden on by bare feet alone.
5. Ferrets outside can climb and there is a danger of falling from a height onto concrete. Ferrets falling onto soft ground or sand rarely break bones as their body 'springs' on impact.
6. With ferrets increasingly being kept in apartments with outside balconies there is a risk of 'high rise syndrome' from getting onto ledges, which must be avoided.
7. The dangers to heavily pregnant jills cannot be overstated. When agitated, they might try to get in or out of places by climbing which can lead to vertebral fractures or disc dislocations.
8. Road accidents concerning ferrets are usually fatal. A fractured pelvis can heal if no drastic bone displacement or severe internal damage has occurred.

Ferret orthopaedic work is finer again than that on rabbit long bones. Studying the ferret skeleton (see Fig. 2.9) it can be seen that the long ferret bones are matchstick-sized (Fig. 19.3).

CHAPTER NINETEEN
Ferret vasectomy, orthopaedics and cryosurgery

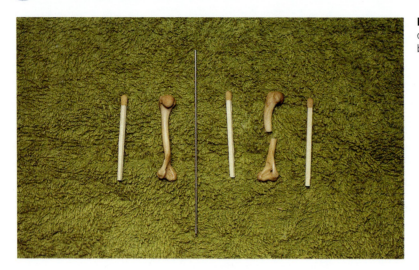

Figure 19.3 Ferret long bones compared with matchsticks and a bone pin.

Fracture treatment

The basic principles of fracture treatment apply to ferrets, with the use of bandages/plaster splinting and use of intramedullary pinning favoured for long bones. The use of plating is not applicable but external skeletal fixation (Kirschner–Elmer-type apparatus) using K-wire may be possible.[4,5]

External coaption

One has to improvise sometimes to adapt the material available to ferret limbs in fracture repair. Vet-Lite (USA) thermoplastic casting material is possible for splints/casts, also for connecting bars for external fixation. Two plaster materials in Australia are Plast-O-Fit (Orfit Industries) and Vet-Lite (DLC Australia Pty Ltd). Modified types of Robert Jones bandages can be used on ferrets but will require thin orthoplastic or Hexalite bars in them (A. Kapatkin, pers. comm. 1999). Before considering light plastic-like casts for limbs, consideration should be given to the extent of soft tissue damage, bone loss or damage and type of fracture. Treatment will depend on the specific bone involved and location of fracture and any presence of infection.

Surgery on even a small site on a ferret might require more extensive attention. Any external splint treatment of limb fractures on ferrets will require monitoring for pad swelling or other complications. Many materials can be adapted as splints for small-limbed animals, e.g. broken-down pop sticks, tongue depressors, plastic syringe cases, etc. The splint or bandage/plaster coaption should be done under a general anaesthetic to prevent pain and also because ferrets would rarely stay still for a good job to be done, at least without strong sedation. Any splint should be kept light in relationship to the weight of the ferret and the ferret would have to be cage-confined for the duration of treatment.

Internal coaption

Intermedullary pinning with K-wire

This is a satisfactory way of treating simple fractures in ferret long bones as with dogs and cats. Due to the matchstick size of ferret long bones, K-wire is used. In one veterinary hospital in the USA, a number of ferret long bone pinnings were done in closed fractures in cases of 'high rise' accidents (A. Kapatkin, pers. com. 1999).

There can, however, be complications with pinning ferret bones, as in any animal. A list of K-wire available in Australia for use with ferrets is given in Table 19.2.

Pinning dog and cat legs will be familiar but I am including an example of a ferret foreleg fracture, as it was the first time I had come across the injury in these animals. It also illustrates the circumstances, owner opinion at the time and final outcome.[6]

A later case occurred where I was asked to assist with a pet sable jill ferret, Lina, which had a suspected left femur fracture from being trodden on (Fig. 19.7). The jill was treated with a 1.6 mm K-wire and a perfect first intention healing was obtained (Fig. 19.8).

Table 19.2 K-wire sizes suitable for ferrets (available in Australia)

(mm)	0.8	1.0	1.2	1.4	1.6	1.8	2.0
(inches)	0.028	0.035	0.045	0.056	0.062	0.072	0.078

Author's clinical example

A ferreter's tale!

A working hob ferret was brought in with a suspected right humerus fracture, sustained possibly by a back kick from a rabbit while out ferreting. The owner was very dubious about the ferret being any good again for ferreting. After some discussion, the ferret was given over to me to operate on it and keep as a pet. I had never done orthopaedics of any kind on a ferret!

Use of K wire in ferret orthopaedics

Subject: 2000 g 1-year-old albino working ferret, Hoppy, (1985 primary case).

Note: Other than the obvious lame right foreleg, Hoppy was alert and active. No external fixation of the leg was attempted, as quite frankly this ferret would not have tolerated anything.

From the radiograph, a 1.2 mm K-wire was selected and sterilized along with standard pack and Jacobs chuck. The operating table was set up as standard plus two warm hot-water bottles covered by a towel to give a space for the ferret to lie in lateral recumbency right side up. For the pinning operation, ketamine was used at the time at 20–30 mg/kg with a calculation of 90 mg i.m. for the ferret's weight.

Time sequence:

1.00 p.m. Hoppy held as usual and given 0.5 mL ketamine (50 mg) into the thigh muscle. He was put in a cat basket on floor and he immediately collapsed. He was seen on his side with head arching and licking lips. He was then transferred to operating table.

1.05 p.m. Hoppy was given another 0.5 mL ketamine into the other leg. This resulted in full relaxation with regular breathing and no musk gland release. After preparation of the lateral aspect of the humerus, a generous incision was made with a 15 size surgical blade from the humeral head, proximally, to the lateral epicondyle, following the lateral border of the humerus. Hoppy, being a fit worker, was very muscular so by careful dissection, mostly digital, the brachiocephalicus and pectoral muscles were separated from apposition with the triceps. The cephalic vein was found and the radial nerve, which ran round the humerus was at the fracture site. After difficulty in keeping the radial nerve out of the way, the fracture site was fully exposed and the K-wire was inserted retrograde from the site into the proximal humeral shaft and out of the body in the standard pinning procedure. The fracture site was reduced and the wire driven into the distal humerus and another radiograph taken (Fig. 19.4) The protruding K-wire was then cut off close to the head of the femur.

2.40 p.m. The muscle layers were then secured with 3.0 chromic gut in single sutures and the skin with 0.20 Vetafil in mattress sutures. Hoppy had begun to show signs of shivering and licking lips.

2.50 p.m. The operation finished with the ferret warm but increasingly shivering and licking lips. He was placed in a warm cage with two warm hot-water bottles and covered by a towel. Hoppy had made a complete recovery from the anaesthetic by the evening. Hoppy was confined to a hospital cage and made no attempt to interfere with the wound or sutures. He was given 0.25 mL chloramphenicol i.m. for several days. No wound or bone infection occurred. Initial recovery was complicated with swelling over the operation site. He showed signs of radial paralysis by dragging the leg and had some swelling over the right shoulder at the extruded wire site.

At 5 weeks post-operation, Hoppy was placing the right foreleg but the swelling enlarged around the right shoulder. A radiograph showed that there was a heavy callus but the pin had moved and was 1.5 cm out of the humerus (Fig. 19.5). Thus a disappointing non-union was suspected so the K-wire was left in another 2 weeks.

Then Hoppy was anaesthetized again with ketamine and the pin removed. A radiograph had shown the humerus with a heavy callus distorted with massive reaction over the shoulder, where the pin had extruded from the bone. Two weeks on and Hoppy was placing the right foreleg well and his leg action improved from that point. Later another radiograph showed the re-modelling of the right humerus into a more natural shape (Fig. 19.6).

Radiological progress of 'Hoppy'

In hindsight, the K-wire was too thin but at the time I feared fracturing the bone more with a tighter fit. However, Hoppy went on to be used for breeding and went back to ferreting, with me!

Lesson ... A larger pin or use of more than one pin would have given more stability.[4]

Intramedullary pinning of ferret long bones with K-wire is a good possibility for fractures though complications can arise as seen with Hoppy. Here, however, we had no post-traumatic osteomyelitis which is possible in both human and animals with poor surgical technique leading to infection.[7] We did have a delayed union situation, which is indicated as a complication in any orthopaedic surgery.[8]

CHAPTER NINETEEN
Ferret vasectomy, orthopaedics and cryosurgery

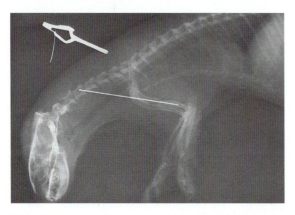

Figure 19.4 Hoppy's right humerus with 1.2 mm K-wire pin (in 1980).

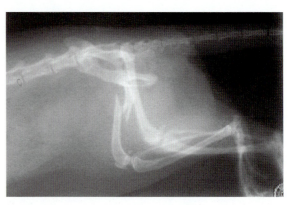

Figure 19.7 Spiral fracture of left femur (in 1986). (Courtesy of Dr D. Baynham, Karrinyup Small Animal Hospital, Perth.)

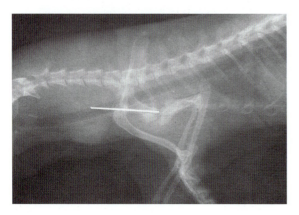

Figure 19.5 Humerus with massive callus and pin movement.

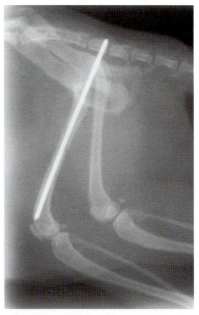

Figure 19.8 Fracture aligned with 1.6 mm K-wire pin. (Courtesy of Dr D. Baynham, Karrinyup Small Animal Hospital, Perth.)

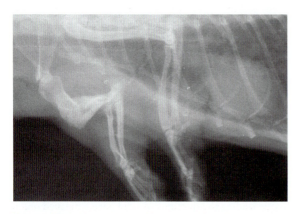

Figure 19.6 Remodelling of humerus after pin removed.

The terminology of bone union, malunion, delayed union or non-union relates to any orthopaedic operation and can also be a feature of ferret surgery. Union means that the bone fracture has healed to bear weight as seen in Hoppy in time but true histological healing can take approximately 18 months to remodel a bone to full strength. Malunion[9] implies that the fracture has healed but the alignment is not compatible with the normal

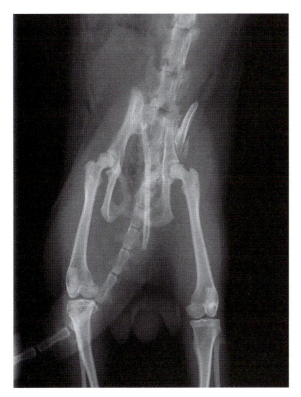

Figure 19.9 Ferret 'Clint' with fractured pelvis. (Courtesy of Lynn Mathison, Coreen Ave Veterinary Clinic, Penrith, NSW.)

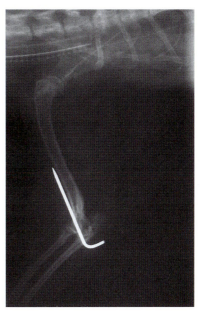

Figure 19.10 Ferret elbow with transarticular pin. (Courtesy of Dr A. Kapatkin, University of Pennsylvania School of Veterinary Medicine.)

function of the bone while a delayed union is considered a vague term to a fracture which has taken a longer amount of time to heal. There are many reasons for this and in our surgical case was the inability of the K-wire chosen to secure the fracture site. This fracture was complicated as it was a spiral fracture and I was afraid of shattering the fragile bone.

It was not a non-union situation because the bone did heal and remodel even though it was primarily out of alignment. The leg came back to normal function in the end but the case stands as a warning to others unfamiliar with ferret orthopaedics. In the case of a dog/cat with a similar fracture a cerclage wire could have been used[10] for a spiral fracture[6] or perhaps use of a Kirschner–Ehmer-type apparatus (K–E) with K-wire could have been tried instead of pinning.

It is interesting that in the USA biodegradable pins made of polydioxine materials are being trialled; these are biochemically stiff enough to allow fracture healing and then resorb gradually by 24 weeks when the bone is remodelled and will not longer need support.[5] Thus there is no need for a second surgery to remove the medullary pin. The use of plastic (polypropylene) rods as intramedullary devices as used in birds has been described.[4]

In the case of Hoppy, the outcome was eventually satisfactory but even a malunion can be corrected with further surgery.[9]

There are cases of ferrets healing themselves, with help, as shown in Figure 19.9, of a ferret Clint who was bitten by a dog around the pelvis. Clint, a 1250 g, 2-year-old albino hob, was given emergency treatment at one clinic and radiology, and then transferred to another clinic, which dealt with NSW Ferret Welfare Society cases. Clint had a purulent bite over the sacrum and lung contusions on radiology. He had deep pain sensation present in both hind legs, slower in the LHL and tail than the RHL. The left ileum was fractured and displaced. There was concern about the L1–L2 alignment, possible vertebral body separation and nerve damage.

It was decided to treat the bite wounds and keep in hospital for a few days under antibiotic (Clavulox 0.1 mL s.c. s.i.d.) and pain killer (methadone 0.02 mL s.c. given b.i.d. or q.i.d. as needed). Over 4 days a remarkable improvement occurred. Initially help was given to express Clint's bladder. On day 2, the ferret was urinating and defaecating and using hind legs though still lame. He was eating but not wanting to attempt walking. He had deep pain and proprioception in both hind legs. Wound on back was improving but lung had some emphysema. On day 3, Clint was placing hind legs, had deep pain perception and withdrawal action with both hind legs. The wound was still good and his mucous

CHAPTER NINETEEN
Ferret vasectomy, orthopaedics and cryosurgery

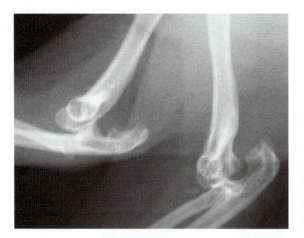

Figure 19.11 Bilateral elbow dislocation. (Courtesy of C. Johnson-Delaney 2005.)

membranes were moist and pink. On day 4, he was still eating, urinating and defaecating. Physiotherapy found Clint attempting walking and placing hind legs, which splayed laterally a bit. The wound was healing. He was sent home on Clavulox medication and required strict cage rest before being re-checked in 2 weeks.

On re-check, Clint was moving well and bowel and urinary system were normal. He was admitted for castration under ACP/methone/atropine pre-med with mask isoflurane anaesthesia. Clint recovered fully after the operation.

This case is an example of the 'box' mending of a fractured pelvis, where the spine is not involved and invasive surgery was not needed.

Elbow luxations can occur with ferrets and can be treated by transarticular pinning as shown in Figure 19.10. (A. Kapatkin, pers. comm. 1999).

A bilateral elbow luxation in an 8-month-old jill ferret, which could not walk, was dealt with by tape wrapping/immobilizing for 3 weeks (Fig. 19.11). The bandage was gradually loosened over 5 weeks by which time she had formed a false joint and became totally ambulatory and pain-free. It would be difficult to know she had a problem unless the leg was palpated at the elbow. The real elbow was solid and bent distal to it. It was theorized that the condition had been a congenital defect as the owner reported that the jill had always limped and not kept up with her housemate (C. Johnson-Delaney, pers. comm. 2005).

Examples of fractured ferret long bones are also given in Figure 19.12a,b; these can be treated with K-wire pinning.

Hydrobathing helps with rehabilitation. I found it useful in 2004 when my ferret kitten Pip broke a humerus when he was accidentally stepped on. I was able to set it quickly manually. Using a washing-up bowl of warm

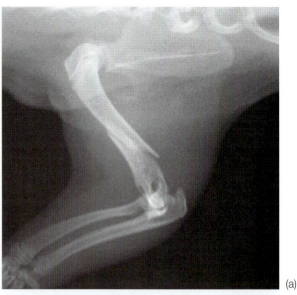

(a)

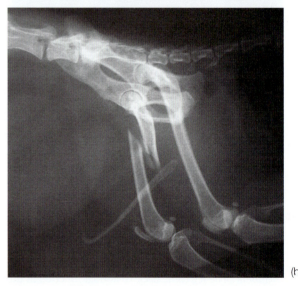

(b)

Figure 19.12 (a) Fracture humerus. (b) Fracture femur. (Courtesy of C. Johnson-Delaney.)

water, he was held gently under the chest/abdomen and gained exercise in the water. Ferrets I find are not too keen to stay long in water, unlike their otter cousins.

Use of Kirschner–Ehmer-type apparatus (K–E) for ferret long bones

This technique has been used in very small animals and has the advantage of providing better stability than coaption splinting.[4] It also maintains the long bone to its normal length and allows for adjustment for correct alignment of fragments. With small animals like ferrets there is the problem of the weight and it is desirable that the device be kept to a minimum and must be placed as close to the skin as possible. The configurations available and the advantages/disadvantages have been discussed by McCoy with regards to birds and can be adapted to ferrets.[11]

One veterinarian considered that the K–E technique avoids disturbance of limb blood supply and uses type 1 configuration small K-wire smooth pins and having closed reduction with nonsterile polymethylmethacrylate as the connecting bars. The lower limb bones are aligned by feel or under fluoroscopy if available after pins are in place. Fractures of the humerus and femur usually have to be aligned by open reduction to get a good alignment. Types of K–E splints other than type 1 are too bulky for ferrets (A. Kapatkin, pers. comm. 1999).

The technique thus carried out requires small K-wires and a size 0.6 mm (0.25 inch) is available in the USA. It is suggested that the pins used should not be larger than 20% of the diameter of the ferret bone or else there is a danger of shattering the bone. I was very aware of the bone fragility when pinning but have had no experience with the K–E apparatus in ferrets so would be even more cautious.

Pins are placed using a low speed drill close to the joint and should be parallel to the joint surface. The stability of fixation can be increased with more pins. However, the pins should be placed at least half of the bone diameter away from the fracture line. The pins must penetrate both cortices fully and the fixation pins should be at 45° to one another in each fragment to prevent them backing out. The best technique in the USA appears to be using K-wire with an acrylic cast (Egger, Colorado State University, 1998). In Australia, the Vet-Lite material would do with the K-wire.

To make the epoxy connecting bars many types of tubular material are available such as plastic tubing, drinking straws, Penrose drain tubing, etc. They must be placed over the fixation pins in each fragment. Clamps are used to give temporary alignment while radiographs are taken to assess the situation[4] but may be too big to hold the bones in good alignment. The tubular material should be positioned just above the skin so that a pin cutter can be used for removal. This will also keep the heat of the exothermic reaction of any epoxy from damaging the underlying structures. The epoxy glue is then injected into the tubular material and allowed to set. The K-wire can also be inserted here for extra strength if needed. This forms a so-called biphasic connecting bar which in the USA has been replaced by Hexcelite and by Vet-Lite in Australia. Once the glue has cured, all the fixation pins are trimmed as close as possible to the cured tube.

Damage to ferret spinal cord

A UK review of the methods suitable for the evaluation of behavioural recovery of animals with spinal cord injuries, ether in a clinical or laboratory situation, has been recorded.[12] The basic concern is about dogs and cats, with about 1–2% of dogs getting intervertebral disc disease with damage to the spinal cord. The authors cite concussion, compression and laceration of the spinal cord as major damage in dogs and cats and this would follow for mustelid types, e.g. ferrets, otters, badgers, etc. in road trauma. Other possibilities of damage include congenital vertebral instability, penetrating or non-penetrating injuries and acquired damage causing stenosis of the vertebral canal. Odd conditions like neoplasia, intraspinal synovial and ganglion cysts and arachnoid cysts are listed.[12] The potentially life-threatening condition of autonomic dysreflexia is cited but not seen in dogs and cats. References are listed to the increased interest in the various therapies for spinal cord injury specifically designed for veterinary use. In time, treatments might include pet ferrets if microsurgery advances in the species. It is noted that animals tend to recover a fair amount of locomotory ability after a spinal cord injury.

Early on in my ferret breeding days I had a heavy post-whelping jill suffering a spinal injury trying to get out of the top of a whelping box and getting caught. She hung over and her weight led to the injury. After many weeks of attempted treatments with prednisolone and rest, there was no improvement and she was euthanized.

In humans, the only clinically-approved treatment for spinal injury according to the authors is high doses of methylprednisolone sodium succinate, which *must* be given within 8 hours of the injury to be effective. Most dogs, and my ferret, are not treated within this time frame.

Useful drugs for spinal treatment are listed as naloxone or tirilazad mesylate, used in humans, which may aid animals. The anti-inflammatory cytokine interleukin 10 (IL-10), the transplantation of olfactory ensheathing glia and monoaminergic cells have been found useful in rats but not checked in other animals. A table of 15 points scoring for evaluation of spinal injury in the dog was added and could be adapted to the ferret.[12]

A hemilaminectomy to decompress the spinal cord was carried out on a ferret with success and was recorded in 2004.[13] A 7-month-old ferret had a 3-week history of acute onset of paraplegia and initial X-rays showed six lumbar vertebrae instead of the usual five. The intervertebral space between the second and third lumbar vertebrae was narrowed. Also there was subtle lucency with indistinct margins affecting the adjacent vertebrae (Fig. 19.13a,b). *Note* there had been no apparent neurological improvement after cage rest with treatment using 1 mg prednisolone and 5 mg marbofloxacin given once daily.

CHAPTER NINETEEN
Ferret vasectomy, orthopaedics and cryosurgery

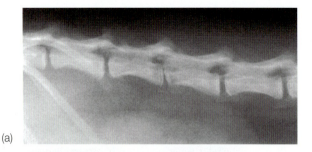

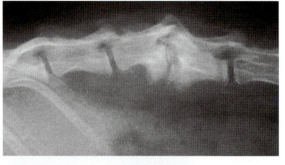

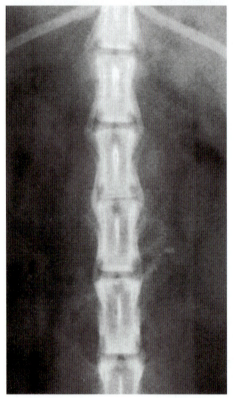

Figure 19.13 (a) Lateral showing intervertebral space between L2 & L3 narrowed. (b) Dorsoventral view showing subtle lucency with indistinct margins affecting adjacent vertebral bodies. (Courtesy of D. Lu, C. Lamb, J.C. Patterson-Kane and R. Capello.)

Figure 19.14 (a) Lateral showing subluxation at L2/3 with ventral displacement of L3. A relatively well-defined lucent zone in the cranial aspect of the body of L3 separates dorsal part of the cranial end plate from the vertebral body. (b) Dorsoventral view showing large osteophytes with indistinct margins on lateral (and ventral) aspects of L2 & L3. (Courtesy of D. Lu, C. Lamb, J.C. Patterson-Kane and R. Capello.)

The ferret showed paraplegia with increased muscle tone in the hind limbs and intact withdrawal reflexes but reduced deep pain sensation on both sides. There was a normal panniculus reflex. On palpation in the midlumbar region, two dorsal articular facets were found raised suggesting they had become displaced or enlarged. The whole midlumbar region was hyperaesthetic. A suspicion of a spinal lesion affecting the upper motor neurons to the hind limbs was made.

Further radiographs showed a subluxation at L2/3 (Fig. 19.14a,b). The caudal articular facets of L2 looked normal but were out of alignment with the remainder of the lumbar spine because L3 was displaced ventrally. The body of L3 had a mostly well-defined lucent zone in the cranial part of its body. On the ventral and lateral aspects of L2 and L3 were large osteophytes with indistinct margins. From lumbar myelography the cord was found displaced dorsally and slightly to the right by the extradural lesion at L2/3 (Fig. 19.15a,b).

Ferret orthopaedics

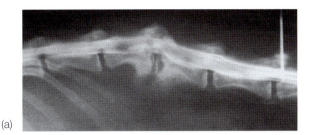

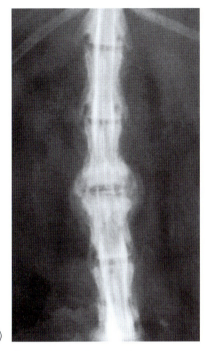

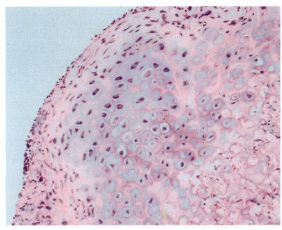

Figure 19.16 Histology section of articular facets. (Courtesy of D. Lu, C. Lamb, J.C. Patterson-Kane and R. Capello.)

Figure 19.15 (a) Lateral lumbar myelogram showing spine displaced dorsally. (b) Dorsoventral lumbar myelogram showing indication of right displacement of spine. (Courtesy of D. Lu, C. Lamb, J.C. Patterson-Kane and R. Capello.)

Note: myelography is done on the anaesthetized ferret in sternal recumbency by a lumbar approach. Under aseptic conditions a 20 or 22 gauge spinal needle is placed through the space between the lumbar vertebrae L5 and L6. For this procedure, the ferret's legs are extended forward to open up the intervertebral space. As an alternative, the needle could be placed in the atlanto-occipital joint. Cerebrospinal fluid samples can be collected for analysis.[14]

It was considered that the outcome of the damage was prolapse of the intervertebral disc at L2/3 and fracture of the cranial endplate of the L3 with the added complication of discospondylitis.

Surgery was performed with a hemilaminectomy, where the left articular facets of L2/3 were found enlarged and removed using rongeurs. Bleeding was controlled by electrocautery. The spinal cord was seen displaced dorsally by firm pale extradural matter on the ventral aspect of the vertebral canal. The material was extruded intervertebral disc and osteophytes. The spinal cord was then decompressed by removing the material with a dental scraper and curette. The wound was then closed and stitched up. For pain relief buprenorphine was given i.m. at 0.02 mg/kg t.i.d. for 48 hours. Enrofloxacin was given intraoperatively at 10 mg/kg and once daily thereafter for 2 months.

Histology of the articular facets revealed lamellar bone fragments with transition to small amounts of woven bone or disorganized chondro-osseous matrix on some surfaces. There were active osteoblasts lining the lamellar bone and Howship's lacunae showed increased osteoclast numbers demonstrating bone remodelling (Fig. 19.16).

A resulting post-operation radiograph (Fig. 19.17a,b) showed a successful fusion of the second and third vertebrae and also smooth well-defined exostosis obliterating the intervertebral joint. Because of the ventral displacement of L3, there was kyphosis and the vertebral canal at L2 appeared to be narrower on the lateral radiograph.

The ferret regained voluntary movement at 10 days post-surgery and became able to walk 1 month after surgery. The ferret continued to improve and a neurological examination was done 5 months after surgery. There was residual mild pelvic limb ataxia, reduced postural reaction with increased muscle tone and exaggerated withdrawal reflexes but the ferret was able to maintain the normal raised back stance of the Mustelidae. Deep pain perception was normal and there was no sign of spinal pain. (No cause for the disc prolapse could be ascertained but ferrets can get into some awkward situations as with my jill ferret with spinal trouble.)

CHAPTER NINETEEN
Ferret vasectomy, orthopaedics and cryosurgery

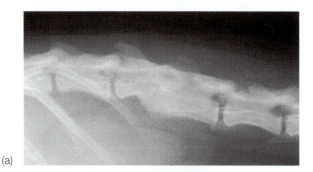
(a)

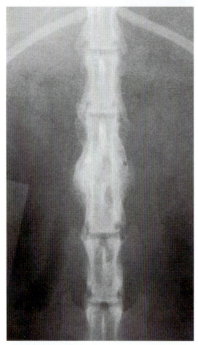
(b)

Figure 19.17 (a) Follow-up image showing fusion of 2nd and 3rd lumbar vertebrae with smooth well-defined exostoses obliterating the intervertebral joints. There is kyphosis, increased curvature, due to L3 displacement. The vertebral canal is narrower at L2. (b) Dorsoventral view of healed L2/L3 fusion. (Courtesy of D. Lu, C. Lamb, J.C. Patterson-Kane and R. Capello.)

It was considered when examining the progression of radiograph signs, that the ferret could have had a situation analogous to discospondylitis in the dog. However, there were no histological signs of inflammation in the ferret case. The remodelling of the articular surfaces as observed could have occurred secondary to spinal instability. The overall recovery of the ferret was remarkable with normal motor function and urinary function regained.

Postoperative care of ferret orthopaedic cases

Spinal cases require special attention and soft bedding with constant attention over the critical period postoperation. Ferrets with limb fractures are also confined initially postoperatively and restricted until splints or pins, etc. are removed. This requires further hospitalization or strict owner compliance. Attention must be given to the state of the ferret feet, especially to where constricting bandages/casts are applied to the leg. Once the limb is clear of pins, etc., physiotherapy for the ferret can commence allowing it to paddle in water by being held with a hand support in a bath, but not freed, so that the injured appendage can be exercised. Advise on prevention of further accident situations with active ferrets!

The question of pain

The subjects of vasectomy and orthopaedics, along with general surgery and trauma, require attention to pain relief. The extent of anticipated pain levels in cats and dogs has been described[15] and can be related to ferrets.

- Mild to moderate pain: De-sexing young ferrets, small soft tissue surgeries, cystitis and otitis
- Moderate pain: Soft tissue surgery without inflammation or external tissue damage, de-sexing older ferrets and enucleation
- Moderate to severe pain: Fracture repairs, joint surgery, peritonitis, pancreatitis, osteoarthritis, thoracotomy, laparotomy (high incision, extensive tissue damage), multiple trauma, ear canal ablation and cancer pain
- Severe pain: Extensive inflammation, e.g. septic peritonitis, multiple fracture repair, bone cancer and meningitis.

In this list, I have replaced 'animal' with 'ferret' so does that make a difference? It should not but regular injection of a separate pain killer on top of anaesthetic may not be warranted in, e.g. cases of sterilizations. If the ferret is under an anaesthetic during recovery, e.g. ketamine/xylazine, when they 'sleep it off' over time, I am of the opinion that the initial pain of surgery has gone on their recovery. *Note*: ketamine is recommended for moderate to severe pain in cats and dogs.[15] Medetomidine (Domitor) also has analgesic properties (Table 19.1). Usually the normal ferret recovers quickly without the use of analgesics. In some cases, the toxicity of any drug on the ferret has considered.

However, analgesia is the absence of pain and drug use for analgesia is to make the pain as tolerable as possible without depressing the patient.[15] It is said that there are three ways of giving analgesia: (a) as needed which might involve the ferret becoming distressed or in pain when receiving the dose and often it requires a higher dose to re-establish analgesia. (b) A fixed schedule is better than 'as needed', as long as the dose interval is tailored for the ferret needs and not over a long time. (c) It is considered that the best way to administer analgesia is by CRI (constant rate infusion), at least in cats and dogs, whereby pain is prevented rather than treated.

Thus, the prophylactic use of analgesic drugs is possible where pain is likely to occur, as in surgery of any kind, and it will prevent animal wind-up, reduce anaesthesia, reduce the need for analgesia postoperatively and decrease overall morbidity.[15]

One ferret vet uses Buprenex (buprenorphine) routinely as a preoperative analgesic for ferrets. Another ferret vet never uses preoperative analgesics but sometimes uses butorphanol postoperatively for major surgery, such as adrenalectomies, exploratory operations, etc. She maintains that butorphanol (1 mL (10 mg/mL) diluted to 1 mL with sterile water with the ferret given 0.1 mL) works quite well with the ferret pretty sedated and works for a few hours unlike with cats and dogs when it only lasts a couple of hours. (I confess I did not use an analgesic with Hoppy. He was given a high ketamine dosage. With my adrenalectomy operation on Josie, I relied on the ketamine and halothane, see Ch. 14). Another ferret vet suggests that ferrets are stoic animals and will mask signs of pain so it is best to give them the benefit of the doubt and give analgesics routinely pre-and postoperatively.[14]

To continue with this concept, some authors have evaluated the use of epidural analgesia in ferrets.[16] They maintain that epidural opioid analgesics do result in longer duration of pain relief than the usual i.m. or s.c. routes. There are fewer side-effects such as motor impairment, sedation or cardiopulmonary depression. They suggest the epidural route for any abdominal, limb or perineal surgery and thus propose it for ferret sterilization and anal sacculectomy as the routine operations carried out on pet ferrets. The authors considered practitioners may scoff at the idea of epidural injections in the ferret but insist that the technique is possible, safe and easy to learn.

Location of the landmarks for epidural administration requires palpation of the cranial wings of the ilea. One visualizes an imaginary transverse line connecting the two points. Thus, the lumbosacral junction would lie midway between these points and at right angles to it. The authors consider the ferret might have 5, 6, or 7 lumbar vertebrae. Figure 2.10 shows the ferret skeleton indicating five, which Howard Evans asserts was the total for the Marshall Farms strain at the time (Evans, pers. comm. 2005). The spinal cord is seen to terminate just before the caudal end of the last lumbar vertebra. It is suggested that the last lumbar vertebra may or may not be palpable in some ferrets. *Note*: this contradicts some suggestions that the dorsal spinous process of the last lumbar vertebra is taller than that of S1. This is true in some ferrets. The three vertebrae making up the sacrum have dorsal spinous processes of which the first is easily palpable. Moreover, the space between S1 and S2 dorsal spinous processes is larger that that between S2 and S3.

The procedure requires the ferret in sternal recumbency with the hips flexed, which opens up the lumbosacral space where the overlying hair must be clipped for about 4 × 5 cm. Under sterile hospital prep precautions, a 25 gauge needle is placed exactly on the midline at the lumbosacral junction with the bevel facing craniad. The needle is advanced perpendicular to the plane of the skin. An empty 1 mL syringe is attached to the needle and 0.1 mL of air is slowly injected to check the site. A negative for blood and lack of resistance to the air injection confirms the correct placement of the needle. If there is resistance, or if the injection of air causes the skin to bulge, then advance the needle until it fully penetrates the ligamentum flavum. The check for resistance should be repeated. The distinct 'popping' sensation of larger animal epidurals does not occur. *Note*: a tail twitch may occur as confirmation of the correct needle placement.

Replace the empty syringe with one with morphine (dosage 0.1 mg/kg or ≈0.1 mL). Two people will be required for the syringe change procedure to keep the needle steady. The authors have treated over 40 ferrets with this technique. There have been good results for analgesia and no signs of morphine-induced nausea. The analgesics useful for ferret medication are given in Table 19.1.

Clinical use of epidural anaesthesia

One Spanish veterinary practice has seen close to 300 ferrets (both sexes) over 4 years. Epidural anaesthesia is used for neutering routinely and also for some other surgery. It is considered that neutering surgeries need to be fast, safe and cheap. They are done under ketamine (5 mg/kg) plus medetomidine (0.08 mg/kg males or 0.1 mg/kg females) plus butorphanol (0.1 mg/kg). These drugs are given as one i.m. injection. *Note*: the butorphanol is diluted as needed. They also give 0.3 mg/kg meloxicam (NSAID). Because the k + m + b has a hypoxaemic effect, they give the ferret oxygen by facemask. No isoflurane is used. It is considered that with the combination, more than 50% of ferrets feel pain when you touch the testicular duct. Using epidural lidocaine the analgesic effect is stronger and it is not

CHAPTER NINETEEN

Ferret vasectomy, orthopaedics and cryosurgery

necessary to infiltrate lidocaine in the deferent duct. The ferret seems more comfortable.

The effect of lidocaine is almost instantaneous and lasts 45 minutes. The neutering operations usually take 30 minutes. The ferret is unable to stand during rest of the 45 minutes but is pain-free. *Note*: the lidocaine has a relaxing effect over the anal (scent) glands, which are removed in the hob, so this procedure comes first. (I can only comment that on my own operations. I never removed the scent glands and never had them expressed during an operation. Of course, I never went to such lengths for analgesia as this procedure does. Techniques have moved on! (see Ch. 16).)

With the female spays, plus orthopaedics, insulinoma operations and abdominal surgeries of other kinds, that practice used higher doses of medetomidine, isoflurane and epidural analgesia. The latter is considered a good choice for the time factor and for pain relief (A. Montesinos, pers. comm. 2005).

Ferret cryosurgery

The speciality of cryosurgery has been proposed as revolutionary with regard to adrenalectomy operations in ferrets, especially on the right adrenal, after being introduced by Weiss in 1999.[17] However, like any new techniques, there are those for and against the idea. Cryosurgery is a difficult procedure and some might question the ability to control the depth of freezing accurately. The proponents of cryosurgery maintain that the effect on the blood vessel wall is minimal due to the flow of blood. The situation might be different with large adrenal tumours occluding the majority of flow through the vena cava. With traditional surgery one knows whether one has removed all the gland or not and bleeding from the vena cava is usually immediately apparent. Those who do not endorse cryosurgery for adrenal disease at present have several queries: whether all the adrenal gland is frozen, whether the vessel wall gets frozen and necroses to give bleeding later, whether there has been invasion of the vena cava by adrenal tumours, or whether large tumours are left to necrose in the body (G. Pye, pers. comm. 2005).

Dr D. Johnson has used cryosurgery for over 2 years and found it compared favourably with standard surgical adrenalectomy and mast cell tumours. He has given a precise account in the Exotic DVM magazine of the procedure with emphasis on removal of the dreaded right adrenal gland tumour which sits on the vena cava.[18] He considers that surgical removal of the whole right adrenal tumour is near impossible and haemostasis is a challenge.

Johnson believes the process offers shorter surgical time for small tumours, better haemostasis, and with

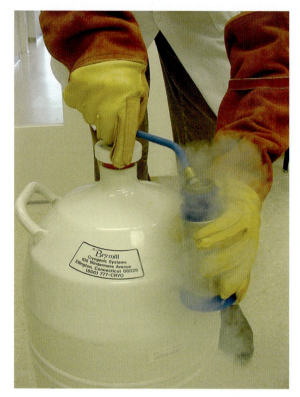

Figure 19.18 Liquid nitrogen storage. (Courtesy of D. Johnson.)

large tumours, he suggests the operative time is comparable to excision.

Theory of cryosurgery

Cell death occurs by intracellular ice crystals damaging the cell wall and organelles; extracellular ice crystals draw water from within the cell causing toxic electrolyte levels, while membrane lipoprotein complexes are damaged resulting in cell wall permeability and lysis. Then vascular stasis occurs leading to ischaemia and cell mediated immunity is enhanced as tumour-specific antigens are exposed.

The most efficient cryogen is liquid nitrogen, which has a boiling point of −196°C. It works faster and penetrates deeper than other agents and thus caution must be taken not to injure healthy tissues.

The cryosurgery procedure

Stock liquid nitrogen is stored in a 20 L size Dewar, which is enough for 4–6 months use (Fig. 19.18). The nitrogen is transferred to the Cryogun using a with-

Ferret cryosurgery

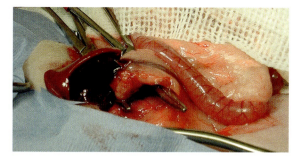

Figure 19.19 The right adrenal gland is located at the junction of the vena cava and the caudate lobe of the liver. (Courtesy of D. Johnson.)

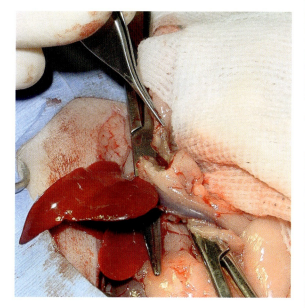

Figure 19.20 The adrenal gland rotated. (Courtesy of D. Johnson.)

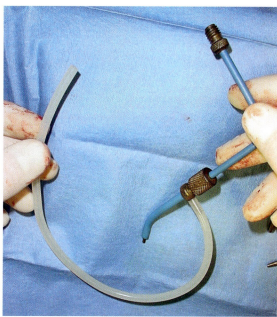

Figure 19.21 Autoclaving cryoprobe and angled extension. (Courtesy of D. Johnson.)

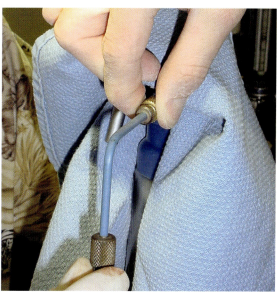

Figure 19.22 The cryoprobe is connected. (Courtesy of D. Johnson.)

drawal tube with appropriate safety measures. *Note*: a loaded Cryogun will remain stable for several hours after filling.

At the operation site of the right adrenal gland, the gland and associated vena cava must be dissected free from the surrounding tissues so that they may be lifted away from the body slightly when the tumour is frozen (Fig. 19.19). The adrenal gland is rotated ventrally to make it accessible and a histological sample can be taken before cryosurgery (Fig. 19.20).

The cryoprobe and angled extension would be autoclaved (Fig. 19.21). The liquid nitrogen can travel through the extension down to the probe tip and then back up and out through the vent when in action. In preparation for surgery, the Cryogun is covered with a sterile towel. Beginning the procedure, the surgeon holds the probe assembly, while an assistant connects them together (Fig. 19.22). Then the area is packed off

455

CHAPTER NINETEEN
Ferret vasectomy, orthopaedics and cryosurgery

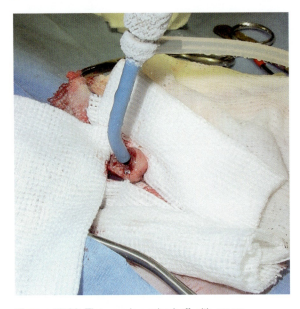

Figure 19.23 The area is packed off with gauze. (Courtesy of D. Johnson.)

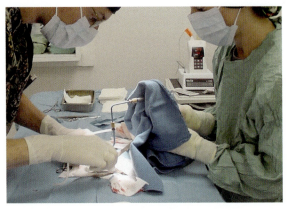

Figure 19.24 Checking the cryoprobe. (Courtesy of D. Johnson.)

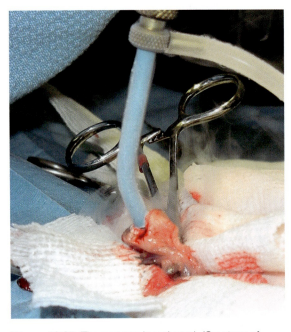

Figure 19.25 The cryogen is activated. (Courtesy of D. Johnson.)

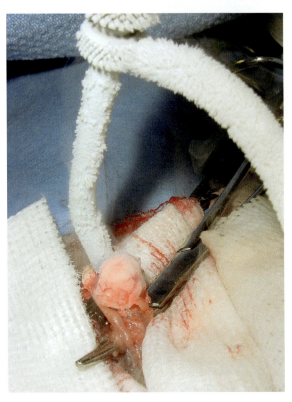

Figure 19.26 Freeze of −20°C to −30°C on tumour. (Courtesy of D. Johnson.)

with dry gauze for insulation and protection (Fig. 19.23). The surgeon then inserts the probe into the affected tumour and checks once more that the probe is not accidentally in contact with other tissue (Fig. 19.24).

Finally, the Cryogun is activated and as soon as freezing is detected, the surgeon applies a gentle upward traction (Fig. 19.25). Elevating the gland protects other tissues from freezing and provides a faster, deeper freeze.

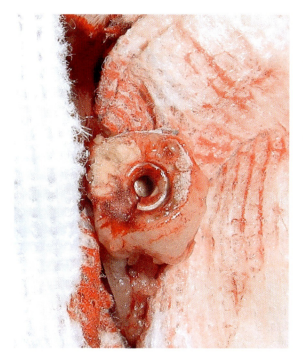

Figure 19.27 Thaw of the adrenal tumour. (Courtesy of D. Johnson.)

To minimize the risk of thrombosis, blood flow through the vena cava is allowed to continue uninterrupted.

Note: when the tumour embedded in normal tissue is frozen, the temperature of the probe tip approaches −196°C but remarkably, the edge of the ice ball reaches only 0°C (Fig. 19.26). The tumour cells must be frozen to a temperature of −20°C to −30°C, thus a freeze margin of 5–10 mm around the target tissue may be warranted. For the ferret, freeze margins of this size would be excessive and dangerous.

Note: dissection and elevation of the adrenal gland overcomes this problem according to Johnson by eliminating the warming effects of nearby tissues. Therefore, using the technique, the entire mass can be deeply frozen without affecting the normal tissue around it.

The adrenal tumour should be allowed to thaw gradually and the temptation to flush with sterile saline must be resisted (Fig. 19.27). In addition, the probe tip should not be removed from the tumour prematurely. Target tissue must go through 2–3 freeze/thaw cycles. *Note*: to completely treat a large tumour, freezing at 2 or 3 more sites may be necessary.

After freezing is completed, the gland is returned to its original position so that the blood flows normally through the vena cava and the body cavity is lavaged with warm sterile saline before the final closure.

References

1. Lewington JH. Anatomical guidelines to the vasectomy operation in the male (hob) ferret Control and therapy. University of Sydney: Postgraduate Foundation 1991; 161:348.
2. Evans HE, An NQ. Anatomy of the ferret. In: Fox J, ed. Biology and diseases of the ferret. Baltimore: Williams & Wilkins; 1998.
3. Crouch JE. Textbook of cat anatomy. Philadelphia: Lea & Febiger; 1969.
4. Cannon M. Orthopaedic surgery in small exotic pets: mammals. In: Bryden D, ed. Internal medicine, small companion animals proceedings. University of Sydney: Postgraduate Foundation 1998; 306:271–277.
5. Kapatkin A. Orthopaedics in small mammals. In: Hillyer E, Quesenberry K, eds. Ferrets, rabbits, and rodents: Clinical medicine and surgery. Philadelphia: Saunders; 1997:364–357.
6. Lewington JH. Orthopaedic surgery with ferrets, Vade Mecum Series. University of Sydney: Postgraduate Foundation 1988; C10:30–31.
7. Braden TD. Post-traumatic osteomyelitis. Vet Clin North Am Small Anim Pract 1991; 21:781–811.
8. Sumner-Smith G. Delayed unions and non-unions. Vet Clin North Am Small Anim Pract 1991; 21:745–759.
9. Anson LW. Malunions. Vet Clin North Am Small Anim Pract 1991; 21:761–780.
10. Schrader SC. Complications associated with the use of Steinmann intramedullary pins and cerclage wires for fixation of long-bone fractures. Vet Clin North Am Small Anim Pract 1991; 21:687–703.
11. MacCoy DM. Treatment of fractures in avian species. Vet Clin North Am Small Anim Pract 1992; 22:225–238.
12. Webb AA, Jeffery ND, Olby NJ, et al. Behavioural analysis of the efficacy if treatment for injuries to the spinal cord in animals. Vet Rec 2004; 155:225–230.
13. Lu D, Lamb CR, Paterson-Kane JC, et al. Treatment of a prolapsed lumbar intervertebral disc in a ferret. J Small Anim Pract 2004; 45:501–503.
14. Lloyd MH. Veterinary care of ferrets, common clinical conditions. Practice 2002; March:145.
15. McAlees T. Treating pain in cats and dogs. Veterinarian 2002; November:28–30.
16. Harms CA, Sladky KK, Horne WA, et al. Epidural analgesia in ferrets. Exot DVM 2002; 4:31–33.
17. Weiss C. Cryosurgery of the ferret adrenal gland. Exot DVM 1999; 1:27–28.
18. Johnson D. Clinical use of cryosurgery for ferret adrenal gland removal. Exot DVM 2002; 4:71–73.

CHAPTER 20

Ferret emergency techniques

Anthony Lucas

'We miss more for not looking, than not knowing.'

Anon

This is never truer than in emergencies involving small companion animals, such as ferrets. However, by applying basic emergency medicine methodology and techniques, many unfamiliar emergency situations can be treated effectively.

The calm and efficient management of emergency situations is assisted by easy access to emergency equipment, medications and diagnostic procedures. Set aside an 'emergency area' in the veterinary practice and ensure that all the required equipment is easily accessible, with the most urgently required items easiest to access. Maintain a list of all the equipment and drugs kept in the emergency area and regularly check stock levels, drug expiration dates and equipment function. The emergency area must have good general lighting and a beam light for increased light intensity on small areas. Train all veterinary staff in emergency procedures so as to allow them to actively anticipate, and assist, in the most efficient manner.

The initial approach to any emergency

All emergency patients should have their critical physiological parameters (heart rate, respiratory rate, temperature etc.) assessed immediately on presentation. A thorough history and complete physical examination should only be performed after any immediately life-threatening conditions have been corrected.

Baseline laboratory tests require minimal cost input by the client and only take several minutes to complete. Packed cell volume (PCV), total serum solids, blood urea nitrogen (BUN) and blood glucose tests can be performed on the blood collected from the hub of an intravenous catheter stylet or 25 G needle. The results of these tests provide important information on the ferret's physiological status, may directly assist in a diagnosis (i.e. renal failure, insulinoma), or identify problems that, when corrected, may significantly improve the ferret's prognosis (i.e. anaemia, dehydration, hypoglycaemia).

Use the remaining blood in the hub of the stylet or needle to produce a pre-treatment blood smear. This smear provides a semi-quantitative assessment of red and white blood cell numbers, predominant white blood cell type(s), changes in cell morphology and platelet count. The platelet count can be accurately determined using a haemocytometer or commercial laboratory; but as a rough guide, determine the average number of platelets per high-power field from ten high-power fields on the blood smear (100×-oil immersion). For each average number of platelets per high-power field, there are approximately 15 000 platelets/mL. Platelet counts under 50 000/mL may lead to spontaneous bleeding. Low platelet counts occur due to failure of production (oestrogen-induced bone marrow suppression) or increased consumption (systemic inflammatory response syndrome, neoplasia, immune-mediated etc.).

An extremely common coagulopathy in the ferret is vitamin K-dependent anticoagulant poisoning (i.e. warfarin). Activated clotting time (ACT), prothrombin time (PT) and activated partial thromboplastin time (APTT) can all be used to assess clotting cascade; however, only the ACT will be available in many practice emergency situations, as PT and APTT usually must be performed at a commercial laboratory. It is important to remember that the ACT requires 2 mL of blood and that the blood volume of an adult ferret is only 30–60 mL. Therefore, the potential benefit of performing the ACT test must be weighed against the risk of taking 2 mL of blood from a suspected coagulopathy patient.

Tissue oxygen delivery

Basic survival depends upon the delivery of oxygen to the tissues of the body. Many emergency conditions result in reduced tissue oxygen delivery (DO_2) and it should therefore come as no surprise that many of the procedures performed on emergency patients are to directly improve DO_2.

DO_2 is dependent upon cardiac output and total arterial blood oxygen content. Cardiac output can be increased by fluid administration. Since most of the oxygen in the blood is reversibly bound to haemoglobin, the total amount of oxygen carried by the blood is proportional to the haemoglobin concentration and degree of saturation (SaO_2). Blood haemoglobin concentration can be increased by blood transfusions and increasing the inspired oxygen concentration can increase SaO_2. Therefore, the quickest ways to optimize DO_2 are to increase the ferret's inspired oxygen concentration, administer intravenous fluids and normalize the PCV.

Oxygen supplementation

The provision of supplemental oxygen to emergency and critical care patients may be life-saving. SaO_2 is normally around 98–100% and a SaO_2 of <80%, and particularly <60%, for a prolonged period of time, will reduce patient survival. Many conditions may cause a reduction in SaO_2, i.e. reduced alveolar ventilation, ventilation/perfusion mismatch, circulatory failure, reduced haemoglobin affinity for oxygen, etc.

Arterial blood gas analysis is the most accurate measurement of SaO_2, but routine collection of arterial blood samples from ferrets is not practical. Pulse oximetry is a reasonably cheap, accurate and reliable alternative and the probe of the oximeter can be easily placed on the ferret's tongue, lip, ear or whole paw.

The available routes of oxygen administration to ferrets include flow past, nasal catheter, mask and oxygen cage. Simply holding the end of an oxygen supply tube (1 L/min) in front of the ferret's nostrils provides flow-past oxygen. While this method rapidly increases the inspired oxygen concentration, it is labour-intensive and many ferrets struggle excessively, making the procedure counterproductive. This method is therefore usually only used on semi-recumbent or recumbent ferrets until a more permanent method of oxygen administration can be arranged.

Mask oxygen is provided by placing a 5 or 10 cm Elizabethan collar over the ferret's head and tying it around the animal's neck. The open front of the collar is covered with clear plastic food wrap and an oxygen tube (1 L/min) is secured, so that the end of the tube is inside the collar. To allow the escape of warmed humid air, a 2–3 cm hole is made in the plastic food wrap (Fig. 20.1). This method is best suited for use on semi-recumbent or recumbent ferrets.

Nasal oxygen administration requires the placement of a nasal catheter. In ferrets, a 3.0 or 3.5 French red rubber catheter is used. First, instil 0.2 mL of 2% lidocaine into the nostril. Insert the catheter to the level of the medial canthus in the ventral nasal meatus and secure the catheter in place with sutures or superglue. Infuse oxygen at 0.1 L/kg per min.

The oxygen cage involves placing the ferret in a well-sealed cage with an in-flowing 100% oxygen supply. It is important that the cage is made of clear material to allow examination of the animal without opening the cage and releasing the additional oxygen. Oxygen is delivered at a rate that will provide an oxygen-enriched environment while preventing a build up of carbon dioxide, humidity and heat inside the cage. The rate of oxygen delivery will depend upon the size and design of the cage. To allow the temperature inside the cage to be monitored, place an easily visible thermometer in the cage.

It is important to note that none of the above methods of oxygen delivery is likely to produce problems with oxygen toxicity.

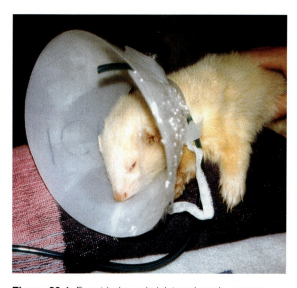

Figure 20.1 Ferret being administered mask oxygen.

CHAPTER TWENTY
Ferret emergency techniques

Fluid administration

Choice of the fluid type depends upon the ferret's requirements; one fluid type is not appropriate for all situations. For maximum effectiveness, all fluids should be given intravenously (i.v.) or intraosseously (i.o.).

Shock-rate fluids

The objective of shock-rate fluid administration is to normalize the ferret's intravascular volume as quickly as possible, by infusing a volume of replacement fluid equal to the normal blood volume of the ferret (60 mL/kg) i.v. or i.o. in the first hour of treatment. A replacement fluid has a sodium level close to that of normal plasma and a low potassium concentration, i.e. Hartmann's or 0.9% sodium chloride.

As it is easy to overestimate the weight of a ferret, weigh all ferrets before starting on shock-rate fluids and use an infusion pump or paediatric giving set to control the rate of fluid administration. Normal gravity drip giving sets (20 drops/mL) are definitely not recommended for ferrets. While shock-rate fluid administration rarely causes complications, it is important to monitor the ferret and reduce the infusion rate if there are any signs of intravascular overload, i.e. new crackles on pulmonary auscultation.

Shock-rate fluids: 60 mL/kg i.v. or i.o. for the first hour.

Maintenance fluids

In addition to normal daily fluid losses (100 mL/kg), sick ferrets may have additional fluid losses i.e. vomiting, diarrhoea, polyuria, etc. The sum of the normal daily fluid losses and additional fluid losses determines the total daily fluid replacement requirement.

Maintenance fluids have sodium and potassium concentrations close to that which the animal is losing in the combination of urine, sweat, respiration and faeces (sodium concentration of 70 mEq/L or less; potassium concentration of around 20 mEq/L). Commonly used maintenance fluids are half-strength sodium chloride (0.45% NaCl + 2.5% glucose, in a 50/50 v/v ratio) or Plasmalyte M supplemented with potassium chloride to give a final potassium concentration of around 20 mEq/L. *Note* that Hartmann's alone is not a suitable maintenance fluid.

It is critical that these high potassium solutions are not infused too rapidly, since potassium will produce life-threatening cardiac arrhythmias, even over very short periods. The rate of maintenance fluid infusion must be controlled with an infusion pump or paediatric giving set. If a paediatric giving set is used, divide the total daily volume into a 4-hourly volume. Place the 4-hour volume into the burette and infuse at the predetermined rate. Refill and repeat every 4 hours.

Maintenance fluids: 100 mL/kg per day i.v. plus any additional fluid losses.

Intravenous catheterization

Intravenous catheters may be placed in ferrets into the cephalic, lateral saphenous and jugular veins. Catheterize the cephalic and lateral saphenous veins as for dogs and cats, using a 22 or 24 G i.v. catheter.

The jugular vein is very deep in the ferret, but may be accessed by making a small cut in the skin with a scalpel blade or 18 G needle, which will help prevent burring of the catheter and assist with visualization of the vein. An 18–20 G i.v. catheter may be used for hobs and a 20–22 G i.v. catheter for jills. Light anaesthesia may be required in some ferrets to permit successful catheterization. A technique for collecting multiple blood samples from the jugular vein has been described.[1]

Intraosseous catheterization

The blood pressure of many ferret emergency patients is too low to allow reliable catheterization of peripheral veins without ruining the vein in the attempt. In these cases, it is advisable to use an intraosseous catheter.

The greater trochanter of the femur is the most common site of catheter placement, followed by the greater tubercle of the humerus. A commercial intraosseous catheter or 18 G needle can be used. As soon as possible, replace the intraosseous catheter with an intravenous catheter.

Blood transfusions

The normal PCV for a ferret is 35–60%. While a PCV of <20% may be life-threatening if the drop has been acute, some ferrets with chronic anaemia can tolerate a PCV as low as 10% with few clinical signs. However, it has been recommended that all ferrets with a PCV below 15% should be transfused.[2] To maintain the ferret's PCV following blood loss, the spleen contracts and blood is drained from the venous system into central circulation. It may take up to 12 hours for the ferret's PCV to accurately reflect the extent of the blood loss, so it is important to always check the ferret's PCV on admission and again 12–24 hours later if haemorrhage is suspected or known to have occurred. It is also important to note that increasing the PCV above the normal range is dangerous, as this will increase vascular resistance and significantly reduce DO_2.

Urine output and urine collection

In some emergencies, the haemoglobin content of the blood may be normal but its affinity for oxygen reduced. Causes of this include paracetamol or carbon monoxide poisoning, acidosis, hypercapnia and hyperthermia. Correction of any acid–base imbalance, normalization of the patient's temperature and treatment of the underlying disease will improve haemoglobin oxygen carrying capacity.

Since ferrets do not have detectable blood group antigens, multiple transfusions from one or more donors are possible without the risk of a transfusion reaction occurring[3] and no pre-transfusion medications need to be given, i.e. antihistamines or corticosteroids. However, in countries where Aleutian and heartworm disease are prevalent, it is prudent to screen the donor before blood collection.

Due to the large volume of blood required from the donor, anaesthesia and placement of a jugular catheter (18 G) will assist in rapid blood collection. Cardiac puncture has also been described for large volume blood collection, using a sternal approach to avoid injury to the donor.[4]

Suitable donors are usually large hobs; however small hobs and jills may be used if necessary. Predetermine the amount of blood to be collected, i.e. 6, 9 or 12 mL from jills, small and large hobs, respectively. Collect whole blood into a syringe containing citrate-phosphate-dextrose adenine at the volume ratio of 1 blood : 9 citrate-phosphate-dextrose adenine (0.66, 1 or 1.33 mL for jills, small and large hobs, respectively). Heparin is not a suitable anticoagulant, as excess heparin may inhibit coagulation in the recipient. To prevent hypotension in the donor ferret, i.v. administer a volume of warmed replacement fluid equal to four times the volume of the blood removed (four times volume required as replacement fluids distribute equally between the vascular and extracellular fluid spaces, which have a volume ratio of 1:3, respectively).

As soon as is possible, transfuse the blood at 37°C i.v. or i.o. into the recipient. The whole transfusion volume is usually infused over 10–15 min, in 1 mL boluses every minute until the transfusion is complete (Fig. 20.2).

Most patients with a coagulopathy require both red blood cells and coagulation factor-rich plasma. However, some coagulopathy patients, i.e. early anticoagulant poisonings, may not have suffered excessive red blood cell loss and only require the coagulation factors found in plasma. To perform a fresh plasma transfusion, centrifuge or let the donor blood settle for 30 min in the refrigerator (4°C). When the plasma has separated from the red blood cell component, draw off the plasma, warm it to 37°C and transfuse i.v. or i.o. Avoid transfusing more than 20 mL/kg of plasma in any 24-hour period.

When fresh ferret blood is not available, Oxyglobin may be used as an alternative to blood transfusion. It has been reported that the administration of 11–15 mL/kg over 4 hours was without apparent adverse effect.[5] Oxyglobin is a colloid and administration to normovolemic ferrets should be monitored to avoid volume overload. Dose-dependent yellow–orange discolouration of the skin, mucous membranes and sclera is possible and will resolve in 3–5 days.[5]

Urine output and urine collection

DO_2 is dependent on cardiac output, but is it is difficult to assess cardiac performance in the ferret using techniques such as systemic arterial blood pressure, central venous pressure, right ventricular pressure or pulmonary capillary wedge pressure. However, urine output is an indicator of cardiac output that can be easily measured.

The placement of a urinary catheter is important in any ferret where ongoing cardiovascular or renal compromise is suspected. Normal minimum urine output is 1 mL/kg per hour, with 2 mL/kg per hour preferred. Monitor urine output and tailor fluid administration to maintain at least this rate.

Urinary catheters may be placed in all hobs and most jills. Despite having a 'J' shaped os penis, urethral catheterization of the hob is easy (Fig. 20.3). If the hob is uncooperative, exteriorize the penis under sedation or light anaesthesia. Clip and disinfect around the prepuce before introducing the catheter. The urethral orifice is

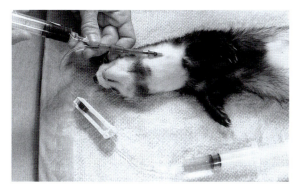

Figure 20.2 Blood transfusion technique showing a simple process of giving blood to recipient ferret using the jugular vein with infusion line to catheter. Another infusion line allows for flushing the catheter with 0.9% sodium chloride solution. (Photograph courtesy of D. Manning, Department of Medical Microbiology, University of Wisconsin Medical School, Madison, USA.)

CHAPTER TWENTY

Ferret emergency techniques

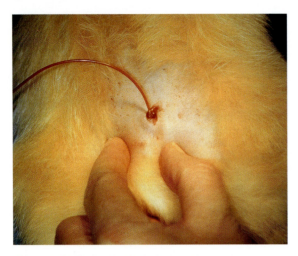

Figure 20.3 Urethral catheterization of the hob ferret. Note the 'J' shaped os penis to the top right of the catheter. The urethra does not bend around inside the os penis.

Nutrition of the critical ferret

'Early and aggressive nutritional support' will improve patient survival and shorten recovery times.[7] The goal is to provide one-third of the ferret's normal daily energy and protein requirements within 12 hours of admission and then increase to supply the ferret's normal requirements within 72 to 96 hours.[7] Although total parenteral nutrition is possible, it is very difficult to maintain catheter patency and sterility in the ferret. It is far superior to use as much of patient's gastrointestinal tract as possible.[7]

Resting energy requirements (RER) in kcal/day
= $70 \times$ (body weight in kg)$^{0.75}$

Energy requirements for emergency and critically ill patients have an included fudge factor depending upon the severity of the disease: mild stress = 1.2 times RER, moderate stress = 1.5 times RER, and major stress/sepsis = 2.0 times RER.

located on the ventral surface of the penis and is not at the distal-most point of the os penis. In cases where the urethral orifice is not obvious, a small amount of urine may be expressed from the bladder to assist in locating it. Urinary catheterization in the jill is more difficult and is best performed on very depressed individuals or under general anaesthesia. The ferret is placed in ventral recumbency. The hindquarters are elevated and a vaginal speculum or otoscope is used to visualize the urethral opening, which is around 1 cm cranial to the clitoral fossa.[6]

For both hobs and jills, a 3.5 French catheter is recommended. Measure and mark the catheter at the point where it is expected to leave the prepuce or vagina. Gently insert the catheter into the urethra to the measurement mark, with or without the assistance of a stylet. Use surgical adhesive tape to create a tab on the catheter where it leaves the animal. Using a 22 G i.v. needle, place a 2/0 Vetafil suture between the tab on the catheter and the skin. Firmly tie the catheter in place.

To measure urine output, attach a gravity line giving set and empty fluid bag to the end of the catheter. To prevent urine backflow into the bladder, always keep the fluid bag lower than the patient. Disconnect the bag at regular intervals, at least every 4 hours, and measure the volume of urine produced. For patients where urine output is so small that the urine produced is lost in the giving set, attach an injection port to the end of the urinary catheter. At regular intervals (hourly), aspirate the urine produced with a needle and syringe.

Nursing

Various methods may be used to increase caloric intake in ferrets: careful food handling, warming of the food, hand feeding, the use of aromatic food, providing a secure environment, petting and vocal reassurance etc. Cleaning the nares may also assist in ferrets with nasal discharges.

Try to feed the ferret foods that it likes and consider getting the owners to bring in the ferret's favourite food and try to feed the animal. Minimizing stress may improve food intake, so consider hospitalizing the ferret on its own in a quiet room.

Water and electrolyte solutions

These solutions are used to assist in the correction of mild fluid and electrolyte abnormalities or to test gastrointestinal motility. Quarter-strength Hartmann's supplemented with 25 g/L glucose or commercial electrolyte solutions with additional glucose may be used. If these solutions are tolerated without vomiting for 6–12 hours, then feeding may be commenced.

Paste consistency or gruel diets

Ferrets with reduced prehension capability and some that are able to eat and swallow normally, will not eat normal food, but will eat paste or gruel diets. These diets are relatively cheap and easy to prepare by mixing commercial recovery diets or normal pet food mixed with water or glucose solutions.

Naso-oesophageal tube

Placement of a naso-oesophageal tube is possible in ferrets. Naso-oesophageal tubes are particularly useful for nutrition in depressed animals and immediately post-surgery, however they are not recommended in vomiting patients or those with functional or mechanical gastrointestinal obstruction. Successful placement of a naso-oesophageal tube in the ferret either requires anaesthesia or a severely depressed animal.

The naso-oesophageal tube is inserted so that its end is in the distal oesophagus. Placement in the stomach is not preferred as possible complications include gastric perforation and oesophagitis secondary to reflux of gastric contents.

Using a 3.0 or 3.5 French, 30 cm nasal catheter, place the end of the catheter at about the ninth rib (Fig. 20.4) and mark the catheter at the point where it will leave the nares. This will ensure that the catheter is inserted to the correct position. Instil 0.2 mL of 2% lignocaine into one nostril. Using a water-soluble obstetrical lubricant, lubricate the tip of the catheter. Insert the catheter into the nares in a medial direction leaving the nasal planum in the normal position. If the end of the catheter is found to be too soft then freeze it for several minutes before use. Initially the catheter may deviate dorsally, but at the level of the canine teeth the catheter passes into the ventral nasal meatus of the nasal cavity (see Fig. 2.13). Advance the catheter into the oesophagus. A guide wire may be required to advance the catheter over the heart (see Fig. 2.19b). When the catheter is inserted to the predetermined mark, confirm the correct position of the catheter by auscultation of the abdomen whilst instilling air into the tube or by radiology (Fig. 20.4). Superglue the catheter close to the point where it exits the nose; between the eyes; on top of the head and at on the dorsum of the neck (Fig. 20.5). An Elizabethan collar may be required to prevent removal of the catheter.

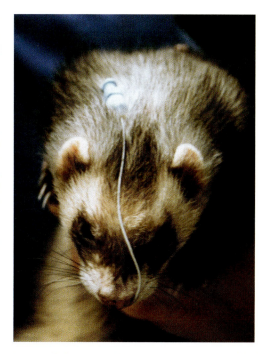

Figure 20.5 A correctly secured nasogastric catheter.

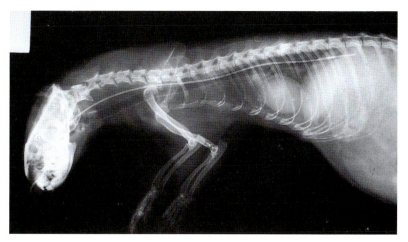

Figure 20.4 Radiograph of a hob, checking the position of the catheter in the distal oesophagus before securing the catheter in place. *Note* that it is obvious that the catheter is in the oesophagus and not the trachea by checking its position in the mid-neck. Pictured is a 3 French ferret nasogastric feeding tube supplied by Cook Veterinary Products, Australia (Cat. No: V-PU3.0-CE-30-P-1S-0-MVP1915).

Nasogastric feeding may be by bolus or slow drip infusion. The infusion is generally started at 0.5–1.0 mL/kg per hour and may be slowly increased up to 10 mL/kg per hour over 12–24 hours.[7] To minimize the possibility of the hypertonicity of the food resulting in diarrhoea, start at one-third strength and one-third of the daily requirement. Feed frequently during the first 24 hours and increase feeding to 75–80% of the ideal intake over 2–3 days as the patient permits.[7] Liquid diets are generally the only foods that will get through these small tubes. When bolus feeding, ensure the food is warmed to room temperature and the tube is flushed with water or an electrolyte solution after use to prevent tube blockage. Always strain liquid diets through several layers of gauze before use to remove any small lumps that may block the tube.

Oesophagostomy and gastrostomy tubes

Methods for the placement of oesophagostomy[8] and gastrostomy tubes[9] in ferrets have been described. Both tube types are relatively easy to insert under general anaesthesia and have a number of benefits over naso-oesophageal tubes in that the tube internal diameter is larger allowing for the use of gruel diets and these tubes can potentially remain in place for longer periods of time.

References

1. Mesina JE, Sylvina TJ, Hotaling LC, et al. A simple method for chronic jugular catheterisation in ferrets. Lab Anim Sci 1988; 38:88–90.
2. Quesenberry KE, Orcutt C. Basic approach to veterinary care, includes sugar gliders and hedgehogs. In: Quesenberry KE, Carpenter JW, eds. Ferrets, rabbits and rodents: Clinical medicine and surgery. Philadelphia: WB Saunders; 2003:13–24.
3. Manning D, Bell JA. Lack of detectable blood groups in domestic ferrets: implications for transfusion. J Am Vet Med Ass 1990; 197:84–86.
4. Fox JG. Anaesthesia and surgery. In: Fox JG, ed. Biology and diseases of the ferret. Philadelphia: Lea and Febinger; 1988:289–302.
5. Orcutt C. Oxyglobin administration for the treatment of anemia in ferrets. Exot DVM 2000; 2:44–46.
6. Marini RP, Esteves MI, Fox JG. A technique for catheterization of the urinary bladder in the ferret. Lab Anim 1994; 28:155–157.
7. Crowe DT Jr. Nutritional support in the seriously ill or injured patient. In: Bryden DI, ed. Anaesthesia, emergency and critical care. University of Sydney: Postgraduate Foundation in Veterinary Science 1995; 254:113–125.
8. Fisher PG. Esophagostomy feeding tube placement in the ferret. Exot DVM 2000; 2:23–25.
9. Benson K, Carr A, Steinberg H, Paul-Murphy J. Nonendoscopic percutaneous gastrostomy tubes in ferrets. Lab Anim 2000; 29:44–46.

Part Four

Special Anatomy

CHAPTER

21 Ferret dentition and pathology by Bob Church 467

CHAPTER 21

Ferret dentition and pathology

Bob Church

'We each day dig our graves with our teeth.'

Samuel Smiles, Duty, 1880

Dentes

Synonyms: teeth, dentition, upper and lower dental arches or arcades, complete dental arcade.[1]

Ferret dentition follows the general mustelid pattern with teeth modified for a highly predacious lifestyle.[2-4] Permanent teeth in ferrets are reduced in number and size from the dentition of the hypothetical eutherian ancestor (i3:c1:m4 = 32 and I3:C1:P4:M3 = 44) and are modified for the necessary slicing, cutting and piercing required of a primary, obligate carnivore.[5] Wild polecats eat less than 5% non-animal foods, categorizing them as primary carnivores.[6-9] The ferret dentition lacks appreciable tooth area dedicated to crushing and grinding when compared with areas reserved for cutting; ferrets are therefore classified as hypercarnivores, lacking the ability to efficiently process significant amounts of plant foods.[10] Additionally, ferrets are obligate carnivores, requiring essential fatty and amino acids only found from animal sources.[11] In three independent studies comprising 372 British polecats, dietary analysis of faecal and gut contents showed the purposeful ingestion of fruits and vegetables was statistically insignificant and the percentage considered zero.[8] Ferrets possess other anatomical adaptations that reflect adaptation to a highly carnivorous diet (i.e. lack of caecum, high stomach pH, short bowel, fast bowel-content transit times, etc.), each dependent upon a specialized dentition designed to capture, kill, render and consume animal prey.

Dental adaptations to this highly carnivorous lifestyle include specialized tooth form and function. Incisors are diminished with chisel-like contacting surfaces for holding and pulling. Canines are sharp-pointed and rounded to an oval in cross-section to safely pierce the skull and vertebrae of prey species. Cheek teeth – the premolars and carnassials – are transformed into shears for tearing and cutting bone and tissue. The diminutive molars no longer grind food, but, like a nutcracker, are designed for cracking bones, insect carapaces and snail shells. Similar to most other mammals, ferrets are diphyodont, having two distinct dental arcades. Initially, the deciduous arcade is utilized during the weaning period when the jill periodically supplements her milk with food items. Subsequently, the permanent arcade erupts after the kits have been weaned off milk and is designed to last the lifespan of the ferret. Dental eruption and exfoliation sequences for the permanent and deciduous dentition of the domesticated ferret are detailed in Table 21.1[12-18] and depicted in Figure 21.1.

Ferret deciduous dental formula

$$di^{3-4}/_3 : dc^1/_1 : dm^3/_3 = 28{-}30$$

Dentes decidui

Synonyms: Deciduous dentition, baby teeth, deciduous arches or arcades, deciduous dental arches or arcades, deciduous teeth, dentes decidui, milk teeth, primary dentition, temporary teeth.[1]

CHAPTER TWENTY-ONE
Ferret dentition and pathology

Table 21.1 Ferret dental eruption and exfoliation sequence

Location	Tooth	Eruption (days postpartum)	Exfoliation
Maxilla	i^1	Embedded at birth; does not normally erupt	Intragingivally resorbed
Mandible	i_1	Embedded at birth; does not normally erupt	Intragingivally resorbed
Maxilla	i^2	Embedded at birth; does not normally erupt	Intragingivally resorbed
Mandible	i_2	Embedded at birth; does not normally erupt	Intragingivally resorbed
Maxilla	i^3	Embedded at birth; does not normally erupt	Intragingivally resorbed
Mandible	i_3	Embedded at birth; does not normally erupt	Intragingivally resorbed
Maxilla	i^4	0 to 3 days	Exfoliated or retained
Maxilla	c^1	19.8 days (± 0.5)	66.0 days (± 4.9)
Mandible	c_1	20.5 days (± 0.9)	61.6 days (± 4.7)
Maxilla	m^3	21.2 days (± 1.5)	67.0 days (± 4.3)
Mandible	m_4	21.6 days (± 1.4)	71.1 days (± 3.7)
Mandible	m_3	21.7 days (± 1.4)	70.2 days (± 3.0)
Maxilla	m^4	22.0 days (± 1.6)	54.8 days (± 2.9)
Mandible	m_2	27.4 days (± 2.5)	61.0 days (± 1.7)
Maxilla	m^2	29.5 days (± 1.2)	61.4 days (± 2.1)
Mandible	I_1	42.5 days (± 0.6)	–
Mandible	I_2	44.1 days (± 1.7)	–
Maxilla	I^1	44.6 days (± 2.0)	–
Maxilla	I^2	44.6 days (± 2.0)	–
Mandible	M_1	50.2 days (± 3.0)	–
Maxilla	I^3	52.4 days (± 3.1)	–
Maxilla	PM^4	54.7 days (± 3.2)	–
Mandible	C_1	55.2 days (± 4.1)	–
Mandible	I_3	55.7 days (± 3.6)	–
Maxilla	C^1	56.0 days (± 4.1)	–
Maxilla	M^1	56.4 days (± 3.2)	–
Mandible	M_2	61.2 days (± 2.4)	–
Mandible	PM_2	61.7 days (± 2.0)	–
Maxilla	PM^2	62.9 days (± 1.6)	–
Maxilla	PM^3	65.6 days (± 2.5)	–
Mandible	PM_3	66.0 days (± 2.6)	–
Mandible	PM_4	71.6 days (± 3.9)	–

Compiled from Berkovitz, 1968,[12] 1973,[13] Berkovitz and Silverstone, 1969,[14] Evans and An, 1998,[15] He et al., 2002,[16] Mazák, 1963,[17] and Shump and Shump, 1978.[18]

Ferret deciduous dentition consists of incisors, canines and molars; premolars are not found in the deciduous arcade. Ferret dental eruption sequences follow the general carnivore pattern for the most part, however, the timing of gingival emergence is sped up to reflect a highly carnivorous lifestyle. Male and female tooth growth and replacement patterns are sexually dimorphic, with female dentition erupting sooner and teeth exfoliating slightly faster than males.[16] Deciduous incisors are natal teeth and are in place at birth – although gingival eruption is uncommon.[5,12] Deciduous canines and molars start erupting at around 20 days, i.e. about when the jill starts offering solid foods.[18] Near the end of the 4th week when all deciduous teeth are in

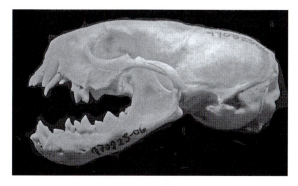

Figure 21.1 Dental eruption at 8.5 weeks of age.

place, the blind, deaf and helpless kit is capable of eating solid food while still suckling the jill's milk.[14,15]

At about 6–7 weeks, the secondary dentition begins to erupt and rapidly replaces the milk teeth, which exfoliate when the permanent crowns are nearly in place.[16] Near 8 weeks, the permanent canines erupt to replace the deciduous ones and both are often in position at the same time; this pseudopolyodontia is sometimes misinterpreted to be a twinned or pathological tooth, but as the adult canine settles into place, the milk canine is shed (Fig. 21.1). Within 2 weeks, the permanent teeth have erupted to replace the deciduous teeth.[15,16]

The timing of the eruption of the two dental arcades is significant. The deciduous arcade is in place and being utilized at a time when the neurological system is still developing. Exposures to various prey and food smells are significant influences in the development of that system.[19-22] Obvious among these influences are olfactory stimulation and environmental enrichment. In the first case, the exposure of olfactory neurons to specific odours strengthens their synaptic connections, helping to preserve them from withering away – the basis of olfactory imprinting.[22,23] In the later case, enrichment from exposure to varied stimuli including, but not limited to olfactory, tactile, taste and neuromotor stimuli, is known to increase the number and complexity of synaptic connections within the cerebral cortex, directly influencing intelligence and curiosity.[24-26] (Also see Vargas and Anderson[27] for effects in closely related black-footed ferrets.) Thus, to maximize olfactory development, the kit should be exposed to as many foods (and associated food odours) as possible, starting when the deciduous teeth have erupted at week 4 and continuing throughout juvenile development until adulthood.

Likewise, the timing of the eruption of the secondary dentition signals a period of high growth in the ferret.[18,28] The brain is still developing and olfactory imprinting continues to take place, so the enriching nature of a varied diet remains of great importance to the immature ferret.[29]

The ferret's nutritional status is extremely influential during this time, impacting dental and skeletal development, body size and muscle to fat ratios in the adult animal.

Deciduous incisors (dentes incisive decidui)

Deciduous incisors in ferrets are laterally compressed, single-rooted teeth with a diminutive crown possessing a chisel-like cutting edge. The upper deciduous incisors are rooted in the right and left premaxillary (incisive) bones, while the lower deciduous incisors are rooted in the proximal right and left mandibles. Deciduous incisors are natal teeth and are generally present at birth. However, deciduous incisors rarely erupt and are only infrequently noted on gross examination or are rarely noted in those atypical occasions immature kits are X-rayed. Natal incisors are generally resorbed prior to emergence, although some could be shed as the permanent incisors erupt. Natal incisors are considered functionless, even if erupted. However, it is possible the teeth provide some support to the gingiva while the kit is suckling or being weaned on solid foods. Commonly an extra deciduous maxillary incisor is present in either or both of the upper quadrants, increasing the number of upper incisors from six to seven or eight. In some ferrets a deciduous maxillary incisor is retained into adulthood as a supernumerary tooth (see Table 21.3).[30,31]

Deciduous canines (dentes canini decidui)

Deciduous canines in ferrets are slightly curved, single-cusped teeth with a relatively long single root. They are the longest teeth in the primary dental arcade and are rounded to an oval in cross-section to increase tooth strength for killing bites.[32] Upper deciduous canines are longer than their mandibular counterparts and have correspondingly longer roots. The crowns of the mandibular canines are more hook-shaped than in the maxillary canines. The upper deciduous canines are rooted in the right and left maxillary bones, while the lower deciduous canines are rooted in the proximal right and left mandibles. Deciduous canines erupt at about 20 days and have a more gracile and shorter appearance than the permanent canines. The maxillary deciduous canine is longer than the other teeth and has a slight lateral deflection that helps it to fit over the mandibular deciduous canine. The tip of the maxillary deciduous canine will often extend beyond the margin of the upper lip. The mandibular deciduous canine fits into a diastema or gap in the maxillary dental arcade. In the permanent dentition, the maxillary diastema is readily apparent between the maxillary incisors and canine, but it is not as evident in the deciduous dentition because the incisors are generally not erupted. Deciduous canines are retained until the permanent canines are nearly fully erupted, providing the kit with the uninterrupted means to render and consume solid prey foods throughout their period of accelerated growth.

Deciduous molars (dentes molars decidui)

Deciduous molars in ferrets are sectorial in nature, similar in shape and form to their later replacements although somewhat smaller in size. Excluding the carnassial, they have relatively simple cusps and are highly compressed buccolingually – taking the form of sharp, thin blades.[2] Taken as a whole, the tooth row of the cheek teeth resembles a serrated knife or saw. The last molars (m_4 and m^4) in the lower and upper deciduous arcade are modified into carnassials, which are thicker and possess a more complex cusp pattern than the adjacent deciduous molars. There are no molariform teeth in the deciduous dentition. The upper deciduous molars are rooted in the right and left maxilla, while the lower deciduous molars are rooted in the proximal right and left mandibles behind the canines. The deciduous molars begin to erupt between 20 and 28 days, but the carnassials are not exfoliated until after the permanent carnassials are almost in place.[16]

Permanent dental formula

$I^3/_3 : C^1/_1 : PM^3/_3 : M^1/_2 = 34$

Dentes permanentes

Synonyms: Permanent dentition, accessional teeth, adult teeth, dentes permanentes, permanent arches or arcades, permanent dental arches or arcades, permanent teeth, secondary dentition.[1]

The permanent dentition in ferrets begins to erupt about 42 days after birth, starting with the permanent incisors, followed by the carnassials and then the remainder of the dental arcade.[14,16] Excluding deciduous incisors that typically do not erupt, the deciduous predecessor is retained until the permanent replacement has almost erupted. The replacement of the deciduous dentition, although similar in sequence between the sexes, is generally faster in females compared to males.[16,33,34] This sexual dimorphic development is most likely correlated to the morphological sexual dimorphism of the dental arcade: female teeth probably develop slightly faster simply because they are smaller and take less time to develop.[35]

The permanent dental arcade is similar to the deciduous one with a notable exception: the presence of premolars. In ferrets, the first premolar is absent, following the evolutionary pattern of tooth loss in mammals where premolars are lost in the rostral-to-caudal direction, while molars are lost in the caudal-to-rostral direction.[5,36] As with other extant members of the Mustelidae, ferrets have a single post-carnassial molar in the maxillary and mandibular arcades.[37] In comparison to the hypothetical eutherian dentition, ferrets have lost three molars on each side of the maxillary dentition, leaving a single molar behind each carnassial in the upper arcade. They have also lost two molars on each side of the mandibular arch; of the two remaining, one has transformed into a carnassial and one is a diminutive molariform tooth. Both premolars and molars are termed cheek teeth. Ferrets have four cheek teeth in the permanent maxillary dentition and five in the mandibular. Tooth size and spacing is relatively uniform in ferrets, however, male skulls and teeth display sexual dimorphism and are significantly larger than those found in typical females (Fig. 21.2).[38]

Permanent incisors: (dentes incisive permanentes)

Ferrets, like most of the members of the Order Carnivora, have six upper and lower incisors in their permanent arcade (sea otters, *Enhydra lutris*, only possess

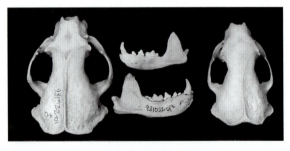

Figure 21.2 Ferrets are extremely sexually dimorphic, with males ranging from 10–40% larger than females. Because one of the factors influencing dental wear is the size of the tooth, smaller teeth will wear faster than larger ones, all other factors being equal. In this study, dental wear in female ferrets was more pronounced than that seen in males. *Note* the avulsed 2nd premolar, 1st molar and the worn carnassial in the female mandible; these individuals were from the same litter and died within days of each other from canine distemper.

four lower incisors). While the deciduous incisors do not erupt, the permanent ones erupt lingual to their embedded precursors and are somewhat larger. The permanent incisors erupt between 42 and 56 days postpartum and are in position soon after. Permanent incisors possess a single, simple cusp with laterally compressed roots. The maxillary incisors overlap the mandibular ones when the jaws are closed.

Maxillary incisors have laterally compressed, slightly recurved roots and are linearly arraigned in the premaxillary bone. The first or medial incisors (I^1) are smaller than the other two pairs, but all are generally larger than those in the mandible. They are medial to the other incisors, adjacent to the suture between the right and left premaxillary bones. The second or intermediate incisors (I^2) are slightly larger than the first. The third or lateral incisors (I^3) are larger and more caniniform than the others and possess a crown that is somewhat laterally deflected. A space or diastema, several millimeters wide exists between the third incisor and the adjacent canine, providing space for the mandibular canine to fit into the tooth row when the jaws are closed, insuring proper occlusion.

Mandibular incisors are notably smaller than their maxillary counterparts and have short, straight, laterally compressed roots. They are irregularly spaced in the mandible, with the second incisor displaced lingually. The first incisor (I_1) is smaller than the others and is rooted adjacent to the mandibular symphysis. The third incisor (I_3) is rooted immediately adjacent to the canine and is approximately the same size as the second incisor (I_2). The second incisor (I_2) is lingually displaced, but has a slight labial tilt in comparison to the others, bringing the surfaces of the cusps into alignment for proper occlusion with the maxillary set.

Permanent canines: (dentes canini permanentes)

Ferret canines are rounded in cross-section to form an ovaloid shape, a characteristic designed to increase tooth strength for piercing the skull and neck bones of their prey, as well as to stand up to the forces exerted by a strong muscled bite.[32,39,40] A ferret can generate bite forces up to 48.8 N (Newtons), which – when normalized for body mass – makes their bite one of the stronger among the mammalia.[41] Species that evolved the hunting technique of using a killing bite to the back of the head or neck of prey animals tend to have rounded canines which reduce drag during piercing, while still possessing a high strength-to-size ratio.[5,32] Ferret permanent canines erupt at about 55–56 days postpartum, mediorostral to their deciduous precursors that remain in place for roughly another week until the adult canines are nearly in position. Ferret permanent canines are slightly recurved, with roots longer than the crown. The crown possesses a single, sharply pointed cusp, more hook-shaped in the mandibular canines. Because canine roots are larger compared to the other teeth in the ferret dentition, they are frequently sectioned to determine age by counting the annular seasonal deposits of cement – generally more accurate than using tooth wear estimates (Table 21.2).[2,42,43]

Maxillary canines are larger than the mandibular ones. They generally project beyond the oral cavity and are visible jutting against the lower lip. Because oral tissues (lips and cheeks) do not insulate the tips of the canines from traumatic injuries caused by falls or collisions, they are frequently chipped or broken in pet ferrets (see Table 21.4).

When the jaws are closed, the mandibular canine fits into the diastema between the corresponding maxillary canine and third incisor. While the mandibular dental arcade sometimes has two small diastemata separating the premolars, it lacks a diastema designed to seat the maxillary canine. It fits buccally over the anterior premolars immediately caudal to the mandibular canine. The fit is sometimes snug and in those cases, the lower

Table 21.2 Ferret ageing techniques

Technique	Reliability	Time frame
Deciduous gingival emergence[a]	Excellent	20–28 days
Permanent gingival emergence[a]	Excellent	46–74 days
Cranial and epiphyseal fusion[b]	Good	1st year
Dental wear and attrition[c]	Fair	Lifespan
Translucence of canines[c]	Poor	Lifespan
Cementum annuli[d]	Good	Lifespan
Os penis[e]	Good	Male lifespan
Body condition[f]	Poor	Lifespan
Activity patterns[f]	Poor	Lifespan

[a]Absolute ageing technique: Can be off 2–4 days (±) depending on individual development, nutrition and neutering. [b]Absolute ageing technique: Can be off 4–6 months (±) depending on neutering, individual development and nutrition. Requires analysis of the skeleton or X-rays. [c]Relative ageing technique: Can be off 1–3 years or more (±). Only accurately comparable within a specific group living under similar conditions and not applicable to ferrets with unknown backgrounds. [d]Absolute ageing technique: Can be off 1–2 years (±) depending on seasonal factors, individual development and nutrition. Requires sectioning of teeth. [e]Absolute ageing technique: Can be off 1–3 years (±) depending on neutering, individual development and nutrition. Males only, requires analysis of the skeleton or X-rays. Fair results can be obtained on live ferrets by estimating the size of the base of the baculum using external manipulation. [f]Relative ageing technique: Can only be used to determine basic life stages, such as neonate, kit, juvenile, subadult, adult, aged adult, geriatric. When reporting absolute ages, report estimated age followed by the degree of error: 3 years (± 1–2 years) or 46 days (± 2–4 days). When reporting relative ages, only report the basic life stage: neonate, kit, juvenile, subadult, adult, aged adult and geriatric.

canine will lightly rub against the upper one, creating wear facets on the buccal side of the mandibular canine and the lingual side of the maxillary canine.

Permanent premolars: (dentes premolars permanentes)

Premolars are only found in the adult dentition, having no deciduous precursors. Premolars are sectorial in nature, compressed buccolingually into blade-like crowns designed to provide a vice-like grip to the bite to help prevent the escape of prey, as well as to transform the jaw into a cutting instrument to reduce prey into pieces small enough to safely swallow. Compared with the incisors and canines, premolars have a more intricate cusp pattern, becoming more intricate proceeding towards the carnassial (the sectorial tooth or dens sectorius). Premolars have two or three roots, depending on the location and tooth. Premolars begin to erupt at 54 days postpartum when the maxillary carnassial (PM^4) emerges to replace its deciduous precursor (the mandibular carnassial, M_1, has already erupted about 4 days prior). The rest of the premolars begin to erupt between 61 and 71 days, starting at the rostral end of the jaw and working caudally. Two small diastemata spacing the premolars are occasionally found.

There are three maxillary premolars (p^2, p^3, p^4) in each quadrant of the dental arcade, the first premolar (P^1, P_1) being lost from the dentition. In the maxillary arcade, the fourth premolar is modified into the upper carnassial. In the mandibular dentition, all three premolars are bladed cutting teeth that are situated rostral to the lower carnassial (M_1).

The second premolar in the maxillary dentition is the smallest of the three and in some ferrets only the tip of the crown is visible in the mouth. Usually there is a small space between P^2 and the maxillary canine, but in some ferrets the second premolar is in direct contact with the canine. The second premolar generally erupts medially to the deciduous 1st molar at about 63 days. It normally has two roots, although on occasion the roots are fused.

The maxillary third premolar is approximately twice the size of the second premolar, erupting rostral and slightly medially to the deciduous carnassial (m^3) at about 65 days postpartum. It also has two roots, although root fusion is less commonly seen. In crowded jaws, the upper-third premolar can twist buccolingually within the maxillary arcade; however, in most ferrets there is a small space between P^3 and P^4.

The fourth upper premolar is a large sectorial tooth-the maxillary carnassial. It is the largest cheek tooth and has three roots. It erupts caudal to the deciduous carnassial (m^3) at 54 days postpartum, but the deciduous precursor is not exfoliated until the adult tooth has almost completely erupted.

Mandibular premolars have two roots and are sequenced in size from small to large starting from the canine. Mandibular premolars erupt lingually to their deciduous precursors at 61 days postpartum for the second permanent premolar, the third at 66 days and the forth at 71 days. The crowns of the mandibular premolars are buccolingually compressed into sharp blade with a pointed cusp.

Permanent molars: (dentes molars permanentes)

Like all mustelids, ferrets only have a single post-carnassial molariform tooth in each dental quadrant – a trait of the Family Mustelidae.[2,37] The maxillary dentition has a single molar, while the mandibular dentition has two: the carnassial and a diminutive peg-like molar. Molariform teeth in the ferret are not used for the type of grinding seen in herbivores or omnivores, but are rather used for powerful compression, similar to the actions and types of force seen in the jaws of pliers. The ferret TMJ (temporomandibular joint; Figs 21.1, 21.3–21.5) prevents side-to-side grinding motion; it only allows the jaw to move dorsoventrally. This allows for more force to be placed into each jaw compression, making the bite stronger without forcing the animal to increase muscle mass.[41,44,45] It is the most efficient way for a subterranean hunter to increase the power of their hunting tools (the teeth) without building mastication muscles so large the animal's head cannot easily go down into the burrow. This force is made all the more powerful by the location of the molars at the very rear of the jaw; the upper molar is located at the very end of the

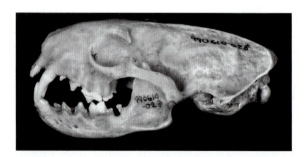

Figure 21.3 The most commonly lost tooth in the ferret is the mandibular second molar. Typically, it is lost as a combination of extreme wear and periodontal disease, including abscesses and food impactions. In this skull, bone loss from periodontal disease is evident, as is an abscess adjacent to the mandibular second molar. Reactive bone and dental calculus are present.

palatine bone, while the lower molar is adjacent to the mandibular ramus. These locations place the molars at the location of the greatest leverage force in the jaw – the best locations for cracking hard objects or crushing tissues. Molariform teeth in the ferret are designed to crush thick tissues for subsequent carnassial cutting and also to crack hard objects, including snail shells, insect carapaces and bones.

The ferret has a single three-rooted molar in the upper jaw. The maxillary first molar (M^1) is a distinctive tooth characteristic of most mustelids, being wider in the buccolingual breadth when compared to the mesiodistal length, giving it the appearance of being rooted at right angles to the rest of the teeth in the row. The molar has a narrow depressed waist separating the lingual side of the crown from the buccal side, with two small cusps on the buccal part and a single cusp on the lingual part. The mandibular molar is seated next to a cone-like cusp at the posterior aspect of the mandibular carnassial and works in conjunction with it. This double-cone structure is situated at right angles to the molar in the upper dentition and rarely comes into contact with it. The upper molar occludes with the combination of carnassial cusp and molar in the mandibular dentition, but because they are at right angles to each other, they do not strike, but rather interlock. The function of this interlocking configuration is a study of elegant simplicity; objects – such as bones – are anchored in the bottom cusps and held in place as they are squeezed against the top cusps, crushing them longitudinally. While this arrangement is suited perfectly for the role of a bone or carapace cracker, its ability to masticate plant foods is limited. The gripping action of these crisscrossing molars may also be useful in stabilizing softer tissues so less effort is used while utilizing the carnassials for cutting. The maxillary molar erupts caudally to the deciduous dentition at 56 days.

There are two molars in the mandibular arcade. The first molar (M_1) is modified into a carnassial and is the largest tooth in the mandible. The crown has three distinct cusps; two forming the blades of the carnassial and a smaller and lower cusp that – in conjunction with the second molar (M_2) – interlocks with the cusps of the maxillary molar (M^1). The first molar has two roots (sometimes an accessory slender central root is present) and erupts caudal to the deciduous carnassial at 50 days postpartum.

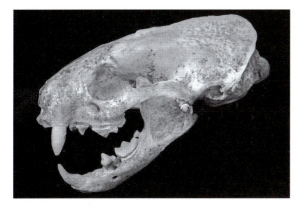

Figure 21.4 The age of the ferret is not necessarily correlated with the risk of periodontal disease and associated infections. The wear on the teeth of this skull indicated a young individual (dental cement analysis suggests 3 years of age ± 1 year), yet already the mandibular premolars have been lost or in the process of being lost due to abscessing and severe periodontal disease. The left maxillary canine shows a great deal of wear, probably due to fabric chewing.

As the jaws occlude, the blades of the mandibular carnassial (M_1) slide lingually past the blades of the maxillary carnassial (PM^4), creating an effective shearing action. The two sets of blades lightly strike the other in passing, creating a wear facet on the buccal side of M_1 and the lingual side of PM^4. Because of the angle of the crowns at the strike point, the wear facets work to maintain a sharp cutting edge on the carnassials; they are – in effect – self-sharpening teeth.

The second mandibular molar (M_2) is a diminutive tooth with a single root and a simplistic oval crown having a minor ridge and cusplets. The second mandibular molar erupts caudal to M_1 about 61 days postpartum. The molar does not occlude with any maxillary teeth, but enhances and supports crushing functions for the caudal cusp of the first mandibular molar (M_1). It is commonly avulsed in pet ferrets due to tooth attrition from a diet of hard kibble,[46] but is also infrequently missing because it never erupted (see Table 21.4). Because of size and occlusion issues, as well as a simplistic root and the occasional congenital absence, the second mandibular molar may be

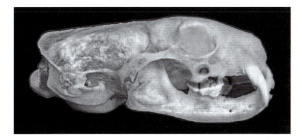

Figure 21.5 Periodontal disease can result in extensive loss of bone that supports the teeth. In this skull, bone loss is extensive, resulting in the exposure of roots and the loss of teeth. There is also a large abscess into the alveolus of the right maxillary carnassial, exposing the root.

Ferret dentition and pathology

Table 21.3 Ferret supernumerary dentition

	n	Maxillary incisor	(%)
Andrews et al., 1979; (British ferrets)[48]	350	27	7.7
Bateman, 1970; (European polecats)[30]	116	9	7.8
Berkovitz and Thomson, 1973; (British ferrets)[31]	54	16	29.6
Berkovitz and Thomson, 1973; (European polecats)[31]	23	6	26.1
Berkovitz and Thomson, 1973; (British ferrets)[31]	40	8	20.0
Glas, 1977; (European polecats)[49]	385	3	0.8
He et al., 2002; (Swedish ferrets)[16]	16	2	12.5
Ruprecht, 1978; (European polecats)[50]	801	14	1.8
This study (Pet domesticated ferrets)	202	10	4.95

in the process of become lost or vestigial (see Chiasson[47] for a similar evolutionary process in fur seals).

Pathological conditions found in ferret teeth

A randomized sample of 202 pet ferrets was collected between 1998 and 2003 from private individuals, breeders, shelters and rescues and veterinarians (Table 21.3). The sampled pet ferrets originated from large and small commercial and hobby breeders (18% from Marshall Farms) and were collected from widely separated geographic locations. The sampled pet ferrets were representative of albinos as well as all basic color types. Analysis of these samples provided the data for the proceeding dental disease rate discussion (Church, unpublished data).

Supernumerary teeth

Supernumerary teeth (Table 21.3[16,30,31,48–50], Fig. 21.6) are somewhat common in adult ferrets and while they may be found in any position in the dental arcade, they are most frequently found between the first and second maxillary incisors. Supernumerary incisors appear to have a genetic element, occurring more frequently in male ferrets than female.[31,50] The Mustelidae have one of the lower rates of extra teeth among the Carnivora, with a rate reported to be 1.1%; they generally have fewer teeth than normal instead of more.[5] Of the genus *Mustela*, reported rates of supernumerary teeth in polecats were 1.9%,[50] but extra teeth in domesticated ferrets, while not numerically quantified as a percentage, are significantly higher; perhaps in some subpopulations as high as 10%.[5,12,30] The rate of supernumerary upper incisors found in ferret skulls randomly culled from Swedish fur farms was reported to be about 12.5%. Within the studied sample, ferrets had a supernumerary tooth rate of 4.96%.

Dental disease

The identification of dental disease (Table 21.4) in the studied population followed standard zooarchaeological procedures for the identification of bone changes associated with disease.[51–54] In cases where ambiguity made identification unreliable, the data were discarded. Because of the small size of the ferret dentition, stereoscopic microscopes were used for identification of pathology.

Dental disease is rampant in pet ferrets, impacting up to 94.1% within a sample of 202 randomly collected

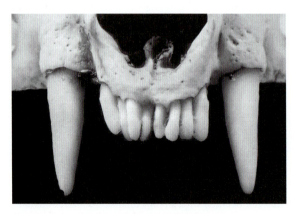

Figure 21.6 Supernumerary incisors are common in ferrets, occurring in 5–10% of the population. In this individual, there are a total of eight maxillary incisors, the two medial incisors being supernumerary; only a single supernumerary incisor is typically found. *Note* the fractured tip of the right canine, probably the result of a high-energy impact, such as a fall.

Pathological conditions found in ferret teeth

Table 21.4 Ferret dental pathology

	Pet ferrets (%)	Feral ferrets (%)
Population (*n*)	202	88
Crowded dental arcade	2.0	0.0
Congenitally absent teeth	1.0	0.0
Avulsed teeth	46.5	0.0
Fractured teeth	30.0	4.5
Dead teeth	15.8	1.1
Dental abrasion (cage bite wear)	23.8	0.0
Dental abrasion (tooth wear)	85.2	3.4
Dental calculus	94.1	2.3
Reactive bone at tooth line	72.3	1.1
Dental abscess	12.4	0.0
Palatine bone erosion	3.0	0.0

'Feral Ferret' data were collated from cleaned skeletons in private possession (R. Church). Two separate assemblages of feral ferret skeletons were randomly collected from various locations in New Zealand and combined here for comparison. 'Pet Ferret' data were collated from cleaned skeletons in private possession (R. Church). Individual pet ferrets were randomly collected from diverse locations in the USA and Canada, donated by private individuals, shelters and rescues, veterinarians and breeders.

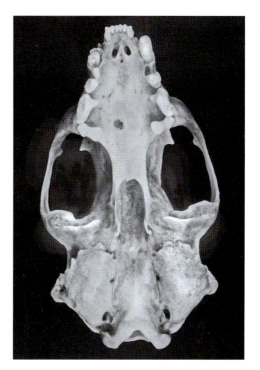

Figure 21.7 Fractured teeth were commonly noted in the study, but only a single instance of a canine broken at the gum line was recorded. *Note* the erosion of the palatine bone, extensive build-up of dental calculus and the missing left premolar, removed for ageing studies.

specimens (Table 21.4). Ferrets within the sample suffer from significant dental calculus (94.1%), reactive bone generally associated with chronic inflammation and infection (72.3%), avulsed teeth lost from various disease processes (46.5%), fractured teeth (30.0%), dead teeth (15.8%), tooth wear from cage biting (23.8%), tooth wear from diet (85.2%) and dental abscesses (12.4%). These dental disease rates are not reflected in feral ferret populations from New Zealand, animals that originated from the same genetic pool (European working ferrets) at about the same time (1880s) as American ferrets. Historic documents from the time period suggest many of the ferrets released in New Zealand originated from American stock (Anonymous 1888),[55] so their genetic differences may be less profound than some might expect.

In 88 feral ferrets sampled from New Zealand, dental disease rates were significantly lower or non-existent, with only 2.3% showing significant dental calculus, 1.1% exhibiting reactive bone associated with chronic inflammation and infection, 4.5% having fractured teeth, 1.1% possessing a dead tooth and 3.4% with measurable tooth wear. These specimens were true feral animals, evading predation, obtaining prey and surviving in an environment made hazardous by traps, motor vehicles and humans seeking eradication of ferrets as environmental pests. Each one of these factors could potentially cause damage or injury to the dentition, such as injuring a tooth while consuming bone-containing foods, in falls or during the act of predation.

Fractured teeth

Vilà et al (1993)[56] reported tooth fracture rates in wild wolves to be 12.8% (Fig. 21.7). However, fracture rates were higher in wolves eating large animals compared to fracture rates in environments where wolves exploit smaller prey. Van Ballenberghe et al[57] reported 46% of wolves caught in traps had broken teeth, a rate more-or-less duplicated by Kuehn[58] that found a 44% fractured tooth rate in trapped wolves. In non-trapped animals where presumably the attempts at escape are not as common (which drive up the frequency of dental fractures), Schlup[59] reported 14.0% of Swiss pet cats had fractured teeth. Capík et al[60] described 5370 pet dogs as having a tooth fracture rate of 2.6%. Van Valkenburgh[61] found a population of large carnivores (*Felidae, Hyaenidae, Canidae*) living in the wild had a mean fracture rate of 25.4% ($n = 729$).

One study of great interest is Andrews,[48] where over a period of 4 years, 350 British ferrets were examined for disease states. This population of ferrets was fed dead rats and tinned dog food, yet had a very low rate of dental disease. Despite careful observation of the oral cavity for disease and abnormal anatomy, the only pathological condition mentioned were three ferrets with broken canines, representing a 0.9% fracture rate.

In the study reported here, feral ferrets had a 4.5% tooth fracture rate and pet ferret fracture rates were 30.0%. Obviously, something is happening to pet ferrets that is driving the tooth fracture rate to higher levels than seen in the wild. The reports of fracture rates in wolves probably provide a clue to the problem; both pet ferrets and trapped wolves respond to entrapment by attempting to escape from confinement. In doing so, they use their teeth during the attempt, increasing damage and driving fracture rates upward. It is likely the high fracture rates of teeth in ferrets are in part due to attempts at escape from a caged confinement (Figs 21.8, 21.9); however, falls, kicks, swinging doors and other objects within a ferret's environment can obviously be a factor in the rates of fractured teeth (Table 21.4, Fig. 21.7).

Avulsed teeth

Rates of tooth avulsion (Figs 21.2, 21.4, 21.9–21.21, Table 21.4) in carnivores are poorly reported; the rates are

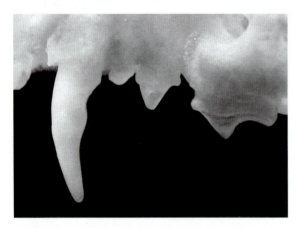

Figure 21.8 Ferrets will frequently bite or tug at cages, which will frequently result in damage to the teeth, especially the maxillary canines and second premolar. In this instance, the ferret used the canines to tug at the cage, wearing a semi-lunar notch in the canines, seriously weakening them. The adjacent premolar is heavily worn down from cage biting. Other dental pathologies include reactive bone, dental calculus, alveolar bone loss exposing tooth roots and dental attrition.

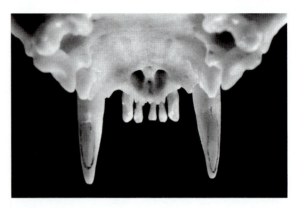

Figure 21.9 While most ferrets tend to pull at cage bars, some will rock or slide their teeth on the wire in an attempt to bite through. This significantly increases the scope of the tooth damage, removing enamel from the posterior of the tooth. *Note* the avulsed left medial incisor, dental calculus and flattened cusps on the premolars.

either not reported or subsumed within fractured tooth rates or those of missing teeth. Verstraete et al[62] reported a 6.5 tooth loss rate in feral cats from Marion Island. In the study reported here, there were no avulsed teeth noted in the 88 feral ferret skulls examined and pet ferret tooth avulsion rates were 46.5% (Table 21.4). The most commonly lost teeth in pet ferrets were the mandibular second molars (M_2), followed by both maxillary and mandibular incisors. In a few cases, a premolar was lost and in a single case, an avulsed canine was noted. In all cases, avulsed teeth are probably due to advanced periodontal disease, dental abrasion or a combination of both. Frequently, ferrets with avulsed teeth also had other dental pathologies, including dental abrasion, reactive bone tissue, moderate or extreme dental calculus and dental abscesses and all probably are symptoms of a greater problem – severe periodontal disease secondary to diet.[63]

Dental abrasion

Teeth wear down in three basic ways, each occurring simultaneously: wear from one tooth striking another, wear from non-food objects and wear from food objects. To reduce misunderstanding, convention references the wear from one tooth striking the other as 'dental attrition', while wear from food or non-food sources are termed 'dental abrasion' (Figs 21.14, 21.18, 21.22, 21.23). While there are many references to the use of dental wear in ageing studies, few actually report the problem in terms of abrasion and what drives the process. Heran[64] reports dental wear in *Mustelae* species to be minimal in wild populations, approximately the same (or lower) seen in the feral ferrets observed (3.4%).

Pet ferrets have dental abrasion of 85.2%, a significantly higher figure than seen in wild animals (Table 21.4). Berkovitz and Poole,[46] reported ferrets consuming a pelleted diet had teeth with more wear than those of polecats consuming a diet of wild prey. In the study reported here, pet ferrets that were fed a hard, crunchy kibble diet had significantly more tooth wear (85.2%) than feral ferrets consuming animal foods (3.4%). Most of this wear was confined to the cheek teeth and the molars. It was common to see the blades of the carnassials flattened or the molars ground down to gum level (Figs 21.14, 21.18, 21.22, 21.23). For comparison with a relatively unworn, sharp carnassial, see Figures 21.1–21.3, 21.10.

The tooth wear problem is probably attributable to a diet of hard kibble. Kibble is popular – at least in part – because it has low moisture levels that prevent the food from spoiling. Those low moisture levels also cause the food to become quite hard, which is a selling point for combating tartar build-up (which in ferrets it fails to do – see the section on dental calculus). It is probably the hardness and abrasive quality of kibble that is causing the high rate of dental abrasion seen in pet ferrets.[46] Kibble-mediated dental wear is common to all species of animals consuming the diet. However, the relative rate of wear in teeth appears to be higher in ferrets. This is probably not due to significant structural differences in the teeth, but more likely a function of Surface Law[65] (see discussion below).

Dental calculus

Dental calculus (Figs 21.3, 21.4, 21.8, 21.11, 21.16, 21.17, 21.19, 21.20–21.24), commonly termed tartar,

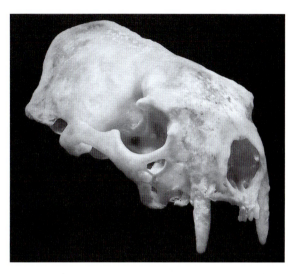

Figure 21.11 Advanced periodontal disease due to a long-term build-up of dental calculus can lead to tooth loss, reactive bone, multiple abscesses and loss of alveolar bone. *Note* the large abscess chambers in the right zygoma, with local destruction of bone tissue.

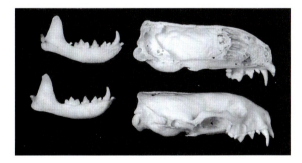

Figure 21.10 The interior of the ferret skull showing a shark-like dentition specialized for rendering animal tissues. *Note* the large dedication of space to the olfactory sense and the lack of ability to grind or chew food. The front third of the skull, literally everything above the teeth, is dedicated to detecting odour. *Note* the missing second molar in the right mandible; the tooth was not avulsed, but never erupted.

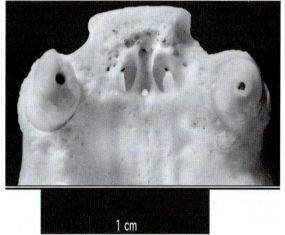

Figure 21.12 Ferrets tend to chew objects in their environment, including cloth bedding and toys. If not provided with a suitable alternative, such as 'ChewWeasels' or 'N-bones', prolonged chewing on cloth can cause significant dental damage to their teeth. In this skull, the maxillary incisors and front premolars have been lost and the wear damage to the canines is extensive, opening the pulp cavities to the external environment. *Note* the slab fracture on the right canine, probably the result of a fall after the canines had been worn flat. Reactive bone, dental calculus and small abscesses are present.

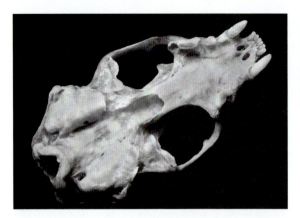

Figure 21.13 Ferrets will naturally attempt to break kibble on their rear molars, which are designed to crack bones and insect carapaces rather than grinding food. This increases the rate of wear significantly and frequently causes the loss of the maxillary molars. Generally, the molars wear down until a crack develops between the roots, then each root fragment is independently lost. In this skull, a small fragment of enamel can be seen on the buccal side of the right maxillary molar, but the remaining tooth, as well as the left maxillary molar, is completely lost. Dentine is exposed in the cheek teeth due to severe dental attrition and reactive bone and dental calculus are evident.

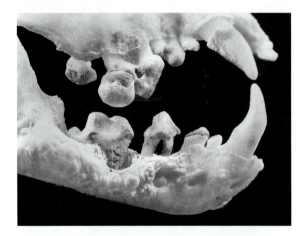

Figure 21.14 In the study, approximately 1% of the skulls displayed signs of acute osteomyelitis, secondary to advanced periodontal disease (this skull represents the worst case seen). Reactive bone, abscesses, severe dental calculus, profound tooth wear and other oral pathology are readily apparent.

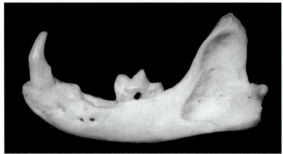

Figure 21.15 Commonly lost teeth on the mandible include the front premolars and the molar, often leaving the carnassial alone in the lower arcade. Tooth loss is often accompanied by the presence of abscesses, as seen in this mandible. The only teeth remaining in this left mandible are the canine and carnassial, all others were lost to the effects of periodontal disease.

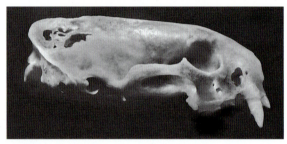

Figure 21.16 Evidence of infection in ferret teeth is often associated with other, more serious problems. In this skull, multiple dental abscesses are associated with extensive skull lesions.

is the buildup of mineralized plaque on tooth surfaces. Berkovitz and Poole[46] reported dental calculus to be insignificant in polecats eating a wild diet and ferrets eating whole mice, but 'heavy' in ferrets fed a pelleted diet, a finding duplicated in this study comparing pet ferrets with New Zealand feral ferrets. This close correlation between periodontal disease and diet has been investigated by many researchers who have reported dental calculus will form in ferrets regardless of the type of food consumed (see Gorrel[66]). Multiple studies have shown wild mammals generally have minor accumulations of dental calculus, while pet and wild animals housed as pets show significant amounts of tartar (see Miles and Grigson[5]). In the study reported here, 94.1% of pet ferrets had dental calculus, while only 2.3% of the feral ferret population suffered from the problem (Table 21.4).

The primary cause of dental calculus (and ultimately periodontal disease) is the presence of plaque that adheres to all exposed tooth surfaces. Plaque is composed of saliva, bacteria, cellular and food debris, various cells and bacterial by-products and it rapidly accumulates on tooth surfaces and below the gum line. Plaque accumulates

Pathological conditions found in ferret teeth

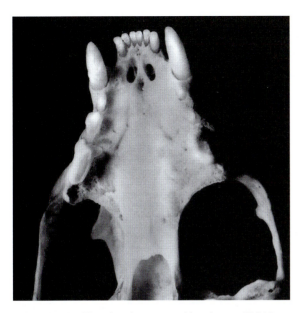

Figure 21.17 The abrasiveness and hardness of kibble grinds the enamel from tooth surfaces, speeding their wear and loss. In this skull, the underlying dentine – here stained with disclosing solution – is evident in the carnassials, showing the enamel has been worn away. As the maxillary molar is worn away, it will fragment and avulse. In this skull, the left molar has been lost and a small fragment of enamel is all that remains of the right molar.

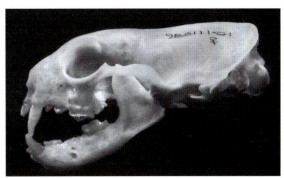

Figure 21.18 Ferret teeth evolved to render animal carcasses into small chunks that can be safely swallowed. While connective tissues and other parts of a prey carcass are tough and will wear teeth down over time, compared with hard kibble their abrasive qualities are limited. The abrasiveness and hardness of kibble speeds tooth attrition, resulting in worn, flattened teeth. This is especially evident in the carnassials and molars. Kibble flattens the blades of the carnassials and as the tooth is worn down towards the roots, fractures become common, which usually results in the loss of the teeth. In this skull, the blades on the mandibular carnassial are almost ground down to the notch, the second mandibular molar has been lost, as well as the third premolar. Mandibular teeth are generally worn down at a faster rate than their maxillary counterparts, in part because they are smaller and with less volume and also because the mandibular teeth move more against the food, increasing wear rates. *Note* the mandibular abscess, extensive dental calculus and reactive bone tissue.

regardless of the food consumed and even forms on teeth when animals are tube-fed.[67] Calculus is mineralized plaque and while it is of itself an irritant, it forms a surface that exacerbates the retention of plaque.[66] Plaque formation is the problem that drives periodontal disease.[68] Plaque formation has long been correlated to periodontal disease, but recent studies indicate the presence of plaque may play a part in other disease states,[66] including cardiovascular ailments[69] and systemic inflammation.[70]

The Rule of Parsimony suggests the difference between the low rate of dental calculus in feral ferrets and the high rate in pet ferrets can be best explained by differences in diet. Since the food consumed has little or no effect on the formation of tartar,[67] then the difference must be in some other aspect of the food. The only real prevention of plaque (and ultimately dental calculus and periodontal disease) appears to be mechanical removal, such as tooth brushing, tartar scaling and polishing.[71] Berkovitz and Poole[46] found ferrets fed whole mice had dental calculus at similar levels found in polecats.

It is probable that rendering a carcass, including administering the killing bite, tearing through the fur and skin, consuming muscles and bones and the general pulling, tugging and gnawing associated with consuming whole prey provides the mechanical abrasion required to clean the surface of the teeth of adherent plaque. The process of rendering a prey animal is also very stimulating to gingival surfaces, increasing blood flow and increasing bacterial resistance.[71] In the absence of whole prey carcasses, the best solution to prevent dental calculus appears to be toothbrushing,[71] combined with a program of veterinary dental care.

Dental abscesses

Pet ferrets examined in the study reported here have a 12.4% dental abscess rate (Figs 21.3–21.5, 21.11–21.23), some associated with extensive bone loss (Table 21.4). In about half the cases, the abscess tended to remain localized and small and generally, some degree of healing had taken place (Figs 21.3, 21.12, 21.13, 21.17, 21.19, 21.22). In some cases, the abscess was active, with little demonstrable healing, but remaining localized (Figs 21.4, 21.18, 21.20, 21.21). However, in at least nine individuals within the study, the abscessing was

CHAPTER TWENTY-ONE

Ferret dentition and pathology

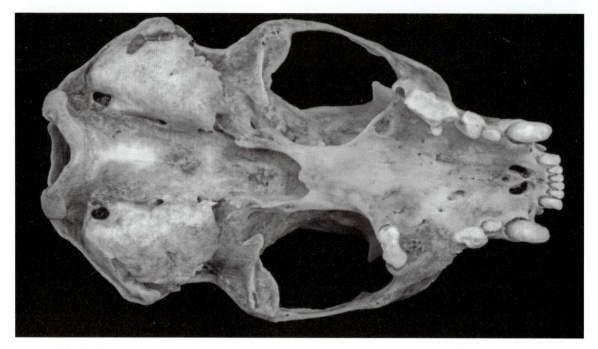

Figure 21.19 It is common to find missing teeth in older ferrets, often more than one. In this skull, the left carnassial has been missing for quite some time and the right molar avulsed more recently. *Note* the extensive build-up of dental calculus, the worn teeth and the presence of pitting in the bone surface, a possible indicator of chronic infection.

extensive, destructive and probably contributed to the death of the animal (Figs 21.5, 21.11, 21.14–21.16, 21.23).

Other pathological dental conditions

There are relatively few changes in the ferret's dentition resulting from domestication. In most cases, there are no dental traits that could be reliable enough to distinguish a wild polecat from a domesticated ferret.[49] About 2% of ferrets had a crowded dental arcade, presumably from a reduction in rostral length (Fig. 21.25).

Reactive bone – that is, new bone recently deposited on the surface of older bone as a result of infection or inflammation – was seen in 72.3% of the ferrets, generally along the gum line (Figs 21.3, 21.17, 21.18, 21.21–21.24), but sometimes extending over the portions of the skull (Figs 21.4, 21.5, 21.11, 21.14, 21.16, 21.20, 21.26). Palatine bone erosion was seen in 3.0% of pet ferrets (Figs 21.7, 21.27). Osteoporosis, not quantified for this portion of the study, was noted in a considerable number of ferret skulls; in some cases the demineralization was extensive and profound (Fig. 21.26).

A single ferret suffered periodontal disease secondary to impaling a canine through a piece of rubber, driving it against the gum line (Fig. 21.20). Dental wear from habitual fabric or toy chewing was apparent, but not separately quantified because of the difficulty of identifying the object causing the damage. However, ferrets that were long time fabric chewers were easily distinguished by a pattern of extensive wear to the canines, worn down as they were dragged across the fabric (Fig. 21.12).

Kibble and dental disease

Arguments that kibble helps to retard the development of dental calculus are somewhat contradictory to the collected data. If 94.1% of ferrets have dental calculus and their diet is primarily kibble, then it is obvious that the role of kibble in preventing or reducing tartar is overstated. In ferrets, this is probably due to the chisel-like cross-section of their cutting teeth; these narrow teeth do not penetrate the kibble enough before it breaks to allow significant abrasive cleaning. It is possible the carbohydrates in kibble can provide nourishment to the bacteria living in the oral cavity and exacerbate the condition. The evidence suggests that in ferrets kibble does not make much of a contribution to preventing periodontal disease and probably contributes greatly towards it.

Pathological conditions found in ferret teeth

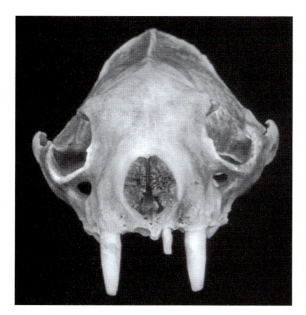

Figure 21.20 Maxillary incisors are commonly lost in ferrets, mostly as a result of periodontal disease or chewing foreign objects. In this skull, there is extensive bone loss secondary to periodontal disease, abscessing and loss of all but one of the maxillary incisors. *Note* the extensive pitting of the bone surface, including the interior floor of the nasal opening, which is probably an indicator of chronic infection. *Also note* the blunted tips of the canines; microscopic inspection suggests they were worn down as a result of chewing foreign objects, such as fabric bedding or toys.

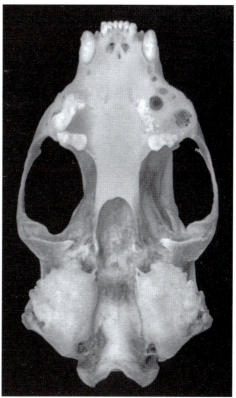

Figure 21.21 If dental calculus is visible, it can be safely assumed that calculus also extends under the gumline. However, the reverse cannot always be held true – just because visible dental calculus is minor, it does not follow that periodontal disease is also insignificant. In this skull, dental calculus is minor. However, there is extensive periodontal disease and the left carnassial has been recently avulsed due to infection and bone loss. The carnassial abscess opened a fistula into the nasal cavity and the left maxilla is inflated, pitted and possessing several small abscess outlets. Several premolars have also been lost; the exception being the left maxillary second premolar, removed for ageing studies. The bright area next to the lost carnassial is newly deposited or reactive, bone.

The abrasiveness and hardness of kibble is most likely the driving force behind the increased wear rates seen in pet ferret teeth. When a ferret uses their carnassials, the sectorial teeth slide past one another, cutting the tissue and forming facing wear facets that help keep the teeth sharp. When the same ferret eats a piece of kibble, only the tips of the carnassial blades contact the food, blunting them and dulling the cutting facets. This process initiates several problems that at first do not seem to be associated with dental wear. First, flat platforms are formed on the teeth that increase the likelihood of catastrophic fractures, such as slab fractures. The rate of wear on the enamel is increased, which exposes the softer dentine underneath. Once the dentine is exposed, the wear rate will increase so that teeth that appeared to be slowly wearing away will suddenly wear down 'overnight'. Also, worn teeth become sensitive to touch, which may help to explain why older ferrets become somewhat anorexic; it simply may be too painful to eat.

Dental wear rates are strongly correlated to the size of the tooth. This is because of Surface Law.[65] The Surface Law governs how the surface area of a three-dimensional object, such as a tooth, increases additively while the volume increases multiplicatively. For example, the formula for determining the surface area of a three-dimensional object is: $SA = 2(L \times W) + 2(L \times H) + 2(H \times W)$, while the formula for determining volume is: $V = L \times W \times H$ (L, length; H, height and W, width). The

CHAPTER TWENTY-ONE
Ferret dentition and pathology

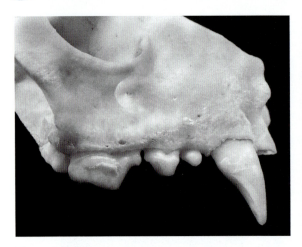

Figure 21.22 Reactive bone changes can be caused by infections or inflammations (among other things). When found in the dental arcade they generally indicate the presence of periodontal or other dental disease. *Note* the presence of a small abscess above the carnassial. Such abscesses are difficult to detect in an animal that is being held, rather than sedated for dental X-rays. Also, the abscess is very small and could be misinterpreted as an artifact. *Note* the dental attrition on the tooth cusps, receding bone and exposed roots and dental calculus.

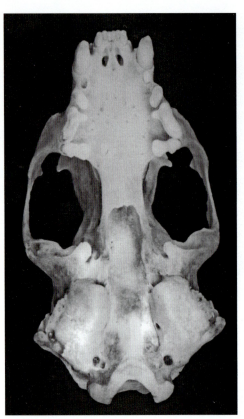

Figure 21.24 While ferrets display many characteristics generalized to domesticated animals, such as behavioural neoteny and coat colour changes, the changes to the skeleton are relatively minor. One change is a slight reduction in the length of the rostrum, resulting in dental crowding. Generally, dental crowding can be present without changing the relative position of the teeth (just the spaces between the teeth are reduced), but in this skull, the third premolars are rotated and slightly displaced medially to their normal position. The right maxillary premolar was lost post mortem.

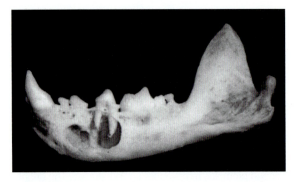

Figure 21.23 On visual inspection, the oral cavity of this ferret appeared more-or-less normal, with some gingivitis present and only moderate wear to the teeth. After skeletal preparation, it was clear a discrepancy was evident and there was more than what appeared to the eye. Bony tissue destruction secondary to abscesses was extensive in both mandibles.

surface area of a cube having three 1 inch sides would be $2(1 \times 1) + 2(1 \times 1) + 2(1 \times 1)$ or 6 square inches. The volume would be $1 \times 1 \times 1$ or 1 cubic inch, giving a ratio of surface area to internal volume of 6:1. Double the size of the cube and the surface area increases to 24 square inches. However, the volume is now $2 \times 2 \times 2$ or 8 cubic inches, resulting in a surface area to volume ratio of 24:8 or 3:1. Double the cube again and the surface area is 96 square inches, with a volume of 64, making the ratio 1.5:1. Double it again and the ratio is 0.75:1.

What this means in terms of dental wear is that smaller teeth have relatively smaller volumes and smaller volumes means there is simply less tooth material to wear away. If all other factors are equal, larger teeth will survive an abrasive diet better simply because they have more tooth

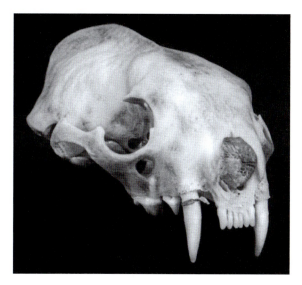

Figure 21.25 Ferrets are 'obligate chewers' and are quite persistent in finding objects to masticate. In this skull, a small fragment of a rubber chew toy was pierced by the right maxillary incisor, trapping it on the tooth at the gum line. This caused a loss of bone at the root of the tooth, as well as localized periodontal disease.

material to abrade. In the study being discussed, female ferrets displayed more profound dental wear than males, which probably reflects sexually dimorphic differences in tooth size. This also allows a rough prediction of tooth wear rates for different-sized animals eating the same size, abrasiveness and hardness of kibble: a small female ferret should have more dental wear than a large male ferret, who should have more wear than a larger cat, who should have more wear than a small dog. Because smaller teeth have proportionately smaller volumes, the probability that kibble will harm the teeth increases as the tooth size decreases.

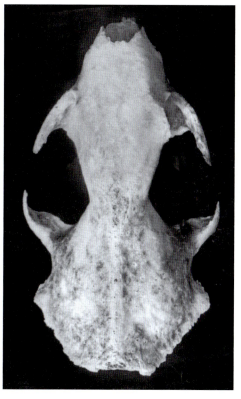

Figure 21.26 Some degree of osteoporosis is a common observation in neutered and caged pet ferrets, which can be exacerbated by other disease and drug therapy. It is especially notable in the vertebral bodies, the pelvis and on the skull. This skull, belonging to a 6-year-old neutered male ferret with severe periodontal disease and unspecified kidney problems, was missing multiple teeth and had been subjected to long-term steroid therapy. The zygomatic arch is deteriorated and missing and the surface of the skull is pockmarked with dissolution features. Bone density is between 40 and 50% of normal.

Recommendations

Ferrets require regular tooth brushing with a non-fluoridated dentifrice, with periodic inspection with probing, cleaning and polishing by a qualified veterinarian or veterinary technician. Cages should be modified to prevent a ferret from using their teeth in an attempt to escape. If a softer diet cannot be provided, kibble should be softened slightly to minimize its abrasive effect on the teeth. If a ferret consistently desires to chew fabrics, they should be removed (shredded paper is a good substitute for cloth bedding). Ferrets with bad breath, facial swellings, loose teeth and bleeding, red or puffy gums should have dental X-rays made to check for abscesses, bad teeth and bone loss. Veterinarians should start regarding periodontal disease as a serious threat to a ferret's long-term health, rather than assuming it is just a minor problem that does not need to be aggressively addressed. Commercially available chewing treats, such as gelatin chews or edible sticks, should be provided for stimulating the gums and satisfying the urge to chew. Research needs to be done on the impact of periodontal disease on ferret health, including its involvement in other organ diseases.

CHAPTER TWENTY-ONE
Ferret dentition and pathology

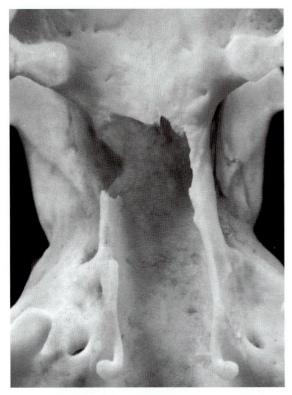

Figure 21.27 Significant erosion of the palatine bones was seen in approximately 1% of the skulls in the study. It is still to be determined what caused the erosion; it may be associated with lymphoma, oral injuries, abscesses or osteoporosis. This female ferret was diagnosed with lymphoma and suffered from severe osteoporosis.

References

1. Harty FJ. Concise illustrated dental dictionary, 2nd edn. Oxford: Wright; 1994.
2. Hillson S. Teeth. Cambridge manuals in archaeology. Cambridge: Cambridge University Press; 1986.
3. Popowics TE. Ontogeny of postcanine tooth form in the ferret, *Mustela putorius* (Carnivora: Mammalia) and the evolution of dental diversity within the Mustelidae. J Morphol 1998; 237:69–90.
4. Popowics TE. Postcanine dental form in the Mustelidae and Viverridae (Carnivora: Mammalia). J Morphol 2003; 256:322–341.
5. Miles AW, Grigson C, eds. Colyer's variation and diseases of the teeth of animals, revised edition. Cambridge: Cambridge University Press; 1990.
6. Lodé T. Trophic status and feeding habits of the European polecat *Mustela putorius* L. 1758. Mammal Rev 1997; 27:177–184.
7. Lodé T. Sexual dimorphism and trophic constraints: prey selection in the European polecat (*Mustela putorius*). Ecoscience 2003; 10:17–23.
8. McDonald RA. Resource partitioning among British and Irish mustelids. J Anim Ecol 2002; 71:185–200.
9. Weber D. The diet of polecats *Mustela putorius* L. in Switzerland. Z Saügetierkd 1989; 54:157–171.
10. Holliday JA, Steppan SJ. Evolution of hypercarnivory: the effect of specialization on morphological and taxonomic diversity. Paleobiology 2003; 30:108–128.
11. Fox JG, McLain DE. Nutrition. In: Fox JC, ed. Biology and diseases of the ferret, 2nd edn. Baltimore: Williams & Wilkins; 1998:149–172.
12. Berkovitz BKB. Supernumerary deciduous incisors and the order of eruption of the incisor teeth in the albino ferret. J Zool, London 1968; 155:445–449.
13. Berkovitz BKB. Tooth development in the albino ferret (*Mustela putorius*) with special reference to the permanent carnassial. Arch Oral Biol 1973; 18:465–471.
14. Berkovitz BKB, Silverstone LM. The dentition of the albino ferret. Caries Res 1969; 3:369–376.
15. Evans HE, An NQ. Anatomy of the ferret. In: Fox JC, ed. Biology and diseases of the ferret, 2nd edn. Baltimore: Williams & Wilkins; 1998:19–69.
16. He T, Friede H, Kiliaridis S. Dental eruption and exfoliation chronology in the ferret (*Mustela putorius furo*). Arch Oral Biol 2002; 47:619–623.
17. Mazák V. Eruption of permanent dentition in the Genera *Mustela* Linnaeus, 1758 and Putorius Cuvier, 1817 with a note on the Genus *Martes* Pinel, 1792 (Mammalia, Mustelidae). Vestn Cesk Spol Zool Acta Soc Zool Bohemoslov 1963; 27:328–334.
18. Shump AU, Shump KA. Growth and development of the European ferret (*Mustela putorius*). Lab Anim Sci 1978; 28:89–91.
19. Apfelbach R. Imprinting on prey odors in ferrets *Mustela putorius* f. *furo* and its neural correlates. Behav Processes 1986; 12:363–382.
20. Denisov EI. Experimental study of ferret *Putorius furo* biology during the raising of their young. Izv Sib Otd Akad Nauk SSSR Ser Biol Nauk 1985; 2:89–93.
21. Miller B, Biggins D, Wemmer C, et al. Development of survival skills in captive-raised Siberian polecats (*Mustela eversmanni*) I. Locating prey. J Ethology 1990; 8:89–94.
22. Rehn B, Breipohl W, Mendoza AS, et al. Changes in granule cells of the ferret *Mustela putorius furo* olfactory bulb associated with imprinting on prey odors. Brain Res 1986; 373:114–125.
23. Kelliher K, Baum M, Meredith M. The ferret's vomeronasal organ and accessory olfactory bulb: effect of hormone manipulation in adult males and females. Anat Rec 2001; 263:280–288.
24. Kusak J, Huber D. Curiosity in the Carnivores. Veterinarski Arch 1991; 61:395–409.
25. Passineau MJ, Green EJ, Dietrich WD. Therapeutic effects of environmental enrichment on cognitive function and tissue integrity following severe traumatic brain injury in rats. Exp Neurol 2001; 168:373–384.
26. Stiles J. Neural plasticity and cognitive development. Dev Neuropsychology 2000; 18:237–272.
27. Vargas A, Anderson SH. Effects of experience and cage enrichment on predatory skills of black-footed ferrets (*Mustela nigripes*). J Mammal 1999; 80:263–269.
28. Fox JG, Bell JA. Growth, reproduction and breeding. In: Fox JC, ed. Biology and diseases of the ferret, 2nd edn. Baltimore: Williams & Wilkins; 1998:211–227.
29. Apfelbach R. Wild animal-domesticated animal-experimental animal: changes in the brain during early ontogeny depend on environmental conditions. Tierarztl Umsch 1996; 51:157–162.

30. Bateman JA. Supernumerary incisors in mustelids. Mamm Rev 1970; 1:81–86.
31. Berkovitz BKB, Thomson P. Observations on the aetiology of supernumerary upper incisors in the albino ferret. Arch Oral Biol 1973; 18:457–463.
32. Valkenburgh B Van, Ruff CB. Canine tooth strength and killing behaviour in large carnivores. J Zool (London) 1987; 212:379–397.
33. Gittleman JL, Valkenburgh B Van. Sexual dimorphism in the canines and skulls of carnivores: effects of size, phylogeny and behavioural ecology. J Zool, London 1997; 242:97–117.
34. Lawes INC, Andrews PLR. Variation of the ferret skull (*Mustela putorius furo* L.) in relation to stereotaxic landmarks. J Anat 1987; 154:157–171.
35. Buchalczyk T, Ruprecht AL. Skull variability of *Mustela putorius* Linnaeus, 1758. Acta Theriologica 1977; 22:87–120.
36. Hall ER. Supernumerary and missing teeth in wild mammals of the Orders Insectivora and Carnivora, with some notes on disease. J Dent Res 1940; 19:103–143.
37. Romer AS. Vertebrate paleontology, 2nd. edn. Chicago: University of Chicago Press; 1962.
38. He T, Friede H, Kiliaridis S. Macroscopic and roentgenographic anatomy of the skull of the ferret (*Mustela putorius furo*). Lab Anim 2001; 36:86–96.
39. Dayan T, Simberloff D, Tchernov E, et al. Inter- and intraspecific character displacement in mustelids. Ecology 1989; 70:1526–1539.
40. Dayan T, Simberloff D. Character displacement, sexual dimorphism and morphological variation among British and Irish mustelids. Ecology 1994; 75:1063–1073.
41. Dessem D, Druzinsky RE. Jaw-muscle activity in ferrets, *Mustela putorious furo*. J Morphol 1992; 213:275–286.
42. Klevezal GA. Recording structures of mammals: determination of age and reconstruction of life history. [translated by Mina MV and Oreshkin AV] revised and updated edition. Brookfield: AA Balkema; 1996.
43. Thome H, Geiger G. Comparison of two age determination methods in wild carnivores of known age using tooth wear. Anatomia, Histologia, Embryologia: Veterinary Medicine Series C 1997; 26:81–84.
44. Greaves WS. A functional analysis of carnassial biting. Biol J Linn Soc 1983; 20:353–363.
45. Greaves WS. The generalized carnivore jaw. Zool J Linn Soc 1985; 85:267–274.
46. Berkovitz BKB, Poole DFG. Attrition of the teeth in ferrets. J Zool, London 1977; 183:411–418.
47. Chiasson RB. The dentition of the Alaskan fur seal. J Mammal 1957; 38:310–319.
48. Andrews PLR, Illman O, Mellersh A. Some observations of anatomical abnormalities and disease states in a population of 350 ferrets (*Mustela furo* L.). Z Versuchstierkd 1979; 21:346–353.
49. Glas GH. Numerical variation in the permanent dentition of the polecat, *Mustela putorius* (Linnaeus, 1758), from the Netherlands. Z Säugertierkd 1977; 42:256–259.
50. Ruprecht AL. Dental variations in the common polecat in Poland. Acta Theriologica 1978; 23:239–245.
51. Baker J, Brothwell D. Animal diseases in archaeology. New York: Academic Press; 1980.
52. Lyman RL. Vertebrate taphonomy. Cambridge: Cambridge University Press; 1994.
53. Reichs KJ. Forensic osteology: advances in the identification of human remains. Springfield: Charles C. Thomas; 1986.
54. Reitz EJ, Wing ES. Zooarchaeology. Cambridge: Cambridge University Press; 1999.
55. Anonymous. Ferrets by the thousand. N Y Times 1888; December 15:2.
56. Vili C, Urios V, Castroviejo J. Tooth losses and anomalies in the wolf (*Canis lupus*). Can J Zool 1993; 71:968–971.
57. Ballenberghe V Van. Injuries to wolves sustained during live-capture. J Wildl Manage 1984; 48:1425–1429.
58. Kuehn DW, Fuller TK, Mech LD, et al. Trap-related injuries to gray wolves in Minnesota. J Wildl Manage 1986; 50:90–91.
59. Schlup D. Epidemiologische und morphologische am katzengebiß I. Mitteilung: epidemiologische untersuchungen. Kleintier Prax 1982; 27:87–94.
60. Capík I, Ledecky V, Sevcík A. Tooth fracture evaluation and endodontic treatment in dogs. Acta Vet Brno 2000; 69:115–122.
61. Van Valkenburgh B. Incidence of tooth breakage among large, predatory mammals. Am Nat 1988; 131:291–302.
62. Verstraete FJM, Aarde RJ Van, Nieuwoudt BA, et al. The dental pathology of feral cats on Marion Island, Part II: periodontitis, external odontoclastic resorption lesions and mandibular thickening. J Comp Pathol 1996; 115:283–297.
63. Gorrel C, Robinson J. Periodontal therapy and extraction technique. In: Crossley DA, Penman S, eds. Manual of small animal dentistry, 2nd edn. Cheltenham: British Small Animal Veterinary Association; 1995:139–149.
64. Heran I. Some notes on dentition in Mustelidae. Vestn Cesk Spol Zool 1971; 35:199–204.
65. Schmidt-Nielsen K. Scaling: why is animal size so important? Cambridge: Cambridge University Press; 1984.
66. Gorrel C. Periodontal disease and diet in domestic pets. J Nutr 1998; 128:2712–2714.
67. Egelberg J. Local effects of diet on plaque formation and gingivitis development in dogs.III Effect of frequency of meals and tube feeding. Odontol Revy 1965; 16:50–60.
68. Lang NP, Mombelli A, Attström A, et al. Dental plaque and calculus. In: Lindhe J, ed. Clinical periodontology and implant dentistry, 3rd edn. Copenhagen: Munksgaard; 1997:102–137.
69. Joshipura KJ, Ward HC, Merchant AT, et al. Periodontal disease and biomarkers related to cardiovascular disease. J Dent Res 2004; 83:151–155.
70. D'Aiuto F, Parker M, Andreou G, et al. Peridontitis and systemic inflammation: control of the local infection is associated with a reduction in serum inflammatory markers. J Dent Res 2004; 83:156–160.
71. Ingham KE, Gorrel C, Blackburn JM, et al. The effect of toothbrushing on periodontal disease in cats. J Nutr 2002; 132:1740–1741.

Appendix

Physiological data on blood cells, blood chemistry and urine constituents have been tabulated for research ferrets (Table A.1a–c).[1] Normal haematological values are given in Table A.2 and it can be noted that the haematocrit for ferrets is relatively high compared with the dog, cat and rat. The ferret has a negligible erythrocyte sedimentation rate, so haematocrit samples need to be spun longer. The presence of Howell–Jolly bodies is a feature in about 5% of both sexes.[1] The blood picture is otherwise very like the cat except for a higher erythrocyte count and presence in the ferret of a higher percentage of reticulocytes. There is a naturally lower platelet and leukocyte count in the jill in heat.

Blood chemistry

The blood chemistry of the ferret corresponds with those of the dog and cat and is shown in Table A.3. The ferret shows an age-related decrease in alkaline phosphatase, like other species, due to the bone isoenzyme decreasing after the end of the rapid bone growth period.[1]

Note that with clinical pathology, there can be variations of values between laboratories and in Australia we have to relate to American data as Table A.3. A more

Table A.1a Basic ferret data

Ferret life span	6–10 years (some worker ferrets to 13 years)
Mature ferret body weight	
Jills	500 g–1.2 kg
Hobs	1–2 kg
Sexual maturity	6–9 months
Breeding life	Up to 6 years
Breeding season	
Southern hemisphere (SH)	August to January of following year
Northern hemisphere (NH)	March to August same year
Usual peak of mating	From September (SH) *or* March (NH), with hobs' testicles maximum weight and jills with maximized swollen vulva corresponding with jill fertility in lengthened daylight periods
Ovulation stimulus	Induced by coitus; jill becomes anoestrous 1 week after fertilization
Gestation period	Usually 42 days
Litter sizes	4–14 kittens (baby ferrets). Numbers reduce after 5 years of age
Kitten birth weights	Usually 10 g, range 6–12 g
Kitten hearing function	At 32 days
Kitten eyes open	Between 4 and 5 weeks of age
Kitten weaning	From mother between 6 and 8 weeks of age
Ferret diploid chromosome number	40
Structural anatomy	Ch. 2
Dental anatomy and pathology	Ch. 21

Table A.1b Metabolic values for laboratory ferrets

Semi-moist food consumption	140–190 g/24 h (compare feeding pet and working ferrets in Ch. 4)
Water intake	75–100 mL/24 h
Urine volume	26–28 mL/24 h
Urine pH	6.5–7.5

Table A.1c Cardiovascular/respiratory and arterial blood pressure standard measurements

Mean systolic (conscious)	
Jill	133 mmHg
Hob	161 mmHg
Mean diastolic (anaesthetized)	110–125 mmHg
Heart rate	200–400 bpm
Cardiac output	139 mL/min
Circulation time	4.5–6.8-s
Blood volume (5–7% of body weight)	
Jill	40 mL
Hob	60 mL
Respiration	33–36/min
Body temperature	38.8°C (range 37.8–40°C)

Table A.1a–c adapted from Fox JG, ed. Biology and diseases of the ferret, 2nd edn. Baltimore: Williams and Wilkins; 1998:184, 1998, with permission.

Appendix

Table A.2 Haematological values for normal ferrets

Normal values		Albino ferrets Male	Female	Fitch ferrets Male	Female
PCV (L/L)	Mean	0.55	0.49	0.43	0.48
	Range	0.44–0.61	0.42–0.55	0.36–0.50	0.47–0.51
Haemoglobin (g/L)	Mean	178	162	143	159
	Range	163–182	148–174	120–163	152–174
RBC ($\times 10^{12}$/L)	Mean	10.23	8.11		
	Range	7.3–12.18	6.77–9.76		
Platelets ($\times 10^9$/L)	Mean	453	545		
	Range	297–730	310–910		
Reticulocytes (%)	Mean	4.0	5.3		
	Range	1–12	2–14		
WBC ($\times 10^9$/L)	Mean	9.7	10.5	11.3	5.9
	Range	4.4–19.1	4.0–18.2	7.7–15.4	2.5–8.6
Differential (%) Bands	Mean			0.9	1.7
	Range			0–2.2	0–4.2
Neutrophils	Mean	57.0	59.5	40.1	31.1
	Range	11–82	43–84	24–78	12–41
Lymphocytes	Mean	35.6	33.4	49.7	58.0
	Range	12–54	12–50	28–69	25–95
Monocytes	Mean	4.4	4.4	6.6	4.5
	Range	0–9	2–8	3.4–8.2	1.7–6.3
Eosinophils	Mean	2.4	2.6	2.3	3.6
	Range	0–7	0–5	0–7	1–9
Basophils	Mean	0.1	0.2	0.7	0.8
	Range	0–2	0–1	0–2.7	0–2.9

Tables A.2–A.4 adapted from Moody et al., 1985.[1]

recent tabulation of the reference ranges of haematology and blood chemistry values of pet ferrets from Antech Diagnostics, Farmingdale, New York, gives similar ranges except for creatinine (K. Rosenthal, pers. comm. 1999). The newer creatinine values are 8.8–35.4 mmol/L; the previous values are now considered to have been too high.

Urinalysis

For urine checks on ferrets, urine can be collected by manual bladder expression under a sedative, use of a clean scats tray or by catheterization. There will be blood contamination with jills on heat. It is known that proteinuria occurs in most normal ferrets and may be due to the relatively high systolic blood pressure in the ferret and thicker intrarenal arterial walls. Interestingly the usual dark hob urine may give false positive values for ketonuria as the urine colour matches the reagent test strip colour.[1] Urinalysis details are given in Table A.4.

Drug formulary 2006

The range of drugs I have used on ferrets is relatively small and was used empirically in the 1970s. There are still very few drugs on the market specifically tailored for ferrets (2006). Human drugs have been commandeered for ferrets with FADC (Ch. 14). A number of dog and cat drugs have been used at lower dosage for heartworm and fleas and suggested for rare gastrointestinal parasites in ferrets.[2] The possibility of drug toxicity in ferrets from antibiotics has been pointed out.[3] My use of antibiotics in ferrets has been recorded.[4] When dealing with ferrets it is essential to weigh them accurately for drug dosage, keep the drugs used to a minimum and start from a low dosage if unsure of effects.

The USA Food and Drug Administration in 1996 approved the use of human or animal drugs for ferrets, in spite of the fact that such drugs had not been safety tested for ferrets. It therefore falls to the veterinarian to be cautious and inform the client of the facts.

Table A.3 Serum chemistry values for normal ferrets

		Albino ferrets	Fitch ferrets
Sodium (mmol/L)	Mean	148	152
	Range	137–162	146–160
Potassium (mmol/L)	Mean	5.9	4.9
	Range	4.5–7.7	4.3–5.3
Chloride (mmol/L)	Mean	116	115
	Range	106–125	102–121
Calcium (mmol/L)	Mean	2.3	2.32
	Range	2.0–2.94	2.15–2.62
Inorganic phosphorus (mmol/L)	Mean	1.91	2.1
	Range	1.29–2.94	1.81–2.81
Glucose (mmol/L)	Mean	7.55	5.61
	Range	5.22–11.49	3.47–7.44
BUN (nmol/L)	Mean	7.85	10.0
	Range	3.57–16.06	4.28–15.35
Creatinine (mmol/L)	Mean	53	35
	Range	35–79	17–53
Total protein (g/L)	Mean	60	59
	Range	51–74	53–72
Albumin (g/L)	Mean	32	37
	Range	26–38	33–41
Total bilirubin (µmol/L)	Mean	<17	
Cholesterol (mmol/L)	Mean	5.63	
	Range	1.65–7.64	
SAP (U/L)	Mean	23	53
	Range	9–84	30–120
ALT (U/L)	Mean		170
	Range		82–289
SGOT (U/L)	Mean	65	
	Range	28–120	

Table A.4 Urinalysis results in normal ferrets based on a 24-hour check (mean value)

	Male ferret	Female ferret
Volume (mL/24 h)	26	28
Sodium (mmol/24 h)	1.9	1.5
Potassium (mmol/24 h)	2.9	2.1
Chloride (mmol/24 h)	2.4	1.9
pH	6.5–7.5	6.5–7.5
Urine protein (mg/L)	70–330	0–230

Veterinarians treating pet ferrets would do well to record their use of drugs in these animals and pass on their experience in actual drug treatment and results, especially of any suspect toxicity. The Ferret Drug Formulary should be filled with safe ferret drugs. As stated, drugs are checked for safety for human use but not for ferret use, though ferrets are one of the mainstays still of medical research. There are some drugs which have been found to be essential for treating ferrets but have been withdrawn from the market for various reasons unrelated to the species, e.g. ProHeart 6 (moxidectin) (see Ch. 10).

The MUMS (Minor Use and Minor Species) Act of the USA Congress in 2004 is a way of making drugs legally available for large numbers of animal species for which few drugs are currently approved (FDA Newsletter May/June 2004). Animal drug companies have been reluctant to seek costly Food and Drug Administration (FDA) approvals for animal drugs that have a limited market. The Act allows 'conditional approval' which allows drug sponsors to make a drug available on the market before the company has collected all the necessary effectiveness data on the drug. Also 'indexing'

Appendix

Table A.5 Antibiotics used for ferrets

Antibiotic	Dose and administration	Comments
Chloramphenicol palmitate liquid	50 mg/kg b.i.d., p.o.	Drug of choice but now restricted use (children)
Chloramphenicol succinate	30–50 mg/kg b.i.d. i.m. s.c.	Can be given orally but with sugar solution as it is bitter
Clavulanic acid (12.5 mg/mL) Amoxicillin liquid (50 mg/mL)	12.5 mg/kg b.i.d. p.o. (1 mL/5 kg); I have used 0.25 mL b.i.d. without toxicity problems	Good wide spectrum and has pleasant taste. Very safe useful drug for ferrets
Doxycycline 100 mg/g paste	(10 mg/g paste no longer made)	Drug as paste useful if prepared to be empirical
Enrofloxacin (Baytril) (50 mg/mL)	3–5 mg/kg s.c. i.m. Note: injection might cause site necrosis. Not for young ferrets due to potential to erode joint cartilage	Broad spectrum drug for hepatitis especially. Use low dosage. Injectable form can be given orally mixed in syrup
Enrofloxacin 25 mg/mL liquid	5–15 mg/kg b.i.d. p.o.	Considered drug over-used and may result in resistance. Also be wary of long-term toxicity
Gentamicin common base antibiotic for ear infections	5 mg/kg s.i.d. i.m. s.c.	Potentially nephrotoxic and ototoxic. Avoid long usage
Neomycin common base antibiotic for ear infections	10 mg/kg q.i.d, p.o.	Potentially nephrotoxic and ototoxic. Also possible neuromuscular blockage. Avoid long use
Metronidazole	50 mg/kg s.i.d. p.o. or 10–25 mg/kg b.i.d. p.o.	Used for anaerobic infections. Neurotoxicity seen in dogs. May be used with chloromycin
Oxytetracycline	20 mg/kg t.i.d. p.o.	Can get renal disease in geriatric ferrets. Also teeth discolouration in neonatals
Tetracycline	20 mg/kg t.i.d. p.o.	Same problems as oxytetracycline
Sulfadimethoxine	30–50 mg/kg s.i.d. or b.i.d. p.o.	Renal disease in geriatric ferrets is possible
Sulfamethazine	1 mg/mL water	Same problems as sulfadimethoxine
Trimethoprim-sulfadiazine Trimethoprim-sulfamethoxazole	20–30 mg/kg b.i.d. s.c. p.o.	Used for urinary and respiratory infections. Same problems as sulfadimethoxine
Tylosin	10 mg/kg t.i.d. p.o. or 5–10 mg/kg b.i.d. i.v. i.m.	Used for Gram +ve bacteria plus spirochaetes, large viruses and some Gram −ve plus mycoplasma. No toxicity indicated
Clindamycin hydrochloride. Drug derived from *Streptomyces lincolnensis* but not apparently immediately toxic unlike streptomycin which is toxic to ferrets	Aquadrops have 25 mg/mL, dog dose is 5.5 mg/1000 g, approx. 6 mg/0.25 mL for ferrets	Used personally at 0.25 mL for 23 days on 600 g BEW jill with severe mammary gland abscess with no apparent toxicity. Bitter taste so use with sugar/honey bolus before and after
Amoxicillin	10–25 mg/kg s.i.d. or b.i.d. p.o., s.c.	Useful in combination drug dose, with metronidazole and bismuth subsalicylate, also with enrofloxacin
Ampicillin	5–30 mg/kg b.i.d. s.c., i.m., p.o.	Broad-spectrum
Cefadroxil	15–20 mg/kg b.i.d. p.o.	First-generation cephalosporin
Cephalexin (Keflex)	15–25 mg/kg b.i.d. p.o.	Good for urinary and respiratory infections
Cephaloridine	10–15 mg/kg s.i.d. s.c., i.m.	Broad-spectrum
Clarithromycin	50 mg/kg s.i.d., b.i.d. p.o.	Useful with amoxicillin or with metronidazole/bismuth subsalicylate for *Helicobacter mustelae*
Ciprofloxin	5–15 mg/kg b.i.d. or 10–30 mg/kg s.i.d. p.o.	Use as enrofloxacin
Penicillin G (sodium and potassium)	40 000 IU/kg s.i.d. i.m. or 20 000 IU/kg b.i.d. i.m.	
Amikacin	8–10 mg/kg s.c. i.m., i.v. at q. 8–12 h	

s.i.d., once daily; b.i.d., twice daily; t.i.d., three times daily; q.i.d., four times daily; p.o., per os (by mouth, orally); s.c., subcutaneous; i.v., intravenous; i.m., intramuscular.

Table A.6 Drugs for external and internal ferret parasites

Drug	Dose and administration	Comments
External parasites		
Fleas		
Carbaryl	50 g/kg	In powder form. Use on ferret coat or bedding but use sparingly once weekly. Superseded by sprays?
Piperonyl butoxide and pyrethrins together in shampoos	10 g/L and 1 g/L	Use only puppy/kitten concentration. Possibly once weekly. Superseded by sprays?
Fibronil (Frontline)	2.5 g/L 2–3 sprays per ferret	No toxicity seen. Easy to use with colony ferrets. (Do not use on pregnant jills)
Imidacloprid (Advantage)	0.4 mL/ferret of 9.1% solution applied topically monthly	Appears safe. Actually approved drug for ferrets/rabbits
Lufenuron (Program)	30 mg/kg monthly p.o.	
Selamectin (Revolution)	As for heartworm prevention	Appears safe. Expense factor for single ferrets?
Foot mange		
Lime sulphur (Sarcoptic)	Diluted 1:40	Safe old-type weekly wash for ferrets
Ivermectin (Sarcoptic)	1% solution, 0.05–0.1 mL p.o., s.c. Three doses at 2-week intervals	Safe drug
Ear mange		
Ivermectin (Otodectic)	1% solution mixed 1:20 with propylene glycol. Place 0.2–0.3 mL (10–15 mg) in each ear	Repeat in 4 weeks. Safe drug
Demodex: Amitraz (3% sol)	Possible to apply to skin at 14-day intervals for 3–6 treatments	Amitraz and malathion can be used for mange but I consider ivermectin safer
Malathion (2% sol)	Possible to use as dip every 10 days for 3 treatments	
Ivermectin	Use at 600 μg/kg daily	For at least 30 days
Internal parasites		
Pyrantel embonate 90 mg/g plus niclosamide monohydrate 264 mg/g	Felex paste. Lower cat dose to 1 kg possible for ferrets	Worms in ferrets are rare Most antihelminth drugs for dogs and cats are combinations of drugs
Pyrantel embonate alone 14.4 mg/mL	Canex Puppy Suspension, 0.5 mL/500 g weight	
Piperazine alone	50–100 mg/kg once; repeat dose in 2 weeks, p.o.	
Praziquantel alone	12.5 mg once; repeat dose in 2 weeks, p.o.	
Metronidazole	20 mg/kg s.i.d., b.i.d. p.o., for 5–10 days	For protozoan intestinal infections
Fenbendazole (Panacur)	50 mg/kg s.i.d. p.o., for 3 days	More effective than metronidazole
Sulfadimethoxine	50 mg/kg p.o., then 25 mg/kg once daily for 5 days	For coccidiosis
Heartworm prevention		
Ivermectin for microfilaria and 3–4 weeks post adulticide treatment	0.006 mg/kg every 30 days p.o.	Use minimal dose. *Note* 0.3 mL ivermectin in 10 oz (28 mL) propylene glycol makes 100 μg per mL. Give 0.1 mL/lb *or* 0.2 mL/kg monthly
Selamectin (Revolution)	6 mg/kg topically monthly	Drug appears non-toxic like ivermectin to ferrets
Ivermectin products	Heartgard 30: 68 μg ivermectin Heartgard 30 FX: 55 μg ivermectin	Chewable tablets most useful for ferrets. Monthly
Heartworm treatment Thiacetarsamide (D. Kemmerer-Cottrell advises use of this drug)	2.2 mg/kg b.i.d. i.v. for 2 days	Immiticide not used on ferrets as it kills adult worms too quickly and they cause thrombosis

Appendix

Table A.6 Drugs for external and internal ferret parasites – *cont'd.*

Drug	Dose and administration	Comments
Antifungal drugs		
Griseofulvin	25 mg/kg once daily p.o.	Requires dissolving as human tablets. Used as per cat
Lime sulphur dip	Use weekly	In combination with griseofulvin
Ketoconazole	10–50 mg/kg s.i.d., b.i.d. p.o. or 10–30 mg/kg t.i.d. p.o.	Quarter of 200 mg tablet in suspension
Itraconazole		Quarter capsule daily for ferret. (cryptococcosis: see Ch. 12).
Itraconazole (transdermal gel)	5 mg/kg on the ear s.i.d. until 4 weeks after negative fungal growth	Made up with 100 mg/cc concentration
Fluconazole	100 mg capsule per 4 kg cat daily 50 mg/kg p.o. b.i.d., for 2–6 months for cats for CNS infections. Adjust to ferret weight	Long-term treatment. CNS infections in ferrets need early diagnosis and long treatment
Amphotericin B	Possibly 0.4–0.8 mg/kg i.v. given weekly	High toxicity of drug and only given i.v., so not practicable for treatment of fungal diseases in ferrets

which allows legal marketing of an unapproved drug that a qualified expert panel determines to be safe and effective and 'designation', basically a designated drug, at the time of approval or conditional approval, will be given a granted 7 years of marketing exclusivity. A present range of antibiotics for use with ferrets is given in Table A.5.

Note that with all drugs likely to be toxic in ferrets, it is advisable to make sure the animal is hydrated during treatment.

Some selected drugs used for external and internal parasites of ferrets are given in Table A.6.

Note: There is an ongoing problem of resistance to drugs and Reynoldson[5] stated in February 1999 that there were no new drugs in the pipeline to replace the presently available antiparasitic drugs. A few antiflea drugs have surfaced but not registered for ferrets though some might try them out (Ch. 10). Useful drugs for general medication for ferrets are shown in Table A.7.

The types of tranquillizers, anaesthetics and analgesics are shown in Table A.8.

My differential diagnosis ideas are seen in Table A.9.

General treatments for ferret wounds, Table A.10.

An example of the percentage constituents in ferret, cat, dog and cow milk is shown in Table A.11.

The types of milk supplements are shown in Table A.12.

The ferret owner should be able to make up a rehydration salts formula for use in dehydration in cases of ferret *heat stress* as in Table A.13.

The insulinoma elixir suggested by Mary Van Dahm in Chapter 14, is shown on page 499.

Pet food additives

The following is a list of additives to the general processed pet food, by Mary Van Dahm *Pet Food Exposed?* USA FAIR Report January/February 2001, with permission: Anticaking agents, antimicrobial agents, antioxidants, colouring agents, curing agents, drying agents, emulsifiers, firming agents, flavour enhancers, flavoring agents, flour treating agents, formulation aids, humectants, leavening agents, lubricants, non-nutritive sweeteners, nutritive sweeteners, oxidizing and reducing agents, pH and control agents, processing aids, sequestrants, solvents/vehicles, stabilizers/thickeners, surface-active agents, surface finishing agents, synergists, texturizers.

Feeding kittens by hand

The following are recipes for feeding kittens by hand (USA) as done by Amy Flemming of Flemming Farms, Hartun, Brighton, MI, USA.

A. Ferret formula

(from *Zoologic – Ferret-specific*)
Mix together:

Zoologic Milk Matrix $^{30}/_{55}$ at 63% (11.4 volume) and Zoologic Milk Matrix $^{25}/_{13}$ at 37% (4.9 volume).

Table A.7 General ferret drugs

Drug	Dose and administration	Comments
Cardiac drugs		
Furosemide	1–4 mg/kg b.i.d., t.i.d. p.o., s.c., i.m.	First drug of choice for heart disease, also as diuretic. Can use higher dose to treat and then reduce after 24–48 h
Digoxin elixir	0.005–0.01 mg/kg s.i.d., b.i.d., p.o., for maintenance	Requires monitoring
Enalapril	0.25–0.5 mg/kg p.o. daily. Start q. 48 h dosing for 2 weeks to allow ferret to adapt to drug	Vasodilator for congestive (dilated) cardiomyopathy, requires monitoring, i.e. avoid anorexia and lethargy of high dosage
Lanoxin tablets	Use 1/8th of 0.125 mg tablet given once every other day	Needs to be in solution
Propranolol (Inderal)	0.2–1.0 mg/kg p.o. b.i.d., t.i.d.	For hypertrophic cardiomyopathy
Atenolol with either DCM or HCM, providing the contractility of heart is not too weak	6.25 mg/ferret s.i.d. p.o. 1.0 mg/kg s.i.d. p.o. (lower dose)	Beta blocker. Reduces frequent ventricular premature contractions (VPCs). Caution with severe congestive heart failure
Theophylline	5–10 mg/kg p.o., b.i.d.	Heart rate artificially increased
Metaproterenol	0.5–1.0 mg/kg b.i.d.	Ditto above. Can be used as gel
Nitrol ointment	Use 1–6 mm of ointment on shaved skin s.i.d. *or* b.i.d.	
Antihistamines		
Chlorpheniramine tabs	1–2 mg/kg b.i.d., t.i.d. p.o.	For sneezing and coughing. Only injectable available in Australia (tablet form only combined with prednisolone)
Diphenhydramine	0.5–2 mg/kg q. 8–12 h i.v. *or* i.m.	Used for vaccination reactions in USA
Shock therapy		
Dexamethasone sodium phosphate	4–8 mg/kg i.m., i.v.	
Dexamethasone	0.5 mg/kg. p.o., s.c., i.m., i.v.	
Anti-toxicity		
Atropine sulfate	5–10 mg/kg s.c., i.m.	For organophosphate poisoning
Activated charcoal	Mixed with water p.o.	Toxic substance binding
Bronchodilator		
Aminophylline	4 mg/kg b.i.d., p.o., i.m., i.v.	
Theophylline elixir	4.25 mg/kg b.i.d., t.i.d. p.o.	Useful smooth muscle relaxant for lung and heart stimulation
General GI disease/chronic IBD		
Ensal: phthalylsulfathiazole/kaolin base	Cat dose 2.5–5.0 mL q.i.d. Use up to 1 mL q.i.d. according to ferret size	Safe drugs for ferrets. Soothes the bowel mucosa
Peptosyl: bismuth salicylate 17 mg/mL bentonite	0.25–0.5 mL/kg	Not antibiotic
Bismuth subsalicylate	0.5 cc p.o., b.i.d.	As above
Sucralfate (Carafate) suspension	25 mg/kg up to 125 mg/ferret t.i.d., q.i.d., p.o. (4–7 days)	Use for GI ulcers on empty stomach. Can use with acid blockers
Loperamide (Imodium)	0.2 mg/kg p.o., b.i.d.	For diarrhoea
Cisapride	0.5 mg/kg p.o., b.i.d.	For oesophagitis
Acid blockers		
Ranitidine (Zantac)	3.5 mg/kg p.o., b.i.d.	Lasts 12 hours
Famotidine (Pepcid)	0.25–0.5 mg/kg p.o., s.i.d.	Lasts 24 hours
Omeprazole (Prilosec)	0.7 mg/kg p.o., s.i.d.	Ditto
Misoprostol (Cytotec)	1–5 mg/kg p.o., t.i.d.	Helps heal gastric ulcers.
Metoclopramide (Reglan)	0.5–1.0 mg/kg p.o., b.i.d.	Encourages gastric emptying
Cobalamin (Vitamin B_{12})	20–50 mg weekly	Helps gut healing
Azathioprine (Imuran)	0.9 mg/kg p.o., q. 48 h	Anti-inflammatory superior to corticosteroids

Table A.7 General ferret drugs – cont'd.

Drug	Dose and administration	Comments
Useful corticosteroids		
Prednisolone: glucocorticoid	0.10–2.5 mg/kg s.i.d., b.i.d. p.o.	Wide spectrum of uses for insulinoma, eosinophilic
Prednisone: synthetic glucocorticoid	Anti-inflammatory and anti-allergic agents	gastroenteritis, etc.
Apnoea emergency		
Doxapram hydrochloride 20 mg/mL	I have used 0.10 mL/kg i.v. (0.28–0.55 mL/kg for dogs/cats)	Should be operating room standard
Jill heat suppression		
Proligestone 100 mg/mL (Covinan, Intervet) (long-acting progestogen)	Give 50 mg s.c., if no response, give 25 mg at 7 days. Repeat at further 7 days (should not be necessary)	Use all heat suppression drugs on the jill 10 days in heat. Consider blood profile re anaemia if jill in oestrous 21 days
Human chorionic gonadotropin (Chorulon, Intervet) 1500 IU	100 IU per ferret i.m.	Repeat in 14 days
Buserelin acetate (Receptal, Hoechst)	0.25 mL i.m.	As above
Whelping aid		
Oxytocin	0.2–10 USP units/kg s.c., i.m.	For assisting kitten delivery and stimulating lactation
Blood sugar stabilization		For diabetes mellitus
Insulin NPH	0.5–6.0 IU/kg s.i.d., b.i.d. *or* to effect	Also for glucagonoma or post-surgical diabetes after insulinoma removal
Prednisolone	2.5 mg per day decreasing	Insulinoma cases
Diazoxide	10–20 mg/kg s.i.d. p.o.	Insulinoma cases. Use with prednisolone
CNS disturbances		Used for controlling fits.
Phenobarbital elixir	1–2 mg/kg b.i.d., s.i.d. p.o.	Dose will require adjustment for maintenance
Chemotherapy drugs (combinations vary with protocols, Ch. 13)		
Vincristine	0.07–0.12 mg/kg	i.v.
Cyclophosphamide	10 mg/kg	p.o.
Prednisone	1–2 mg/kg	p.o. b.i.d.
Asparaginase	0 2 mg/kg	i.p. but once only
Methotrexate	0.5 mg/kg	given s.q.

The dry powder may be blended together and stored in a closed container following label directions. This allows the blended milk replacer to be reconstituted more quickly when needed.

Mix 23.5 g of mixed powder with 76.5 g water

or

Mix 1 volume of powder to 1.5 volumes of water, to make a milk containing 23.5% solids.

B. Weasel/mink formula

(from *Rehabilitation of North American Wild Mammals: Feeding and Nutrition* by Debbie Marcum)
Full-strength formula – mix together:

1 part Esbilac or Zoologic Milk Matrix $^{33}/_{40}$ (powder)
1 part KMR or Zoologic Milk Matrix $^{42}/_{25}$ (powder)
3 parts water.

Start with $^3/_4$ water to $^1/_4$ of this formula, move to $^1/_2$ and $^1/_2$, then to $^1/_4$ water to $^3/_4$ formula, then full-strength formula. Full-strength formula should not be started any earlier than 24 hours after the first feeding. An oral electrolyte solution can be substituted for water if dehydration is a concern.

C. Striped skunk formula

(from *Rehabilitation of North American Wild Mammals: Feeding and Nutrition* by Debbie Marcum)

Table A.8 Tranquillizer, anaesthetic and analgesic drugs for ferrets

Drug	Dose and administration	Comments
Acepromazine	0.1–0.3 mg/kg i.m. *or* s.c.	Promex 2 Australia
Alfaxalone	8–12 mg/kg i.v.	Alfaxan CD Jurox
Ketamine	20–30 mg/kg i.m.	Very safe drug. Longer recovery
Xylazine	1–2 mg/kg i.m.	Safe used at low dose
Ketamine + xylazine	20–30 mg/kg + 1–2 mg/kg i.m.	Take xylazine into syringe first
Ketamine + acepromazine	20–30 mg/kg + 0.25 mg/kg	Use for intubating ferret
Halothane	Induction 3.0–3.5% Maintenance 0.5–2.5%	Oxygen rate of 500 mL/kg per min
Isoflurane	Induction 2.5–5% Maintenance 0.5–3%	As above *Note* Table 16.8 (Ch. 16)
Atropine used especially with isoflurane	0.04 mg/kg i.m., s.c., *or* i.v.	Anticholinergic; gives prolonged dilated pupils
Sevoflurane	Use to effect	
Diazepam	1–2 mg/kg i.m.	Usually combined with ketamine
Midazolam	0.25–0.5 mg/kg s.c. *or* i.m.	Usually combined with ketamine
Ketamine + diazepam	25–35 mg/kg + 2–3 mg/kg i.m.	For minor procedures
Ketamine + midazolam	5–10 mg/kg + 5 mg/kg i.m.	Premed before gas anaesthesia
Medetomidine (Domitor)	0.050 mL/1250 g ferret i.m.	See Clinical use Ch. 16
Atipamezole (Antisedan) reverses medetomidine	0.05–0.1 mL s.c. *or* i.m.	Works with no adverse effects
Ketamine + medetomide	10 mg/kg + 120 µg/kg i.m.	See Table 16.10
Ketamine + medetomide + Butorphanol	5 mg/kg + 80 µg + 100 µg i.m. *or* s.c..	Hypoxia can occur if the 100 µg butorphanol exceeded
Tiletamine + zolazepam	22 mg/kg *or* 25 mg/kg i.m.	Zoletil 20 now discontinued. Telazole USA
Butorphanol	0.05–0.5 mg/kg q. 4 h s.c. *or* i.m.	
Buprenorphine	0.01–0.03 mg/kg q. 8–12 h s.c., i.m.	
Pentazocine	5–10 mg/kg q. 4 h s.c., i.m.	
Oxymorphine	0.05–0.2 mg/kg q. 6–12 h s.c., i.m	
Meperidine (pethidine)	5–10 mg/kg q 2–3 h s.c., i.m.	
Morphine	0.5–2.0 mg/kg q 12–24 h	The basic analgesic
Nalbuphine	0.5–1.5 mg/kg i.m., i.v. every 2–3 h	Potent synthetic (UK)
Naloxone structurally related to oxymorphine	40 µg/kg s.c., i.m., i.v.	Reverses the effects of administered narcotics
Flunixin	0.5–2.0 mg/kg q. 12–24 h i.m.	Must be given i.m.
Glycopyrrolate	0.1 mg/kg i.m.	Anticholinergic
Pentobarbitone	25–30 mg/kg i.m., s.c., i.v.	Mostly used for euthanasia

Appendix

Table A.9 Differential diagnosis for ferret problems

Clinical signs	Differential diagnosis
Not eating/reluctance to chew	Oral gingivitis disease Bleeding gums Teeth root abscess (dental odour) Broken teeth (sign of 'chattering')
Respiratory distress: Sneezing, cough, snuffles hyperventilation suggesting…	House dust allergy Urine vapour irritation (scat trays) 'Snuffles', bacterial rhinitis 'Kennel cough' Human viral influenza Canine distemper Bacterial pneumonia Cryptococcosis Anterior thorax neoplasia Heartworm disease Cardiomyopathy Thoracic neoplasia
Vomiting/regurgitation	Gastroenteritis Oesophageal obstruction Bowel obstruction Megaoesophagus (kitten) Insulinoma Metabolic disturbance
Diarrhoea	Dietary Gastroenteritis GI foreign body Epizootic catarrhal enteritis *Helicobacter mustelae* gastritis Proliferative bowel disease Eosinophilic gastroenteritis Intestinal parasites
Hypersalivation	Grass seed in tongue Frog skin excretions Gum sores (poisons) Dental injury Gastroenteritis GI foreign body Hypoglycaemia (insulinoma)
Lymphadenopathy: generalized or localized	Neoplasia Cryptococcosis Disseminated idiopathic myositis
Abdominal enlargement	Splenomegaly Polycystic kidneys GI foreign body Neoplasia Ascites Renal cyst
Chronic wasting	Aleutian disease Megaoesophagus Dental disease Chronic bowel foreign body (plastic) Internal parasites Proliferative bowel disease

Table A.9 Differential diagnosis for ferret problems – cont'd.

Clinical signs	Differential diagnosis
	Gastroenteritis Mycotic disease Neoplasia
Alopecia	Hyperoestrogenism (post-oestrous anaemia) Seasonal coat change (especially tail) Ferret adrenal gland complex (FADC) External parasites Dermatomycosis Mast cell tumour
Swollen vulva	Normal oestrous Post-oestrous anaemia (POA) Ferret adrenal gland complex (FADC) Ovarian remnant Vaginitis
Pruritus	External parasites (fleas/ear mites) Ferret adrenal gland complex (FADC) Mast cell tumour
Neurological signs	Rabies virus Canine distemper virus Meningitis (cryptococcosis) Insulinoma Toxin Trauma Proliferative bowel disease Neoplasia Pseudohypoparathyroidism
Paraparesis	Trauma Ventral disc trauma/disease Insulinoma Hypocalcaemia Poisoning Myelitis Thromboembolism Aleutian disease Primary and secondary neoplasia
Weakness	Aleutian disease Post-oestrous anaemia Anaemia from injury Anaemia from parasites, e.g. fleas Cardiomyopathy Insulinoma Lymphosarcoma Metabolic disease
Heart murmurs	Heart enlargement Other cardiomyopathy Heartworm disease

Appendix

Table A.10 General treatments for ferret wounds

Chemical	Action	Comments
Lavage: Chlorhexidine diacetate	Good antimicrobial action, not systemically absorbed easily. Works in presence of exudates	0.05% dilution kills bacteria and lasts for 2 days
Lavage: Povidone-iodine	Good against bacteria, viruses, fungi and yeasts. Exudates impair its action. Scrubbing wound not recommended	*Note* iodine absorption can initiate a transient thyroid dysfunction
Lavage: Tris EDTA addition	Increases bacterial susceptibility to antibiotics and antiseptics	Good against Gram –ves, – with chlorhexidine increases efficiency by 100%
Aloe vera: source of gel, useful agent for sores and burns	Has antiprostaglandin and antithromboxane effects	Acemannan in aloe vera promotes wound healing, allantoin stimulates epithelial growth

After Pilny AA, Hess L. Ferrets: wound healing and therapy. Vet Clin Exotic Anim 2004; 7.

Table A.11 Comparison of constituents of ferret, cat, dog and cow milk

	Ferret	Cat	Dog	Cow
Protein	6.0%	7.0%	7.5%	3.3%
Fat	8.0%	4.8%	10.0%	4.0%
Lactose	3.8%	4.8%	3.8%	5.0%

Table A.12 Milk supplements

Constituent	Esbilac	Ensure Plus[a]	Feedmilk	Animalac	Biolac	Di-Vetelact
Crude protein, min.	4.5%	9 g	25%	29.7%	6%	24%
Crude fat, min.	6%	6 g	25%	10%	7%	29%
Crude fibre, max.	0%	0 g	0%			
Moisture, max.	85%					2%
Ash, max.	1%					6%
Salt, max.			1.7%			
Ash + V + M					3%	
Carbohydrates		40 g			4%	
Lactose			29%			<2%
Galactose						16%
Lactose + dextrose				49.2%		

Ash + V + M, Ash + vitamins + minerals; min., minimum; max. maximum. [a]Ensure Plus is a human supplement recommended for prevention of pregnancy toxaemia in ferrets. Label data given relates to 237 mL of prepared mixture (J.A. Bell, pers. comm. 1998).

Table A.13 Formula for rehydration salts

Constituent	Quantity	Kitchen measures
Clean water	1.0 L	1 pint
Glucose	20 g	1 tablespoon
Sodium chloride (table salt)	3.5 g	½ teaspoon
Sodium bicarbonate (baking soda)	2.5 g	½ teaspoon
Potassium chloride (Lite salt)	1.5 g	¼ teaspoon

Full-strength formula – mix together:

1 part Esbilac or Zoologic Milk Matrix $^{33}/_{40}$ (powder)
1 part Multi-Milk or Zoologic Milk Matrix $^{30}/_{55}$ (powder)
2 parts water.

Proceed as for Formula B.

Weaning formula for kittens

Formula 1

Milk formula, either **A**, **B** or **C**
Hill's Prescription Diet a/d canned food.

Mix together and serve to kittens warm, by syringe, from finger or from low bowl. Consistency should be of a thick gravy. Discard unused mixture. Opened AD canned food can be stored as per label. Unused milk formula should be discarded.

Formula 2

Milk formula either **A**, **B** or **C**
AD canned food
Chicken or turkey baby food.

Mix and serve as for Formula 1.

Formula 3

Completely softened kibble soaked in milk formula either **A**, **B** or **C**
AD canned food and/or chicken or turkey baby food.

Mix and serve as for Formula 1.

Insulinoma Elixir recipe

2 cups	High protein (derived from meat, not plant protein) dry kitten or ferret food
2 cups	Water
1–2 jars	Meat baby food (all meat – no vegetables) adds to flavour and improves texture
1 tsp.	Shark cartilage powder
100 mg	Echinacea powder (¼ of a 400 mg capsule)
17 mg	Sylimaryn milk thistle powder (¼ of a 70 mg capsule)
½ tsp.	Brewer's yeast (a natural source of chromium)
1 tsp.	Ensure (powdered) *or* 1 mL Karo syrup
1 tsp.	Lecithin granules or soy concentrate power (helps to keep mixture bound)
3200 IU	Vitamin E (d-α-tocopherol) *Note*: dry vitamin E powder mixes best
7500 IU	Vitamin A (not required if fatty acid supplement has high vitamin A content)
2 oz	Fatty acid supplement, from blend of soybean, cod liver oil, and wheat germ oil
4 tablesp.	Butter (optional, for flavour and extra calories for underweight ferrets)
3–4 cups	Extra water

Note: commercial brands of fatty acid supplement are Ferretone and Linotone.

Instructions: Mix ferret food with 2 cups water and let stand until soft (3–4 hours or overnight in fridge). Mix in blender until smooth. Add shark cartilage, milk thistle, echinacea, brewer's yeast and Ensure. Let the mixture sit for 20–30 min to allow yeast to 'wake up' and eat some of the sugars in the Ensure. Blend in the lecithin, vitamin E and oils. Melt butter and add to mixture. Add more water to bring volume to half a gallon.

This makes 32 servings (2 oz each). Serve 1 serving per ferret as a preventative measure or 2–3 times a day as needed for active insulinoma control. More or less water may be added to make the consistency more palatable for the ferret. The portions are adjusted to ferret size accordingly. Many ferrets like the mixture served slightly warm.

From Mary van Dahm, 2005, with permission.

Appendix

Table A.14 Coat, eye and nose features

Colour	Coat (guard hairs)	Eyes	Nose
Albino	White	Red	Pink
Black	Black	Black	Black
Black sable	Black/brown	Black or Brown	Black/brown
Champagne	Light tan or diluted chocolate	Brown or burgundy	Pink, may have tan outline
Chocolate	Warm milk chocolate brown	Brown	Pink, may have brown outline
Dark eyed white	White	Black or burgundy	Pink
Sable	Medium warm brown	Brown	Brown or pink with freckles

From American Ferret Association, 2005, with permission.

Table A.15 Coat pattern description and mask type

Pattern	Description	Mask
Point	Distinct difference in colour concentration between the body colour and the colour points (legs and tail)	Thin V-shaped mask
Standard	Moderate colour contrasts between points (legs and tail) and the body	Full mask
Solid	No colour contrasts between points (legs and tail) and the body. Solid colour from mask to tip of tail	T-bar mask
Blaze	Wide white stripes from forehead to shoulder, white mitts or toe tips, white knee patches, may be speckled	Colour rings around eyes or colour smudges below eyes
Panda	Full white head, including neck and throat, speckled belly, white knee patches, mitts and toe tips	May have colour rings around eyes
Roan	50% colour guard hairs (any colour) and 50% white guard hairs create the salt and pepper look.	Colour smudges below eyes

From American Ferret Association, 2005, with permission.

External features of American pet ferrets

As mentioned in Chapter 2, the external features of American pet ferrets are shown here, in Tables A.14, A.15 (Courtesy of the American Ferret Association).

Ferret family tree

As mentioned in Chapter 5, a family tree for Teddy has been drawn up by Christina Bernard (Fig. A.1).

Ferret family tree

Teddy, whose picture appears on page 8, is a brown ferret with white mitts, obtained by Christina and Klaus Bernhard from Val Hutcheon. The family tree, which gives the phenotypes is as follows:-

Figure A.1 Family tree for ferret 'Teddy'.

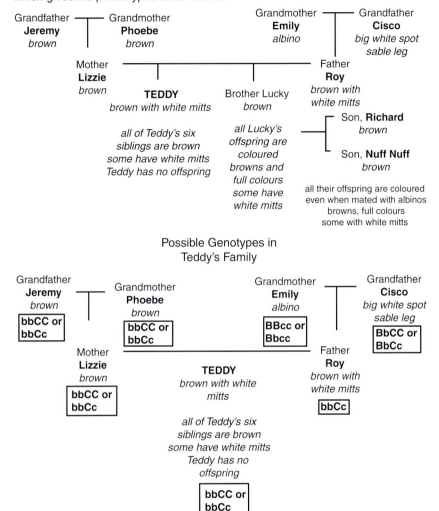

Grandfather Cisco is an interesting case. He is not a white ferret with a sable leg, but rather a sable (full colour) ferret with a very big white spot. Were it not for the coloured leg he would be a dark-eyed white (DEW)

References

1. Moody KD, Bowman TA, Lang CM. Laboratory management of the ferret for biomedical research. Lab Anim Sci 1985; 35:272–279.
2. Smith DA, Burgmann PM. Formulary. In: Hillyer EV, Quesenberry KE, eds. Ferrets, rabbits and rodents: Clinical medicine and surgery. Philadelphia: WB Saunders; 1997:392–395.
3. Collins BR. Antimicrobial drugs in use in rabbits, rodents and other small mammals. Antimicrobial Therapy North American Veterinary Conference. Orlando: Bayer; 1995.
4. Lewington JH. Review of antibiotics in use with ferrets. Control and therapy. University of Sydney: Postgraduate Foundation 1996; 193:901–902.
5. Reynoldson J. Prophylactics and therapeutics. Pets, people and parasites. Contin Vet Edu Perth: Murdoch University 1999; 1/99:63–75.

Index

A

abdominal organs 25, 27–8, 29, 30–2
    palpation 155, 156
abscesses
    dental 196
    grass seed 197
    Staphylococcus infections 196
Absidia corymbifera (syn. *ramosa*) 197, 291
accommodation 34–56
    bedding 45
    cages
        breeding 35–6
        laboratory 52
        Lewington ferret cage 44, 45–6
        standard 44–5
    dangers
        indoor 48, 49, 50, 55–6
        outdoor 36, 53–5
    and foot mange 254
    hospital 160
    indoors
        breeding cages 35–6
        darkness 49, 50, 374
        house ferrets 48–51
        hutches 42
    laboratory ferrets 51
    outdoors 35–48
        boltholes 38–9, 41
        cooling 45, 46
        ferret courts 47–8
        ferret garden ground plan 37
        ferret-proofing the garden 36–40
        ferretaria 39
            ferretarium 1 40–2
            ferretarium 2 42–4
        hutches 43
        Lewington ferret cage 44, 45–6
        sheds 46–7
        standard cages 44–5
    in pregnancy 45, 46, 91
    size recommendations 45–6
    Swiss regulations 7–8
    veterinary hospital 52
    whelping cage 91
acepromazine 398, 399, 495

acetaminophen toxicosis 385–6, 388
achondroplastic dwarfism 119
ACTH challenge 349
activated charcoal 493
acute renal failure (ARF) 266–8, 269
    blood investigation 267
    treatment 268
additives/preservatives 81, 82–3, 492
adenocarcinomas 319, 328
    duodenal 415
    gastric 336
adenomas 328, 329, 330
    anal 333
adrenal gland disease 7, 8, 273
    see also ferret adrenal disease complex (FADC)
adrenal glands 28, 30, 350–1, 433
    enlarged 164
    neoplastic *vs* normal 353
    neuroendocrine pathway 347
    partial resection 435
    removal 350–2, 353, 433–5
        cryosurgery 454, 455–7
adrenal tumours 28, 32, 329, 330, 331, 336
    adrenal gland carcinoma 352, 361
    adrenocortical adenomas 351
    removal 434
    teratoma 329–30
    ultrasonography 424, 425–6
adrenalectomy *see* adrenal glands, removal
Advantage (imidacloprid) 249, 251–2, 491
Aelurostrongylus abstrusus 238, 239
agalactia 95
age determination 471, 474
aggression 35
agouti 110
Agway Marshal Ferret Diet 57
albino ferrets 6, 15, 132
    crosses 112–13
    genetics 108–9
Aleutian disease 12, 180–5, 216
    diagnosis 181, 182
    and myocarditis 283
    signs 182
    testing 183–4
    treatment 182–3
alfaxalone 495

Index

allergy to ferrets 159
alphaxalone 410
American ferrets 12–13
    coat colours 16–17
    neoplasia 318–35
    nutrition 57–66, 69
        commercial foods 59–60, 62–6
amikacin 199, 490
aminoglutethimide 357
aminophylline 493
amitraz 254, 255, 491
amoxicillin 490
    bacterial diseases 186, 190, 199, 262
        gastrointestinal 206, 208, 209, 215, 216
        hepatic 220
    cryptococcosis 309
    ear infections 294
    heartworm 245
    parasitic diseases 227
    renal disease 271, 274
amphotericin B 198, 310, 492
ampicillin 189, 190, 271, 490
amprolium 229–30
anaesthesia 393–411
    for bronchoalveolar lavage 192
    cardiac arrest 405
    cardiac irregularities 404–5
    Cathy Johnson-Delaney (C J-D) protocol 403–4
        operative procedure 404–5
    drugs used 495
    early protocols 395–6
    and hypothermia 394
    induction times 395
    intubation 400, 402
    pre-anaesthetic check 394–5
    premedication drugs 398
    preparation 394
    recovery scoring 409–10
    recovery times 393–4
    reversible 394
    and stress 393
anal adenomas 333
anal glands *see* musk glands
anal sacculectomy (descenting) 18, 431–2
anal sphincters 25
analgesia 443
    drugs used 495
    epidural 453–4
    level 452–3
    in orthopaedics 452–4
    prophylactic 453
anastrozole 357
anatomy 18–32
    brain 21–2
    ear 290–1
    eye 295–6
    skeleton 18–19
    skull 19–21
Ancyclostoma spp. 237–8
Angiostrongylus cantonensis 238
Angora ferrets 119
Animalac 63, 106, 498
anorexia 204, 269
anti-prostaglandin 263–4
anti-toxicity 493
antibiotics 490
anticoagulant poisoning 384, 458–9
antihistamines 493
Antinoff Treatment Protocol 244
Antisedan (atipamezole hydrochloride) 404, 405, 406, 495
Apex ear drops 294
apocrine tumours 328, 332–4
Archetype Diet 69
artificial respiration 380
asparaginase 323, 324, 326, 494
atenolol 282, 493
atipamezole hydrochloride (Antisedan) *see* Antisedan (atipamezole hydrochloride)
atropine 398, 402, 403, 493, 495
auditory system 130, 131, 289–91
    diseases 291–5
    disorders affecting otic nerves/brain stem 293
    ear anatomy 290–1
Australian Bat Lyssavirus 173
Australian ferrets 8–9
    brain size 21–2
    coat colours 16, 17
    neoplasia 336–8
    nutrition 66–70
        commercial foods 69–70
        natural feeding 66–9, 70
        non-commercial food 66–9
    temperature/outdoor life 34–5, 37
aviary, converted 38
azathioprine 212, 213, 215, 493
azotaemia 267

B

bacterial diseases 185–97
    anaerobic 195–7, 216
    bacterial overgrowth/enteritis 215–16
    Bacteroides infections 196
    Bordetella bronchiseptica 179–80, 185–6, 189
    botulism 189–90
    colibacillosis 195

enterotoxaemia 216
Fusiformis infections 195
hepatitis 165
leptospirosis 190–1
listeriosis 194
Mycobacteria spp.
    diagnosis 193–4
    non-tuberculous 191–4
    treatment 192–3
    tuberculosis 191
Mycoplasma 189
pneumonia 188–9
Pseudomonas aeruginosa 188
salmonellosis 194–5
snuffles 154
'snuffles' 154, 186–8
Staphylococcus infections 196–7
Streptococcus infections 196
susceptibility of carnivores 171
vaginitis 262
Bacteroides infections 196
basal cell tumours 332, 334
bedding 45
behaviour
    and domestication 132–3
    group behaviour 35
    and mating 88–90
    problems 119
Belgian ferrets 7
    Aleutian disease 184
    feeding 79
benzene hydrochloride 254
betamethasone 291, 299
bicalutamide 357
biliary carcinoma 221
biliary cysts/cystadenomas 220, 221
biopsies
    bowel 210, 212
    lymph node 211, 212
biotin deficiency 72
bismuth salicylate 208
biting/nipping 151
black-eyed whites (BEW) 115–16
    galactose-induced cataracts 303, 304
black-footed ferret (*Mustela nigripes*) 6, 57, 124
    binocular vision 296
    classification 4, 127, 128, 129
    toxoplasmosis in 225
bladder 30, 31
    stones 272, 273
        removal 438
    ultrasonography 422, 423
Blastomyces dermatidis infection 198–9

bleomycin 327
blood sampling 156–9, 382
blood/serum chemistry 487–8, 489
blood smear, pre-treatment 458
blood transfusions 460–1
boarding 226
body weight 61, 71, 72
    kittens 101–3
    obesity 78
boltholes 38–9, 41
bonding 151–2
bone(s)
    reactive 480, 482
    sizes of 443–4
    'soft bone' syndrome 106
    see also fractured bones
bone marrow transplant 158–9
bone tumours 339–43
Bordetella bronchiseptica 179–80, 185–6, 189
botulism 189–90
brain size 21–2, 130, 131
bread dough toxicosis 384
bromethalin poisoning 384–5
bronchoalveolar lavage 192
Brugia spp. 245
buprenorphine 443, 453, 495
buserelin acetate 494
butorphanol 403, 407–10, 443, 495
    as analgesic 453–4

C

C-cell carcinoma 327, 329
caesarean section 96–7
cages *see* accommodation
calcitrol 270
calcium oxalate 387
Campylobacter jejuni 96
Canadian ferrets, FADC in 362
cane toad poisoning 54
canine distemper 24, 53, 174–9
    treatment 175–6
    vaccination 176–9
    vs influenza 176
canine teeth 467
    deciduous 468, 469–70
    permanent (secondary) 471–2
Capillaria spp. 236, 237
Capstar (nitenpyram) 249
carbamates 250, 251
carbaryl 252, 491
carcinomas 328, 330
cardiac neural crest 117

Index

cardiovascular disease 275–84
    and anaesthesia 403
Carparsolate 241, 243
castration 30, 32, 430
    under ketamine 397
cataracts 301–6
    aetiology 302–3
    family relationships 304, 305
catheterization
    intraosseous 460
    intravenous 381, 402, 460
    naso-oesophageal 463–4
    oesophagostomy/gastrostomy tubes 464
    urinary 461–2
cats and ferrets 50
caudal artery blood sampling 158
cefadroxil 490
central nervous system diseases 284–7, 309
    neoplasia 343, 344
cephalexin 490
cephalic vein blood sampling 156–7
cephaloridine 490
Chastek paralysis 72
Chediak–Higashi syndrome 180
chemotherapy 321, 322
    administration protocols 325–7
    drugs used 494
    efficacy 337
    nutritional supplements 325
    protocols 323–7
children 151
chloramphenicol 490
    bacterial diseases 189
    ear infections 293
    eye infections 301
    parasite infections 196
    renal disease 271–2
Chloroint 301
chlorpheniramine 493
Chlorsig drops 301
chocolate 383
cholangiohepatitis 219
cholecalciferol poisoning 385
chondrosarcoma 335
chordoma 328, 334
    cervical 335
    removal 438
chorioptic mange 255
chromosomes 107
chronic interstitial nephritis (CIN) 268–9
chronic renal failure (CRF) 268–71
    protein restriction 269, 270–1
    treatment 269–71

cimetidine 385–6
ciprofloxin 490
cirrhosis 220
cisapride 205
clarithromycin 192, 208, 209, 490
classification 3–5, 124, 127, 128–9
    family tree 4
clavulanic acid 490
    bacterial diseases 186, 262
    cryptococcosis 309
    ear infections 294
    renal disease 271, 274
Clavulox palatable drops 301, 309
clindamycin 226, 490
clofazimine 192
Clostridium spp. 216
    C. botulinum 189–90
coat colours 16–18, 500
    breeding for 107–8
    and deafness 289
    and domestication 130
    family tree 501
    Italian ferrets 115
    patterns/masks 500
cobalamin 493
coccidioidomycosis 199
coccidiosis 214, 228–30
Coccidioides immitis infection 195, 198
congestive heart failure 277
conjunctivitis 298–300
    treatment 299–300
'Coolgardie meat safe technique' 45
corneal irritation 300
corneal ulcers 300–1
coronavirus
    coronavirus enteritis 214–15
    SARS coronavirus (SCV) 170–1
corticosteroids 212–13, 241, 494
    after adrenalectomy 352
cortisol values 365
cranial vena cava blood sampling 158
Crenosoma lungworms 238
cryosurgery 454–7
    procedure 454–7
    theory 454
cryptococcosis 22, 308–16
    diagnosis 308–9
    epidemiology 313–15
    infection methods 315
    infections/tissues affected 312
    pathology 309–10
    prevention 315–16

prognosis 316
treatment 310–12, 313
Cryptococcus spp. 284
   C. bacillisporus 198, 308, 311, 315
   C. gatti 308, 312, 313
   C. neoformans 154, 308, 313, 314
      var. *grubii* 312, 314
   viability 313–14
Cryptosporidium parvum 230–1
Ctenocephalides felix 248
Curl restraint device 158
cyclophosphamide 323, 324, 494
cystitis 274
cystotomy 273, 438
Cytosar/Cytoxan 326
Czech ferrets 8

D

dark-eyed whites (DEW) *see* black-eyed whites (BEW)
darkness, need for 49, 50
   see also photoperiodism
deafness 289–90
demodectic mange 255
demodex 491
dental care 483
dental disorders 63, 155, 196, 474–83
   abrasion 476–7
   abscesses 478, 479–80, 482
   avulsed teeth 476
   calculus 477–9, 480, 481
   chewing-associated 481, 483
   dental disease 474–5
   fractured teeth 475–6
   kibble-associated 478, 479, 480–3
   periodontal disease 477, 478
   pet *vs* feral ferrets 475
   plaque 478–9
   prevalence 474–5
   supernumerary teeth 474
   tooth abscesses 298
   wear 478, 479, 480–3
dentistry 21
   anaesthesia 396
dentition 20–1, 467–74
   adaptations 467, 477
   age determination 471, 474
   crowded 482
   deciduous 467–70
      canines 469–70
      eruption/exfoliation 468, 469
      formula 467

      incisors 469
      molars 470
      synonyms 467
   and diet 77, 78, 467
   and domestication 130, 131
   examination 154–5
   pathological conditions *see* dental disorders
   permanent (secondary) 467, 470–4
      canines 471–2
      eruption 468, 469
      formula 470
      incisors 470–1
      molars 472–4
      premolars 472
   sexual dimorphism 470
   supernumerary 474
deprenyl 357
dermatofibromas 328
deslorelin 355
dexamethasone 245, 370, 387, 493
dexamethasone suppression test 349
diabetes 375, 376–7
diabetic cataracts 303
diarrhoea 204
diazepam 395–6, 398, 495
diazoxide 367, 368, 370, 494
Dichelobacter nodosum see Fusiformis infections
dichlophoren 252
Diet 41 78–9
differential diagnoses 496–7
digestive system 25, 61
digoxin 281, 493
dihydrotachysterol 377
dilated cardiomyopathy 275, 276–81, 283–4
   clinical signs 276–7
   diagnosis 277–80
   heart 276
   treatment 280–1
diltiazem 282
diphenhydramine 403, 493
Diphyllobothrium latum 247
Dipylidium caninum 246–7
Dirofilaria immitis see heartworm
diseases *see* infections
dislocation of elbow 448
disseminated idiopathic myositis (DIM)
   diagnosis 284–5, 286–7
   treatment 286, 287
distribution of domesticated ferrets 6–14
diuresis 382
Dizzy Kitty box 50
dogs and ferrets 50, 56

Index

dolls' houses, converted 38–9
domestication 116–17, 122–50
   archeological record
      geographical issues 122–3
      identification problems 123–4
      lack of evidence 124
      preservation problems 122
   'African domestication' hypothesis 123
   behavioural changes 88–90, 132–3
      fearfulness 133
      gregariousness 133
   cats *vs* ferrets 140
   history 126–9, 133–8
   introgression (hybridization) 124–5, 126
   karyotype studies 125
   mechanism of change 138–40
   morphological changes
      body size 130, 132
      cranial shape 130, 131
      dentition 130, 131
   phylogenetics 124, 125–6
   physiological changes
      coat colour 130
      cranial capacity 130, 131
      hearing 130, 131
      reproduction 129–30
      vision 130–1
Domitor (medetomidine hydrochloride) 404, 405, 406, 407–10, 495
   as analgesic 443, 452, 453–4
doramectin 253–4
doxapram 494
doxorubicin 323, 324, 367
doxycycline 186, 187, 192, 311, 490
   contraindication 195
Dracunculus spp. 245–6
drug formulary 488–92
   anaesthetics/analgesics/tranquilizers 495
   anti-toxicity 493
   antibiotics 490
   antifungals 492
   antihistamines 493
   antiparasitics 491
   bronchodilators 493
   cardiac drugs 493
   chemotherapy 494
   corticosteroids 494
   gastrointestinal disorders 493
   general 493–4
   heat suppression 494
   shock therapy 493
drug resistance 492

drug toxicity 242, 251–2, 309
   chemotherapy 325, 327
   ototoxicity 293, 294–5
dystocia 96

E

ears
   anatomy 290–1
   examination 154
ear diseases 291–5
ear mange 252–3
ear mites 197–8, 291, 292, 293, 294
Echidnophaga gallinacea 154
echocardiography 426–8
   dilated/hypertrophic cardiomyopathy 279
   patient positioning 418–19
   reference values 426
   valvular heart disease 282
Eimeria spp. 228, 229
electrocardiography (ECG)
   before/during anaesthesia 395
   dilated cardiomyopathy 278–9
   normal 278, 279
emergency techniques 458–64
   blood transfusions 460–1
   catheterization
      intraosseous 460
      intravenous 460
      urinary 461–2
   initial approach 458–60
      baseline laboratory tests 458
      fluid administration 460
      oxygen supplementation 459
      tissue oxygen delivery 459
   nutrition 462–4
      gruel diets 462–3
      naso-oesophageal tube 463–4
      water/electrolytes 462
endocrine diseases 346–79
   aetiology 371–7
      diabetes 376–7
      diet 375–6
      genetics 371–2
      photoperiodism manipulation 373–5
      pseudohypoparathyroidism 377
      sterilization, early 348, 372–3
      viral infection 376
endocrine glands 23–4
enalapril 280–1, 282, 283, 493
enrofloxacin 490
   bacterial diseases 186, 206, 215, 216, 220

heartworm 245
  parasitic diseases 227
Ensal 493
enterotomy 432–3
enterotoxaemia 216
entropion 307
eosinophilia 204
eosinophilic gastroenteritis/granulomatous disease 215
epithelioma 328
epizootic catarrhal enteritis (ECE) 214–15
Escherichia coli 195, 299
ethoxyquin 83–4
European polecat (*Mustela putorius*) 3, 4, 5, 6, 124
  binocular vision 296
  classification 128, 129
  external features 15
  hybridization 125
external features 15–18, 500
eyes
  anatomy 295–6
  colour 500
    and deafness 289
  examination 154
  eyesight *see* vision
eye conditions/infections 100–1, 298–307

F

FADC *see* ferret adrenal disease complex (FADC)
family tree 4
famotidine 205, 206, 208, 403, 493
Fasciola hepatica 245
Fascioloides magna 245
Felex Paste 235, 491
fenbendazole 236, 239, 491
fentanyl 405
feral ferrets
  dental disorders 475, 478, 479
  nutrition 74
ferret adrenal disease complex (FADC) 48–9, 153, 155, 346–64
  aetiology 348
  Australian ferrets 336
  clinical signs 348–9
  diagnosis 348–9
  in males 353–4, 356
  markers 347
  oestrogen precursor values 346–7
  risk outside USA 362–4
  steroid assay 347, 360
  synonyms 346
  treatment 347–8
    medical 354–60
    surgical 350–3
  in UK 369
  unusual cases
    female 360–1
    male 361–2
Ferret Complete 76–7
  feeding trial 77–8
ferret (*Mustela furo*)
  binocular vision 296, 297
  classification 3, 4, 5, 127, 128–9
  compared with stoat/weasel 11
  description 3–4
  domestication 124
  genetic history 4–5
ferret paralysis 53
ferretaria 39
  ferretarium 1 40–2
  ferretarium 2 42–4
  ground plan 41
Ferret's Choice 69
ferretting *see* working ferrets
'Ferretville' 12
fertility 93
fever 204
fibrolipoma 328
fibroma 328
fibronil (Frontline) 249, 250–1, 254, 491
fibrosarcoma 320, 328
finasteride 357
fitch farms
  feeding/nutrition 65, 70–2
  mastitis in 99–100
  see also fur farms
fitch-ferret 4, 15
'flattening' 265–6
fleas 88, 153, 248–52
  host range 248
  and POA 258
  'stick-tight' fleas 154, 248
  and tapeworms 246
  treatment 249–52
    drug toxicity 251–2
fluconazole 310, 311, 492
flucytosine 310
fluid therapy 268, 382, 460
  intraosseous catheterization 158, 460
  intravenous catheterization 381, 402, 460
  maintenance fluids 460
  rehydration formula 499
  shock-rate fluids 460
flunixin meglumine 443, 495
flutamide 265, 357

foot mange 154, 253–4
foreign bodies
    gastric 205–6, 432
    intestinal 214, 413, 433
    removal 432–3
foulmart (*Mustela putorius*) 4
fractured bones 19
    causes 443
    complications
        delayed union 445, 447
        malunion 445–6
        non-union 447
    immobilization 442
    initial wound treatment 443
    open 442
    pinning
        biodegradable pins 447
        K-wire 444–7, 448
        for Kirschner–Ehmer-type apparatus 449
    postoperative care 452
    rehabilitation 448
    sites
        baculum 413
        elbow 447
        femur 446
        humerus 445–6
        pelvis 447–8
        spine 449–52
    treatment 444–9
        external coaption 444
        internal coaption 444–8
        Kirschner–Ehmer-type apparatus 448–9
fractured teeth 475–6
Frankie Ferret 78
French ferrets 7
Frontline (fibronil) 249, 250–1, 254, 491
fungal infections *see* mycotic diseases
fur farms 9, 12
    see also fitch farms
furosemide 268, 280, 282, 283, 493
Fusiformis infections 195

G

galactose-induced cataracts 303–6
Galictis spp.
    G. cuja 4
    G. vittata 4
gall bladder 29, 163
ganglioneuromas 343
gardens, ferret-proofing 36–40
gastroenteritis, chronic, sequelae of 211
gastrointestinal diseases/disorders 205–17
    clinical findings 204–5
    drugs used 493
    foreign bodies 205–6
    megaoesophagus 205
    oral ulcers 205
    overview 203–4
    trichobezoars 205–6
gastrointestinal tract, ultrasonography of 423–4
gastrostomy tubes 464
genetics 106–21
    A locus 110
        mutant genes 118–19
    B locus 109, 114–15
        basic concepts 107–8
        behavioural problems 119
    C locus 108–9, 112–13
        and classification 124
        coat colours 107–8
    D locus 109–10
        and domestication 116–17
        domestication studies, problems with 125–6
    E locus 109
        and endocrine neoplasia 371
        endothelial receptor type B 118
        ferret crosses 112
    G locus 111, 113
        genes with multiple effects 117–18
    I locus 110
        inbreeding 119–20
    R locus 111, 113
    S locus 110
    S^{ab} locus 110–11
        sensory defects 116
        star gene 139
        Waardenburg syndrome 118
genitalia *see* reproductive system
gentamicin 199, 299, 490
German ferrets 8, 18, 79
giardiasis 231–2
glaucoma 307
glucose-induced cataracts 303
glycopyrrolate 495
Gnathostoma nipponicum 246
gonadotropin-releasing hormone (GnRH) agonist 347–8
gonadotropin-releasing hormone (GnRH) analogue 355
goserelin 357
granular cell tumour 343
grass awn injury 197, 264
griseofulvin 197, 492
group behaviour 35
growth *see* body weight
Gulo gulo gulo 4
Gulo gulo luscus 4

H

haemangiomas 328, 330
haemangiosarcomas 328, 338, 339
haematological values 488
halothane 399–400, 495
hand-rearing 98–9, 492, 493–4, 498–9
    ferret formula 492, 494
    striped skunk formula 494, 499
    weaning formula 499
    weasel/mink formula 494
handling 19, 151
    in clinic 152–6
    kittens 93
    pregnant jills 153–4
    'scruffing' 89, 155–6
    for ultrasonography 417
heart 24, 26
    dilated cardiomyopathy 276
    examination 155
    normal 275–6
    ultrasonography 422–3
    vagi and sympathetic nerve complex 276
heart rate 380
    before/during anaesthesia 395, 409
heartworm 36, 54, 192, 239–45
    diagnosis 239–45-41
    prevention 241, 242–3, 491
    treatment 241–2, 491
    in USA 243–4
heat stress 53
Helicobacter gastritis 206, 207–9
helminth parasites 233–48
hemilaminectomy 449, 451
Hendra virus (HENV) 169
hepatic diseases 217–21
    biliary carcinoma 221
    biliary cysts/cystadenomas 220, 221
    end stage liver disease 220
    hepatitis
        bacterial 165
        lymphocytic 218
        suppurative 218–19
    hepatocellular adenocarcinoma 221
    hepatoma 221
    lipidosis 219–20
    lymphocytic hepatitis 218
    neoplasia 220–1, 338–9
    overview 204
    suppurative hepatitis 218–19
    vacuolar hepatopathy 219
hepatic lipidosis 219–20
Hepatozoon canis 231

herbal flea remedies 250
heterozygosity 108
'high-rise syndrome' 48
histiocytoma 328
Histoplasma capsulatum infection 198, 199–200
history 5–6
hob (dog) ferrets
    behaviour in mating season 89
    body weight 61, 71, 72, 102
    external features 15
    feeding 71
    photoperiodism 374
    reproductive system 30, 31–2, 87, 88
        problems 93–4
hobbles 89
homozygosity 108
hookworms 237–8
hospitalization 152–6, 159–65
    accommodation 160
    equipment 159–62
        diagnostic 161
        examination 159–60
        laboratory 160
        laparoscopy 161
        surgical 160–1
        treatment 160
    examination 152–6
    pregnant jills 153–4
housing *see* accommodation
human chorionic gonadotropin 494
Hungarian ferrets 8, 79
hutches
    converted 38
    indoor 42
    outdoor 43
hydrocortisone 301
hydronephritis 272
hyperglycaemic cataracts 303
hyperparathyroidism 73, 105
    secondary 269–71
hyperphosphataemia 270
hypertrophic cardiomyopathy 275, 279–80, 281–2
hypervitaminosis 73

I

Iams Kitten Food 59–60
ibuprofen toxicosis 386, 387–8
Ictonyx striatus 4
imidacloprid (Advantage) 249, 251–2, 491
Immiticide 241
immune-complex mediated glomerulonephritis (ICGN) 185
inbreeding 119–20

Index

incisors
   deciduous 469
   permanent (secondary) 470–1
indoor accommodation
   breeding cages 35–6
   dangers 48, 49, 50
      air pollution 56
      electric cables 55
      human feet 56
      washing machines 55
   darkness 49, 50, 374
   house ferrets 48–51
      ferret rooms/cages 50–1
   hutches 42
infections
   of European wildlife 170
   susceptibility of ferrets/dogs/cats 171
   see also bacterial diseases; mycotic diseases; viral diseases
inflammatory bowel disease 209–13
   diet 213
   sequelae 210
influenza 24, 96, 154, 169, 174
   H5N1 169, 174
   vs canine distemper 176
injections 155, 156
insect bites 53–4
insecticides 382–3
insulin
   and diet 376
   normal values 364–5
   therapeutic 377, 494
insulinomas 7, 8, 329, 330, 346, 364–9
   Australian ferrets 336
   clinical signs 364
   debulking 435
   diagnosis 364–5
   endocrine dysfunction 364
   lumpectomy 436
   partial pancreatectomy 436–7
   prognosis 367, 368–9
   recurrence 436–7
   treatment
      medical 367
      post-operative 365–7
      surgical 365
   in UK 369–71
insulinoma elixir 367
   recipe 499
interleukin 10 (IL-10) 449
intraosseous catheterization 158, 460
intravenous catheterization 381, 402, 460
introgression (hybridization) 124–5, 126
   and behavioural changes 132

intubation 400, 402
iopamidol 411
Irish spotting 110
isofluothane 226
isoflurane 399, 400, 403, 454, 495
   assessment 401
   cardiac irregularities 404–5
   cardiopulmonary depression 402
   echocardiography reference values 427
   premedication 402
Isospora spp.
   I. belli 231
   I. hominis 231
   I. laidlawii 228, 229
Italian ferrets 8, 18
   accommodation 35, 51
   feeding 79
itraconazole 310, 311, 314, 492
ivermectin 491
   cryptococcosis 311
   ear infections 294
   heartworm 241–2, 243, 244
   mange 252–3, 254, 255
   toxicity 242
Ixodes holocyclus 54, 255

J

Japanese ferrets 8, 18
   accommodation 35
   Aleutian disease 185
   FADC 362
   feeding 79
   neoplasia 335–6
jaw muscles 23
jill ferrets
   behaviour in mating season 89
   body weight 61, 71, 72, 102
   external features 15
   feeding 71
   photoperiodism 374
   reproductive system 24, 25, 31, 87, 88
      problems 94–8, 99–100
jugular vein 23
   blood sampling 157
juvenile neoplasia 25

K

K-wire
   intramedullary pinning with 444–7
   with Kirschner–Ehmer-type apparatus 449
   sizes for ferrets 444, 445

karyotype studies 125
ketamine 262, 325, 396–7, 406, 407, 495
    + acepromazine 399
    + diazepam 398
    + Domitor 407
        + Antisedan 404, 406
        +butorphanol 453
    + halothane 399–400, 440
    + isoflurane 400, 402
    + midazolam 427
    + xylazine 395–6, 397–8
        + tiletamine/zolazepam 411
    as analgesic 452
    concerns 403
    echocardiography reference values 427
ketoconazole 492
    bacterial diseases 198, 199
    cryptococcosis 309, 310
    parasite infections 198, 291
kidneys 24, 30, 163
    diseases 265–72
    enlargement 265
    failure 265
    ultrasonography 420, 421
kidney tumours 331
Kirschner–Ehmer-type apparatus 448–9
kittens
    accommodation 43, 45, 46
    eye infections of newborns 100–1
    hand-rearing 98–9, 492, 493–4, 498–9
    'swimmers' 105–7
Kolinsky (*Mustela sibirica*) 3, 4

L

laboratory ferrets 13
    accommodation 51
    experimental infections 169
    feeding 78–9
lactation 95
    and accommodation 45
lanoxin 493
laparoscopy 161–5
    equipment 161–2
large intestine 25
    thickened 204
Lawsonia intracellularis 217
leishmaniasis 233
lens luxation 307
leptospirosis 190–1
Leukeran 326
leukocytosis 204
leuprolide acetate 347–8, 355–7, 358, 373

    administration technique 356–7
    dosage 356
levamisole hydrochloride 247
Lewington ferret cage 44, 45–6
lice 255
lidocaine 453–4
lime sulphur 254, 491, 492
limonene 250, 251
lindane 254
lipoma 329
Listeria monocytogenes 194
liver 25, 27, 29, 164
    biopsy 165, 437–8
    ultrasonography 422, 428
liver adenosarcoma 338
liver flukes 245
lufenuron (Program) 249, 491
lungs 24, 26
lungworms 238–9
lymphadenopathy, mesenteric 204
lymphocystosis 205
lymphocytic hepatitis 218
lymphoma 8, 165, 216–17, 319–23
    in adults 322
        thymic 321–2
    Australian ferrets 337
    chest wall 335–6
    clinical signs by age 321
    diagnosis 323
    of footpads 335, 336
    and inflammatory bowel disease 210, 212
    multiple system involvement 330
    and myocarditis 283
    palatine bone erosion 484
    prevalence 329
    T-cell 340–3
    tail 334
    treatment 321, 322, 324
    in young ferrets 321
    see also specific types
lymphoplasmacytic gastroenteritis 209–13
Lyncodon patagonicus 4

M

major histocompatability complex (MHC) 120
Malassezia infection 198, 291
malathion 254, 491
mammary duct ectasia 363
mange 252–5
    demodectic mange 255
    drugs for 491
    ear mange 252–3

Index

mange (contd)
    foot mange 154, 253–4
    notoedric mange 254
    psoroptic mange 255
Marshall Premium Ferret Diet 57, 58, 59–60, 63
    growth of kittens 102, 103
Martes spp.
    M. americana 4
    M. flavigula 4
    M. foina 4
    M. gwatkinsi 4
    M. martes 4
    M. melampus 4
    M. pennanti 4
    M. zibellina 4
mast cell tumours 329, 330, 331–2
    cryosurgery 454
    removal 439
mastitis 196
    acute 99–100
    chronic 100
mebendazole 236
medetomide 495
medetomidine hydrochloride (Domitor) *see* Domitor (medetomidine hydrochloride)
medication 159
megaoesophagus 23, 205
megestrol acetate 262
melaena 204
melanin 108, 109
melarsomine 243, 244
melatonin 357–60
    and breeding cycle 87
meperidine 495
mesenteric lymph nodes 424, 425
    biopsy 438
mesotheliomas 329, 339
metabolism and nutrition 62
metaproterenol 493
methoprene 250, 251
methotrexate 323, 324, 326, 494
metoclopramide 493
metronidazole 208, 233, 490, 491
miconazole 198, 291
midazolam 398, 495
    echocardiography reference values 427
milbemycin oxime 242
milk
    comparison across species 498
    consumption and cataract 305
    supplements 498
mineral deficiencies 300

mink
    Aleutian disease 180
    classification 4, 128
    genetics 107
    melatonin implants 357, 358, 359
    nutrition 58
        influence on ferret feeding 75–6
        requirements 76
misoprostol 386, 387, 493
mitotane 354–5
mitt ferrets 16, 110, 112
Mittendorf's dot 298
molars
    deciduous 468, 470
    permanent (secondary) 472–4
monosulfiram 291
morphine 495
mosquitoes 36, 54
moulting 89
moxidectin (ProHeart 6) 242, 244–5
Mucomyst Formula 3D 301
mucormycosis 197
MUMS (Minor Use and Minor Species) Act 489
muscle wasting 204
mushrooms 387
musk glands 25, 30
Mustela spp.
    M. africana 4
    M. altaica 4
    M. erminea 4, 11
    M. eversmanni 6, 9, 124, 125, 127
        binocular vision 296
        classification 3, 4, 5, 128, 129
    M. frenata 4
    M. furo 4, 124, 127
        binocular vision 296, 297
        classification 3, 4, 5, 127, 128–9
    M. kathiah 4
    M. lutreola 4
        classification 128
    M. lutreolina 4
    M. nigripes 6, 57, 124, 127
        binocular vision 296
        classification 4, 128, 129
        toxoplasmosis in 225
    M. nivalis 3, 4, 11
    M. nivalis rixona 4
    M. nudipes 4
    M. putorius 9, 124, 125
        binocular vision 296
        classification 3, 4, 5, 127, 128, 129
    M. sibirica 4, 5
    M. strigidorsa 4

M. vison 4, 180
M. felipei 4
Mustelidae family
   classification 3, 127
   domestication 3
Mycobacteria spp. 191–2
mycobacterial disease 190–4
   diagnosis 193–4
   treatment 192–3
Mycoplasma 189
mycotic diseases 197–200
   antifungal drugs 492
   blastomycosis 198–9
   coccidioidomycosis 199
   histoplasmosis 199–200
   Malassezia infection 198
   mucormycosis 197–8
   Pneumocystis carinii 200
   ringworm 197
myelography 451
myocarditis 283–4

N

nalbuphine 495
naloxone 387, 449, 495
naphthalene 384
nasal anatomy 307
nasal examination 154
nasal neoplasia 316
nasal worm of weasels 247–8
nausea 204
nematode parasites 233–46
neomycin 291, 490
neoplasia 216–17, 318–46
   adrenal gland 28, 32
   by age/gender 327
   hepatic diseases 220–1
   juvenile 25
   liver 25
   multiple system involvement 330
   nasal 316
   skeletal 334–5
   treatment protocols 323–7
   by type/body sites 328–9
Neosporosium caninum infection 228
Netherland ferrets 7
   Aleutian disease 184
   FADC 362
   feeding 79
neural crest 117
neurofibrosarcomas 343
neuronal ceroid lipofuscinosis 284

neutering *see* sterilization
neutrophilia 205
New Zealand ferrets 9–12
   Aleutian disease 184
   feeding
      commercial breeding ferrets 73–4
      feral ferrets 74
      fitch farms 70–2
niclosamide 247, 491
nicotine 383–4
Nipah virus (NIPV) 169–70
nipping/biting 151
nitenpyram (Capstar) 249
nitroglycerine (Nitrol) 282, 493
notoedric mange 254
nutrition 57–85
   adults 58, 68
   biotin deficiency 72
   breeding ferrets 67, 68
      in lactation 101, 102
      in pregnancy 101, 102
   commercial breeding ferrets 73–4
   deficiencies causing eye conditions 300, 302–3
   dental disease 63
   diet
      additives/preservatives 81, 82–3, 492
      carbohydrates 64
      commercial foods 57–60, 62, 65–6, 69–70, 76–9
         comparison of 59–60
         ingredients 80–3
      and endocrine neoplasia 375–6
      fat 64, 81
      fibre 62, 63, 64, 81
      gruel 462–3
      and insulinomas 366
      low allergen food 83
      maintenance diet 65
      minerals 65–6
      natural feeding 68–9, 70, 83–4, 376
      non-commercial food 66–9
      protein 63–4, 66, 80, 268, 269–70
      and renal disease 268, 269–71
      salt 81–2
      and urolithiasis 272, 274
      vegetarian diet 57, 58
      vitamins 64–5
   emergency 462–4
      nursing 462
      water/electrolytes 462
   excesses causing eye conditions 302–3
   feeding routines 66–7, 68
   feral ferrets 74
   fitch farms 70–2

Index

nutrition (contd)
  food allergy/adverse reactions 79–80, 83
  gruel diets 462–3
  hyperparathyroidism 73, 105
  hypervitaminosis 73
  indoor feeding 50
  intestinal transit time 61–2
  kittens 58, 68, 101–3
    hand-rearing 98–9, 492, 493–4, 498–9
  laboratory ferrets 58, 78–9
  mink diet, influence of 75–6
  naso-oesophageal catheterization 463–4
  outdoor feeding 40, 42
  rickets 73, 105, 106
  and scats 67
  supplements in chemotherapy 325
  support, nutritional 382
  thiamine deficiency 72
  working ferrets 63, 67, 68, 71, 74
    in colony situation 74–5
  yellow fat disease 73

O

octreotide 367
oesophagostomy tubes 464
oesophagus 23
oestrogen and POA 259
oestrus cycle 88
olfactory sense 307–16
olfactory system diseases 308
  see also nasal neoplasia; nasal worm of weasels
omeprazole 206, 208, 493
ophthalmia neonatorum 100–1
optic chiasma 297
oral ulcers 205
organophosphates 250, 251
orthopaedics 442–52
  causes of fractures 443
  complications 445–6, 447
  dislocation of elbow 448
  fracture treatment 444–9
    external coaption 444
    internal coaption (pinning) 444–8
    Kirschner–Ehmer apparatus 448–9
  initial wound treatment 443
  postoperative care 452
  rehabilitation 448
  spinal cord damage 449–52
  transport to hospital 442–3
osteomas 340, 341
osteomyelitis 478
osteoporosis 480, 484

osteosarcomas 339, 340
otitis externa 291
otitis interna 292–5
  idiopathic 292
  and ototoxicity 294
  peripheral vs vestibular 293
  routes of infection 294
  treatment 293–4
otitis media 291–2
Otodectes cynotis 197, 252, 253, 291, 292, 294
ototoxic agents 293, 294–5
outdoor accommodation 35–48
  boltholes 38–9, 41
  cooling 45, 46
  dangers 36
    chemicals 54–5
    climbing/jumping 55
    heat stress 53
    infection 53, 54
    insect bites 53–4
    ponds 53–4
    snakes 53
    toxic plants/animals 54
  ferret courts 47–8
  ferret garden ground plan 37
  ferret-proofing the garden 36–40
  ferretaria 39
    ferretarium 1 40–2
    ferretarium 2 42–4
  hutches 43
  Lewington ferret cage 44, 45–6
  sheds 46–7
  standard cages 44–5
ovarian tumours 336, 337, 338
ovaries 24, 25, 27, 30
  removal 28
  see also spaying
ovariohysterectomy 262, 430, 431
oxygen therapy 459
oxymorphine 443, 495
oxytetracycline 490
oxytocin 494

P

pain
  anticipated levels by procedure 452
  relief see analgesia
pancreas 27, 29, 30, 164, 436
pancreatic beta cell tumours see insulinomas
pancreatic islet tumours 329, 369, 370–1
pancreatic tumours in UK 369–71
panophthalmitis 299

paracetamol toxicosis *see* acetaminophen toxicosis
parasites
    antifungal drugs 492
    external 248–55
        drugs for 491
        fleas 248–52
        lice 255
        mange 252–5
        ticks 255
    internal 221
        drugs for 491
        helminths 233–48
            nematodes 233–46
        protozoan diseases 224–33
            classification 224
parturition (whelping) 91–2
    older jills 97
    problems 95–8
Pasteurella spp. 186
patent ductus arteriosus 282–3
penicillin G 190, 490
pentazocine 495
pentobarbitone 410, 495
Peptosyl 493
peripheral nervous system tumours 343, 344
pet ferrets 7, 8–9, 12–13
    banning 9, 13
    dental disorders 475, 478, 479
    New Zealand 10, 11–12
pethidine 495
pharynx 22
phenobarbital 494
photoperiodism 87, 93
    darkness, need for 49, 50
    and endocrine neoplasia 373–5
    problems 105
phylogenetics 123, 125–6
physiological data 487–9
    basic data 487
    blood/serum chemistry 487–8, 489
    cardiovascular/respiratory 487
    haematological values 488
    metabolic values 487
    urinalysis 488, 489
piloleiomyosarcoma 332
piperazine 491
piperonyl butoxide 252, 491
pipes/pipe mazes 39, 40, 47, 48–9, 50
play 50
pleural effusion 277, 281, 412
pleuropneumonia-like organisms (PPLO) 189
Pneumocystis carinii 198
    pneumonia 200

pneumonia 188–9
    bacterial 189
    chemical-induced 189
    mycotic 200
POA *see* post-oestrus anaemia (POA)
Poecilictis libyca 4
Poecilogale albinucha 4
point pattern 111
poison ticks 255
poisoning *see* toxicoses
poisonous plants 386–7
polecat
    brain size 21
    definition 129
    see also European polecat (*Mustela putorius*)
polecat-ferret 4, 15
polymyxin B 198, 291
post-oestrus anaemia (POA) 153, 155, 195, 258–62
    clinical signs 259–60
    diagnosis 260–1
    and neoplasia 337
    pathology 260
    prevention 261–2
    treatment 262
praziquantel 491
prednisolone 192, 198, 199, 291, 333, 494
    for heartworm 241, 243, 244, 245
    for insulinomas 366, 368, 369
prednisone 213, 323, 324, 326, 367, 368, 494
pregnancy 90–3
    and accommodation 45, 46, 91
    detection 90–1
    examination 153–4
pregnancy toxaemia (PT) 94–5
Premium Ferret Biscuit 69
Premium Ferret Food 69–70
premolars 472
procarbazine 326
proctitis 204, 217
progestogen 494
Program (lufenuron) 249, 491
prohaczik 355
ProHeart 6 (moxidectin) 242, 244–5
proliferative bowel disease/ileitis 217
propranolol 282, 493
prostaglandin 263
prostate disease 435
prostate gland 32
    problems 264–5
    ultrasonography 422, 423, 426
prostatic cysts 32, 264–5
protein 269–71

Index

protozoan diseases 224–33
Pseudamphistomum truncatum 245
pseudohypoparathyroidism 377
Pseudomonas aeruginosa 188
pseudopregnancy 104–5
psoroptic mange 255
puncta, cannulation of 299–300
Purina High Density Ferret 59–60
pyelonephritis 271–2
pyometra 262, 263–4
    stump pyometra, adrenal-induced 350
pyrantel embonate 491
pyrethrins/pyrethroids 250, 251, 252, 491
pyrimethamine 226
pyriproxfen 249

R

rabbit hutch, converted 38
rabies 169
radiology diagnosis 411–15
    abdomen, normal *vs* abnormal 414
    contrast 411–12
ranitidine 205, 206, 208, 209, 493
'raw meaty bone' diet 68
rectal prolapse 204, 217
regurgitation 204
rehydration formula 499
renal cysts 265, 266
    ultrasonography 424, 425
renal disease syndrome 266
renal failure 266–71
renal stones 272
reproduction
    behaviour
        mating 89–90
        in mating season 89
    breeding 86–7
    breeding chart 88
    breeding season 87–9
        heat, signs of 87–8
    and domestication 129–30
    fertility 93
    lactation 92
    parturition (whelping) 91–2
        older jills 97
        problems 95–8
    pregnancy 90–3
        detection 90–1
        examination 153–4
    problems
        hobs 93–4
        jills 94–8, 99–100
        kittens 98–9, 100–1, 105–7
    pseudopregnancy 104–5
    reproductive cycle 88
    and vision 298
reproductive system
    diseases
        female 258–64
        male 264–5
    examination 155
    female 24, 25, 31, 87
    male 30, 31–2, 87, 440, 441
    neoplasia 337–8
resuscitation 405
retina 296
retinal atrophy 306
Revolution (selamectin) 235, 242–3, 249, 491
rickets 73, 105, 106
rifampicin 192
ringworm 197
rotenone 250, 251, 252
roundworms 233–5
Russian ferrets 8, 17–18
    accommodation 35
    FADC, lack of 362
    feeding 79
    neoplasia 336

S

sable ferret *see* fitch-ferret
salivary glands 23
Salmonella spp. 194–5
saphenous vein blood sampling 158
Sarcocystis spp.
    S. hominis 231
    S. muris 227–8
sarcomas 329
    vaccine-associated 179
Sarcoptes scabei 154
    var. *canis* 253, 254
SARS coronavirus (SCV) 170–1
scats trays
    indoors 49–50, 52–3, 56
    kittens and 92–3
    outdoors 39, 41, 42, 45–6
scent gland removal 18, 431–2
schwannoma 329, 343
Science Diet Feline Growth 59–60
'scruffing' 89, 155–6
sedation 157, 325
    drugs 398
    post-vasectomy 442

recovery times 393
scoring 409
selamectin (Revolution) 235, 242–3, 249, 491
self pattern 110, 111
sensory defects 116
serum/blood chemistry 487–8, 489
sevoflurane 402–3, 495
Siberian weasel (*Mustela sibirica*) 3, 4, 5
silica gel packets 383
silvermitts 110–11, 112
silymarin 218
skeletal neoplasia 333–4
    bone tumours 339–43
skeleton 18–19
    dentition 20–1
skin cancers 331
Skrjabingylus spp. 231, 247–8
skull 19–21
small intestine 25, 163
smell, sense of *see* olfactory sense
snakes 53
sneezing 186
'snuffles' 154, 186–8
    antibiotic sensitivity 186
    cryptococcosis-associated 309, 315
    diagnosis 186, 188
    treatment 186–7
'soft bone' syndrome 106
somatostatin 367
South African ferrets 13–14
Spanish ferrets 8
spaying 25, 27–8
    for FADC 350
    for POA 262, 350
    preparation/positioning 394
spinal lymphoma 340–3
Spirometra erinaceieuropaei 247
spleen 27, 30, 164
    biopsy 438
    ultrasonography 420
splenic tumours 330, 336
squamous cell carcinoma 327, 329, 331, 333–4, 336
Staphylococcus infections 196–7
steppe polecat (*Mustela eversmani*) 6, 9, 124
    binocular vision 296
    classification 3, 4, 5, 128, 129
    hybridization 125
sterilization 7, 8, 13
    analgesia 453–4
    early
        embryonic disturbance 348
        and endocrine neoplasia 348, 372–3
    European law 373

'stick-tight' fleas 154, 248
stoat (*Mustela erminea*) 11
straying 34, 152
Streptococcus infections 186, 196
streptomycin 190
streptozotocin 367
Strongyloides stercoralis 235–6
struvite uroliths 272
sucralfate 205, 206, 209, 386, 493
sulfadiazine 226, 490
sulfadimexothine 229, 490, 491
sulfamethazine 490
sulphaquinoxaline 226
'super ferrets' 9
suppurative hepatitis 218–19
suture fracture techniques 436, 437–8
'swimmers' 105–7
Swiss ferrets 7–8

T

T-cell lymphoma 340–3
Taenia spp. 246–7
tail tumours 334, 336
tameness, selection for 139
tamoxifen 357
tapeworms 246–7
taxonomy *see* classification
teeth *see* dentition
temperature (body) 155, 156
    under anaesthesia 394
    taking temperature 152
temperature (environmental) 34
teratoma 329–30
terbutaline 187
testicular tumours 264
tetracycline 199, 490
theobromine 383
theophylline 493
thiabendazole 236, 252, 253
thiacetarsamide 491
thiamine deficiency 72
thoracic organs 24, 25, 27
threadworms 235–6
thymic lymphoma 321–2
thymic lymphosarcoma 336
thymus gland 25
thyroid tumours 319
thyroxine values 365
ticks 255, 314–15
tirilazad 449
tongue 24, 25

Index

Totally Ferret 59–60, 63
   average growth curves 65
Toxascaris leonina 233, 234
toxic plants/animals 54
toxicoses 380–9
   assessment of condition 380
   decontamination 381
   household hazards
      ant bait 382–3
      bread dough 384
      chocolate 383
      cigarettes 383
      human medications 385–6
      liquid potpourri 383
      mothballs 384
      nicotine 383
      pennies 383–4
      rodenticides 384–5
      silica gel packets 383
   poisonous plants 386–7
   supportive care 381–2
   vital function stabilization 380–1
Toxocara spp.
   T. canis 233–4
   T. cati 233, 234
Toxoplasma gondii 225, 226
Toxoplasma-like organisms 225, 283
toxoplasmosis 224–7
tranquilizers 398, 495
travelling 52
triiodothyronine values 365
Trichinella spiralis 236–7
trichobezoars 205–6, 414, 432
   and ultrasonography 418
Trichuris vulpis 236
trimethoprim-sulfadiazine 490
trimethoprim-sulfamethoxazole 189, 200, 271, 274, 490
   cherry flavoured 229
triple phosphate crystals 272
Troglotrema acutum 248
tuberculosis (TB) 191
tumour suppression genes 371–2
tylosin 490

U

ulcers
   bowel 264
   corneal 300–1
   gastric 206–7, 209
   oral 205

ultrasonography 417–29
   abnormalities, assessment of 424
   cardiac *see* echocardiography
   echogenicity of tissues 419
   equipment 417–18
   frequent use 424–6
   guidelines 418–19
   longitudinal plane 419, 420, 421
   paracentesis 424–5
   patient handling 417, 419
   patient positioning 418–19
   patient preparation 419
   routine uses 418
   scanning techniques 419–24
   thoracentesis 426
   transverse plane 419, 420, 421–2
United Kingdom ferrets 6–7
   Aleutian disease 183–4
   feeding 74–9
      working ferrets 74–5
United Kingdom, ferrets in 35
unpalatable medication 229, 230
ureters 30
   trauma to 274–5
urinalysis 488, 489
urinary catheterization 461–2
urinary system 24, 30
   diseases 265–75
urine output 461–2
urolithiasis 63, 95, 272–4
   treatment 273–4
ursodiol 220
uterine horns 24, 28, 30
uveitis 301–2
   cataract-induced 305–6

V

vaccination
   annual check-ups 179–80
   Bordetella bronchiseptica 185
   botulism 190
   canine distemper 176–9
   fleas 249
   rabies 173
vaccine-associated sarcoma 179
vaccine-induced immune response 286
vacuolar hepatopathy 219
vaginitis 262
valvular heart disease 282–3
vancomycin-resistant enterococci 197

vasectomy 30, 32, 430–1
   anaesthesia 440
   incision 441
   procedure 440–2
Vetelar (ketamine) 404
Viadur 357
vincristine 323, 324, 494
viral diseases 169–85
   Aleutian disease 12, 180–5, 216
   Australian Bat Lyssavirus 173
   canine distemper 174–9
      vaccination 176–9
      vs influenza 176
   coronavirus enteritis 214–15
   and endocrine neoplasia 376
   Hendra virus (HENV) 169
   influenza 24, 96, 154, 169, 173, 174
      H5N1 169, 174
      vs canine distemper 176
   Nipah virus (NIPV) 169–70
   nucleic acid differences 172
   rabies 169, 172–3
   SARS coronavirus (SCV) 170–1
   susceptibility of carnivores 171
vision 130–1, 295–8
   of albino ferret 297–8
   binocular 296, 297
   colour 298
   range 296–8
   and reproduction 298
   see also eye conditions/infections
Vitalin 78
vitamins
   deficiencies causing eye conditions 300, 302
   vitamin B_1 injection 190
   see also under nutrition
Vormela peregusna 4
vulva 25

W

Waardenburg syndrome 139
warfarin poisoning 384
washing for fleas 250–2
water availability 65, 68
weaning formula 499
weasel (*Mustela nivalis*) 3, 4, 11
weighing ferrets 159
weight loss 204
whipworms 236–7
white ferrets 5, 6
   black-eyed whites 15
   see also albino ferrets
working ferrets 5–7, 8, 9–10, 12
   feeding 63, 67, 68
      problems 71
   photoperiodism 374
   ratting 13, 14
   'stick-tight' fleas 154, 248
wound treatments 498

X

xylazine 242, 262, 395–6, 411, 495
   reversal 399

Y

yellow fat disease 73
yohimbine (Reversine) 399, 405

Z

zinc toxicosis 383–4, 388
zolazepam/tiletamine (Zoletil) (Telazol) 410–11, 495